Diagnosis and Treatment of Skin Diseases

Diagnosis and Treatment of Skin Diseases

Edited by Derek Kennedy

hayle medical

New York

Hayle Medical,
750 Third Avenue, 9th Floor,
New York, NY 10017, USA

Visit us on the World Wide Web at:
www.haylemedical.com

ISBN: 978-1-63241-575-2

Printed in China.

Cataloging-in-Publication Data

Diagnosis and treatment of skin diseases / edited by Derek Kennedy.
p. cm.
Includes bibliographical references and index.
ISBN 978-1-63241-575-2
1. Skin--Diseases. 2. Skin--Diseases--Diagnosis. 3. Skin--Diseases--Treatment.
4. Dermatology. I. Kennedy, Derek.
RL72 .D53 2019
616.5--dc23

Table of Contents

Preface

This book aims to highlight the current researches and provides a platform to further the scope of innovations in this area. This book is a product of the combined efforts of many researchers and scientists, after going through thorough studies and analysis from different parts of the world. The objective of this book is to provide the readers with the latest information of the field.

The human skin covers on an average an area of two square meters, and constitutes of three distinct layers- the dermis, epidermis and subcutaneous tissue. The medical conditions of the integumentary system, including the hair, skin, nails, muscles and glands are known as skin diseases. It constitutes a range of disorders or dermatoses and many nonpathologic states. The diagnosis of skin diseases follows through a histological examination using a skin biopsy that is then correlated with clinical presentation and laboratory data. Cutaneous ultrasound also allows detection of hair diseases, nail disorders, cutaneous tumors and inflammations. This book attempts to understand the varied types of skin diseases, their diagnoses and treatment strategies. The various studies that are constantly contributing towards advancing the understanding of such diseases are examined in detail. Researchers and students in the field of dermatology will be assisted by this book.

I would like to express my sincere thanks to the authors for their dedicated efforts in the completion of this book. I acknowledge the efforts of the publisher for providing constant support. Lastly, I would like to thank my family for their support in all academic endeavors.

Editor

Skin Lesions on Common Bottlenose Dolphins (*Tursiops truncatus*) from Three Sites in the Northwest Atlantic, USA

Leslie Burdett Hart[1,2]*, Dave S. Rotstein[3,4], Randall S. Wells[5], Jason Allen[5], Aaron Barleycorn[5], Brian C. Balmer[5,6], Suzanne M. Lane[2], Todd Speakman[2], Eric S. Zolman[2], Megan Stolen[7], Wayne McFee[8], Tracey Goldstein[9], Teri K. Rowles[3], Lori H. Schwacke[1,2]

1 Division of Biostatistics and Epidemiology, Department of Medicine, Medical University of South Carolina, Charleston, South Carolina, United States of America, **2** National Oceanic and Atmospheric Administration, National Ocean Service, Hollings Marine Laboratory, Charleston, South Carolina, United States of America, **3** National Oceanic and Atmospheric Administration, National Marine Fisheries Service, Office of Protected Resources, Silver Spring, Maryland, United States of America, **4** Marine Mammal Pathology Services, Olney, Maryland, United States of America, **5** Chicago Zoological Society, c/o: Mote Marine Laboratory, Sarasota, Florida, United States of America, **6** University of North Carolina Wilmington, Department of Biology and Marine Biology, Wilmington, North Carolina, United States of America, **7** Hubbs-SeaWorld Research Institute, Melbourne Beach, Florida, United States of America, **8** Coastal Marine Mammal Stranding Assessments Program, National Oceanic and Atmospheric Administration, National Centers for Coastal Ocean Science, Center for Coastal Environmental Health and Biomolecular Research, Charleston, South Carolina, United States of America, **9** Wildlife Health Center, School of Veterinary Medicine, University of California, Davis, California, United States of America

Abstract

Skin disease occurs frequently in many cetacean species across the globe; methods to categorize lesions have relied on photo-identification (photo-id), stranding, and by-catch data. The current study used photo-id data from four sampling months during 2009 to estimate skin lesion prevalence and type occurring on bottlenose dolphins (*Tursiops truncatus*) from three sites along the southeast United States coast [Sarasota Bay, FL (SSB); near Brunswick and Sapelo Island, GA (BSG); and near Charleston, SC (CHS)]. The prevalence of lesions was highest among BSG dolphins ($P = 0.587$) and lowest in SSB ($P = 0.380$), and the overall prevalence was significantly different among all sites ($p < 0.0167$). Logistic regression modeling revealed a significant reduction in the odds of lesion occurrence for increasing water temperatures (*OR = 0.92; 95%CI:0.906–0.938*) and a significantly increased odds of lesion occurrence for BSG dolphins (*OR = 1.39; 95%CI:1.203–1.614*). Approximately one-third of the lesioned dolphins from each site presented with multiple types, and population differences in lesion type occurrence were observed ($p < 0.05$). Lesions on stranded dolphins were sampled to determine the etiology of different lesion types, which included three visually distinct samples positive for herpesvirus. Although generally considered non-fatal, skin disease may be indicative of animal health or exposure to anthropogenic or environmental threats, and photo-id data provide an efficient and cost-effective approach to document the occurrence of skin lesions in free-ranging populations.

Editor: Tara C. Smith, University of Iowa, United States of America

Funding: Funding for this project was provided by the National Oceanic and Atmospheric Administration's Center of Excellence for Oceans and Human Health at the Hollings Marine Laboratory, Charleston, South Carolina. The funders had no role in study design, data collection and analysis, decision to publish, or preparation of the manuscript.

Competing Interests: The authors have declared that no competing interests exist.

* E-mail: leslie.burdett@noaa.gov

Introduction

Skin lesions in delphinids and other small cetaceans are geographically widespread [1–9]. Reported prevalence estimates for skin lesions among delphinids range between 48% [4] and 100% [3], and 63% to 100% for bottlenose dolphins (*Tursiops truncatus*) specifically [2,3,6,8,10,11]. Tattoo lesions have been studied extensively by Van Bressem et al. [5,9,12], where the reported prevalence of this specific lesion type among bottlenose dolphins ranges from 0% [9] to 71% [12]. Most of these studies used photo-identification (photo-id) data to estimate the population prevalence of skin disease (e.g. [2,3,6,8,10–12]), producing minimum disease prevalence estimates [11] as the detection of lesions are restricted to body parts that are routinely photographed. Although limited for determining skin disease causes, photo-id data provide a relatively inexpensive and non-invasive means of assessing body and skin condition [13], as well as lesion progression, recurrence, or resolution [9,14,15] for free-ranging marine mammal populations. Other studies have relied on by-catch or stranding data [1,4,5,9,16,17], or capture-release health assessment data [3,18,19] to estimate disease burden in wild populations; however, these methods can be limited by small sample sizes or in the case of stranding data, biased towards individuals with compromised health [20].

Microscopic evaluations of skin lesions among cetaceans have revealed a broad spectrum of causes including potentially infectious pathogens such as poxvirus [21] and herpesvirus [22], and lacaziosis (i.e. lobomycosis, [23]), as well as non-infectious causes such as diatom attachment [24] and traumatic scarring [1]. As skin lesions in wild dolphin populations may indicate the emergence [25] or persistence of infectious disease, detection and monitoring of lesions using photo-id data facilitate disease surveillance. Some studies have suggested an association between the presence of skin disease and environmental parameters (eg. salinity and temperature [3,21]) or anthropogenic factors (eg. contaminants and pollutants [5,6,26]); therefore, assessing differences between populations could possibly indicate changes in environmental conditions or exposure to chemical contaminants.

The objective of this study was to use photo-id data to estimate and compare the prevalence of skin lesions and lesion type among dolphins from three U.S. southeast coastal sites: Sarasota Bay and vicinity, Florida (SSB); near Brunswick and Sapelo Island, Georgia (BSG); and near Charleston, South Carolina (CHS)(Figure 1). These efforts provided an assessment of skin lesion occurrence and the distribution of different lesion types among dolphins from different geographic sites, which can serve as a baseline for future surveillance of novel types or changes in overall skin lesion prevalence.

Materials and Methods

Ethics Statement

Samples from stranded animals were collected under NOAA's responsibility to the MMPA 1972 under Section 109(h), and a Stranding Agreement as part of the Marine Mammal Health and Stranding Response Act to respond to and collect samples from stranded marine mammals. Photo-id surveys were conducted under the following NMFS Permit Numbers:

Sarasota Bay: 522–1785; Charleston, SC and Brunswick/Sapelo Island, GA: GA LoC No. 1064-1748 and GA LoC No. 14348.

Study Populations

Sarasota Bay, FL (SSB). The bottlenose dolphin community in Sarasota Bay, FL (Figure 1) is comprised of approximately 160 residents [27], and has been monitored and studied since 1970. Routine photo-id surveys were initiated in 1980 [28] to estimate abundance [29], identify individuals and group composition [30], monitor social structure and life history [31,32], and determine movement patterns [33].

Brunswick and Sapelo Island, GA (BSG). Bottlenose dolphins in estuarine waters near Brunswick and Sapelo Island, GA (Figure 1) have been studied since 2004 [34]. A systematic photo-id study of dolphins in coastal GA waters was conducted during four seasons from 2008 to 2009, resulting in preliminary abundance estimates of less than 100 individuals during fall months to over 230 individuals during the summer in the Brunswick area, and approximately 150–350 individuals in waters near Sapelo Island depending on time of year [35].

Charleston, SC (CHS). Photo-id studies of bottlenose dolphins inhabiting the Charleston, SC (Figure 1) estuarine system have been conducted on a semi-routine basis since 1994 [36]; monthly surveys were initiated in January 2004 [37]. Abundance estimates calculated from post-2004 surveys ranged from approximately 300 dolphins in January to 900 individuals in July due to an influx of animals into the survey area during the spring and summer months [37].

Skin Lesion Detection and Classification

Digital photo-id images for the three sites were obtained across four seasons corresponding to the months of February, April, July, and October, 2009. All images from each dolphin sighting were visually screened for dolphins with skin lesions, based on the detection of a lesion on any dorsal or dorsolateral aspect of the animal's body. Cetacean photo-id projects utilized a standardized and quantifiable methodology [38] to select for the best images of an individual animal's dorsal fin (e.g. [37]). This methodology was modified for this study to detect skin lesions on individual dolphins. Digital images were excluded from lesion screening if distinguishing features of the lesions could not be observed (i.e. dark or backlit, in poor focus). The photographic quality of each sighting was scored as: 1) good – high confidence in determining the presence or absence of skin lesions for all or most animals in the sighting; 2) average – reduced confidence in determining the presence or absence of skin lesions for several animals in the sighting; 3) poor – no confidence in determining the presence or absence of skin lesions for any animal in the sighting. All images scored as 'poor' were excluded from final analyses, as well as images with lesions whose distinguishing features could not be detected.

Once all photos were screened for lesions, each lesion was categorized according to descriptions in previous studies [5,9,11,12]: 1) black; 2) pale; 3) cloudy; 4) lunar; 5) dark-fringed; 6) white-fringed; 7) orange patches; 8) tattoo-like; 9) white velvety; 10) lacaziosis-like; or 11) vesicular. In addition to these lesion types, two new categories, 'spotted' and 'mottled', were added, resulting in 13 possible lesion categories. Spotted lesions were defined as having localized or widespread distribution, were paler in color than the surrounding skin, circular in shape, and did not have a dark border. Mottled lesions were defined as scattered flecks of white, pale gray, or dark gray pigmentation, irregularly shaped, and were usually located laterally.

Dolphin Identification

All dolphins screened for skin lesions were identified as unique individuals and matched to known animals in a photo-id catalog based upon distinctive markings located on the dorsal fin. The methodology for dorsal fin identification has been described elsewhere [39]. Individuals with marginally distinct and non-distinct dorsal fins were excluded from the analysis to avoid inadvertent duplication of records.

Stranding Sampling

To supplement the findings from the photo-id assessment of lesion occurrence and to help examine etiology, lesion samples, categorized according to the aforementioned descriptions, were opportunistically obtained from two stranding organizations in the southeast United States (Coastal Marine Mammal Stranding Assessments Program, Charleston, SC and Hubbs-Sea World Research Institute's Marine Mammal Strandings Program, Melbourne Beach, FL) between 2008 and 2010. These organizations were selected as their stranding response covers geographic areas that are in close proximity to the photo-id study sites (Figure 2); however, overlap of study subjects between the photo-id and stranding assessments was not an intended objective. Lesion sites were swabbed for bacterial culture, and individual lesion biopsies were sub-sampled and preserved in: 1) 10% buffered formalin; 2) viral transport media; 3) RNA Later® (Applied Biosystems/Ambion, Austin, TX); and 4) frozen whole at −20°C. Histological analyses were conducted by a veterinary pathologist, and samples revealing evidence of a viral source were submitted for polymerase chain reaction (PCR) analyses (e.g. [40–42]) to the Wildlife Health Center at the University of California (UC Davis) School of Veterinary Medicine.

DNA was extracted from the skin tissues using a commercial kit according to manufacturer's instructions (DNeasy Blood and

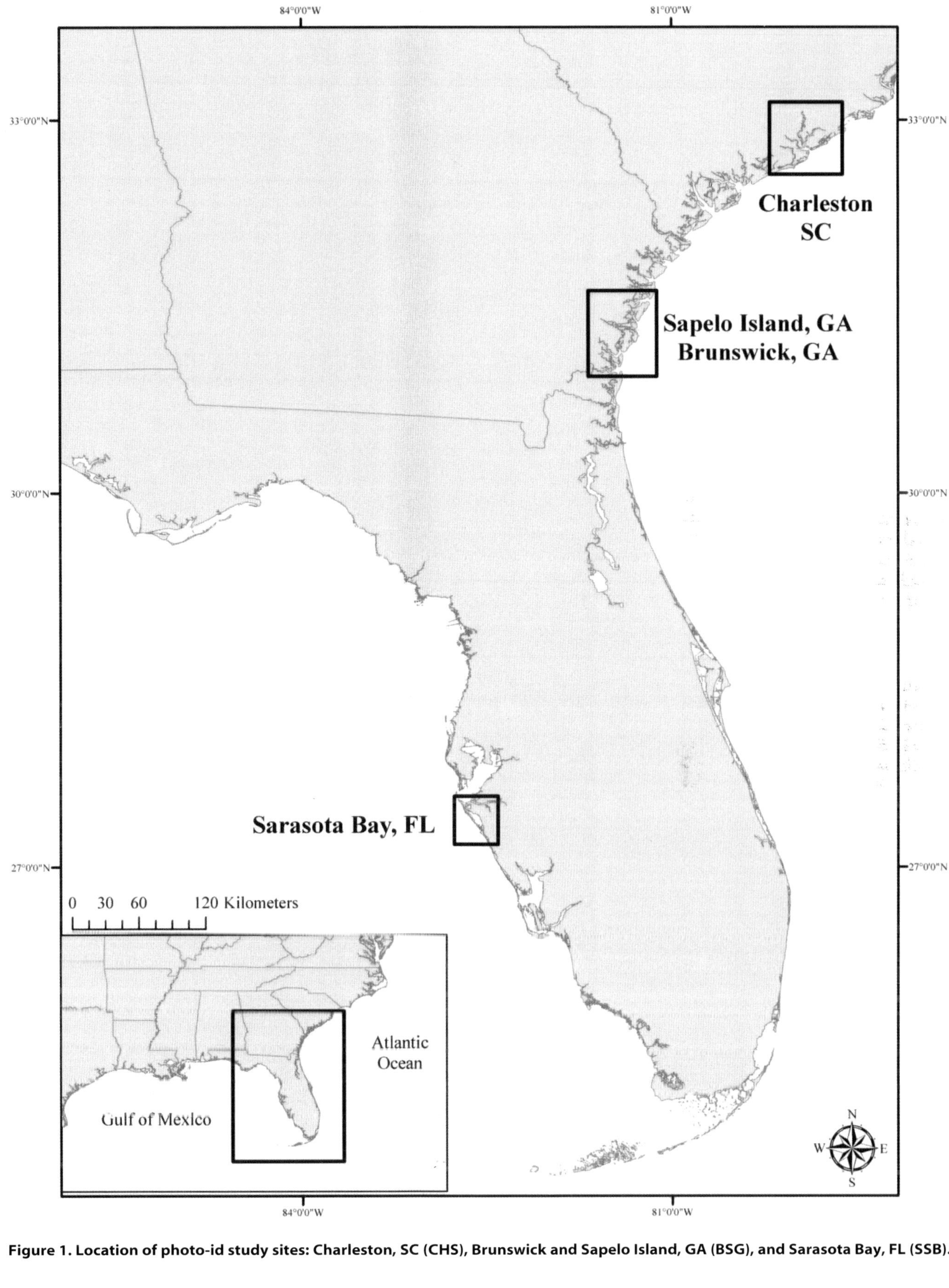

Figure 1. Location of photo-id study sites: Charleston, SC (CHS), Brunswick and Sapelo Island, GA (BSG), and Sarasota Bay, FL (SSB).

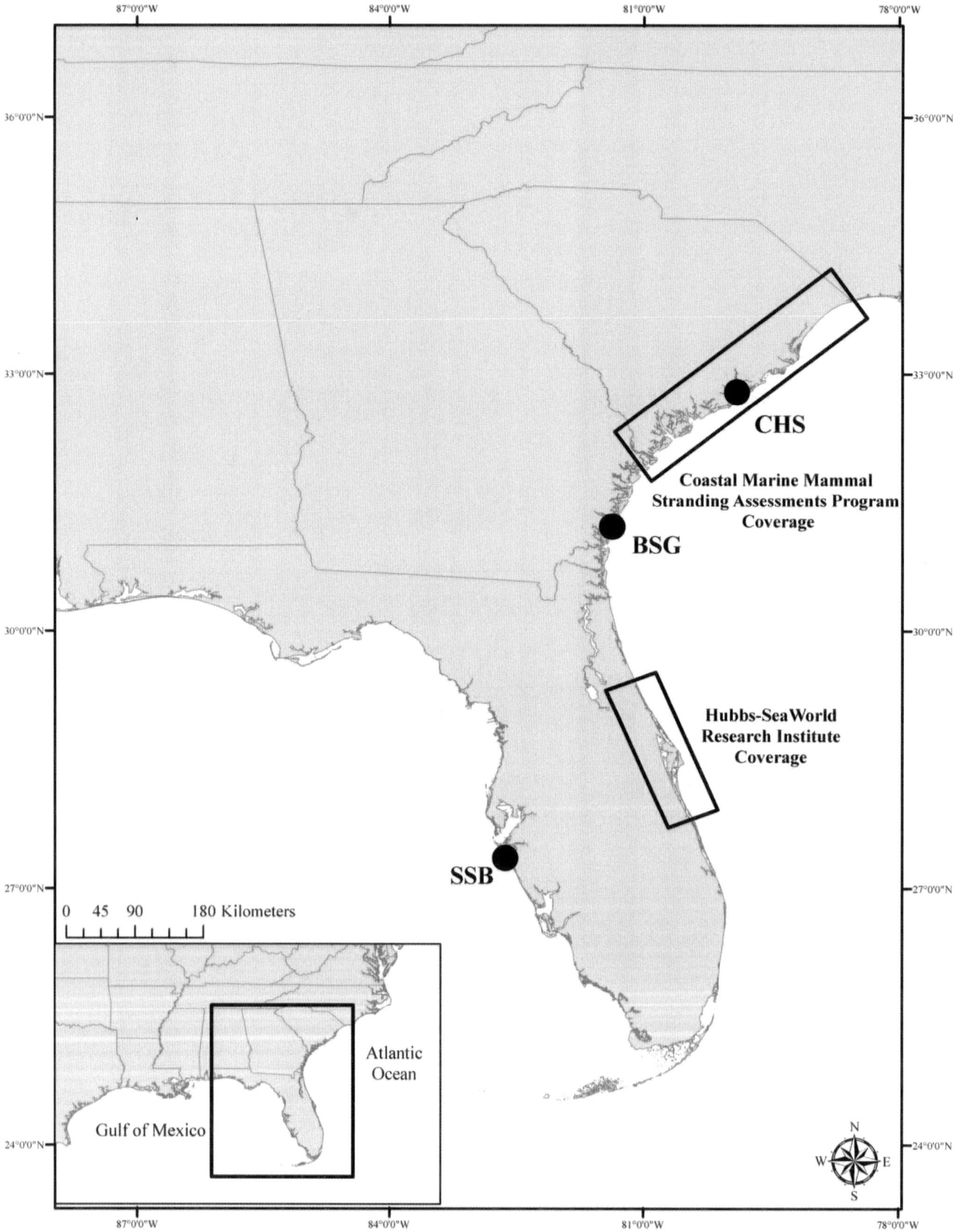

Figure 2. Photo-id study sites [Charleston, SC (CHS); Brunswick and Sapelo Island, GA (BSG); Sarasota Bay, FL (SSB)] and stranding coverage areas for the Coastal Marine Mammal Stranding Assessments Program (South Carolina) and Hubbs-SeaWorld Research Institute (Florida).

Tissue Kit, Qiagen Inc.,Valencia, CA). Multiple primers were used to test for the presence of poxviral DNA. PCR was performed to detect a 594 bp fragment of the genomic region encoding for the virion envelope antigen (p42K) of parapox viruses [42] and a 344 bp fragment of the hemagglutinin (HA) protein of orthopox viruses [40]. PCR to detect herpesviral DNA was performed using primary and nested consensus primers for the DNA-dependent-DNA polymerase (Dpol) gene of herpesviruses to amplify a fragment of 250 bp [41]. Parallel reactions amplifying a 350 bp fragment of the mammalian ferritin gene were performed to control for the PCR amplificability of the DNA sample. PCR products were resolved on 1–1.5% agarose gels. Bands of expected size were excised, purified using the QIAquick Gel Extraction Kit (Qiagen Inc.) and cloned (pCR4-TOPO vector; Invitrogen) and sequenced using the 3730 DNA Analyzer (Applied Biosystems).

Raw sequences were edited with Geneious Pro (version 5.1.4; Biomatters) [43], and the identity of the herpesviral DNA fragments were confirmed with the use of the BLASTn program run on the non-redundant National Center for Biotechnology Information (NCBI) database (http://blast. ncbi. nlm.nih.gov/Blast.cgi). Primer sequences were edited out prior to further analyses and phylogenetic analysis was performed to compare the obtained herpesviral sequences with 23 other herpesviral sequences from all three subfamilies. The nucleotide sequences of the DNA polymerase gene fragments were aligned using MUSCLE [44]. Bayesian analysis of the alignment was performed using Mr. Bayes 3.1 with gamma distributed rate variation [45]. Four incrementally heated Markov Chains were run for 1,100,000 generations, sampling every 200 generations, where 10% of 1,100,000 iterations were discarded as burn in. IgHv-2 (Iguanid herpesvirus-2, Genbank accession number AY236869) was used as the outgroup due to its early divergence from other herpesviruses.

Statistical Analysis

The prevalence of skin lesions was estimated by the proportion of distinct individuals with at least one skin lesion compared to all distinct individuals sighted during the study period (i.e. 2009 overall or each month). Individuals with and without skin lesions during two or more months of the study were only counted once for the 2009 estimate. Similarly, if an individual was sighted with skin lesions twice during the same month, only one occurrence of the lesion was used to estimate the monthly prevalence of skin disease. The overall prevalence of skin lesions was compared between sites using a Chi Square test and Bonferroni correction for multiple comparisons ($\alpha = 0.0167$; [46]), assuming the requirements for a normal distribution approximation [46,47].

Using logistic regression analyses, the occurrence of skin lesions among dolphins from all three sites was examined relative to salinity (ppt) and water temperature (°C) measurements that were collected at each sighting used for lesion screening. Each individual was coded with a "1" (skin lesion present) or "0" (no skin lesion present). If an individual dolphin was sighted on more than one day in the month, salinity and temperature measurements were averaged for the multiple sightings. PROC LOGISTIC in SAS® (SAS Institute Inc., Cary, NC), was used to examine the associations ($\alpha = 0.05$) between lesion occurrence and salinity and temperature where skin lesion status (0,1) was the dependent variable, temperature and salinity were continuous independent variables, and site (CHS, BSG, SSB) was a categorical variable.

Prevalence of different skin lesion types was estimated as the proportion of individuals with a particular lesion type relative to the total number of individuals with lesions, for a given time period (i.e. 2009 overall or by month). In some cases, animals presented with multiple lesion types. Within a single study site, the prevalence of different skin lesion types were compared between months using a Chi Square or Fisher's Exact test depending on expected cell counts [46], and *post-hoc* analyses to determine differences in lesion type occurrence were evaluated using a SAS® macro for multiple comparisons that relied upon arcsine transformation of binomial data ($\alpha < 0.05$; [47]). Major lesion types were also compared between sites using a Chi Square test and the multiple comparisons macro ($\alpha < 0.05$; [47]).

Results

Overall Skin Lesion Prevalence

Digital images of 266 distinct individuals were suitable for lesion screening during the study period in Sarasota Bay (SSB). Of these, 101 animals ($P = 0.380$; 95% CI: 0.321–0.441) had visible skin lesions. In Brunswick and Sapelo Island, GA (BSG), images of 322 distinct individuals were suitable for lesion screening, and 189 ($P = 0.587$; 95% CI: 0.531–0.641) animals were found to have visible skin lesions. Photo-id images were suitable for 351 individuals from Charleston, SC (CHS), and 171 ($P = 0.487$; 95% CI: 0.434–0.541) of these presented with at least one skin lesion (Table 1). Pairwise Chi Square tests with a Bonferroni correction for multiple comparisons ($\alpha = 0.0167$) revealed a significant difference in skin lesion prevalence between all three sites (SSB<BSG $p < 0.0001$; BSG>CHS $p = 0.0107$; CHS>SSB $p = 0.0088$; Table 1). Monthly differences were significant for the comparisons of SSB to the other two sites (Table 1). A consistent seasonal trend in skin lesion occurrence was observed for all three sites with monthly prevalence estimates ranked from highest to lowest: 1) April; 2) February; 3) October; 4) July (Table 1). It's unlikely that this trend was dependent solely on water temperature, as more lesions were observed in April than February. For CHS and BSG dolphins, lower lesion prevalence in the months of July and October could be related to an influx of animals during summer and fall [35,37], assuming that non-residents were largely lesion-free. To better understand the potential effect of influx, dolphin composition in CHS was examined for the month of July. Of the 163 dolphins screened for lesions (Table 1), 47% were considered non-residents. Twenty-five percent of non-residents were observed with at least one skin lesion, while 18% of residents were lesioned, and these proportions were not significantly different based on a Chi-Square test of binomial proportions ($p = 0.3345$). Since one quarter of the non-residents were observed with lesions, and because the proportion of lesioned non-residents was greater than residents, it seems unlikely that the influx of non-resident dolphins to CHS in July was responsible for deflating lesion prevalence.

The minimum, maximum, and mean values for the salinity and temperature measurements were calculated for all three study sites. Mean water temperatures for CHS, BSG, and SSB were 21.1°C, 20.7°C, and 24.4°C, respectively. Mean salinities were 29.9 ppt (CHS), 25.1 ppt (BSG), and 33.1 ppt (SSB). Overall, the largest range in salinity (0.1–33.0 ppt) and water temperature (7.6–30.3°C) occurred in BSG. For all study sites, water temperature was associated with lesion occurrence ($p < 0.05$); however, salinity was significantly associated with lesion occurrence only for the BSG animals. Therefore, the overall environmental logistic regression model for all three sites used water temperature and study site as dependent variables (Figure 3). This model indicated an 8% reduction in the odds of lesion occurrence for each unit increase (°C) in water temperature after adjusting for study site ($OR = 0.92$; 95%CI: 0.906–0.938), as well as significantly increased odds of skin lesions among dolphins in BSG (39%) after adjusting for water temperature ($OR = 1.39$; 95%CI:

Table 1. Skin lesion prevalence and 95% CI for bottlenose dolphins photographed in waters near Charleston, SC (CHS), near Brunswick and Sapelo Island, GA (BSG), and Sarasota Bay, FL (SSB) in 2009.

	2009 Overall	February	April	July	October
Sarasota Bay (SSB)					
Photographed	266	151	127	124	132
AWL	101	40	45	18	20
Prevalence	0.380	0.265	0.354	0.145	0.152
95% CI	(0.321–0.441)	(0.197–0.343)	(0.272–0.444)	(0.088–0.220)	(0.095–0.224)
pvalue (SSB vs BSG)	<0.0001*	<0.0001*	<0.0001*	0.0066*	0.0041*
Georgia (BSG)					
Photographed	322	143	139	195	98
AWL	189	85	96	50	29
Prevalence	0.587	0.594	0.691	0.256	0.296
95% CI	(0.531–0.641)	(0.509–0.676)	(0.607–0.766)	(0.197–0.324)	(0.208–0.397)
pvalue (BSG vs CHS)	0.0107*	0.1296	0.1095	0.0653	0.1009
Charleston (CHS)					
Photographed	351	113	108	163	123
AWL	171	56	74	35	32
Prevalence	0.487	0.496	0.685	0.215	0.260
95% CI	(0.434–0.541)	(0.400–0.591)	(0.589–0.771)	(0.154–0.286)	(0.185–0.347)
pvalue (CHS vs SSB)	0.0088*	<0.0001*	<0.0001*	0.0400	0.0124*

**Indicates a significant difference with a Bonferroni correction for multiple comparisons ($\alpha = 0.0167$).*
"Photographed" - number of dolphins evaluated for lesions with photographs suitable for lesion detection.
"AWL" - number of dolphins photographed with visible skin lesion(s).
"Prevalence" - proportion of 'Photographed' that is 'AWL'.
(p values are reported for comparisons of skin lesion prevalence between sites).

1.203–1.614). It is possible that the site-specific difference in association between lesion occurrence and salinity was a result of the wide salinity range for BSG. Therefore, *post hoc* logistic regression modeling of lesion occurrence in BSG was conducted using both water temperature and salinity, revealing significant associations with both environmental variables (temperature: $OR = 0.92$, *95%CI: 0.895–0.944;* salinity: $OR = 0.96$, *95%CI: 0.938–0.922*).

Skin Lesion Type

Lesions representing 12 of the 13 possible categories were observed on dolphins in CHS, BSG, and SSB (Figure 4). Overall, Sarasota Bay dolphins presented with the greatest number of different skin lesion types ($n = 11$), while the fewest types occurred in Charleston ($n = 9$; Table 2). Approximately one-third of the dolphins from all three sites presented with multiple lesion types ($CHS = 0.38$; $BSG = 0.36$; $SSB = 0.30$). Cloudy lesions were not observed on dolphins from any of the photo-id study sites. Spotted lesions were only observed on BSG dolphins during July, and lacaziosis lesions were only present on SSB dolphins. The most common lesion type observed on dolphins from CHS and BSG were dark-fringed, whereas SSB dolphins were most commonly observed with tattoo-like lesions (Table 2).

Lesion types for which the prevalence among animals from a given site was greater than 15% were considered 'major lesion types' (Table 3, Figure 5). No significant differences in prevalence were observed between sites for black and pale lesions. The proportion of BSG and CHS animals with dark-fringed lesions was significantly higher than dolphins in SSB. Also, dolphins in BSG had a significantly higher prevalence of vesicular lesions than both CHS and SSB. The prevalence of tattoo-like lesions among SSB dolphins was significantly higher than among both BSG and CHS dolphins ($\alpha < 0.05$, Table 3).

Due to the observed geographic disparities in dark-fringed, tattoo-like, and vesicular lesions, associations between these lesion types and environmental parameters were examined using previously described logistic regression methods. Water temperature, after adjusting for study site, was significantly associated ($p < 0.05$) with the occurrence of dark-fringed, tattoo-like, and vesicular lesion types; whereas, salinity was only significantly associated with dark-fringed lesions and therefore not included in subsequent regression models. The regression models for dark-fringed, tattoo-like, and vesicular lesions revealed a respective 12%, 5%, and 16% reduction in the odds of occurrence for each unit increase (°C) in water temperature ($OR_{dark\text{-}fringed} = 0.88$, *95% CI: 0.863–0.905;* $OR_{tattoo\text{-}like} = 0.95$, *95% CI: 0.921–0.986;* $OR_{vesicular} = 0.84$, *95% CI:0.809–0.877*). Also, compared to SSB animals and after adjusting for water temperature, dolphins in CHS and BSG had a significantly increased odds of dark-fringed lesions ($OR_{CHS} = 3.59$, *95% CI: 2.227–5.784;* $OR_{BSG} = 3.47$, *95% CI:2.165–5.576*), a significantly decreased odds of tattoo-like lesions ($OR_{CHS} = 0.07$, *95% CI: 0.026–0.207;* $OR_{BSG} = 0.73$, *95% CI:0.459–1.161*), and BSG dolphins were significantly more likely to have vesicular lesions ($OR = 2.61$, *95% CI: 1.306–5.215*).

Stranding Sampling

Stranded bottlenose dolphins were retrieved from coastal and estuarine shorelines of South Carolina and the central east coast of Florida, which includes the estuarine waters of the

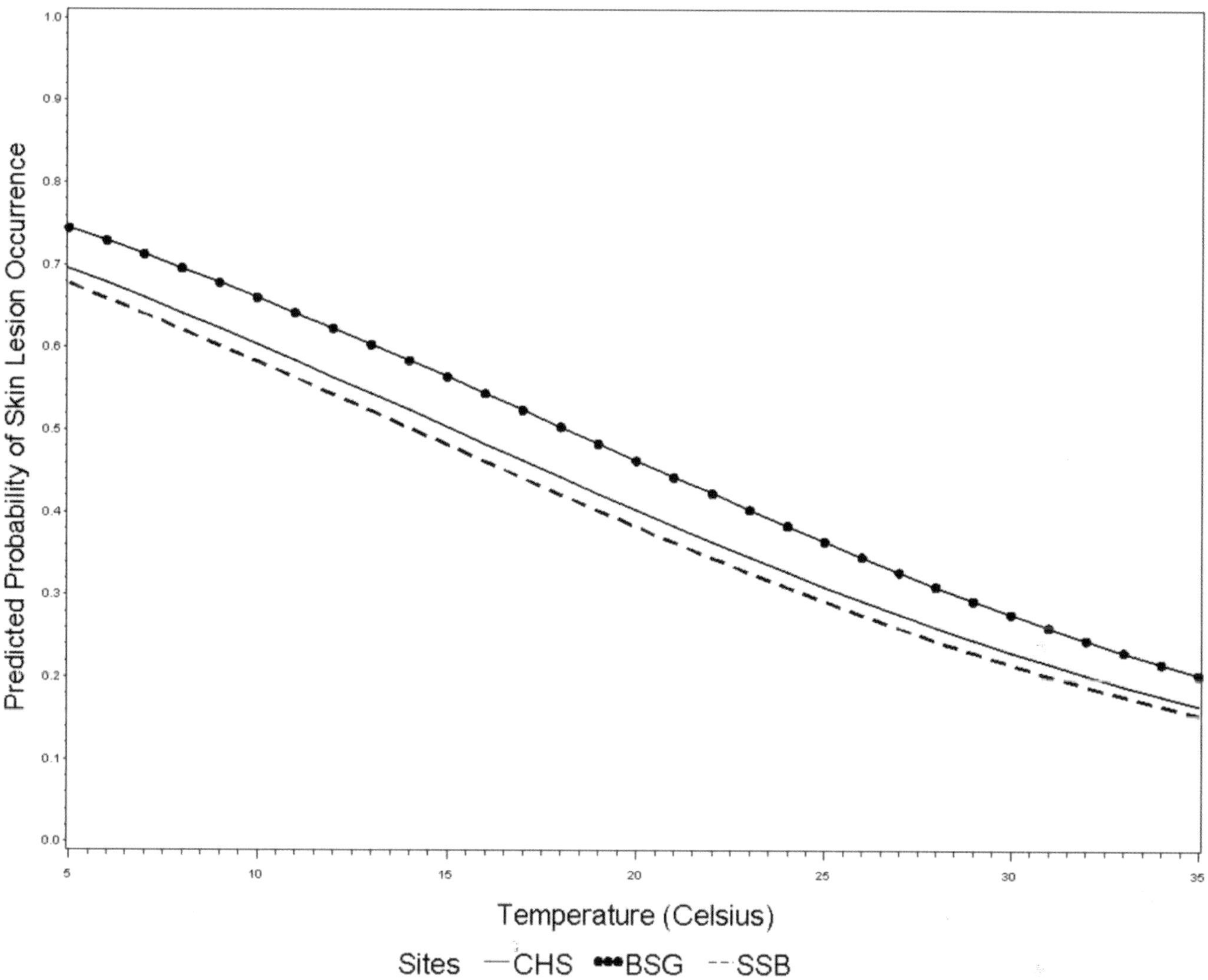

Figure 3. Regression curve for logistic model of the predicted probability of bottlenose dolphin (*Tursiops truncatus*) skin lesion occurrence using water temperature and study site as independent variables [Charleston, SC (CHS); Brunswick and Sapelo Island, GA (BSG); Sarasota Bay, FL (SSB)].

Indian River Lagoon and the oceanic beaches of the Atlantic Ocean (Figure 2). Twenty-nine stranded dolphins presented with at least one skin lesion, and 10 of these animals had multiple lesion types. Based on morphological analyses, none of the stranded animals from Florida or South Carolina were suspected to belong to the offshore ecotype [48]. Forty lesion samples were initially examined by histology, and 11 of the lesions were subsequently analyzed by PCR due to the suspicion of a viral etiology.

Lacaziosis-like disease occurred twice on dolphins from Florida, however, histological examination of biopsies from both animals confirmed infection by *L. loboi* in only one sample. Although histological analyses of lesions categorized as spotted, dark-fringed, and tattoo-like revealed evidence suggestive of a viral infection, all samples were negative for poxvirus and herpesvirus using PCR. Pale lesion histology revealed indications of: 1) healing process due to prior trauma; 2) ectoparasite attachment site; 3) prior viral infection; and 4) inflammation. Three lesion samples tested positive by PCR and sequence analysis of the obtained fragments with the degenerate primers confirmed the presence of herpesviral DNA. Phylogenetic analysis indicated that two sequences (from lesions categorized as pale and cloudy [11]) were identical to each other and to Delphinid Herpesvirus 1 (Genbank accession number AY952779), a gammaherpesvirus previously detected in bottlenose dolphins; and the third (from a white-fringed lesion sample) was identical to Delphinid Herpesvirus 3 (Genbank accession number AY757301), an alphaherpesvirus previously detected in bottlenose dolphins.

Discussion

Environmental and Anthropogenic Influences

These results indicate that geographic differences exist in the prevalence of skin lesions, as well as in the distribution and occurrence of different skin lesion types among dolphins from the three study sites. These differences could potentially be explained by variations in environmental parameters (i.e. temperature, salinity) or disparities in susceptibility due to anthropogenic contaminant exposure. For example, the Altamaha River, the third largest freshwater input into the Atlantic Ocean from North

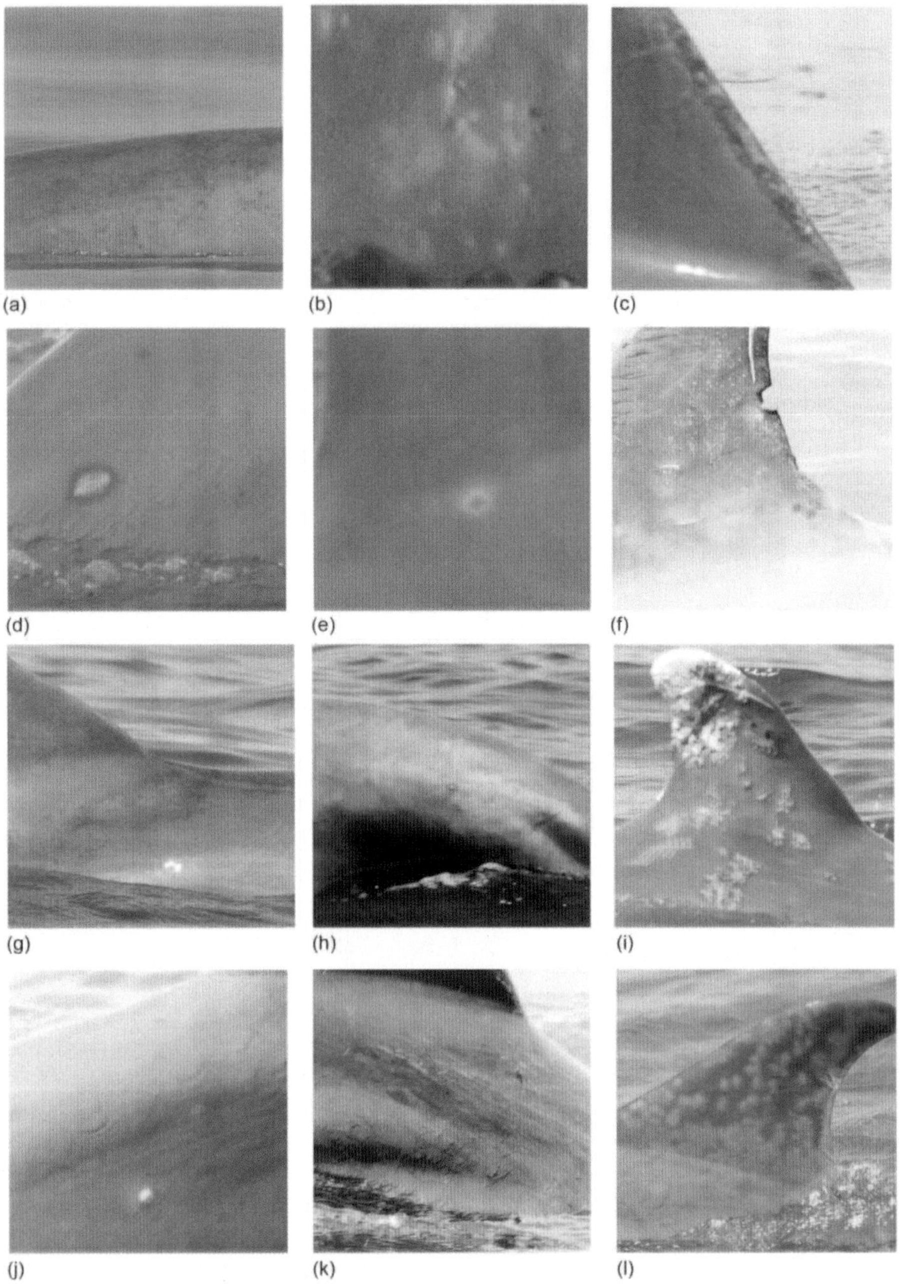

Figure 4. Examples of skin lesion types on free-ranging bottlenose dolphins (*Tursiops truncatus*) photographed in waters near Charleston, SC (CHS), Brunswick and Sapelo Island, GA (BSG), and Sarasota Bay, FL (SSB) in 2009. Lesion types include: black (a); pale (b); lunar (c); dark-fringed spots (d); white-fringed spots (e); orange patch (f); tattoo-like (g); white velvety (h); lacaziosis-like (i); vesicular (j); mottled (k); and spotted (l). (Categories from [3,5,9,12]) Photo credit: B.Balmer, NCCOS/NOS/NOAA, Sarasota Dolphin Research Program.

America [49], bisects the BSG field site. Thus, dolphins sighted predominantly in the waters surrounding the Altamaha River may be more susceptible to skin lesion types associated with freshwater input or runoff. Furthermore, a previous study [3] reported an association between lesion occurrence and environmental factors, where the prevalence of skin lesions decreased with increasing water temperature and salinity. Results from the present study further support the link between the presence of skin lesions and colder water temperatures for all three study sites examined, as logistic regression analyses indicated a decreased odds of lesion occurrence with increasing water temperature. The highest prevalence of skin lesions for all three sites occurred in April, and the mean water temperature for all three sites in April was colder than for the months of July and October; however, February water temperatures were colder than April and the prevalence of skin lesions was lower. These results suggest that skin lesion occurrence is influenced by factors other than just water temperature, that there is a lag time between exposure to colder water temperatures and the clinical manifestation of disease, or that pathogen viability and dolphin susceptibility may be heightened when water temperatures are within a particular range. In this particular study, colder water temperatures in the

Table 2. Prevalence of skin lesion types among lesioned dolphins photographed in waters near Charleston, SC (CHS), near Brunswick and Sapelo Island, GA (BSG), and Sarasota Bay, FL (SSB) in 2009.

Type	Charleston (n = 171)	Georgia (n = 189)	Sarasota Bay (n = 101)
Black	0.263	0.201	0.287
Dark-Fringed	0.550	0.577	0.238
Lunar	0.064	0	0.020
Pale	0.123	0.212	0.158
Tattoo	0.199	0.212	0.426
Vesicular	0.152	0.302	0.109
White Velvety	0.006	0.069	0.040
White-Fringed	0.146	0.116	0.030
Lacaziosis-Like	0	0	0.040
Orange Patch	0	0.069	0.069
Mottled	0.047	0.005	0.129
Spotted	0	0.053	0
Cloudy	0	0	0
Other	0.018	0.021	0.010

northern study sites (CHS and BSG), and freshwater exposure to BSG dolphins could help to explain observed geographic differences in skin lesion prevalence.

As for differences in susceptibility resulting from chemical contaminant exposure, recent analyses of remote and surgical blubber biopsies of dolphins from Brunswick, GA revealed unprecedented levels of polychlorinated biphenyls (PCBs) [34,50]. Previous studies of PCB toxicity among mammalian laboratory animals indicated that skin lesions can manifest from exposure to different contaminant mixtures [51–53]. Anthropogenic contaminants have also been linked to immune suppression in marine mammals [54–56]; therefore, high levels of PCB exposure among BSG dolphins could contribute to the higher prevalence of skin lesions among animals from this site due to an inability to ward off pathogens.

Lesion Identification and Differentiation

Three visually distinctive lesions from stranded dolphins were found positive for herpesvirus by PCR. Furthermore, two of the samples were found positive for identical strains, which suggest that different lesion types are not always representative of different diseases. Histological evidence of poxviral infection has been observed in biopsies of tattoo lesions [17,21], as well as in 'ring lesions' [21,57] and 'round marks' [4], which included dark-fringed spots as described in the current study. Although all dark-fringed and tattoo-like samples in this study were negative for poxviral infection by PCR, histological analyses provided evidence of a prior viral infection (i.e. cytoplasmic swelling, intracytoplasmic inclusion bodies). Results from the current study cannot confirm if poxvirus is associated with dark-fringed or tattoo-like lesions from the sampled dolphins; however, it seems possible that the virus could manifest as both lesion types. These stranding results strengthen the hypothesis that different visual lesion types could be

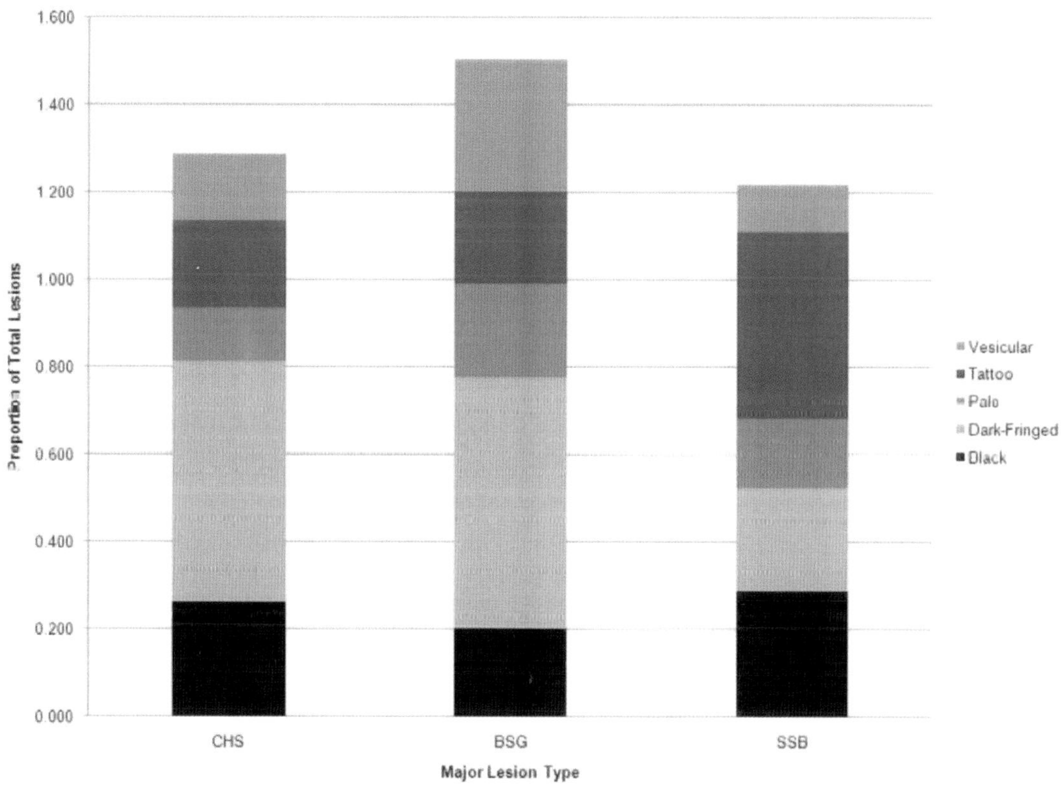

Figure 5. Proportion of major skin lesion types (2009 overall proportion >0.15) for free-ranging bottlenose dolphins (*Tursiops truncatus*) photographed in waters near Charleston, SC (CHS), near Brunswick and Sapelo Island, GA (BSG), and Sarasota Bay, FL (SSB) 2009.

Table 3. Proportion of major skin lesion types (*P*>*0.15*) and study site comparisons for lesioned dolphins photographed in waters near Charleston, SC (CHS), near Brunswick and Sapelo Island, GA (BSG), and Sarasota Bay, FL (SSB) in 2009.

Type	CHS (n = 171)	BSG (n = 189)	SSB (n = 101)	Chi Square (p)	Significant Difference^
Black	0.263	0.201	0.287	0.1964	-
Dark-Fringed	0.550	0.577	0.238	<0.0001*	CHS>SSB BSG>SSB
Pale	0.123	0.212	0.158	0.0757	-
Tattoo	0.199	0.212	0.426	<0.0001*	SSB>BSG SSB>CHS
Vesicular	0.152	0.302	0.109	0.0001*	BSG>SSB BSG>CHS

Indicates a significant difference ($\alpha = 0.05$).

^Indicates a significant difference after post-hoc multiple comparisons tests ($\alpha < 0.05$; Horne and Plaehn 2007).

caused by the same pathogen or may be different stages of the same disease [3,4,11].

Bottlenose Dolphin Skin Lesion Differences between Study Sites

The prevalence of skin lesions among animals from the three study sites ranged from 38% to 59%. These estimates are substantially lower than the prevalence of skin lesions reported in other bottlenose dolphin populations across the globe, which ranged between 63% and 100% [2,3,6,8,10,11]. Skin lesion occurrence has not been previously assessed for the CHS or BSG dolphins, so it is possible that the prevalence values reported here are minimum estimates for animals from these study sites. However, in a previous study, 62.7% of Sarasota Bay dolphins had at least one skin lesion detected on the dorsal fin [3]. The discrepancy between the previous and the current SSB prevalence estimate (38.0%) could be explained by a decreased burden of skin disease among dolphins from the SSB site during the intervening decade, differences in lesion categorization, or differences in photographic quality between studies. The lesion categories for both studies were derived from previous descriptions [11]; however, the current study did not include orange hues as a skin lesion type as the focus was on lesions that may have an infectious disease etiology, and orange hues could be films caused by the external attachment of diatoms [24]. In the Wilson et al. study [3], orange lesions were included in the 'other' category, which comprised 42% of the lesions observed in SSB; therefore, it is possible that the exclusion of animals with orange hues may have contributed to the lower prevalence estimate for skin lesions in SSB. As for differences in image quality between the two studies, higher-resolution digital images that were used for the current study likely improved the discretion of epidermal markings resulting from scarring or trauma that may have previously been classified as a skin lesion in lower resolution photographs. Although the prevalence of skin lesions on SSB dolphins was substantially different than a previous study [3], both estimates of skin lesion prevalence for SSB dolphins was the lowest compared to all other sites examined in either study.

In addition to environmental and anthropogenic influences, differences in skin lesion prevalence among dolphins from the three study sites in this paper could be due to heterogeneous age-class and sex distributions. Several previous studies of skin lesions and cetaceans have indicated differential susceptibility and severity among animals of varying age-class [9,12,17] and sex [8]. Age and sex data were not uniformly available for animals examined in the current study, and analyses that rely upon photo-id data are often limited to images of dorsal body surfaces, which prevent sex determination from genital morphology. Furthermore, age-class identification from photo-id data is often limited to adult or calf distinctions, which may not provide useful information for diseases that commonly occur among sub-adults (e.g. tattoo skin disease [9,17]). To obtain a clear epidemiological understanding of factors influencing the prevalence of skin lesions and different lesion types, age-class and sex information are necessary.

Conclusion

Skin lesions among bottlenose dolphins are geographically widespread and can affect a large proportion of a population. Also, lesion types may be differentially distributed among populations. In the current study, the prevalence of skin lesions was significantly different among dolphins from the three study sites, and differences in the occurrence of lesion types were also observed. The findings suggest that skin disease can vary by population, and that certain disease types may be geographically distinct. These geographic differences may be due to seasonal or environmental fluctuations, exposure to anthropogenic influences, or differences in population demographics; however, more research in these areas is needed to confirm this. This study demonstrates that images from photo-id surveys can be used as a non-invasive and cost-effective approach to study lesion occurrence in wild cetacean populations, and while many skin lesions do not appear to be fatal [2,12,21,57,58], lesions detected on free-ranging animals may serve as an indication of other underlying health concerns or environmental threats.

Acknowledgments

We would like to thank the staff, interns, and volunteers of the Sarasota Dolphin Research Program (SDRP), Charleston Dolphin Abundance and Distribution project (CDAD), Georgia Department of Natural Resources, and the Georgia Dolphin Project for providing crucial photo-id images and dolphin identification data. We would also like to thank Wendy Noke Durden, Teresa Mazza, James Powell, Elise Kohli, and volunteers of the Coastal Marine Mammal Stranding Assessments Program (SC), Hubbs-Sea World Research Institute's Marine Mammal Stranding Program (FL), as well as the other stranding organizations within the Southeast U.S. Marine Mammal Stranding Network who contributed samples and advice to this project. Thank you to Dr. Kathleen Colgrove of the Zoological Pathology Program at the University of Illinois, Urbana-Champaign College of Veterinary Medicine for additional PCR analysis of stranding samples. Thanks also to S. Fire, T. Greig, and K. Moore for reviewing this manuscript.

NOAA Disclaimer

This publication does not constitute an endorsement of any commercial product or intend to be an opinion beyond scientific or other results obtained by the National Oceanic and Atmospheric Administration (NOAA). No reference shall be made to NOAA, or this publication furnished by NOAA, to any advertising or sales promotion which would indicate or imply that NOAA recommends or endorses any proprietary product mentioned herein, or which has as its purpose an interest to cause the advertised product to be used or purchased because of this publication.

Author Contributions

Conceived and designed the experiments: LBH LHS RSW TKR. Performed the experiments: LBH DSR JA AB BCB SML TS ESZ MS WM TG. Analyzed the data: LBH DSR TG LHS JA SML TS BCB. Contributed reagents/materials/analysis tools: DSR TG TKR. Wrote the paper: LBH LHS RSW BCB TG.

References

1. Baker JR (1992) Skin disease in wild cetaceans from British waters. Aquatic Mammals 18: 27–32.
2. Harzen S, Brunnick BJ (1997) Skin disorders in bottlenose dolphins (Tursiops truncatus), resident in the Sado estuary, Portugal. Aquatic Mammals 23: 59–68.
3. Wilson B, Arnold H, Bearzi G, Fortuna CM, Gaspar R, et al. (1999) Epidermal diseases in bottlenose dolphins: impacts of natural and anthropogenic factors. Proceedings from the Royal Society of London B 266: 1077–1083.
4. Van Bressem M-F, Van Waerebeek K, Mones D, Kennedy S, Reyes JC, et al. (2006) Diseases, lesions and malformations in the long-beaked common dolphin Delphinus capensis from the Southeast Pacific. Diseases of Aquatic Organisms 68: 149–165.
5. Van Bressem M-F, Van Waerebeek K, Reyes JC, Felix F, Echegaray M, et al. (2007) A preliminary overview of skin and skeletal diseases and traumata in small cetaceans from South American waters. Latin American Journal of Aquatic Mammals 6: 7–42.
6. Bearzi M, Rapoport S, Chau J, Saylan C (2009) Skin lesions and physical deformities of coastal and offshore common bottlenose dolphins (Tursiops truncatus) in Santa Monica Bay and adjacent areas, California. Ambio 38: 66–71.
7. Kiszka J, Bressem M-FV, Pusineri C (2009) Lobomycosis-like disease and other skin conditions in Indo-Pacific bottlenose dolphins Tursiops aduncus from the Indian Ocean. Diseases of Aquatic Organisms 84: 151–157.
8. Rowe LE, Currey RJC, Dawson SM, Johnson D (2010) Assessment of epidermal condition and calf size of Fiordland bottlenose dolphin Tursiops truncatus populations using dorsal fin photographs and photogrammetry. Endangered Species Research 11: 83–89.
9. Van Bressem M-F, Van Waerebeek K, Aznar FJ, Raga JA, Jepson PD, et al. (2009) Epidemiological pattern of tattoo skin disease: a potential general health indicator for cetaceans. Diseases of Aquatic Organisms 85: 225–237.
10. Maldini D, Riggin J, Cecchetti A, Cotter MP (2010) Prevalence of epidermal conditions in California coastal bottlenose dolphins (Tursiops truncatus) in Monterey Bay. Ambio 39: 455–462.
11. Wilson B, Thompson PM, Hammond PS (1997) Skin lesions and physical deformities in bottlenose dolphins in the Moray Firth: population prevalence and age-sex differences. Ambio 26: 243–245.
12. Van Bressem M-F, Gaspar R, Aznar FJ (2003) Epidemiology of tattoo skin disease in bottlenose dolphins, Tursiops truncatus, from the Sado estuary, Portugal. Diseases of Aquatic Organisms 56: 171–179.
13. Pettis HM, Rolland RM, Hamilton PK, Brault S, Knowlton AR, et al. (2004) Visual health assessment of North Atlantic right whales (Eubalaena glacialis) using photographs. Canadian Journal of Zoology 82: 8–19.
14. Hamilton PK, Marx MK (2005) Skin lesions on North Atlantic right whales: categories, prevalence and change in occurrence in the 1990 s. Diseases of Aquatic Organisms 68: 71–82.
15. Burdett Hart L, Wells RS, Adams J, Rotstein DS, Schwacke LH (2010) Modeling lacaziosis lesion progression in common bottlenose dolphins Tursiops truncatus using long-term photographic records. Diseases of Aquatic Organisms 90: 105–112.
16. Noke Durden W, Leger JS, Stolen M, Mazza T, Londono C (2009) Lacaziosis in bottlenose dolphins (Tursiops truncatus) in the Indian River Lagoon, Florida, USA. Journal of Wildlife Diseases 45: 849–856.
17. Van Bressem M-F, Van Waerebeek K (1996) Epidemiology of poxvirus in small cetaceans from the Eastern South Pacific. Marine Mammal Science 12: 371–382.
18. Reif JS, Mazzoil MS, McCulloch SD, Varela RA, Goldstein JD, et al. (2006) Lobomycosis in Atlantic bottlenose dolphins from the Indian River Lagoon, Florida. Journal of the American Veterinary Medical Association 228: 104–108.
19. Burdett Hart L, Rotstein DS, Wells RS, Bassos-Hull K, Schwacke LH (2011) Lacaziosis and lacaziosis-like prevalence among wild, common bottlenose dolphins Tursiops truncatus from the west coast of Florida, USA. Diseases of Aquatic Organisms 95: 49–56.
20. Gulland FMD, Hall AJ (2005) The role of infectious disease in influencing status and trends. In: Reynolds JE, Perrin WF, Reeves RR, Montgomery S, Ragen TJ, eds. Marine Mammal Research: Conservation Beyond Crisis. Baltimore, MD: Hopkins University Press. pp 47–61.
21. Geraci JR, Hicks BD, Aubin DJS (1979) Dolphin pox: a skin disease of cetaceans. Journal of Comparative Medicine 43: 399–404.
22. Barr B, Dunn JL, Daniel MD, Banford A (1989) Herpes-like viral dermatitis in a beluga whale. Journal of Wildlife Diseases 25: 608–611.
23. Migaki G, Valerio MG, Irvine AB, Garner FM (1971) Lobo's disease in an Atlantic bottle-nosed dolphin. Journal of the American Veterinary Medical Association 159: 578–582.
24. Nemoto T, Brownell RL, Ishimaru T (1977) Cocconeis diatom on the skin of Franciscana. The Scientific Report of the Whales Research Institute 29: 101–105.
25. Rotstein DS, Burdett LG, McLellan W, Schwacke L, Rowles T, et al. (2009) Lobomycosis in offshore bottlenose dolphins (Tursiops truncatus), North Carolina. Emerging Infectious Diseases 15: 588–590.
26. Van Bressem M-F, de Oliviera Santos MC, de Faria Oshima JE (2009) Skin diseases in Guiana dolphins (Sotalia guianensis) from Paranagua estuary, Brazil: a possible indicator of a compromised marine environment. Marine Environmental Research 67: 63–68.
27. Wells RS (2009) Learning from nature: bottlenose dolphin care and husbandry. Zoo Biology 28.
28. Wells RS (1991) The role of long-term study in understanding the social structure of a bottlenose dolphin community. In: Pryor K, Norris KS, eds. Dolphin Societies: Discoveries and Puzzles. Berkeley, CA: University of California Press. pp 199–225.
29. Wells RS, Scott MD (1990) Estimating bottlenose dolphin population parameters from individual identification and capture-release techniques. Report of the International Whaling Commission (Special Issue 12): 407–425.
30. Scott MD, Wells RS, Irvine AB, Mate BR (1990) Tagging and marking studies on small cetaceans. In: Leatherwood S, Reeves RR, eds. The Bottlenose Dolphin. San Diego, CA: Academic Press. pp 489–514.
31. Wells RS (2003) Dolphin social complexity: Lessons from long-term study and life history. In: Waal FBMd, Tyack PL, eds. Animal Social Complexity: Intelligence, Culture, and Individualized Societies. Cambridge, MA: Harvard University Press. pp 32–56.
32. Wells RS, Scott MD, Irvine AB (1987) The social structure of free-ranging bottlenose dolphins. In: Genoways H, ed. Current Mammalogy Vol 1. New York: Plenum Press. pp 247–305.
33. Irvine AB, Scott MD, Wells RS, Kaufman JH (1981) Movements and activities of the Atlantic bottlenose dolphin, Tursiops truncatus, near Sarasota, Florida. Fishery Bulletin 79: 671–688.
34. Balmer B, Schwacke L, Wells R, George R, Hoguet J, et al. (2011) Patterns of persistent organochlorine contaminants in relation to sighting patterns of bottlenose dolphins from coastal Georgia, USA. Science of the Total Environment 409: 2094–2101.
35. Balmer B, Schwacke LH, Wells RS, Adams J, George RC, et al. (In review) Seasonal abundance, site-fidelity, habitat use, and ranging patterns of bottlenose dolphins within the estuaries of southern Georgia, U.S.A. Journal of Wildlife Management.
36. Zolman ES (2002) Residence patterns of bottlenose dolphins (Tursiops truncatus) in the Stono River Estuary, Charleston County, South Carolina, USA. Marine Mammal Science 18: 879–892.
37. Speakman TR, Lane SM, Schwacke LH, Fair PA, Zolman ES (2010) Mark-recapture estimates of seasonal abundance and survivorship for bottlenose dolphins (Tursiops truncatus) near Charleston, South Carolina, USA. Journal of Cetacean Research and Management 11: 153–162.
38. Urian KW, Hohn AA, Hansen LJ (1999) Status of the photo-identification catalog of coastal bottlenose dolphins of the western North Atlantic: report of a workshop of catalog contributors. In: Memorandum NT, ed. 22 p
39. Wursig B, Jefferson TA (1990) Methods of photo-identification for small cetaceans. Report of the International Whaling Commission (Special Issue 12): 43–52.
40. Ropp SL, Jin Q, Knight JC, Massung RF, Esposito JJ (1995) PCR strategy for identification and differentiation of smallpox and other orthopoxviruses. Journal of Clinical Microbiology 33: 2069–2076.
41 Van Devanter DR, Warrener P, Bennett L, Schultz ER, Coulter S, et al. (1996) Detection and analysis of diverse herpesviral species by consensus primer PCR. Journal of Clinical Microbiology 34: 1666–1671.
42. Nollens HH, Jacobson ER, Gulland FMD, Beusse DO, Bossart GD, et al. (2006) Pathology and preliminary characterization of a parapoxvirus isolated from a California sea lion (Zalophus californianus). Journal of Wildlife Diseases 42: 23–32.
43. Drummond A, Ashton B, Buxton S, Cheung M, Cooper A, et al. (2010) Geneious Pro.
44. Edgar R (2004) MUSCLE: multiple sequence alignment with high accuracy and high throughput. Nucleic Acids Research 32: 1792–1797.
45. Huelsenbeck J, Ronquist F (2001) Mr Bayes: Bayesian inference of phylogeny. Bioinformatics 17: 754–755.
46. Rosner B (2006) Fundamentals of Biostatistics, 6th Edition. Belmont, CA: Thomson Brooks/Cole. 868 p.
47. Horne J, Plaehn D Multiple comparisons on 2xc proportions; 2007 September 17–18; Seattle, WA.

48. Hersh S, Duffield D (1990) Distinction between Northwest Atlantic Offshore and Coastal Bottlenose Dolphins Based on Hemoglobin Profile and Morphometry. In: Leatherwood S, Reeves RR, eds. The Bottlenose Dolphin. New York: Academic Press, Inc. pp 129–139.
49. Frangiamore CS, Gibbons W (2004) The New Georgia Encyclopedia. Georgia Humanities Council.
50. Kucklick J, Schwacke L, Wells R, Hohn A, Guichard A, et al. (2011) Bottlenose dolphins as indicators of persistent organic pollutants in the Western North Atlantic Ocean and Northern Gulf of Mexico. Environmental Science & Technology 45: 4270–4277.
51. Vos JG (1972) Toxicology of PCBs for mammals and for birds. Environmental Health Perspectives 1: 105–117.
52. Zinkl JG (1977) Skin and liver lesions in rats fed a polychlorinated biphenyl mixture. Archives of Environmental Contamination and Toxicology 5: 217–228.
53. Kimbrough R, Buckley J, Fishbein L, Flamm G, Kasza L, et al. (1978) Animal toxicology. Environmental Health Perspectives 24: 173–184.
54. Lahvis GP, Wells RS, Kuehl DW, Stewart JL, Rhinehart HL, et al. (1995) Decreased lymphocyte responses in free-ranging bottlenose dolphins (Tursiops truncatus) are associated with the increased concentrations of PCBs and DDT in peripheral blood. Environmental Health Perspectives 103(Suppl. 4): 67–72.
55. De Swart R, Ross PS, Vos JG, Osterhaus AD (1996) Impaired immunity in harbor seals (Phoca vitulina) exposed to bioaccumulated environmental contaminants: review of a long-term feeding study. Environmental Health Perspectives 104: 823–828.
56. Ross PS, Swart RD, Addison R, Loveren HV, Vos J, et al. (1996) Contaminant-induced immunotoxicity in harbor seals: wildlife at risk? Toxicology 112: 157–169.
57. Van Bressem M-F, Van Waerebeek K, Raga JA (1999) A review of virus infections of cetaceans and the potential impact of morbilliviruses, poxviruses and papillomaviruses on host population dynamics. Diseases of Aquatic Organisms 38: 53–65.
58. Flom JO, Houk EJ (1979) Morphologic evidence of poxvirus in "tattoo" lesions from captive bottlenosed dolphins. Journal of Wildlife Diseases 15: 593–596.

2

Health Outcome Measures in Atopic Dermatitis: A Systematic Review of Trends in Disease Severity and Quality-of-Life Instruments 1985–2010

Balvinder Rehal, April Armstrong*

Department of Dermatology, University of California Davis, Davis, California, United States of America

Abstract

Background: A number of disease-severity and quality-of-life (QoL) instruments have emerged in atopic dermatitis (AD) in the last decade.

Objectives: To identify trends in outcomes instruments used in AD clinical trials and to provide a useful summary of the dimensions and validation studies for the most commonly used measures.

Method: All randomized control trials (RCTs) from 1985 to 2010 in the treatment of AD were examined.

Results: Among the 791 RCTs reviewed, we identified 20 disease-severity and 14 QoL instruments. Of these outcomes instruments, few have been validated. SCORAD, EASI, IGA and SASSAD were the most commonly used disease-severity instruments and CDLQI, DFI, DLQI and IDQOL were the most frequently used QoL measures.

Limitations: The small number of RCTs using QoL scales makes identifying trends for QoL instruments difficult.

Conclusion: Overall, there is an increase in the use of disease-severity and QoL instruments in AD clinical trials.

Editor: Lise Lotte Gluud, Copenhagen University Hospital Gentofte, Denmark

Funding: These authors have no support or funding to report.

Competing Interests: The authors have declared that no competing interests exist.

* E-mail: aprilarmstrong@post.harvard.edu

Introduction

Atopic dermatitis is a chronic, inflammatory skin disease that affects patients' physical and psychosocial wellbeing. The burden of atopic dermatitis has been documented in the medical literature [1,2]. Patients suffering from atopic dermatitis often experience embarrassment from the skin lesions, and severe disease can adversely affect social interactions and personal relationships. The symptoms of atopic dermatitis, notably pruritus, can be intractable and lead to significant emotional distress and sleep loss [3].

Despite continuing efforts in developing new treatments for atopic dermatitis, scarce literature exists that evaluates disease-severity and quality of life (QoL) outcome measures in AD [1,5,6,7]. This systematic review examines the trends in outcomes instruments, specifically disease-severity and QoL instruments, in randomized controlled trials (RCT) in the treatment of AD published between 1985 to 2010. We discuss the most frequently used disease-severity and QoL measures in terms of their dimensions (aspects of AD that the instrument measures) and validation studies that have supported their increased use in clinical trials.

Methods

To examine the disease and QoL outcome measures used in atopic dermatitis trials, we conducted a systematic review of RCTs for AD from 1985 to 2010 in the U.S. National Library of Medicine using the Medline search engine and in the electronic database, Scopus, which includes the EMBASE database. In Medline we applied the Medical Subject Headings search terms "atopic dermatitis" and "treatment" and limited the search to human RCTs published in the English language from January 1, 1985 to July 14, 2010. In Scopus, we searched for RCTs in atopic dermatitis using the search "TITLE-ABS-KEY(atopic dermatitis) AND (TITLE-ABS-KEY(randomized control trial*) OR TITLE-ABS-KEY(RCT))."

Results

In Medline, our search identified an initial group of 552 studies published between 1985 and 20010 in AD. Of these 552 studies, 195 were excluded either because they were not RCTs, not pertaining to atopic dermatitis studies, not in English, or no outcome measures were used (Figure 1). In Scopus our search generated 239 studies from 1985–2010. After cross-referencing the list of studies with our Medline search, we were left with 141 articles. Of these, 116 were excluded for the reasons listed above. After exclusion, 382 studies were reviewed from both Medline and Scopus.

A total of 20 disease-severity scales and 14 QoL scales were used in the RCTs for the treatment of atopic dermatitis. We list the

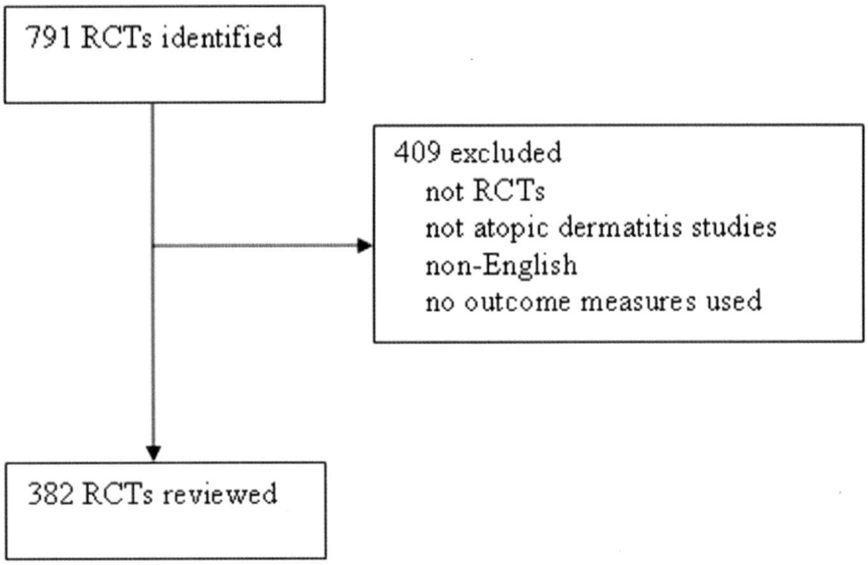

Figure 1. Excluded studies.

disease-severity instruments and QoL measures in Tables 1 and 2, respectively.

The most frequently used disease-severity instruments from 1985 to 2010 were the Severity scoring of atopic dermatitis (SCORAD), Eczema Area and Severity Index (EASI), Investigators' Global Assessment (IGA) and Six Area, Six Sign Atopic Dermatitis (SASSAD) (Table 1). SCORAD was the most frequently used scale; it was used in 113 out of 382 RCTs (30%). The next most frequently used scale was the EASI, which was used in 63 out of 382 RCTs (16%), followed by the IGA that

Table 1. Severity of disease scales.

Scale	Clinical signs						Disease extent	Subjective Sx	# of studies used in
	Erythema	Edema/ papulation	oozing/ crusts	excoriation	lichenification	dryness/ scaling			
Severity scoring of atopic dermatitis (SCORAD)	*	*	*	*	*		*	*	76
Eczema Area and Severity Index (EASI)	*	*		*	*		*		51
Investigators' Global Assessment (IGA)	*	*	*						41
Six Area, Six Sign Atopic Dermatitis (SASSAD)	*		*	*	*	*	*	*	14
Investigators' Global Atopic Dermatitis Assessment (IGADA)	*	*	*	*	*	*	*		4
Costa et al	*	*	*	*	*	*	*	*	3
Leiciester Sign Score (LSS)	*		*	*	*	*	*		2
Visual Analogue Scale (VAS) pruritus								*	2
Total Severity Score (TSS)	*	*	*	*	*		*		2
Physicians Global Assessment (PGA)	*					*	*		2
Intensity Item Score Aggregate (IISA)	*	*	*	*	*	*	*	*	1
Atopic Dermatitis Severity Index (ADSI)	*		*	*	*		*	*	1
Investigators' Static Global Assessment (ISGA)	*	*	*		*	*		*	1
Nottingham Eczema Severity Score (NESS)							*	*	1
Investigators' Global Assessment Score (IGAS)	*	*						*	1
Dry skin are and severity index (DASI)	*					*	*	*	1
Atopic Dermatitis Area and Severity Index (ADASI)	*	*	*	*	*	*	*		1
Total body severity assessment (TBSA)	*	*	*	*		*	*		1

Table 2. Quality of life scales.

Scale	Severity	itching	mood	sleep	dressing/ clothes	leisure activities	treatment	Parent mood	Parent sleep	family disruption/ tension	# Studies used in
Children's Dermatology Life Quality Index (CDLQI)		*	*	*	*	*	*				13
Dermatology Life Quality Index (DLQI)		*	*		*	*	*				8
Infant's Dermatology Quality of Life (IDQOL)	*	*	*	*	*	*	*				7
Dermatitis Family Impact (DFI)				*		*		*	*	*	6
Parent's Index of Quality of Life in Atopic Dermatitis (PIQoL-AD)					*		*	*	*	*	2
Quality of Life Index for Atopic Dermatitis (QoLIAD)			*		*	*					2
Short Form Health Survey (SF-36)			*		*	*					2
Parents of Children with Atopic Dermatitis (PQoL-AD)								*	*		1
German Instrument for the assessment of Quality of Life in Skin Diseases (DIELH)		*	*			*	*				1
Eczema Disability Index (EDI)						*	*				1
Skindex-29		*	*	*		*					1

was used in 48 out of 382 RCTs (13%). SASSAD was used in 18 out of 382 RCTs (5%). The four most commonly used scales, SCORAD, EASI, IGA and SASSAD, were used in the majority of RCTs: 242 out of 382 (63%). The remaining 14 scales were used in 57 out of 382 RCTs (15%).

The trend for disease-severity scales showed that the number of disease-severity instruments used in clinical trials increased dramatically from 1985 to 2010 (Figure 2). Specifically, SCORAD was used in 4% of RCTs from 1985–1997 and 40% RCTs from 1998–2010. SCORAD had its peak usage from 2005 to 2010.

EASI, IGA and SASSAD were also used more commonly from 1985–2010 (Figure 2). From 1985–1997, no RCTs used EASI, IGA or SASSAD. EASI also had its peak usage from 2005 to 2010. To our knowledge, IGA has not been validated to date, but its usage has been nearly identical to that of EASI (Figure 2). Out of the 48 RCTs that used IGA, 32 trials used IGA in conjunction with EASI (67%).

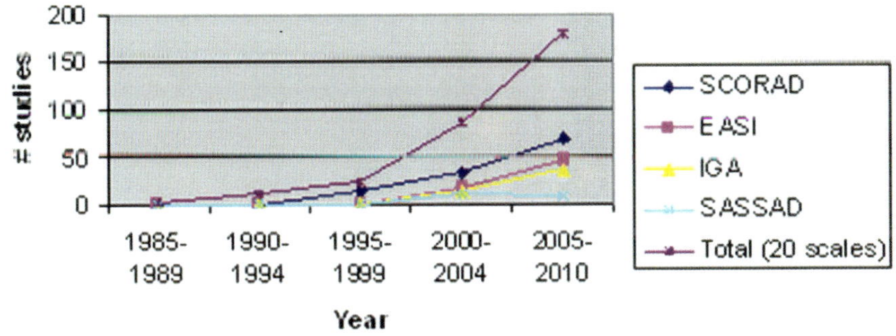

Figure 2. Trends in Disease Severity Instruments 1985–2010.

Among the 382 RCTs, 67 studies employed QoL instruments. Of the studies that used QoL outcomes measures, the Children's Dermatology Life Quality Index (CDLQI) was the most frequently used (33%), followed by the Dermatitis Family Impact (DFI) (15%), the Dermatology Life Quality Index (DLQI) (13%) and the Infant's Dermatology Life Quality Index.

(IDQOL) (12%) (Table 2). Overall, the use of QoL scales in RCTs has increased from 1985 to 2010 (Figure 3). None of the four most commonly used QoL instruments, CDLQI, DFI, DLQI or IDQOL were used between 1985–1997.

Common Disease-Severity Scales in Atopic Dermatitis: Dimensions and Evidence for Validation

Severity Scoring of Atopic Dermatitis (SCORAD). From 1985 to 2010, SCORAD was the most widely used disease-severity scale in atopic dermatitis. SCORAD was used in 113 out of the 382 studies that met our search criteria (30%). It was developed in

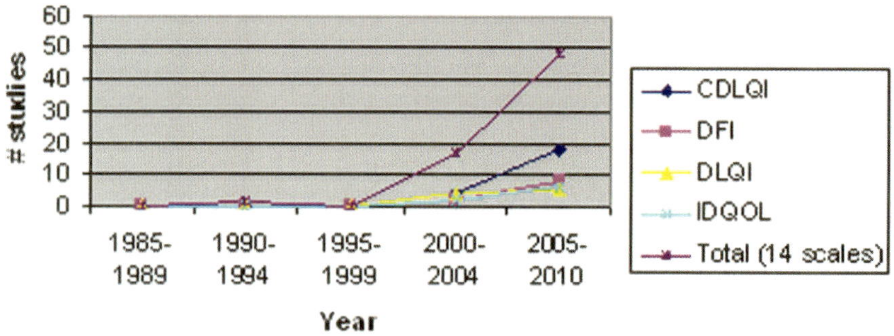

Figure 3. Trends in Quality of Life Instruments 1985–2010.

1993 by the European Task Force on Atopic Dermatitis [8]. The SCORAD index uses the rule of nines to assess disease extent and evaluates five clinical characteristics to determine disease severity: (1) erythema, (2) edema/papulation, (3) oozing/crusts, (4) excoriation and (5) lichenification. SCORAD also assesses subjective symptoms of pruritus and sleep loss with Visual Analogue Scales (VAS) [8]. These three aspects: extent of disease, disease severity and subjective symptoms combine to give a maximum possible score of 103. Although it is a combined score, the three aspects can be separated and used individually if necessary. Of all the severity scales used in atopic dermatitis, it is the most widely validated disease-severity instrument [9]. SCORAD has been found to be valid and reliable, and it has shown excellent agreement with global assessments of disease severity [8,9,10,11,12,13,14,15,16,17,18,19,20,21,22]. However, some studies have shown interobserver variation in scoring lichenification and extent of disease [8,9,10,18,20,23].

Eczema Area and Severity Index (EASI). EASI was the second most commonly used scale in our review of the literature. It was used in 63 out of 382 RCTs (16%). EASI was developed by modifying the PASI (Psoriasis Area and Severity Index), a widely accepted and standardized scoring system for psoriasis [24]. EASI assesses extent of disease at four body sites and measures four clinical signs: (1) erythema, (2) induration/papulation, (3) excoriation, and (4) lichenification each on a scale of 0 to 3. EASI confers a max score of 72 [25]. EASI evaluates two dimensions of atopic dermatitis: disease extent and clinical signs. Unlike the SCORAD, it does not assess symptoms like pruritus and sleep loss. Some investigators express that subjective symptoms may be the most important marker for assessing patient morbidity and they may also be a good indicator for disease severity. In a large validation study with a cohort of 1550 pediatric patients, EASI was found to have excellent validity, internal consistency and sensitivity to change [26]. While EASI is a valid and reliable instrument, most interobserver variability lies in the dimension of induration/papulation [13,21,25,26,27].

Investigators' Global Assessment (IGA). IGA was the third most common scale, used in 48 out of 382 RCTs (13%). IGA allows investigators to assess overall disease severity at one given time point, and it consists of a 6-point severity scale from clear to very severe disease (0 = clear, 1 = almost clear, 2 = mild disease, 3 = moderate disease, 4 = severe disease and 5 = very severe disease) [28]. IGA uses clinical characteristics of erythema, infiltration, papulation, oozing and crusting as guidelines for the overall severity assessment [28]. To our knowledge, IGA has not been validated as an outcome measure [7]. However, IGA has been used to validate other outcome scales as one "gold standard." [9,26] While the combined use of IGA with another validated scale does not make IGA itself a stand-alone, validated instrument, IGA appears to correlate well with the EASI and is considered an instrument with reasonable face validity. Potential weaknesses of IGA include lack of responsiveness and discrimination for disease severity and lack of subjective symptoms.

Six-Area, Six-Sign Atopic Dermatitis (SASSAD). SASSAD was used in 18 out of 382 RCTs (5%), which ranks SASSAD as the fourth most commonly used scale. SASSAD assesses six clinical signs of disease severity (erythema, exudation, dryness, cracking, excoriation, and lichenification) at six body sites (head/neck, trunk, arms, hands, legs and feet). Each clinical sign on a given body site is graded on a scale of 0–3, and the scale confers a maximum score of 108 [29]. SASSAD does not assess subjective symptoms. The SASSAD is sensitive to changes in topical steroid requirements, pruritus, and sleep loss [30,31,32,33,34]. In a small reliability study involving 6 patients, there was interobserver variation for dryness and lichenification [35].

Quality-of-Life Instruments in Atopic Dermatitis: Dimensions and Evidence for Validation

Children's Dermatology Life Quality Index (CDLQI). CDLQI was the most common QoL instrument from our search, used in 22 out of 382 RCTs (6%). Drs. Lewis-Jones and Finlay developed and validated CDLQI in 1995, with the purpose of measuring the QoL in children with skin disease [36]. The questionnaire was designed for children ages 4 through 16. CDLQI is completed by the child with the help of an adult if necessary, preferably a parent. The questionnaire consists of 10 questions that encompass different aspects of a child's life that could be affected by their skin disease. The instrument includes physical symptoms, such as itching and sleep loss, as well as psychosocial questions regarding friendships, bullying, school performance, sports participation, and enjoyment of vacation. The questions are graded from 0–3, with a possible maximum score of 30 with higher scores representing worse QoL. [36]. In the initial validation study, children with atopic eczema accounted for 20% of all patients [36]. To determine test-retest repeatability, CDLQI was used in a population of children without skin disease [36].

Since its validation, CDLQI has been used in numerous studies to determine the effectiveness of interventions in children with AD [37,38]. CDLQI has been translated and validated in Cantonese [39,40,41]. A cartoon version of CDLQI was validated in 2003, which appears to be quicker and preferred by children [42].

Dermatitis Family Impact (DFI). The DFI questionnaire was used in 10 out of 382 RCTs (2.6%), making it the second most common quality of life scale used in our review. It was developed in 1998 by Drs. Lawson, Lewis-Jones, Finlay, Reid and Owens to help measure how family life is affected by a child suffering from atopic dermatitis [43]. It is designed to be completed by a caretaker of the child, usually a parent, and consists of 10 questions related to housework, food preparation and feeding, sleep, family leisure activity, shopping, expenditure, fatigue, emotional distress and relationships [43]. Each question is graded from 0–3 with a maximum possible score of 30. DFI has been found to be valid, reliable, and sensitive to change in multiple studies [6,39,43,44,45,46,47,48]. Two studies that assessed validity of the instrument were based on using separate components of the DFI, as opposed to using the total score as was originally intended by creators of the scale [43,46]. DFI has also been validated in Malay and Portuguese [39,44,45,48].

Dermatology Life Quality Index (DLQI). DLQI was the third most common QoL scale that was used in 9 out of 382 RCTs (2.4%) in our review. DLQI was developed in 1994 by Drs. Finlay and Khan to measure quality of life in routine clinical practice in adults over age of 18 [49]. DLQI is a 10-item questionnaire that inquires about skin symptoms, feelings of embarrassment, and how skin disease has affected day-to-day activities, working and social life. Similar to CDLQI, each question on DLQI is scored from 0 to 3 with a maximum score of 30 and high scores representing worse QoL.

Both DLQI and CDLQI are specialty-specific but not disease-specific QoL instruments. In the original article by Finlay and Khan, patients with atopic dermatitis had the worst QoL as measured by DLQI compared to the other skin diseases assessed in the study [49]. DLQI has been extensively validated in multiple studies [49,50,51]. A 10-year review of the literature found that DLQI is highly specific for assessing decrements in QoL in patients with atopic dermatitis compared with the general population [51]. Specifically, patients with atopic eczema had a mean score of 4.2 compared to 0.3 in a normal population [50,51]. DLQI has high repeatability, internal consistency, and sensitivity to change [51].

Infants' Dermatitis Quality of Life Index (IDQOL). IDQOL was the fourth most common scale found in our review, used in 8 out of 382 RCTs (2.1%) examined. It was developed in 2001 by Drs. Lewis-Jones, Finlay, and Dykes to assess QoL in infants with AD [52]. IDQOL is completed by the parents of infants from birth to 4 years. The instrument consists of 10 questions regarding an infant or young child's difficulties with mood, sleep, bathing, dressing, play, mealtimes, other family activities, and treatment [52]. Each question is graded from 0–3 with a maximum total score of 30. A higher number correlates with a greater impairment of quality of life. An additional question exists that is scored separately on a scale of 0–4 that asks for the parents' overall assessment of eczema severity. In the original article the scale was validated with repeatability and sensitivity to change confirmed [52]. The scale was further validated with sensitivity to change confirmed and has been used in over 15 studies [43,53].

Discussion

Effective management of skin diseases begins with evaluation of both clinical disease severity and health-related QoL. In dermatology, the assessment of disease severity is frequently condition-specific and uses defined, observable parameters [54,55,56,57]. QoL refers to the impact of a disease on a patient's overall function and wellbeing [58]. While disease severity is central for clinical evaluation and monitoring treatment response, QoL measures are as important for determining the effect of a disease or intervention on a patient's general welfare.

In the last 25 years, 20 disease-severity scales and 14 QoL instruments have been used in clinical trials involving patients with atopic dermatitis. Despite the emergence of multiple disease-severity and QoL instruments, few instruments have been validated. The four most commonly used disease-severity scales SCORAD, EASI, IGA, and SASSAD were used in 242 out of the 382 RCTs reviewed (63%). SCORAD, EASI, and SASSAD have been extensively validated [7]. The four most commonly used QoL instruments were DLQI, CDLQI, IDQOL, and DFI. All four scales have demonstrated validity, reliability, and sensitivity to change [36,47,51,52].

The use of four top disease-severity instruments in AD has increased from 1985 to 2010 (Figure 2). For example, when we compared instrument usage patterns between the period from 2000–2004 with that from 2005–2010, we found that SCORAD usage increased by 106%; EASI usage increased by 165%; IGA usage increased by 169%, and SASSAD usage decreased by 20%. Over this ten-year period, IGA had the greatest rate of increase. The greater increased rate of IGA usage may be attributed to its ease of administration. Compared to IGA, EASI also experienced a higher rate of adoption in clinical trials since 1985. The usage patterns of EASI and IGA appear to parallel with each other, which suggests researchers' preference for both scales as objective measures of AD.

The increased usage of disease severity scales appeared to coincide with the publication of validation studies. SCORAD had its peak usage from 2005 to 2010, which corresponded closely to the publication of its validation studies from 2004 to 2006. EASI also had its peak usage from 2005 to 2010, which coincided with the publication of its validation studies in 2004 and 2005.

Among the four most commonly used QoL instruments, all were used more commonly as the years progressed. One possible explanation for this trend is that QoL measures have become as important as disease-severity instruments for patient evaluation and management. Of note, the four most common quality of life scales were developed by the same group of physicians and are similar in format and design. This may limit the diversity of the scale and the variety of characteristics that are used when assessing QoL in patients with atopic dermatitis. Additionally, our search of the literature was limited to randomized controlled trials. Other disease-specific quality of life instruments may exist that have not been used in randomized control trials.

Another limitation of our review is that, out of 382 RCTs examined, we identified 67 RCTs that used QoL measurements (18%), which makes identifying trends for individual QoL instruments difficult.

In this review, we identified trends for disease-severity and QoL outcomes measurements in atopic dermatitis from 1985–2010. We also summarized dimensions of the most commonly used scales and cited evidence for their validation. Although the consistent use of validated measures assessing disease severity and QoL in AD was not observed 20 years ago, this study found a promising trend of increased usage of validated instruments in clinical trials that measure AD disease severity and QoL in the past decade. Outcomes researchers in dermatology are encouraged to select validated outcomes measures that provide accurate measurement of disease dimensions and allow for comparison among studies.

This is the first systematic analysis of trends in the usage of outcomes measures in dermatological research. We anticipate that similar studies will be forthcoming in other disease areas within dermatology that assess the use of outcomes instruments. This type of study depicts the progression of a field's research quality and validity, and it encourages future outcomes researchers to devise instruments that will be streamlined, valid, and reliable.

Author Contributions

Conceived and designed the experiments: AA BR. Analyzed the data: AA BR. Contributed reagents/materials/analysis tools: AA BR. Wrote the paper: AA BR.

References

1. Holm EA, Wulf HC, Stegmann H, Jemec GB (2006) Life quality assessment among patients with atopic eczema. Br J Dermatol 154: 719–725.
2. Chamlin SL, Frieden IJ, Williams ML, Chren MM (2004) Effects of atopic dermatitis on young American children and their families. Pediatrics 114: 607–611.
3. Hanifin JM, Rajka G (1980) Diagnostic features of atopic dermatitis. Acta derm venereol (Stockh). pp 44–47.
4. Dohil MA, Eichenfield LF (2005) A treatment approach for atopic dermatitis. Pediatr Ann 34: 201–210.
5. Finlay AY (1998) Quality of life assessments in dermatology. Semin Cutan Med Surg 17: 291–296.
6. McKenna SP, Doward LC (2008) Quality of life of children with atopic dermatitis and their families. Curr Opin Allergy Clin Immunol 8: 228–231.
7. Schmitt J, Langan S, Williams HC (2007) What are the best outcome measurements for atopic eczema? A systematic review. J Allergy Clin Immunol 120: 1389–1398.
8. Kunz B, Oranje AP, Labreze L, Stalder JF, Ring J, et al. (1997) Clinical validation and guidelines for the SCORAD index: consensus report of the European Task Force on Atopic Dermatitis. Dermatology 195: 10–19.
9. Charman C, Williams H (2000) Outcome measures of disease severity in atopic eczema. Arch Dermatol 136: 763–769.
10. (1993) Severity scoring of atopic dermatitis: the SCORAD index. Consensus Report of the European Task Force on Atopic Dermatitis. Dermatology 186: 23–31.
11. Angelova-Fischer I, Bauer A, Hipler UC, Petrov I, Kazandjieva J, et al. (2005) The objective severity assessment of atopic dermatitis (OSAAD) score: validity, reliability and sensitivity in adult patients with atopic dermatitis. Br J Dermatol 153: 767–773.
12. Ben-Gashir MA, Seed PT, Hay RJ (2004) Quality of life and disease severity are correlated in children with atopic dermatitis. Br J Dermatol 150: 284–290.
13. Breuer K, Braeutigam M, Kapp A, Werfel T (2004) Influence of pimecrolimus cream 1% on different morphological signs of eczema in infants with atopic dermatitis. Dermatology 209: 314–320.
14. Charman CR, Venn AJ, Williams H (2005) Measuring atopic eczema severity visually: which variables are most important to patients? Arch Dermatol 141: 1146–1151; discussion 1151.
15. Hon KL, Kam WY, Lam MC, Leung TF, Ng PC (2006) CDLQI, SCORAD and NESS: are they correlated? Qual Life Res 15: 1551–1558.
16. Hon KL, Leung TF, Wong Y, Fok TF (2006) Lesson from performing SCORADs in children with atopic dermatitis: subjective symptoms do not correlate well with disease extent or intensity. Int J Dermatol 45: 728–730.
17. Hon KL, Ma KC, Wong E, Leung TF, Wong Y, et al. (2003) Validation of a self-administered questionnaire in Chinese in the assessment of eczema severity. Pediatr Dermatol 20: 465–469.
18. Oranje AP, Stalder JF, Taieb A, Tasset C, de Longueville M (1997) Scoring of atopic dermatitis by SCORAD using a training atlas by investigators from different disciplines. ETAC Study Group. Early Treatment of the Atopic Child. Pediatr Allergy Immunol 8: 28–34.
19. Pucci N, Novembre E, Cammarata MG, Bernardini R, Monaco MG, et al. (2005) Scoring atopic dermatitis in infants and young children: distinctive features of the SCORAD index. Allergy 60: 113–116.
20. Schafer T, Dockery D, Kramer U, Behrendt H, Ring J (1997) Experiences with the severity scoring of atopic dermatitis in a population of German pre-school children. Br J Dermatol 137: 558–562.
21. Staab D, Kaufmann R, Brautigam M, Wahn U (2005) Treatment of infants with atopic eczema with pimecrolimus cream 1% improves parents' quality of life: a multicenter, randomized trial. Pediatr Allergy Immunol 16: 527–533.
22. Wolkerstorfer A, de Waard van der Spek FB, Glazenburg EJ, Mulder PG, Oranje AP (1999) Scoring the severity of atopic dermatitis: three item severity score as a rough system for daily practice and as a pre-screening tool for studies. Acta Derm Venereol 79: 356–359.
23. Sprikkelman AB, Tupker RA, Burgerhof H, Schouten JP, Brand PL, et al. (1997) Severity scoring of atopic dermatitis: a comparison of three scoring systems. Allergy 52: 944–949.
24. Fredriksson T, Pettersson U (1978) Severe psoriasis–oral therapy with a new retinoid. Dermatologica 157: 238–244.
25. Hanifin JM, Thurston M, Omoto M, Cherill R, Tofte SJ, et al. (2001) The eczema area and severity index (EASI): assessment of reliability in atopic dermatitis. EASI Evaluator Group. Exp Dermatol 10: 11–18.
26. Barbier N, Paul C, Luger T, Allen R, De Prost Y, et al. (2004) Validation of the Eczema Area and Severity Index for atopic dermatitis in a cohort of 1550 patients from the pimecrolimus cream 1% randomized controlled clinical trials programme. Br J Dermatol 150: 96–102.
27. Belloni G, Pinelli S, Veraldi S (2005) A randomised, double-blind, vehicle-controlled study to evaluate the efficacy and safety of MAS063D (Atopiclair) in the treatment of mild to moderate atopic dermatitis. Eur J Dermatol 15: 31–36.
28. Siegfried E, Korman N, Molina C, Kianifard F, Abrams K (2006) Safety and efficacy of early intervention with pimecrolimus cream 1% combined with corticosteroids for major flares in infants and children with atopic dermatitis. J Dermatolog Treat 17: 143–150.
29. Berth-Jones J (1996) Six area, six sign atopic dermatitis (SASSAD) severity score: a simple system for monitoring disease activity in atopic dermatitis. Br J Dermatol 135 Suppl 48: 25–30.
30. Berth-Jones J, Finlay A, Zaki I, Tan B, Goodyear H, et al. (1996) Cyclosporine in severe childhood atopic dermatitis: A multicenter study* 1. Journal of the American Academy of Dermatology 34: 1016–1021.
31. Granlund H, Erkko P, Sinisalo M, Reitamo S (1995) Cyclosporin in atopic dermatitis: time to relapse and effect of intermittent therapy. Br J Dermatol 132: 106–112.
32. Berth-Jones J, Graham-Brown RA, Marks R, Camp RD, English JS, et al. (1997) Long-term efficacy and safety of cyclosporin in severe adult atopic dermatitis. Br J Dermatol 136: 76–81.
33. Jenner N, Campbell J, Marks R (2004) Morbidity and cost of atopic eczema in Australia. Australas J Dermatol 45: 16–22.
34. Sowden JM, Berth-Jones J, Ross JS, Motley RJ, Marks R, et al. (1991) Double-blind, controlled, crossover study of cyclosporin in adults with severe refractory atopic dermatitis. Lancet 338: 137–140.
35. Charman CR, Venn AJ, Williams HC (2002) Reliability testing of the Six Area, Six Sign Atopic Dermatitis severity score. Br J Dermatol 146: 1057–1060.
36. Lewis-Jones MS, Finlay AY (1995) The Children's Dermatology Life Quality Index (CDLQI): initial validation and practical use. Br J Dermatol 132: 942–949.
37. Emerson RM, Lawson S, Williams HC (1998) Do specialist eczema clinics benefit children with atopic dermatitis? British Journal of Dermatology 139: 46.
38. Harper JI, Ahmed I, Barclay G, Lacour M, Hoeger P, et al. (2000) Cyclosporin for severe childhood atopic dermatitis: short course versus continuous therapy. Br J Dermatol 142: 52–58.
39. Aziah MS, Rosnah T, Mardziah A, Norzila MZ (2002) Childhood atopic dermatitis: a measurement of quality of life and family impact. Med J Malaysia 57: 329–339.
40. Chuh AA (2003) Validation of a Cantonese version of the Children's Dermatology Life Quality Index. Pediatr Dermatol 20: 479–481.
41. Clayton TH, Clark SM, Britton J, Pavlov S, Radev S (2007) A comparative study of the Children's Dermatology Life Quality Index (CDLQI) in paediatric dermatology clinics in the UK and Bulgaria. J Eur Acad Dermatol Venereol 21: 1436–1437.
42. Holme SA, Man I, Sharpe JL, Dykes PJ, Lewis-Jones MS, et al. (2003) The Children's Dermatology Life Quality Index: validation of the cartoon version. Br J Dermatol 148: 285–290.
43. Beattie PE, Lewis-Jones MS (2006) An audit of the impact of a consultation with a paediatric dermatology team on quality of life in infants with atopic eczema and their families: further validation of the Infants' Dermatitis Quality of Life Index and Dermatitis Family Impact score. Br J Dermatol 155: 1249–1255.
44. Lewis-Jones M, Finlay A (2006) Quality of life research. In: Medicine WCo, ed.
45. Alvarenga TM, Caldeira AP (2009) Quality of life in pediatric patients with atopic dermatitis. J Pediatr (Rio J) 85: 415–420.
46. Grimalt R, Mengeaud V, Cambazard F (2007) The steroid-sparing effect of an emollient therapy in infants with atopic dermatitis: a randomized controlled study. Dermatology 214: 61–67.
47. Lewis-Jones MS, Finlay AY, Dykes PJ (2001) The Infants' Dermatitis Quality of Life Index. Br J Dermatol 144: 104–110.
48. Weber MB, Fontes Neto Pde T, Prati C, Soirefman M, Mazzotti NG, et al. (2008) Improvement of pruritus and quality of life of children with atopic dermatitis and their families after joining support groups. J Eur Acad Dermatol Venereol 22: 992–997.
49. Finlay AY, Khan GK (1994) Dermatology Life Quality Index (DLQI)–a simple practical measure for routine clinical use. Clin Exp Dermatol 19: 210–216.
50. Badia X, Mascaro JM, Lozano R (1999) Measuring health-related quality of life in patients with mild to moderate eczema and psoriasis: clinical validity, reliability and sensitivity to change of the DLQI. The Cavide Research Group. Br J Dermatol 141: 698–702.
51. Lewis V, Finlay AY (2004) 10 years experience of the Dermatology Life Quality Index (DLQI). J Investig Dermatol Symp Proc 9: 169–180.
52. Lewis-Jones MS, Finlay AY, Dykes PJ (1999) Measurement of the impact of atopic dermatitis on infant's and their families lives. British Journal of Dermatology 141: 105–106.
53. Department of Dermatology WCoM, Cardiff University The Infant's Dermatitis Quality of Life Index (IDQOL).

54. Chren MM (2000) Giving "scale" new meaning in dermatology: measurement matters. Arch Dermatol 136: 788–790.
55. Williams H (1997) Is a simple generic index of dermatologic disease severity an attainable goal? Archives of Dermatology 133: 1451.
56. Chen SC (2007) Dermatology quality of life instruments: sorting out the quagmire. J Invest Dermatol 127: 2695–2696.
57. Barzilai DA, Weinstock MA, Mostow EN (2007) Practicing evidence-based dermatology: a short guide. Skinmed 6: 122–127.
58. Finlay AY (1997) Quality of life measurement in dermatology: a practical guide. Br J Dermatol 136: 305–314.

3

Clinical Efficacy of Blue Light Full Body Irradiation as Treatment Option for Severe Atopic Dermatitis

Detlef Becker, Elise Langer[¶], Martin Seemann[¶], Gunda Seemann, Isabel Fell, Joachim Saloga, Stephan Grabbe, Esther von Stebut*

Department of Dermatology, University Medicine, Johannes Gutenberg University, Mainz, Germany

Abstract

Background: Therapy of atopic dermatitis (AD) relies on immunosuppression and/or UV irradiation. Here, we assessed clinical efficacy and histopathological alterations induced by blue light-treatment of AD within an observational, non-interventional study.

Methodology/Principal Findings: 36 patients with severe, chronic AD resisting long term disease control with local corticosteroids were included. Treatment consisted of one cycle of 5 consecutive blue light-irradiations (28.9 J/cm^2). Patients were instructed to ask for treatment upon disease exacerbation despite interval therapy with topical corticosteroids. The majority of patients noted first improvements after 2–3 cycles. The EASI score was improved by 41% and 54% after 3 and 6 months, respectively ($p \leq 0.005$, and $p \leq 0.002$). Significant improvement of pruritus, sleep and life quality was noted especially after 6 months. Also, frequency and intensity of disease exacerbations and the usage of topical corticosteroids was reduced. Finally, immunohistochemistry of skin biopsies obtained at baseline and after 5 and 15 days revealed that, unlike UV light, blue light-treatment did not induce Langerhans cell or T cell depletion from skin.

Conclusions/Significance: Blue light-irradiation may represent a suitable treatment option for AD providing long term control of disease. Future studies with larger patient cohorts within a randomized, placebo-controlled clinical trial are required to confirm this observation.

Editor: Carol Feghali-Bostwick, University of Pittsburgh, United States of America

Funding: The authors have no support or funding to report.

Competing Interests: The authors have declared that no competing interests exist.

* E-mail: vonstebu@uni-mainz.de

¶ The authors contributed equally to this work.

Introduction

Atopic dermatitis (AD) is a common inflammatory skin disease affecting approximately 10–15% of all individuals in industrialized countries. A genetic predisposition is well documented. The disease severity can range from infrequent, localized skin affections at predeliction sites to acute exacerbation of the entire skin leading to erythrodermia requiring hospitalization. The patients suffer from significant reductions in their quality of life due to pruritus, sleeplessness and stigmatization [1–3].

The pathogenesis of AD is complex. Apart from genetic factors responsible for a predisposition, several alterations of the skin immune system (e.g. differences in the amount of anti-microbial peptides produced by keratinocytes, alterations in the phenotype and function of epidermal dendritic cells with the appearance of normally absent IDEC) and stromal cells (e.g. filaggrin mutation) are important [1]. Acute exacerbation of disease is characterized by a dense infiltrate of the dermis with CD4$^+$ T cells showing a Th2-phenotype. Under more chronic conditions, the Th2 predominance is shifted towards a Th1 immune response as shown in atopy patch test experiments [1].

Therapy of AD is based on a regular treatment with basic emollients supplemented with intermittent immunosuppressive therapy of exacerbated skin disease. According to (inter)national guidelines, immunosuppression can be achieved either locally by application of corticosteroid- or calcineurin inhibitor-containing ointments or systemically (e.g. using cyclosporine A, reserved for severe AD) [2,3]. In addition, UV irradiation (especially UVA1) has proven to be beneficial in those heavily affected patients in whom the above mentioned interval therapy with local immunosuppression is not sufficient for disease control. However, UV radiation has been shown to be carcinogenic and thus, UV phototherapy is usually not recommended as long-term treatment, and for young and immunosuppressed patients [2–4].

More recently, it was suggested that blue light irradiation may represent a therapeutic alternative for long term control of AD. Krutmann *et al.* showed that blue light irradiation was found to induce a significant clinical improvement of atopic hand and foot eczema [5]. In addition, anecdotal treatment of several patients with severe AD was reported to be helpful for long-term control of disease. Thus, in the present study we assessed the clinical efficacy and histopathological alterations induced by blue light treatment of patients with severe, chronic AD.

Materials and Methods

Patients

Prior to the initiation of the present observational study, the study protocol was approved by the local Ethics Committee of the State Rhineland-Palatinate (Ethik Komission, Landesärztekammer Rheinland-Pfalz), Germany. Between August 1st, 2007, and July 31st, 2008, all adult patients (≥18 years) who received full body blue light irradiation for AD in our Department were asked to participate in this observational, non-interventional study (n = 36). Inclusion criteria were an age ≥18 years, commitment to non-smoking and the inability to provide long term control of their AD with frequently performed interval therapy using class II/III corticosteroids. All patients included gave written informed consent and showed reliable compliance.

Irradiation device and treatment protocol

A photonic irradiation system (Neuroderm®, Spectrometrix Optoelectronic Systems GmbH, Berlin, Germany) was utilized. In this newly-developed full body irradiation device, over 66% of the resulting emission spectrum was between 400 and 500 nm (28.9 J/cm^2) at a total fluence of 43.7 J/cm^2 (see Figure 1). A single treatment consisted of a 24 min exposure of each side of the body. The residual UVA emission per treatment was less than 1 J/cm^2 and the irradiation device therefore fulfilled the criteria for UV-free radiation defined by the International Commission on Non-Ionizing Radiation Protection of the International Radiation Protection Agency (ICNIP/IRA).

Not before 48 hrs after the last treatment within a 5-day treatment cycle, patients were asked to continue treatment with local application of topical corticosteroids, e.g. mometasone 1% cream once daily until their eczema fully disappeared. They were instructed to then discontinue treatment and return to our clinic to receive the next 5-day cycle of irradiation upon reappearance of their AD (flare up).

Clinical and serological information collected

On day 0 (d0), before treatment was started, clinical and serological parameters were obtained. Similar information and material was obtained on day 15 before the 15th irradiation (d15), and again after 3 and 6 months. On initiation visit, genetic predisposition was judged using the Diepgen Score [6]. Clinical response to treatment was assessed using the eczema area and severity index (EASI) [7], clinical photographs of affected body sites were taken and patients were asked questions about additional treatments, well-being, itching, sleep, and their global assessment of response. In addition, patients were handed the Dermatology Life Quality Index (DLQI) [8] for completion at d0, d15 and after 3 and 6 months.

Routine blood tests involved a differential blood count including eosinophils (normal 0–7%), C-reactive protein (normal <5 mg/l), eosinophilic cationic protein (ECP, normal <24 ng/ml), Total IgE (normal <100 IE/ml). ELISAs specific for human TARC (R&D), IL-4 (ImmunoTools), IL-5 (BD), IL-10 (ImmunoTools), IFNγ

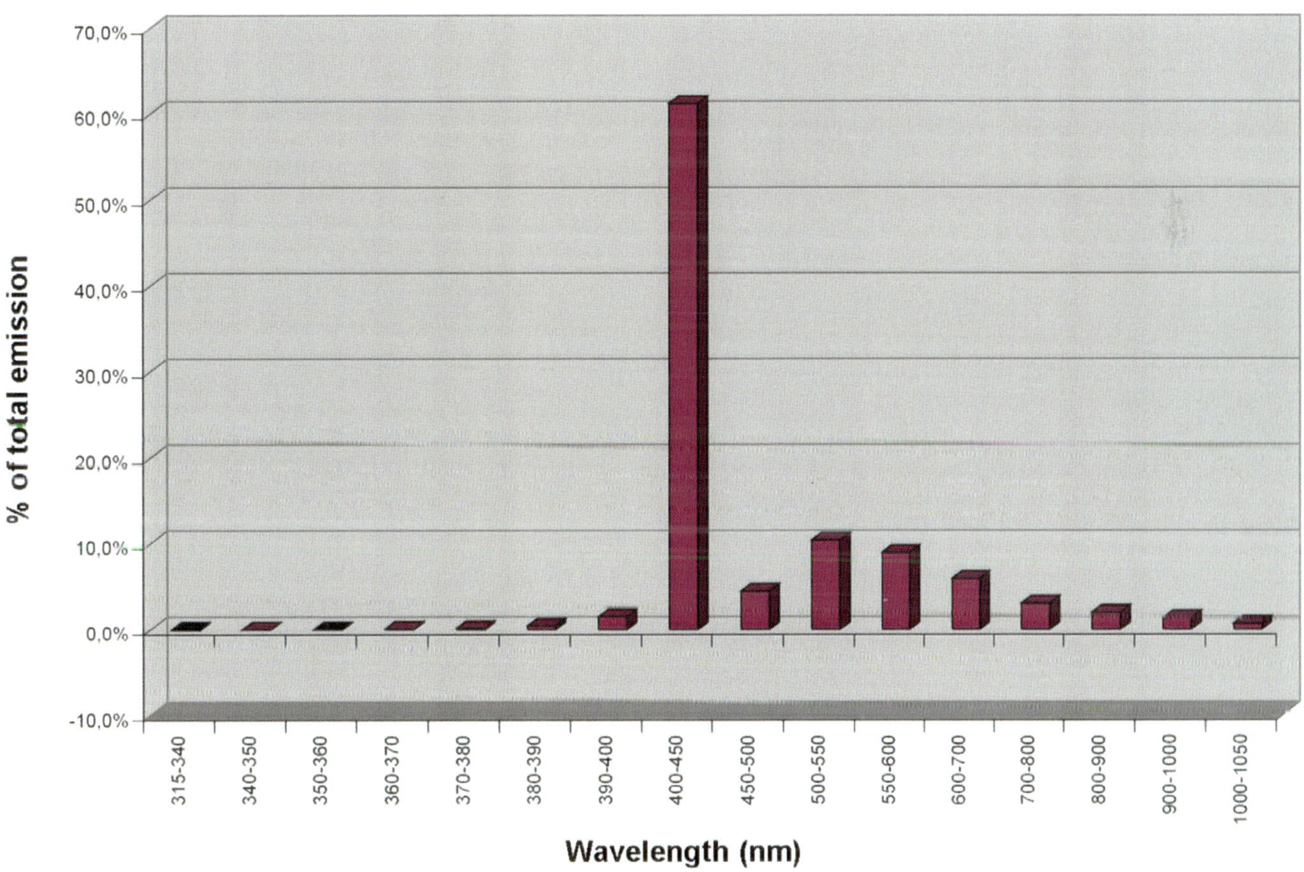

Figure 1. Emission spectrum of the Neuroderm® full body irradiation device.

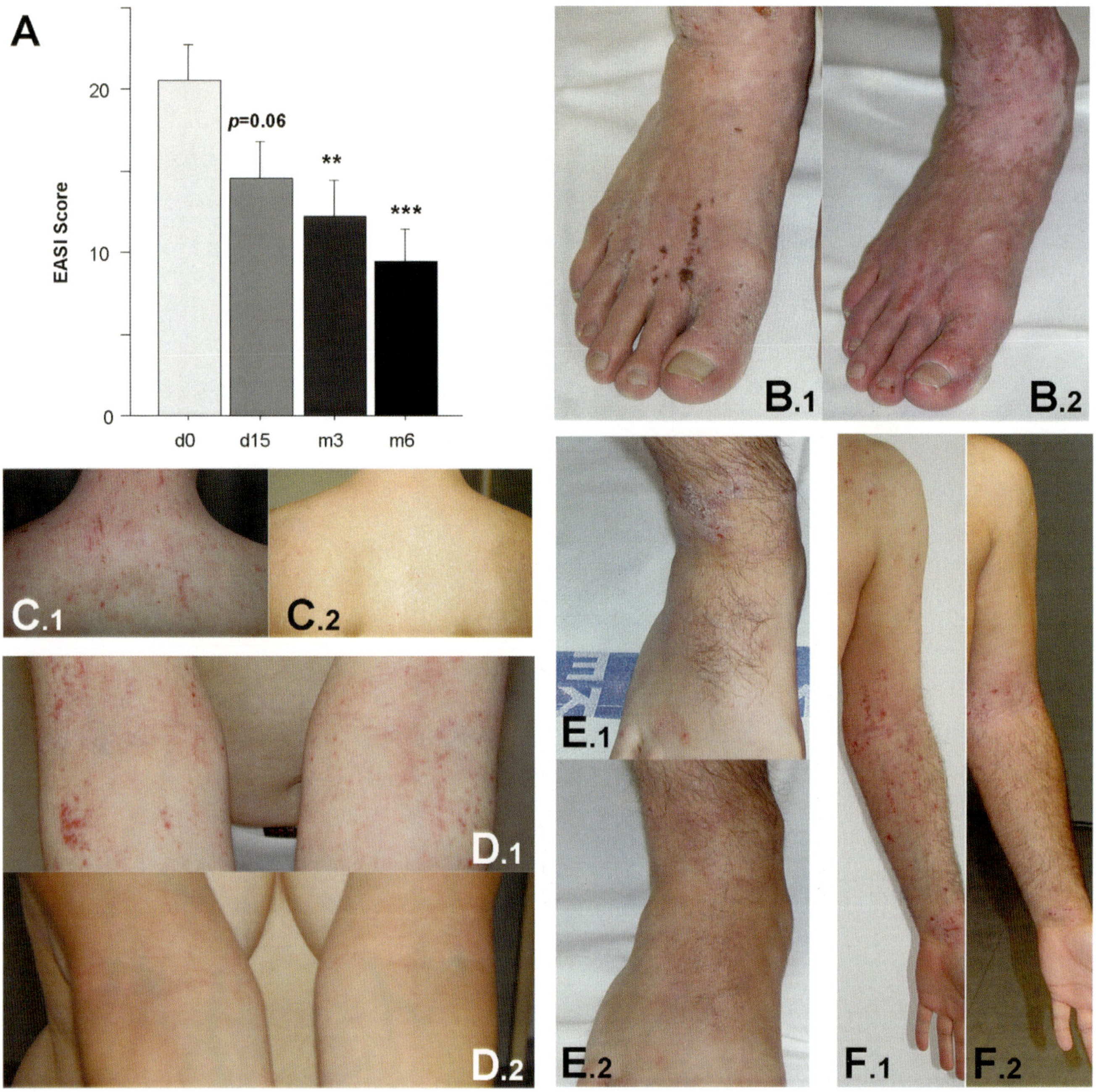

Figure 2. Clinical improvement after blue light irradiation. A, EASI assessment of the severity of skin affection was obtained before treatment (d0), on day 15 (d15), and after 3 and 6 months (m3 and m6, respectively). Data are presented as mean$\pm$SEM (n$\geq$29, * = p$\leq$0.05, ** = p$\leq$0.005, and *** = p$\leq$0.002). **B–F**, Representative clinical pictures from before treatment (.1, d0) and after 6 months (.2). **B+C**: patient #10 – male, 38 years; **D**: patient #15 – female, 41 years; **E+F**: patient #16 – male, 28 years.

(ImmunoTools) and TNFα (ImmunoTools) were performed on serum.

Skin biopsies

Ethical approval was obtained to analyse the effects of blue light irradiation in skin biopsies of 20 patients before, on day 5 before the last irradiation (end of cycle 1) and on d15 before the 15th irradiation. Informed consent was obtained from 19 patients. Skin biopsies were obtained in local anaesthesia from the same body site from each individual (trunk, legs or arms). Biopsies were generally 0.5×1 cm in size and were fixed in formalin. Sections were stained with H&E to confirm the diagnosis for each patient.

Immunohistochemistry was performed using anti-CD1a (clone M3571, dilution 1:100, Dako, Hamburg, Germany), HLA-DR (clone LN3, 1:50), and anti-CD4 (clone 1F6, 1:40; both Novocastra-Laboratories, Newcastle, England) to quantitate antigen-presenting cells and T cell inflammatory responses, respectively. Stainings were developed using the Chem Mate detection kit from Dako, and analysed using an investigator blinded to the patient's identity using light microscopy.

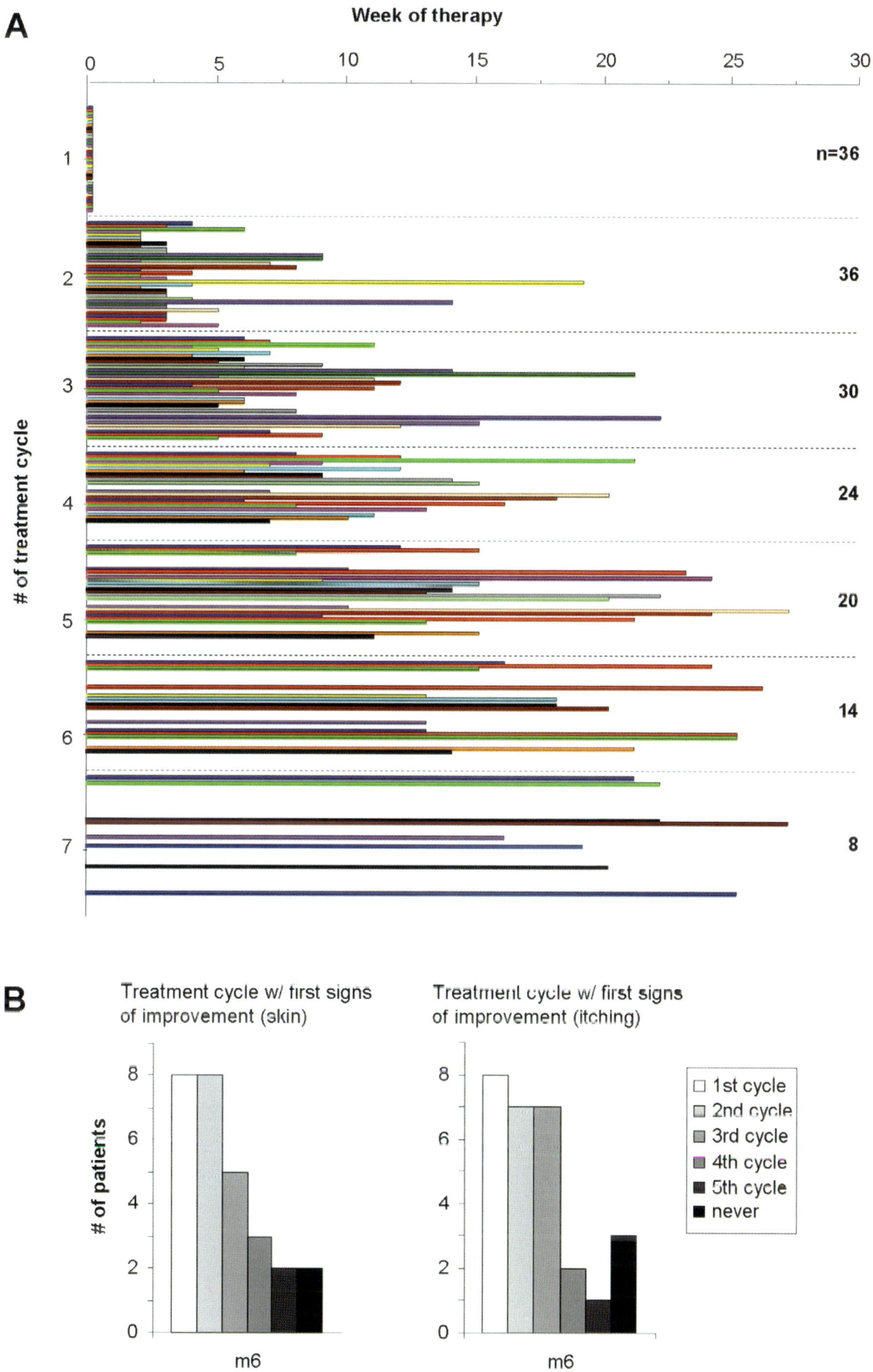
A
Week of therapy
0
5
10
15
20
25
30
# of treatment cycle
1
2
3
4
5
6
7
n=36
36
30
24
20
14
8
B
Treatment cycle w/ first signs of improvement (skin)
Treatment cycle w/ first signs of improvement (itching)
# of patients
0
2
4
6
8
m6
1st cycle
2nd cycle
3rd cycle
4th cycle
5th cycle
never

Figure 3. Number of treatments within 6 months and time of first improvement. A, For each individual patient (n = 36), the time point at which he/she asked for a subsequent irradiation cycle due to disease exacerbation is depicted. **B+C**, After 6 months, all patients were asked to indicate the irradiation cycle in which they first observed improvement of their skin and/or the itching, respectively.

Statistical analysis

Statistical comparisons were performed using Statview for Windows and the Students *t* test for unpaired samples.

Results

Patient collective

Within a year, 36 adult patients with AD received full body blue light irradiation (compare Fig. 1) within an observational, non-interventional study. The mean age was 36.9 (±2, range 20–57, 15 males/ 21 females), the diagnosis had been confirmed 26 years ago (range 2–48), their mean Diepgen score was 21.5 (±0.9, range 9–32). Due to the observational, non-interventional nature of the study, not all patients responded to follow up requests and were willing to donate blood for further analysis at all time points.

Clinical response

The clinical activity of AD was assessed on each visit by a physician. As expected, we noted considerable variations in the baseline level of AD activity. However, the study patient collective consisted of mainly severely affected patients with an EASI [7] of 20.6±2.2 (range 6.8–54) (see Figure 2A). Over time, both the percentage of body surface affected as well as the clinical symptoms erythema, induration, excoriation and lichenification significantly decreased as revealed by an improvement of the EASI: At day 15, 3 and 6 months after treatment initiation, disease severity was decreased by 29%, 41% and 54%, respectively ($n \geq 29$, $p = 0.06$, $p \leq 0.005$ and $p \leq 0.002$, see Figure 2A).

In addition, on each visit, the patients were photographed to document skin involvement. Figures 2B–F depict the clinical response of 3 different patients. One panel (.1) shows typical AD lesions as head/neck dermatitis, involvement of flexures and feet. The same body sites were photographed after 6 months (panel .2). Notably, skin maceration, erythema and scaling were markedly reduced.

Side effects of blue light irradiation were generally mild and consisted of local redness, warmth and itching of the skin within the first few hours after treatment. Systemic side effects (dizziness or head ache) were reported infrequently and disappeared within a few hours.

Next, we assessed the frequency in which the patients received therapy which correlates with the necessity to obtain treatment because of a flare up. As depicted in Figure 3A, all 36 patients asked for a minimum of 2 cycles of irradiation, although each of them after a different time interval. 50% of the patients received at least 5 cycles within 6 months of treatment. Interestingly, the time interval between the last two irradiations increased in the majority of the patients before they did not require additional treatment cycles indirectly indicating that the flare up frequency decreased over time.

Twenty-six of 28 (93%) and 25/28 (89%) of the patients observed improvement of their skin and/or their itching during treatment, respectively; 2 (skin) and 3 (itching) patients did not benefit (see Figure 3B). The majority observed AD resolution as well as a reduction of itching after 2–3 cycles of treatment.

Effects on quality of life

The majority of AD patients suffered from severe itching (7.0±0.3 of maximal 10, mean±SEM, n = 36) and sleeplessness (5.1±0.5 of maximal 10, mean±SEM, n = 36) (see Figure 4A+B). In parallel to disease improvement, the degree of itching was already reduced after 15 days of treatment ($p \leq 0.05$), which became highly significant after 3 and 6 months (~40% reduction, see Figure 4A). In addition, the degree of sleeplessness also decreased significantly over time (see Figure 4B).

Finally, a standardized measure for the life quality was used (see Figure 4C) before treatment (d0), on d15 and after 3 and 6 months [8]. The DLQI consists of 10 questions all scored between 0 (= not relevant) to 4 (= very much affected). The DLQI total score significantly improved during treatment ($p \leq 0.005$) due to

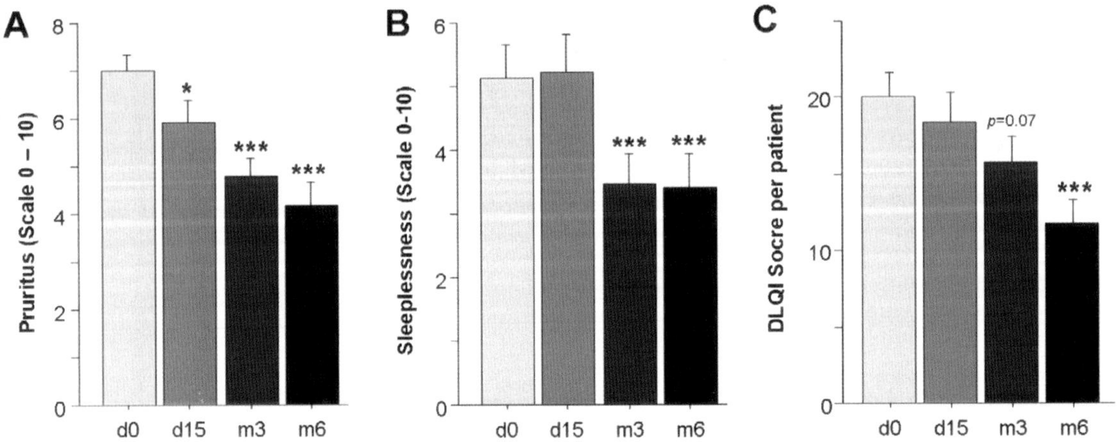

Figure 4. Significant quality of live improvement of blue light-treatment. A+B, At the indicated time points, patients were asked to quantify their degree of itching and sleeplessness on an analogous scale from 0 = none to 10 = severe. **C**, Prior to treatment, on day 15 and after 3 and 6 months, each patient completed the Dermatology life quality index (DLQI) consisting of 10 questions which are scored between 0 = not relevant and 4 = very much affected. Data are presented as cumulative data from all 10 questions. **A–C**, All data are shown as mean+SEM, * = $p \leq 0.05$, and *** = $p \leq 0.002$ as compared to d0.

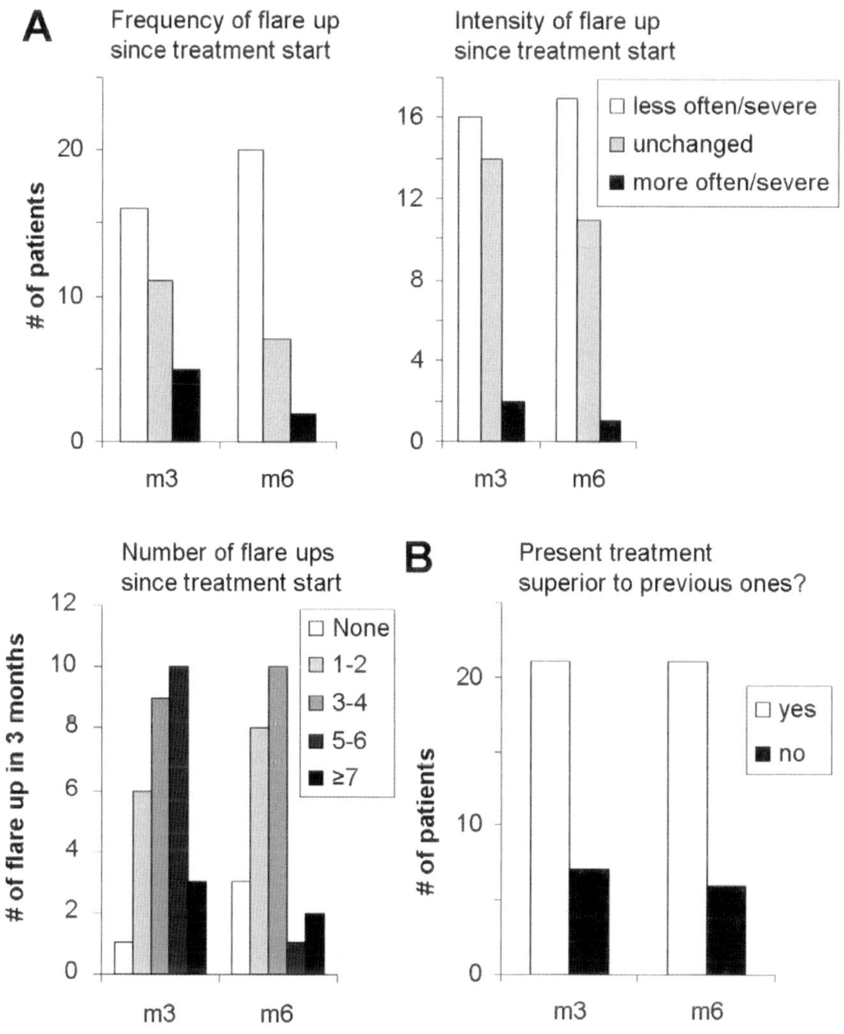

Figure 5. Improvement of severity and frequency of disease exacerbations. A, After 3 and 6 months after blue light therapy initiation, patients were asked about their total number of disease exacerbations within the last 3 months, and about the frequency and intensity of these flare ups since treatment start. **B**, The number of patients that judged this treatment superior to prior treatments at 3 and 6 months post treatment initiation is given.

improvements in all categories. Worsening was not observed in any category. Before blue light irradiation, 18% of patients scored the degree by which their skin condition influences their life quality as 'very much' or 'a lot', but after 6 months of treatment, this percentage was dropped to 21%. At this time, 33% and 46% of the patients stated that their skin influenced their quality of life a little or not at all, respectively.

Patient assessment

After 3 and 6 months of treatment, patients were asked to judge about the total number, the frequency and intensity of disease exacerbations within the last 3 months (see Figure 5A). All three parameters improved significantly. In addition, the question "Is the present treatment superior to previous ones?" was answered with 'yes' in 21 cases (75% and 77%) and with 'no' in 7 and 6 cases after 3 and 6 months, respectively (see Figure 5B). Seven of 27 patients observed no changes or an increase in the topical corticosteroid use, whereas 20/27 (74%) used less or much less local immunosuppressants (see Figure 5C). Systemic antihistamines were not routinely taken by all patients; consequently, 7 patients reported to use less systemic antihistamines, whereas 13 observed no change.

Serological data

Not all patients agreed to give blood upon follow-up visits (64%; n = 23/36 blood samples were analysed). Corresponding with the clinical score, the mean total IgE was significantly elevated in our patient collective at day 0 (7,062±1,999 IE/ml). Over the observation period of 6 months, no alteration of the IgE level was observed (data not shown). CRP levels were not above control levels at any point of time. Eosinophil counts were slightly elevated as compared to controls (9.2±1.2%) and remained the same throughout the observation period. Basic ECP levels were well above normal (56±27 ng/ml). Interestingly, 15 days and after 3 months after irradiation therapy initiation, increased levels of ECP were detected of up to 78 ng/ml, which decreased to baseline by the sixth month. We also assessed the levels of IL-4, IL-5, IL-10, TNFα and thymus and activation regulated chemokine (TARC) in the serum of AD patients. Serum levels of the pro- and anti-inflammatory cytokines TNFα and IL-10 were low and no

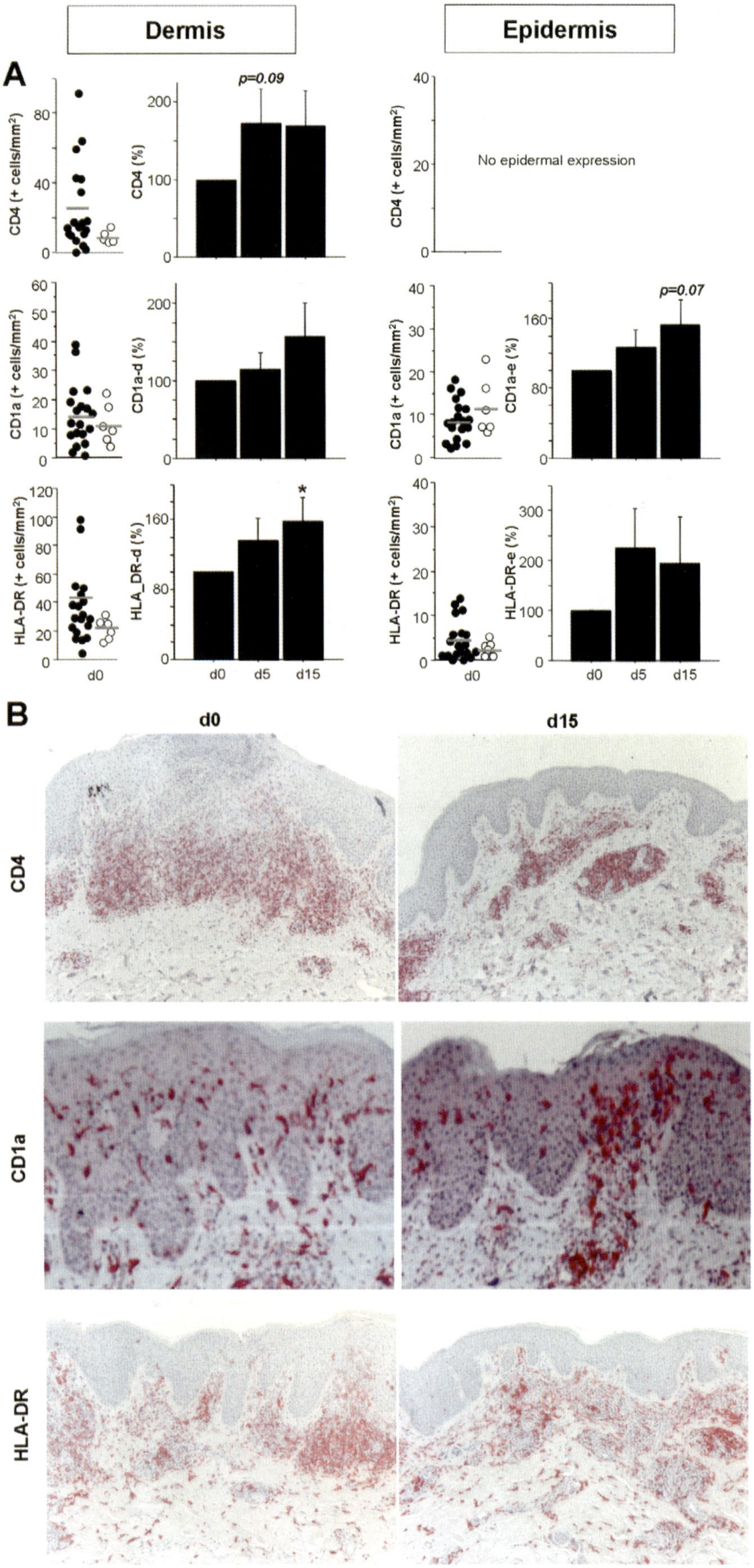
Dermis
Epidermis
A
p=0.09
No epidermal expression
p=0.07
*
CD4 (+ cells/mm²)
CD4 (%)
CD1a (+ cells/mm²)
CD1a-d (%)
CD1a-e (%)
HLA-DR (+ cells/mm²)
HLA_DR-d (%)
HLA-DR-e (%)
d0
d5
d15
B
d0
d15
CD4
CD1a
HLA-DR

Figure 6. Blue light treatment does not act though similar mechanisms as UV light irradiation. Skin biopsies of AD patients were obtained before treatment (day 0, d0), on day 5 before irradiation and on day 15 before the last irradiation in the third cycle. Formalin-fixed skin was sectioned and immunohistochemistry performed with anti-CD4, anti-CD1a, and anti-HLA-DR. **A**, The number of positive cells/mm^2 was counted in 5 representative fields per patient both in the epidermis and the dermis. Left panels indicate the mean baseline number for each individual patient (black dots) on d0 with bars showing the mean value of all patients. White dots represent results of healthy control skin from unrelated patients. Right panels contain cumulative data in which the percent change on d5 and d15 to baseline was calculated. Data are shown as mean±SEM (n≥16, * = p≤0.05 as compared to d0). **B**, Representative stainings for CD4, CD1a and HLA-DR are presented for baseline day 0 and day 15 (x100 magnification for CD4 and HLA-DR, x400 for CD1a).

significant changes observed. IL-4 and IL-5 were negative. Serum TARC was elevated in our AD patient collective at day 0 (1,286±142 ng/ml), but obvious alterations over time were not observed.

Histological findings

To assess blue light-mediated alterations in the specific skin inflammatory infiltrate of AD patients, we obtained skin biopsies from 19 patients on day 0, day 5 and day 15 post therapy initiation.

First, because mast cells (MC) have been implicated in the pathogenesis of AD, MC numbers in lesional tissue were assessed in Giemsa-stained sections. We observed no alterations of the MC numbers or their degranuation status upon irradiation with blue light (data not shown).

Next, we assessed if blue light therapy resulted in alterations in the inflammation induced by skin-infiltrating T cells (see Figure 6). AD has been shown to be induced by (antigen-specific) CD4$^+$ T cells that in the acute phase resemble Th2 cells, whereas chronic AD is characterized by infiltrating Th1 cells. Interestingly, when comparing the number of CD4$^+$ cells in skin, unlike UV-mediated effects [8], we did not observe a decrease in the number of T cells infiltrating the skin. In contrast, we observed a relative increase in the number of lymphocytes. In addition, histomorphological signs of lymphocyte apoptosis were not found in H&E stained sections (data not shown).

Finally, antigen presenting cells (APC) were characterized using anti-CD1a (epidermal Langerhans cells (LC), dermal DC), and anti-HLA-DR (see Figure 6). A relative increase in the number of CD1a$^+$ DC was observed for both dermal DC as well as Langerhans cells (p = 0.07). Since the staining intensity of the LC for CD1a appeared increased as well (compare Figure 6), we performed additional stainings for HLA-DR, expressed by APC as well as activated T cells (see Figure 6A+B). Both dermal DC and LC expressed more HLA-DR. Thus, in summary, unlike effects of UV, blue light therapy did not lead to a DC depletion from skin.

Discussion

Atopic dermatitis is a common disease with high socioeconomic impact. In the present study we assessed the efficacy and potential mechanism of action of blue light irradiation therapy of patients with severe, chronic AD. In line with a prior report about treatment of atopic hand- and foot eczema [5], both the clinical response and the patient assessments showed that full body blue light irradiation may serve as attractive treatment alternative for AD providing long term control of disease.

Interestingly, one of the first signs of a clinical response was a decrease in the pruritus as reported by the patients. The overall clinical response was determined as a ~50% improvement after 6 months as assessed by using the EASI [7]. Other important parameters such as the frequency and intensity of disease exacerbation, topical corticosteroid use and the total quality of life were also improved. Interestingly, the majority of patients observed AD resolution as well as a reduction of their pruritus after 2–3 cycles of treatment (10–15 single irradiations), thus decisions about a continuation of treatment can be made early.

Comparisons with regard to the effectiveness of blue light irradiation as compared to e.g. UV-based treatment regimens are not appropriate. However, it appears that classical first-line treatment of acute AD with UVA1 leads to a more rapid improvement that does not last as long [9–13]: improvement based on reductions of the clinical response were ~30% after 1 week [10], ~67% and 40% after 3 weeks of cold-light UVA1 and medium-dose UVA1, respectively [11], ~35% after 3 weeks of medium-dose cold-light UVA1 [12], and ~32% and 47% after 2 and 4 weeks of bath PUVA compared to 24% and 45% after 2 and 4 weeks of UVB [13]. The improvement observed in our patients who were selected based on their unresponsiveness to classical interval therapy with class II-III topical corticosteroids may thus be comparable to that of classically used UVA1 irradiation [2,3]. However, improvement of long term disease control and not the ability to provide rapid, acute intervention for disease exacerbation may be the main feature of blue light therapy. The overall effectiveness of UV treatment on AD is well accepted. However, UV is one of the main risk factors for the development of epidermal or melanocytic skin tumors [14]. Thus, the development of UV-free irradiations with proven therapeutic effect is beneficial.

All patients included in the present study were suffering from long-lasting AD with no response to standard interval treatment using topical class II-IV corticosteroid application. Thus, blue light treatment can be considered an "add on" therapy as compared to their prior treatment protocol. However, the contribution of the combinatory therapeutic approach to the overall efficacy of the treatment needs to be evaluated further.

Due to the non-interventional, observational nature of the present study, not all patients agreed to complete all questionnaires and came to follow up assessments. Because of the study design, patients were usually re-evaluated when they experienced a flare up just before they received another cycle of irradiation, so the assessments may in some cases underestimate the overall clinical response. In addition, since treatment cycles are offered only when disease worsening is observed, not all patients received the same amount of irradiation. To better estimate the degree of response in relation to established therapies such as other UV-light treatments, clinical trials with proper control groups need to be conducted.

Using skin biopsies and serological analyses, we have started to investigate the mechanism of action of blue light irradiation in AD. Similar to other treatment modalities, a visible effect of this treatment on serum parameters (i.e. total IgE, ECP, etc.) was not obvious [2,3]. As described previously, despite the observation that a certain Th1/Th2 ratio in the skin correlates with disease severity, serum levels of pro- and anti-inflammatory cytokines were low and no significant changes observed. Serum TARC was elevated in our AD patient collective prior to the study as reported [15], but alterations were not achieved by therapy.

The blue light-mediated alterations in the inflammatory infiltrate of the skin involved the absence of signs of lymphocyte or DC/LC apoptosis. Our findings are in line with a recent publication demonstrating that application of visible blue light did not cause DNA damage or early photo-ageing; the biological effects observed on normal skin were transient melanogenesis and cellular vacuolization without resulting apoptosis [16]. Thus, the authors concluded that (short-term) utilization of visible blue light in dermatological practice may be safe [16]. Our observations are in stark contrast to the well known effects of UV-light on skin inflammation, which include T cell apoptosis, and depletion of LC from skin [9,17]. In addition, UV-induced $CD4^{+}CD25^{+}$ regulator T cells (Treg) are expanded by UV-exposed cutaneous LC [18]. Both the induction of apoptotic cell death, and the induction of Treg producing IL-10 results in UV-mediated local immunosuppression [9,19]. In aggregate, even though in retrospect the time points chosen for obtaining the biopsies may not have been optimal and futures studies should attempt to analyse skin responses also at later time points, the effects of blue light on skin inflammation appear to be mediated by a mechanism different from that of UV light. With regard to the molecular targets of blue light irradiation, oxidative stress is potentially relevant. In addition, the degree of DNA damage and/or immune modulatory mechanisms need to be analysed.

In summary, despite this highly selected patient collective with high disease activity and severity, our data strongly suggest that blue light irradiation may represent a suitable treatment option for AD providing long term control of disease. In addition to very few side effects, a good clinical outcome was observed together with a high patient satisfaction. Our data together with more information on a possible mechanism of action will have to be confirmed and extended in a larger patient cohort within a randomized, placebo-controlled clinical trial.

Acknowledgments

This work is part of the dissertations of Elise Langer and Martin Seemann.

Author Contributions

Conceived and designed the experiments: EvS DB JS SG. Performed the experiments: EvS DB MS GS EL. Analyzed the data: EvS DB JS. Contributed reagents/materials/analysis tools: EvS DB SG. Wrote the paper: EvS DB. Designed the study, performed analysis: DB EvS. Performed study: EL MS GS IF JS.

References

1. Boguniewicz M, Leung DY (2010) Recent insights into atopic dermatitis and implications for management of infectious complications. J Allergy Clin Immunol 125: 4–15.
2. Hoare C, Li W, Williams H (2000) Systematic review of treatments of atopic eczema. In: Health Technology Assessment 4: 1–191.
3. Werfel T, Claes C, Kulp W, Greiner W, Graf von der Schulenburg JM (2006) Therapie der Neurodermitis. In: Health Technology Assessment 4: 1–176.
4. Werfel T, Aberer W, Augustin M, Biedermann T, Fölster-Holst R, et al. (2009) Atopic dermatitis: S2 guidelines. J Dtsch Dermatol Ges 7: S1–46.
5. Krutmann J, Medve-Koenigs K, Ruzicka T, Ranft U, Wilkens JH (2005) Ultraviolet-free phototherapy. Photodermatol Photoimmunol Photomed 21: 59–61.
6. Diepgen TL, Fartasch M, Hornstein OP (1989) Evaluation and relevance of atopic basic and minor features in patients with atopic dermatitis and in the general population. Acta Derm Venereol Suppl (Stockh) 144: 50–4.
7. Hanifin JM, Thurston M, Omoto M, Cherill R, Tofte SJ, et al. (2001) The eczema area and severity index (EASI): assessment of reliability in atopic dermatitis. EASI Evaluator Group. Exp Dermatol 10: 11–8.
8. Finlay AY, Khan GK (1994) Dermatology Life Quality Index (DLQI) – a simple practical measure for routine clinical use. Clin Exp Dermatol 19: 210–16.
9. Schwarz T (2008) 25 years of UV-induced immunosuppression mediated by T cells-from disregarded T suppressor cells to highly respected regulatory T cells. Photochem Photobiol 84: 10–8.
10. Meduri NB, Vandergriff T, Rasmussen H, Jacobe H (2007) Phototherapy in the management of atopic dermatitis: a systematic review. Photodermatol Photoimmunol Photomed 23: 106–12.
11. von Kobyletzki G, Pieck C, Hoffmann K, Freitag M, Altmeyer P (1999) Medium-dose UVA1 cold-light phototherapy in the treatment of severe atopic dermatitis. J Am Acad Dermatol 41: 931–7.
12. Polderman MC, Wintzen M, le Cessie S, Pavel S (2005) UVA-1 cold light therapy in the treatment of atopic dermatitis: 61 patients treated in the Leiden University Medical Center". Photodermatol Photoimmunol Photomed 21: 93–6.
13. Der Petrossian M, Seeber, A, Hoe H, Nigsmann H, Tanew A (2000) Half-side comparison study on the efficacy of 8-methoxypsoralen bath-PUVA versus narrow-band ultraviolet B phototherapy in patients with severe chronic atopic dermatitis. Br J Dermatol 142: 39–43.
14. Greinert R (2009) Skin cancer: new markers for better prevention. Pathobiology 76: 64–81.
15. Saeki H, Tamaki K (2006) Thymus and activation regulated chemokine (TARC)/CCL17 and skin diseases. J Dermatol Sci 43: 75–84.
16. Kleinpenning MM, Smits T, Frunt MH, van Erp PE, van de Kerkhof PC, et al. (2010) Clinical and histological effects of blue light on normal skin. Photodermatol Photoimmunol Photomed 26: 16–21.
17. Grundmann SA, Beissert S (2009) Regulation of cellular immunity by Photo(chemo)therapy. Front Biosci 14: 4326–36.
18. Loser K, Beissert S (2009) Regulation of cutaneous immunity by the environment: an important role for UV irradiation and vitamin D. Int Immunopharmacol 9: 587–9.
19. Weichenthal M, Schwarz T (2005) Phototherapy: how does UV work? Photodermatol Photoimmunol Photomed 21: 260–6.

4

Interferon and Biologic Signatures in Dermatomyositis Skin: Specificity and Heterogeneity across Diseases

David Wong[1], Bory Kea[1], Rob Pesich[2], Brandon W. Higgs[3], Wei Zhu[3], Patrick Brown[2], Yihong Yao[3], David Fiorentino[1]*

1 Department of Dermatology, Stanford University School of Medicine, Stanford, California, United States of America, **2** Department of Biochemistry, Stanford University School of Medicine, Stanford, California, United States of America, **3** MedImmune, Translational Sciences, One MedImmune Way, Gaithersburg, Maryland, United States of America

Abstract

Background: Dermatomyositis (DM) is an autoimmune disease that mainly affects the skin, muscle, and lung. The pathogenesis of skin inflammation in DM is not well understood.

Methodology and Findings: We analyzed genome-wide expression data in DM skin and compared them to those from healthy controls. We observed a robust upregulation of interferon (IFN)-inducible genes in DM skin, as well as several other gene modules pertaining to inflammation, complement activation, and epidermal activation and differentiation. The interferon (IFN)-inducible genes within the DM signature were present not only in DM and lupus, but also cutaneous herpes simplex-2 infection and to a lesser degree, psoriasis. This IFN signature was absent or weakly present in atopic dermatitis, allergic contact dermatitis, acne vulgaris, systemic sclerosis, and localized scleroderma/morphea. We observed that the IFN signature in DM skin appears to be more closely related to type I than type II IFN based on in vitro IFN stimulation expression signatures. However, quantitation of IFN mRNAs in DM skin shows that the majority of known type I IFNs, as well as IFN g, are overexpressed in DM skin. In addition, both IFN-beta and IFN-gamma (but not other type I IFN) transcript levels were highly correlated with the degree of the *in vivo* IFN transcriptional response in DM skin.

Conclusions and Significance: As in the blood and muscle, DM skin is characterized by an overwhelming presence of an IFN signature, although it is difficult to conclusively define this response as type I or type II. Understanding the significance of the IFN signature in this wide array of inflammatory diseases will be furthered by identification of the nature of the cells that both produce and respond to IFN, as well as which IFN subtype is biologically active in each diseased tissue.

Editor: Serge Nataf, University of Lyon, France

Funding: The authors have no support or funding to report.

Competing Interests: The authors have declared that no competing interests exist.

* E-mail: fiorentino@stanford.edu

Introduction

Dermatomyositis (DM) is a chronic inflammatory disorder that can affect the skin, muscle, and other organs and is associated with significant morbidity and mortality. The prevalence of DM is not well-defined, as it is historically grouped together with polymyositis (PM) and inclusion body myositis (IBM) in most epidemiologic studies. The estimated incidence of DM is approximately 1 per 100,000 per year [1]. There are two forms of DM, juvenile and adult, that have overlapping but some distinct clinical features [1]. DM is considered an autoimmune disease, as it is associated with specific autoantibodies, and its prevalence is associated with particular HLA alleles [2].

Currently classified as an idiopathic inflammatory myopathy (IIM), much of the work in understanding DM has been focused on the muscle pathology that accompanies this disorder. Some authors have suggested that the muscle disease is due to an immune-mediated vasculopathy, with resultant ischemic damage to the muscle fibers resulting in myocyte death and muscle atrophy [3]. However, the precise mechanism of either endothelial cell or myocyte damage is unclear [3]. Inflamed muscle shows infiltration with B lymphocytes, T lymphocytes, and dendritic cells, and the contribution of each to the disease is not well understood [4,5]. Cytokines and chemokines are also postulated to be important in disease pathogenesis [6]. DM muscle expresses large amounts of type I interferon (IFN)-inducible genes [7]. It is possible that these gene products might themselves be causing the vascular and parenchymal cellular damage [7]. In addition, an IFN signature that correlates with overall disease activity is observed in peripheral blood of most DM patients, including patients with juvenile DM [8,9,10]. Thus, much as with other autoimmune diseases such as Systemic Lupus Erythematosus and Sjogren's syndrome, DM is emerging as a potentially type I IFN-driven autoimmune disease.

The pathogenesis of skin inflammation in DM is not well-studied and its pathologic mechanisms may or may not overlap with those causing DM muscle disease. The typical cutaneous histopathologic changes in DM include pathologic apoptosis/necrosis of keratinocytes, perivascular and lichenoid inflammation, increased dermal mucin deposition, endothelial cell damage with loss of capillaries, and vascular dilatation [11,12]. Similarities to muscle disease exist in the skin: first, vasculopathy and vascular deposition of complement components can be detected in cutaneous DM skin [13,14]; second, there is damage to the parenchymal cells (e.g. keratinocytes) [11]; third, DM skin appears to be characterized by increased abundance of several gene products that are known to be upregulated by IFN [15,16] as well as by increased numbers of plasmacytoid dendritic cells [17,18]. It has been proposed that some of these gene products, such as CXCL9/10/11, act as chemoattractrants for CXCR3-bearing T lymphocytes which can then perpetuate inflammation and keratinocyte necrosis [16]. In addition, there appears to be a topographical relationship between the site of cell injury, inflammation, and the basement membrane that is shared by both skin and muscle disease in DM [19]. However, there are certain differences between muscle and skin disease in DM patients: clinically, the course of skin and muscle disease is often discordant between patients [20], suggesting different mechanisms of disease pathogenesis; in addition, there are important histopathologic differences between skin and muscle—for example, B lymphocytes are rarely found in the skin disease [21], in contrast to their common perivascular location in DM muscle. Current therapies for DM skin disease include immunosuppressive medications, which are not uniformly efficacious and can be associated with significant morbidity [20]. A better understanding of molecular pathogenesis of DM could potentially unveil better molecular markers for this disease and more effective targets for therapy.

In this study, we performed global gene expression analysis of skin from DM patients and healthy controls. Our results reveal a gene expression signature that is unique to skin inflammation in both DM and lupus, but distinct from other inflammatory skin diseases. Within this signature, we also identify a characteristic IFN-driven expression pattern in DM and lupus that partially overlaps with the pattern seen in other lichenoid dermatoses as well as psoriasis.

Results

Defining expression signature in skin of individuals with DM

In order to understand the molecular characteristics of DM, we hybridized RNA from skin biopsies from patients with active DM ($n = 16$) and healthy patients ($n = 10$) (total of 32 independent biopsies, with 12 technical replicates for total of 44 arrays) to HEEBO oligonucleotide arrays. The baseline characteristics of these patients are listed in Table S1. Using significance analysis of microarrays (FDR$<$0.05), we identified 946 unique genes that were differentially regulated at least 2-fold in DM skin relative to healthy skin: we term this the "DM gene module" (Table S2). Over two-thirds (646 of 946) of the genes identified were up-regulated and 300 were down-regulated in DM skin relative to healthy skin. Two-dimensional hierarchical clustering using these 946 genes segregated all healthy controls and DM patients into 2 distinct clusters (Fig. 1A). The 3 DM patients (4 samples) that segregated with the healthy controls formed a separate sub-cluster unto themselves. There was no apparent clustering with regards to age, gender, or site of biopsy (not shown). When patients with inactive skin disease were included in the cluster analysis, we found that 6 of 7 of the inactive DM patients clustered with the healthy controls (Fig. S1).

We noted that the DM gene module contained groups of genes that are known to function in several distinct biological pathways (Figs. 1A and S2). For example, a group of 13 genes associated with keratinocyte/epidermal activation (S100A7/8/9, SERPINB3/4, and FABP5) was upregulated in DM (yellow bar, Figs. 1A and S2). In addition, genes involved in epidermal differentiation, including IVL, TGM, SPRR2A/B/E/G, SERPINB7/8, are induced in DM (red bar, Figs. 1A and S2), which have also been shown to be elevated in other inflammatory skin diseases, such as psoriasis and atopic dermatitis [22,23]. A large cluster of genes upregulated in DM are involved in T cell (IL2RB, CD2, TRAC, CD3D, CTLA4), cytotoxic/NK cell (NKG7), macrophage (CD68), and dendritic cell (CD83) function (green bar, Figs. 1A and Fig. S2), which is consistent with previous observations regarding T cell and macrophage infiltration in DM skin [21]. The overexpression of the cell surface marker CD83 is consistent with previous studies that showed with immunostaining that mature dendritic cells are present in DM skin (either myeloid or plasmacytoid) [16,18]. In addition, skin from patients with DM had induction of markers of endothelial cell activation (VCAM1, SEL-L). A subset of the DM samples showed elevated immunoglobulin expression, indicative of infiltrating mature B lymphocytes and/or plasma cells, the former of which have been shown to be present in low and variable amounts in DM skin (lavender bar, Figs. 1A and S2) [21].

A striking observation in DM skin was the over expression of genes that were induced by IFN (light blue bar, Figs. 1A and S2). In fact, 21 of the top 25 most upregulated genes are known or presumed to be upregulated by IFN [24,25,26] (Table S3). These genes included CXCL10, IFIH1, ISG15/UBE2L6, C1S/R, IRF7, IDO1, MXB and CHN1. Notably this cluster of IFN genes was generally not overexpressed in the skin of DM patients with inactive skin disease (Fig. S1), suggesting that they are induced preferentially in active skin lesions.

Of the downregulated genes in DM, many were involved in either ribosomal synthesis (brown bar, Figs. 1A and S2) or lipid metabolism (dark purple bar, Figs. 1A and S2). The latter group of genes included MVD, MGST1, GCS1, FADS1/2 and GAL. Many of the genes involved in lipid metabolism have been previously reported to be downregulated in other inflammatory skin disorders such as psoriasis and atopic dermatitis [22,27].

To validate our findings from these microarrays, we performed TaqMan quantitative real-time reverse-transcriptase PCR-(QRT-PCR-) based assays on several genes from two of the enriched gene modules, the IFN and lipid gene modules (Fig. 1B). As suggested by the arrays, TaqMan QRT-PCR confirmed that two IFN-induced genes (IFIT3 and OAS2) were upregulated, and two genes involved in lipid metabolism (FADS, HMGCS1) were downregulated in the skin of DM patients. Across patient samples, there was a good correlation between microarray and QRT-PCR values for each of the four genes (Spearman $\rho = 0.76$ to 0.88).

In order to systematically investigate the biological processes that are altered in DM skin, we constructed a gene module map ($p<0.05$, FDR$<$0.05) to look for enrichment of gene sets associated with various biologic pathways and/or functions, based on either Gene Ontology (GO) and KEGG pathway annotations and on data derived from publicly available gene expression studies (Figs. 2 and S3). Biologic functions and pathways found to be enriched in the upregulated genes in DM skin included antigen processing, complement activation, MHC I/II receptor activity, T cell function, chemokine activity, antiviral and immune responses and epidermal differentiation (Fig. 2). Besides the IFN signaling pathway, TNF-alpha, IL-1, IL6, IL17 and VEGF pathway activation was also observed in the skin of DM patients (Fig. S3). Downregulated processes in DM skin included fatty acid

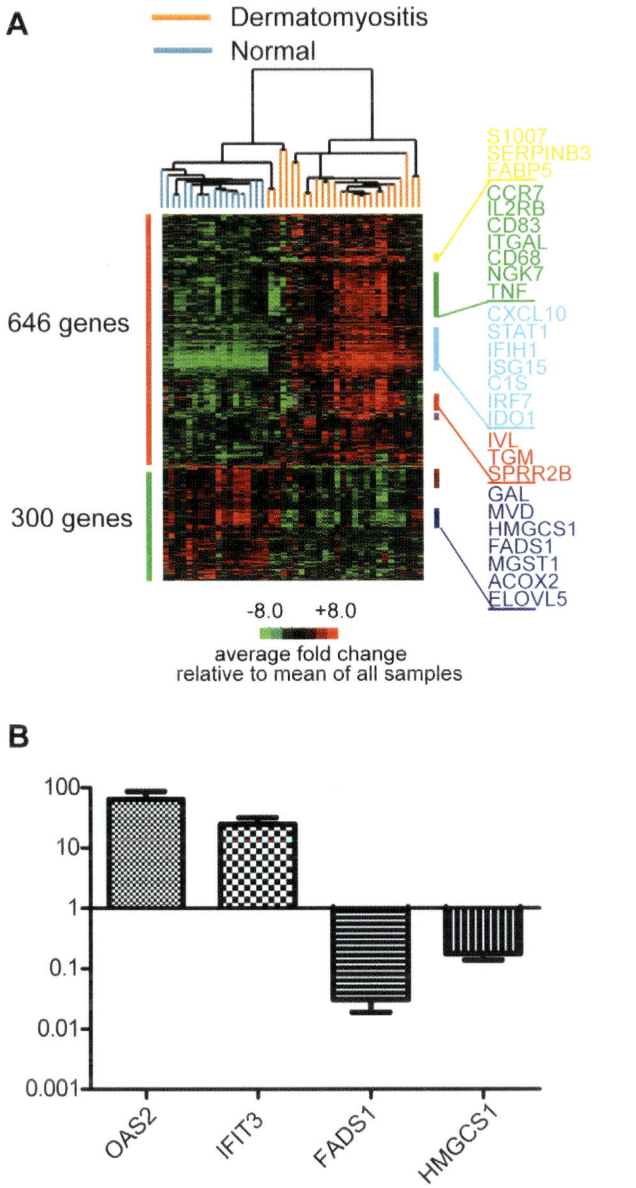

Figure 1. Visualization and validation of DM gene expression on HEEBO oligonucleotide arrays. RNA was prepared from skin biopsies as detailed in Methods, and the same source was used for both gene expression array (**A**) and QRT-PCR experiments (**B**). **A.** Experimental hierarchical clustering dendrogram. Two-dimensional hierarchical clustering was performed on gene expression data from active DM skin lesions and skin from healthy controls. A set of 946 genes whose average expression significantly differed between DM and healthy controls (the "DM module) was used to group sample expression data; 646 genes were upregulated (red bar on left) and 300 genes were downregulated (green bar on left) in DM patients relative to control biopsies. All values are in $\log_2$ space and are mean-centered across each gene. Colored bars on right indicate gene clusters evident on dendrogram: yellow bar epidermal activation; green bar leukocyte function; light blue bar—IFN signature; red bar—epidermal differentiation; lavender bar—immunoglobulin; brown bar—ribosome; dark purple bar-lipid metabolism. A larger view of the dendrogram and more complete lists of genes in these clusters can be found in **Supplementary Figure S2. B.** Validation of array data using TaqMan QRT-PCR of selected transcripts. QRT-PCR was performed (see Methods) on 9 DM skin RNA samples and 8 control skin RNA samples for four selected transcripts that were either found to be upregulated (OAS2, IFIT3) or downregulated (FADS1, HMGCS1) in DM skin. Shown are the mean values (with SEM) for each transcript in DM skin relative to the mean value in control skin. Relative transcript values for each of the 4 genes across the 9 DM samples showed a high correlation (Pearson's r = 0.71 to 0.86) between the HEEBO array and QRT-PCR.

metabolism, lipid biosynthesis and metabolism, mitochondrial function (electron transport and pyruvate metabolism), peroxisome and ribosomal function.

Mapping the DM gene module across different skin diseases

We next sought to study the specificity of these gene expression changes across various inflammatory skin diseases. With the exception of the cutaneous lupus samples (which were internally collected and processed along with the DM samples), we used publicly available gene expression sets, and all disease data were normalized to internal healthy controls within each study. We examined the expression of genes in the DM gene module across the different diseases (Fig. 3; see also Fig. S4 for a full pairwise correlation matrix). Due to the use of different array platforms in this analysis, only 490 genes of the original 946 genes of the DM module were contained in all of the experimental datasets analyzed and could thus be used for the analysis. Although the data were generated by different investigators on different microarray platforms, diseases for which more than one dataset existed (psoriasis and atopic dermatitis) showed remarkably similar expression patterns between datasets (Spearman $\rho = 0.77$ to 0.82). A similar correlation analysis between DM samples analyzed using HEEBO arrays and an independent set of DM samples analyzed using Affymetrix arrays demonstrated high correlation (Spearman r = 0.76) (Fig. 3). This suggests that the differences observed between diseases were primarily driven by biological disease-specific characteristics rather than platform or laboratory differences.

The gene expression profiles in DM and lupus skin samples were remarkably similar (Spearman r = 0.87; Fig. 3), suggesting that skin from individuals with DM and lupus, which are both autoimmune interface dermatitis processes, have a common pathophysiology. Interestingly, the upregulated genes in the DM gene module were similarly induced in the muscle of DM patients (Spearman r = 0.56; Fig. 3). DM skin also showed similarity to samples from (herpes simplex-2) HSV-2 infection (Spearman r = 0.64; Fig. 3). The rest of the inflammatory skin diseases appeared to have a small subset of similarly regulated genes as in DM, but overall the pattern was quite different. The epidermal activation genes, such as S100 and SERPIN genes appear to be generally upregulated across most of the skin diseases except for localized and systemic scleroderma (yellow bar, Fig. 3). In addition, many of the inflammatory genes were variably expressed across different diseases, with the highest expression observed in cutaneous lupus and HSV-2, moderately high expression in DM skin and muscle, and modest increase in expression in other diseases (green bar, Fig. 3). Genes involved in the complement cascade (C1S, C1R, C1QB, and C2) were only upregulated in DM skin/muscle, cutaneous lupus, and HSV-2 skin (not shown). IFN-inducible genes were very highly overexpressed in DM skin/muscle, lupus skin, and HSV-2 skin; and to a lesser degree in psoriasis, and the blood of DM and lupus patients (light blue bar, Fig. 3). Genes of lipid metabolism were generally repressed not only in cutaneous DM and lupus but also psoriasis, atopic dermatitis, and morphea, and to a variable extent in other inflammatory skin diseases (dark purple bar, Fig. 3). Of note, this repression of lipid metabolism genes is not found in DM muscle, DM blood, or

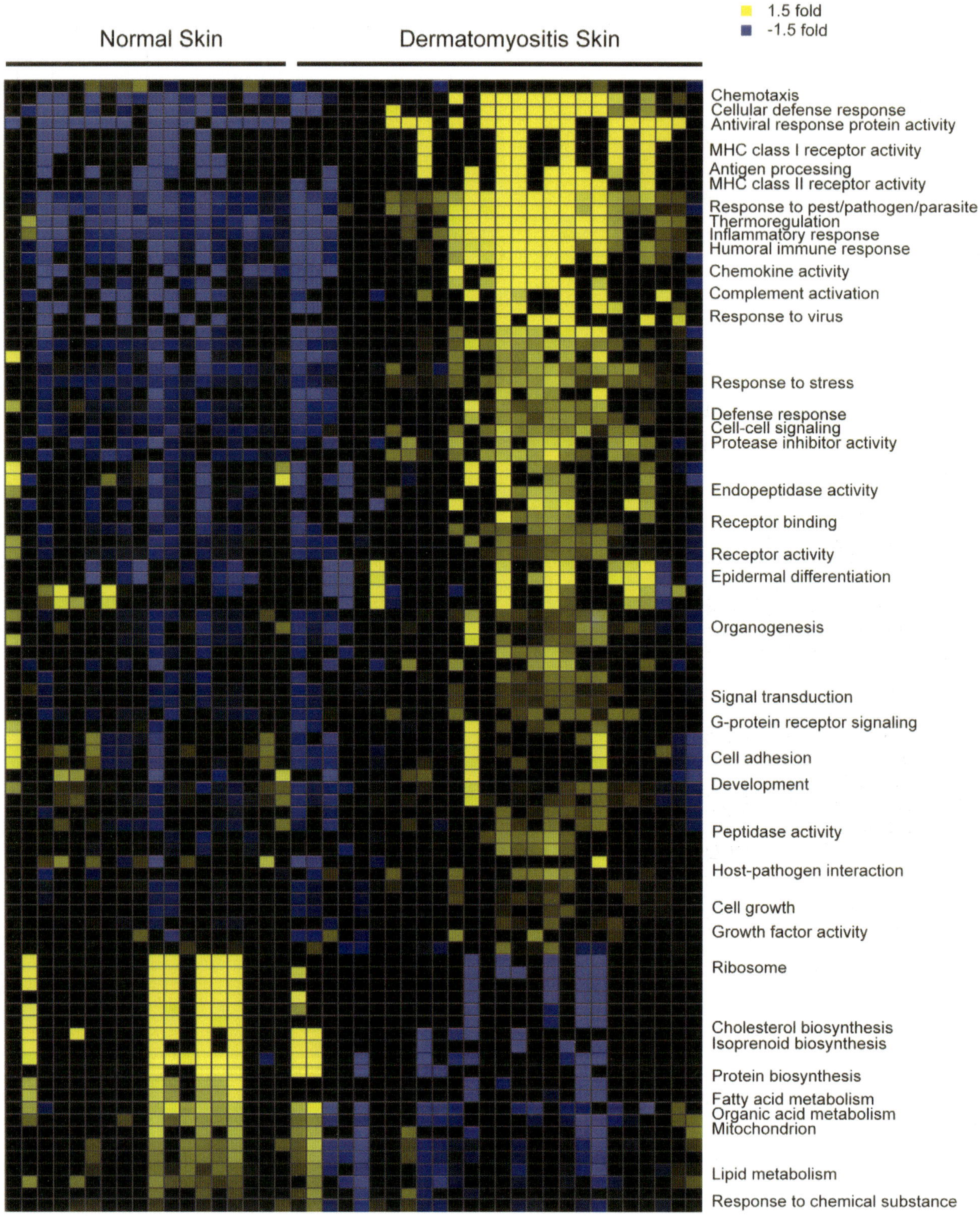

Figure 2. DM skin module map. Module map of the Gene Ontology (GO) and Kyoto Encyclopedia of Genes and Genomes (KEGG) Biological Processes differentially expressed among the active DM samples is shown. Each column represents a single microarray (e.g. patient) and each row represents a single GO or KEGG biological process. Only modules that were significantly enriched (minimum 2-fold change, p = 0.05) on at least 4 microarrays are shown. The average expression of the gene hits from each enriched gene set is displayed here. Only gene sets that show significant differences after multiple hypothesis testing were included. Selected GO or KEGG biological processes are shown. The entire figure with all biological processes can be viewed in Supplementary Figure S3.

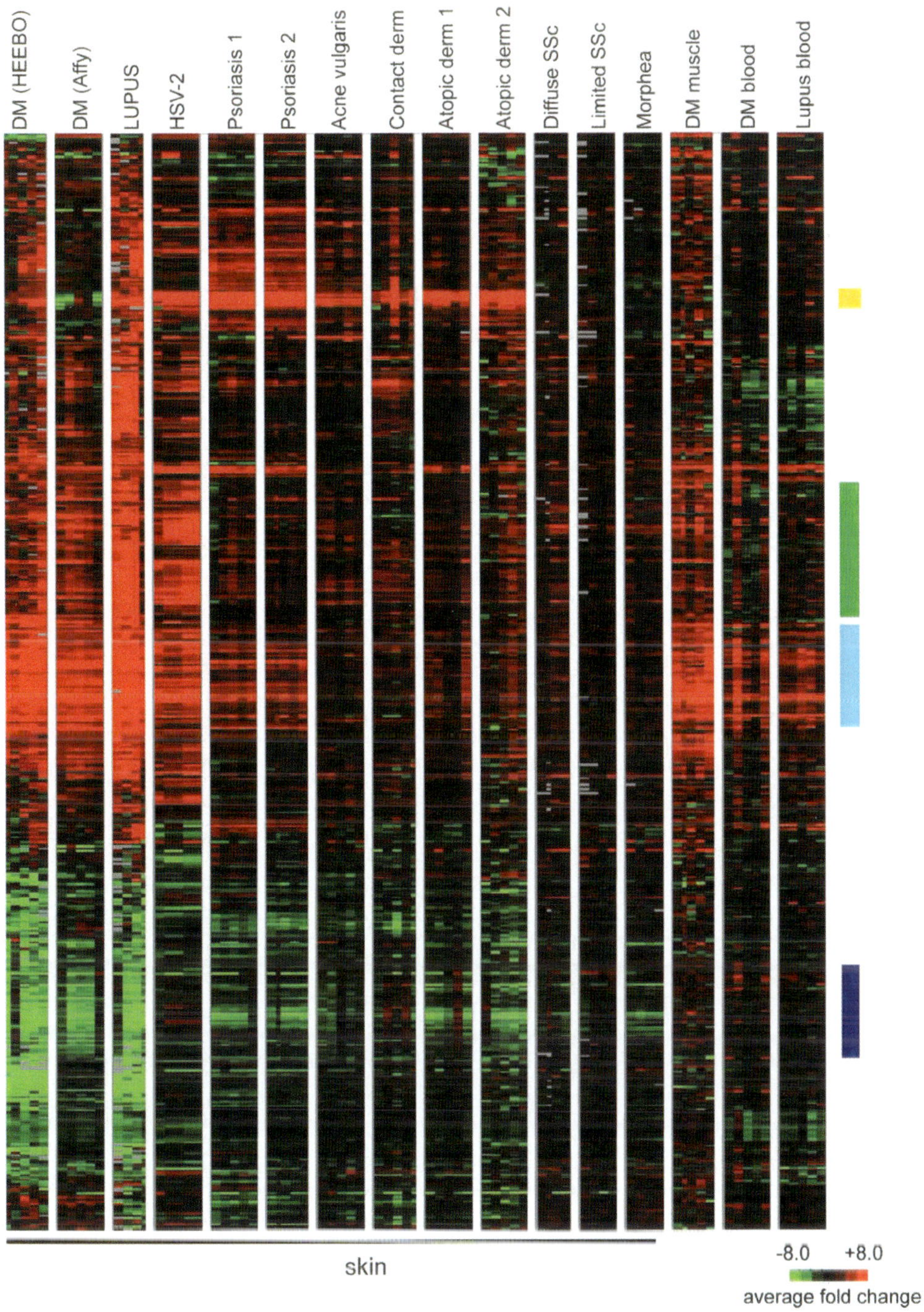

Figure 3. Mapping the DM module across different inflammatory disease tissues. Shown is a hierarchical clustering dendrogram of gene expression data from DM and multiple other diseases. The genes visualized represent all of the genes of the DM module that are common to all of the array platforms used to generate the data shown. The expression pattern of this set of 490 genes across all of the disease states shown was clustered using average linkage clustering, while the columns (samples) were not clustered and grouped by disease and experimental dataset. Expression data for each gene is relative to the mean expression level for all healthy controls (red = upregulated, green = downregulated) within each dataset, with the exception that HSV-2 data is relative to uninvolved skin of *diseased* HSV-2 patients (see Methods). Each disease state is composed of five columns, representing five representative examples (patients) of each disease. DM (HEEBO) and DM (Affy) represent data from independent DM skin biopsies run on either HEEBO or Affymetrix arrays, respectively. The remaining datasets were obtained from publicly available GEO omnibus data (see Methods). All data are derived from skin biopsies with the exception of the three diseases on the right, as indicated. Colored bars on right indicate gene clusters of the DM module that were discussed in the text for Figure 1: yellow bar—epidermal barrier; green bar—leukocyte function; light blue bar—IFN signature; dark purple bar-lipid metabolism.

lupus blood, and may thus be a skin-specific phenomenon. Thus, a cross disease comparison reveals that some gene expression changes may be more commonly seen in inflammatory skin diseases, while other (e.g. IFN signature) are more specific, and overall, DM and lupus skin share a highly unique gene expression signature.

Measuring the IFN signature across different skin diseases

Although many IFN-inducible genes were upregulated in our DM module, we wished to determine in more detail how expression of a pre-defined module of IFN-inducible genes was regulated in DM and several other inflammatory skin diseases. A consensus list of 117 IFN-stimulated genes (Table S4) was derived by using publicly available data from in vitro stimulations of various cell types with either type I or II IFNs (see Methods). The expression pattern of these IFN-inducible genes was then surveyed across both the *in vitro* IFN stimulation data as well as diseased skin expression data. Some variation exists in the *in vitro* response upon IFN stimulation, depending on the cell type, IFN type, and the independent labs that generated the data (Fig. 4A, left panel). Again it appeared that DM skin and muscle, lupus skin, and HSV-2 skin infection had the most robust overexpression of IFN-inducible genes (Fig. 4B, right panel; also see Fig. S5 for a full pairwise correlation matrix). As was the case for the entire DM module, the expression patterns of IFN-inducible genes in skin of DM and lupus patients appeared almost indistinguishable, and similar to those in DM muscle and HSV-2. DM blood and lupus blood had a weaker induction of IFN genes, which is likely due to the fact that the IFN module was constructed using data from cell types present in skin and not blood. Interestingly, psoriasis demonstrated induction of a subset of IFN-inducible genes. In contrast, most of the skin samples of acne vulgaris, contact dermatitis, atopic dermatitis, allergic contact dermatitis, systemic sclerosis, and morphea did not appear to show significant induction of IFN-driven genes.

We next quantified the strength of the IFN-signature across different disease states. Similar to previous studies, we selected the top 25 most highly IFN-inducible genes from our "core IFN signature", based on the *in vitro* studies that were used to define this signature (Table S4) [28]. We found that the scores calculated these 25 genes versus the full 117 gene module display a high correlation (Spearman's $r = 0.96$; not shown). We then calculated the median expression value (relative to healthy controls) of these 25 genes for each sample, which constituted the "IFN score" (Fig. 4B) [28]. DM and lupus skin had the highest average median IFN scores of 20 and 44, respectively. DM muscle and HSV-2 skin had high IFN scores (9.5 and 8.1, respectively), while the two psoriasis datasets yielded mean scores of 2.5 and 2.8. In contrast, all other skin diseases had scores of 1.7 or less.

In addition to the differences in overall IFN score, we were intrigued with the different patterns of IFN-induced genes in the various skin inflammatory diseases (Fig. 4A). These different patterns of IFN signature could be due to multiple factors, including: 1) a difference in cell types responding to IFN stimulation, 2) a difference in IFN subtypes (e.g. type I or II) that are present among the diseases, or 3) the presence of other cytokines that may induce a subset of genes in our "core IFN set". To further investigate the differences in these patterns, we performed principal components analysis of the various disease samples as well as the samples obtained using in vitro IFN stimulations (Fig. 4A) using the *in vitro*-defined core IFN signature genes (Fig. 5A). We observed that the horizontal component tends to correlate with the strength of IFN signature, specifically in the skin (Figs. 4B and 5). Thus, DM muscle, DM and lupus skin, and HSV-2 are furthest to the right, while psoriasis, DM and lupus blood, and selected systemic sclerosis and atopic dermatitis samples all are modestly displaced to the right from all other skin diseases that are clustered together on the left—this is in general agreement with our IFN scoring data (Fig. 4B). On the other hand, the vertical component (component 2) appears to at least partially distinguish type I versus type II IFN (see *in vitro* stimulation data towards the right of Fig. 5). Additionally, the disease samples tend to be more positively positioned along this component, suggesting that DM, lupus and psoriasis all have signatures more consistent with type I IFN than with type II IFN.

IFN gene expression in DM skin

In order to further characterize the IFN response in DM skin, we performed QRT-PCR analysis of the selected IFNs, including IFN-alpha (subtypes 1,2,4,6,8,14 and 21), IFN-beta, IFN-kappa, IFN-omega, and IFN-gamma. Due to unavailability of RNA from samples in our original dataset, these data were derived from skin biopsy samples from an independent cohort of 39 DM patients (see Methods). Importantly, these samples showed similar gene expression patterns to our original dataset (Fig. 4A and S5). We found that expression levels of all IFN transcripts, with the exception of IFN-α4, were elevated in DM skin compared to healthy controls, although there was considerable variation between patients (Fig. 6A). Noting this variation, we next wished to clarify if any of the IFN transcripts were coordinately regulated by performing average linkage hierarchical clustering of the QRT-PCR data for the IFN transcripts across the 39 samples. The IFN-alpha transcripts (with the possible exception of IFN-a21 and IFN-a4) as well as the IFN-omega transcripts were coordinately regulated (Fig. 6B). IFN-beta and IFN-gamma were more closely correlated with one another than any of the other transcripts, while IFN-kappa had the most distinct pattern of expression across the samples.

Our previous data suggested that the IFN signature in DM skin was more similar to the pattern seen with type I rather than type II IFN (Fig. 5). We reasoned that another independent method of identifying the dominant IFN subtype(s) generating the *in vivo* IFN signature in DM skin was to perform a correlation analysis between the level of each particular IFN family transcript and the IFN score for all of the available samples. Strikingly, IFN-beta transcript level was very highly correlated with IFN signature strength in the skin (Spearman $r = 0.82$; $p<0.0001$) (Fig. 6C). Interestingly, IFN-gamma also demonstrated a high correlation with IFN signature score (Spearman $r = 0.72$; $p<0.0001$), while none of the IFN-alpha subtypes (as well as IFN-omega) were significantly correlated with the strength of the IFN signature (Fig. 6C; data not shown).

Discussion

This is the first study of global gene expression in the skin of DM patients. We demonstrate an expression signature (the "DM module") in the skin of 16 DM patients relative to skin from 10 normal, unaffected individuals using whole genome HEEBO oligonucleotide arrays. This DM signature was validated in an independent set of DM skin samples on a different microarray platform (Affymetrix). In addition, examination of this signature across multiple different inflammatory skin diseases demonstrated that this signature is unique to DM and lupus, suggesting that cutaneous DM and cutaneous lupus have a similar underlying pathogenetic mechanism. This signature was characterized by up-regulation of genes involved in antigen processing, complement activation, MHC I/II receptor activity, T cell function, chemokine activity, antiviral and immune responses and epidermal differentiation, and down-regulation of genes involved in fatty acid metabolism, lipid biosynthesis and metabolism, mitochondrial function, and ribosomal function.

One might argue that these gene expression changes are simply a function of increased immune cell infiltration in DM skin. Thus,

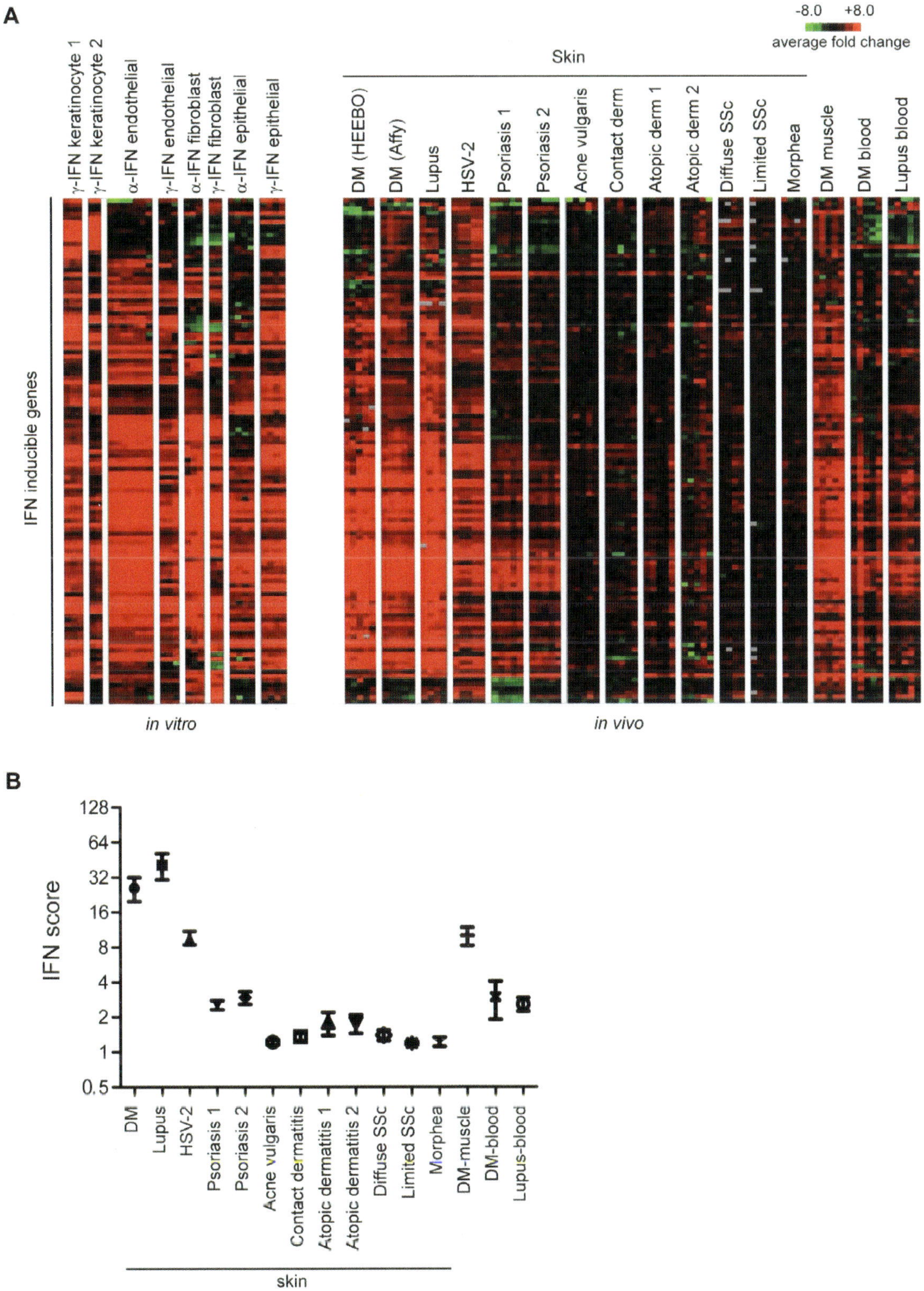

Figure 4. Visualizing the pattern and strength of the IFN signature expression across multiple disease states. A. Heatmaps of gene expression of the IFN inducible genes both *in vitro* and *in vivo* across diseases. The expression of a set of 117 genes comprising the "core IFN signature" (labeled as "IFN inducible genes" in the figure) is shown following one-way hierarchical clustering (genes only) using the entire *in vitro* and *in vivo* dataset. The left panel shows the expression patterns of this IFN signature following various *in vitro* stimulations with IFN-alpha or IFN-gamma on different responding cell types, as indicated. The right panel shows the expression patterns of the IFN signature across multiple disease states. The data from the disease states were derived from publicly available data as described in Figure 3 and Methods. **B.** Comparing the strength of the IFN signature across disease states using an IFN score. The top 25 expressed IFN-inducible genes (a static list) was derived from the same *in vitro* data used to generate the core IFN signature as described in Methods. The median expression value (in linear space) of this set of 25 genes within each

disease sample was defined as the IFN score for that sample. Shown is the mean and SEM for IFN scores calculated for each disease dataset represented in panel A.

we performed a study across multiple inflammatory skin diseases to address the specificity of the altered transcriptional modules seen in DM skin. This cross-disease comparison suggests that, while several gene expression patterns are shared more commonly across inflammatory skin diseases, many of the gene expression patterns are not found uniformly across inflammatory skin diseases. For example, upregulation of genes typically associated with epidermal activation was seen in all skin diseases except scleroderma. In addition, we observed downregulation of a large number of genes involved in lipid metabolism across most of the skin diseases we studied. The only disease in which this was not apparent was HSV-2, and this may actually reflect the fact that this dataset used non-lesional skin from patients (rather than skin from healthy volunteers) as a control—downregulation of lipid genes has been seen in non-lesional skin of psoriasis patients [27] and we have also seen this in the uninvolved skin from DM patients (data not shown). Downregulation of genes involved in lipid metabolism has been previously reported in psoriasis and atopic dermatitis [22,27,29], but our data suggest that it is a more general feature of many inflammatory skin diseases. It is unclear what cell types are being affected to cause these observed changes, although this lipid regulation could indicate the presence of a defective epidermal barrier, as suggested previously [22]. However, we found other signatures, notably the interferon signature as well as others, that appear to be more characteristic of only selected inflammatory skin diseases, despite the fact that many conditions lacking these signatures (e.g. atopic dermatitis, acne vulgaris) are known to be characterized by inflammatory infiltrates in the skin. Of course, it is still possible that the transcriptional changes seen in DM skin are a direct result of a unique type(s) of infiltrating cell. For the interferon signature, one possible cell type would be the plasmacytoid dendritic cell, and experiments to correlate the strength of various transcriptional responses with infiltrating cell types would be important to perform in the future.

Our data show conclusively that a genuine IFN signature is seen in DM skin, similar to that found in the blood and muscle of DM patients [9,10,30,31]. It is important to look at a complete set of IFN-inducible genes and not simply one gene product, as this can lead to erroneous conclusions of an IFN signature being present. For example, focusing only at MxA, a protein classically characterized as type I IFN-specific, would have led to the conclusion that both atopic dermatitis datasets showed an average of 2.9-fold overexpression relatively to healthy controls (data not shown); this could be misconstrued as evidence of type I IFN activation in the skin of atopic dermatitis, which is clearly not the case. Thus, our results confirm and extend previous reports that demonstrated upregulation of a few selected, IFN-inducible proteins (MxA, CXCL9, CXCL10) in DM skin [15,16]. This signature was found in all patients in which active skin disease was biopsied, but was found at low or absent levels in biopsies from

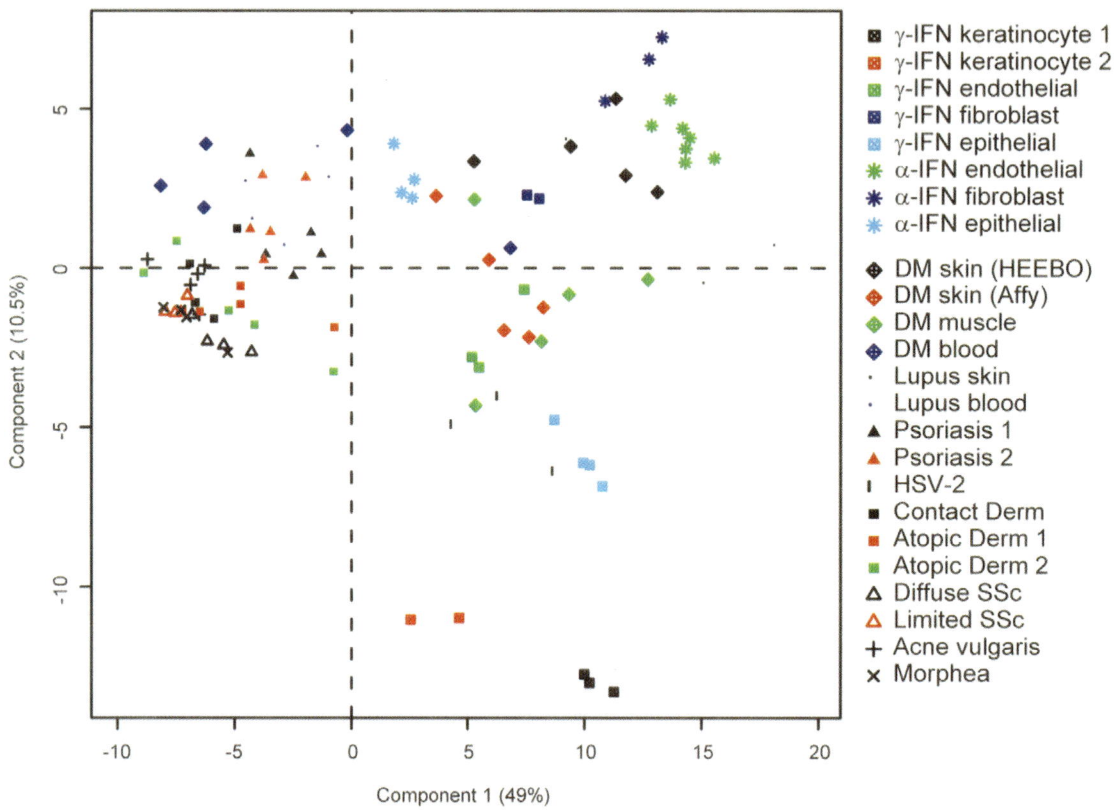

Figure 5. Distinguishing between type I and II IFN expression patterns across disease states. Two-dimensional PCA plot is shown using expression data derived from our data (DM, lupus) and publicly available datasets across the 117 gene "core IFN gene set" as described in Methods. Approximately 60% of the total data variation is summarized in these first two principal components.

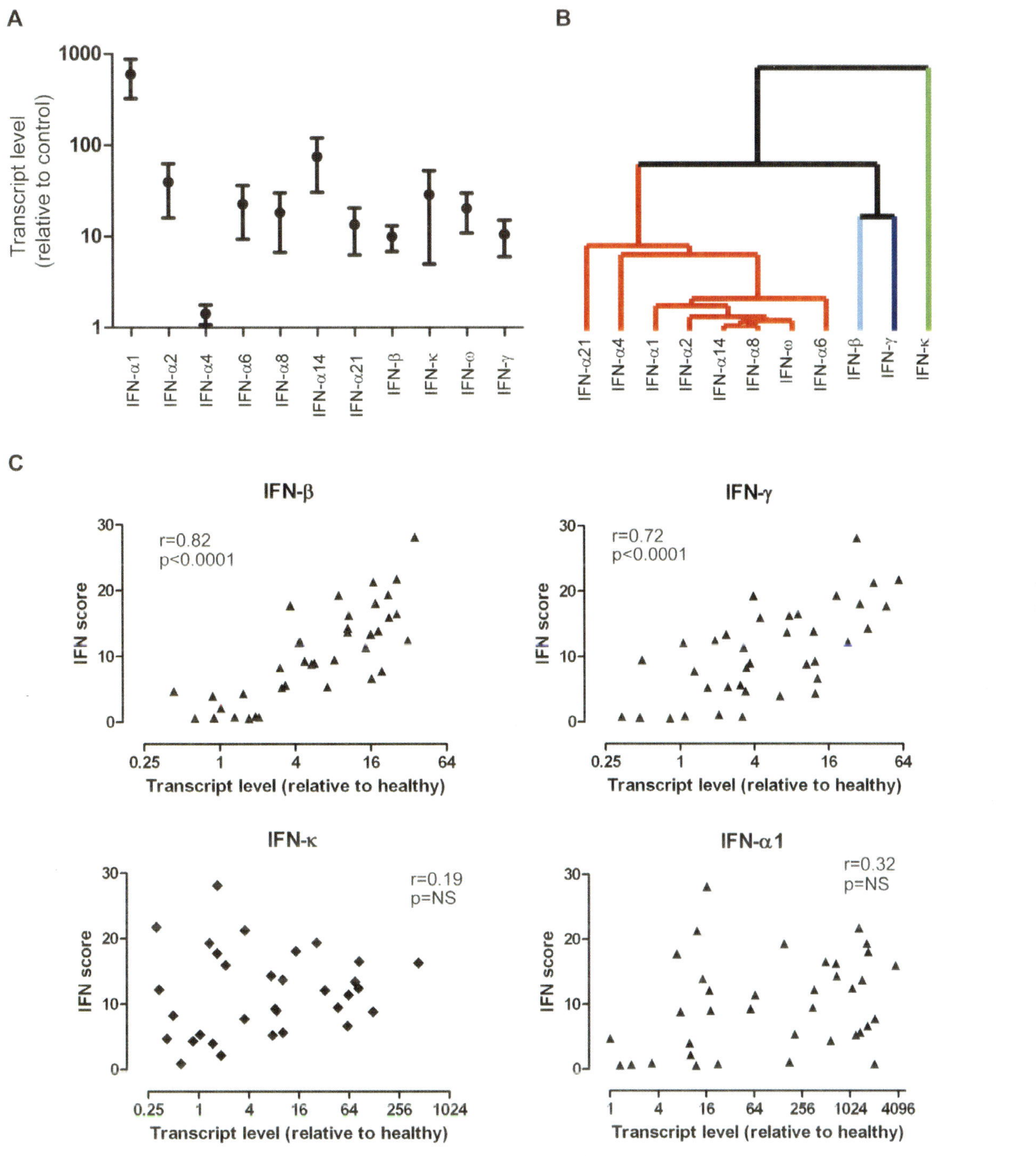

Figure 6. Expression of IFN transcripts in DM skin and correlation with downstream response. A. Upregulation of most IFN transcripts in DM skin. QRT-PCR analysis of different IFN transcripts in DM skin samples. TaqMan PCR was performed (see Methods) on 39 DM skin RNA samples and 4 control skin RNA samples for selected IFN transcripts. Shown are the mean values (with SEM) for each transcript in DM skin relative to the mean value in control skin. **B.** IFN transcripts are not co-regulated across DM skin samples. Hierarchical clustering dendrogram is shown for relative IFN transcript expression levels (using QRT-PCR) across 39 DM samples. Average linkage clustering was performed using correlation (uncentered) similarity metric. Similarity branches (length is inversely correlated with similarity of expression patterns) for IFN-α and IFN-ω are shown in red, IFN-beta in light blue, IFN-gamma in dark purple, and IFN-κ in green. **C.** IFN-beta and IFN-gammacorrelate most closely with the IFN score in DM skin. For each RNA sample made from 39 independent DM skin biopsies, an IFN score was calculated based on transcript levels of downstream IFN-inducible genes from array data (as described in Figure 4B and Methods) as well as a relative transcript level (using QRT-PCR) for several IFN transcripts (see panel A). Shown are correlation plots (for each of the 39 samples) of the IFN score and IFN transcript levels for IFN-a1, IFN-beta, IFN-gamma, and IFN-kappa.

patients with inactive skin disease, despite the presence of active myositis in the latter group. Thus, the IFN signature in the skin might serve as a useful marker for cutaneous disease activity in DM.

This study also provides information regarding the specificity of the IFN signature across many inflammatory skin diseases. We found that DM, lupus, and HSV-2 skin, and to a lesser degree, psoriasis, had moderate-to-robust IFN signatures, whereas atopic dermatitis, contact dermatitis, systemic sclerosis, and acne vulgaris had relatively weak or absent IFN signatures. Psoriasis was characterized by induction of a large subset of the IFN "core" genes whose expression pattern appeared to correlate with a type I IFN response, in agreement with prior observations [32]. The subtle differences between the IFN signatures of DM and lupus compared with psoriasis may be due to a different source of IFN in the two diseases, different population of responding cells, or modulating cytokines. It is curious that psoriasis appears to have an IFN signature, as all other skin diseases that we found to have this signature are characterized by a predominance of keratinocyte injury and/or death. Indeed, it has been suggested that the IFN signature is characteristic of the lichenoid skin reaction [33], but, given the fact that keratinocyte death is not associated with psoriasis, it is clear that the significance of an IFN signature in skin disease may be more complicated. However, it should be noted that the IFN score was much lower in psoriasis skin than in the other lichenoid disorders, and thus may not reach a threshold required to initiate pathways involved in keratinocyte death.

Our data have highlighted the difficulty in assigning an IFN signature as being "type I" or "type II", especially in tissue that contains multiple cell types and cannot be easily modeled *in vitro*. Although a type I IFN signature has been suggested to be present in multiple inflammatory skin diseases, this has yet to be shown conclusively [32,33,34]. Many genes thought to be specifically induced by type I IFN can also be induced by type II IFN, and this relationship is highly dependent on responding cell type and IFN dose. We have employed two methodologies to address this question in DM skin. First, we used various methods of comparing patterns of IFN-inducible gene expression with those obtained from various *in vitro* stimulations using recombinant type I or type II IFN. Although these comparisons suggest that DM skin is more characteristic of Type I IFN rather than type II IFN activity (see Fig. 5), it is difficult to draw firm conclusions from these data. One weakness of this approach is that it is difficult to compare patterns of gene expression obtained under in vitro conditions in cell lines and that which occurs in a dynamic tissue with multiple responding cell types and unknown concentrations of various IFN proteins. Our data certainly could be consistent with activation of either the type I or II IFN pathways in DM skin.

We also performed a correlation analysis between specific IFN transcript levels and a composite measurement of IFN-activity, namely the IFN gene score. We found that IFN-beta and IFN-gamma levels most closely correlate with activation of IFN-induced genes (see Fig. 6C), also suggesting that either type I or II IFNs could be driving the IFN response. Although we did not find a correlation between the IFN-alpha (and other type I) transcripts we measured, this does not rule out a role for these interferons in DM skin disease. It is possible that a threshold level of IFN-alpha is required for the IFN response, which may then be modulated by varying levels of other interferons. The involvement of specific interferons in disease activity will only be conclusively answered by treating patients with specific IFN inhibitors. An alternative interpretation of these data is that IFN-betaand IFN-gamma) are regulated in the same manner as the other IFN-induced transcripts in DM skin, although this is unlikely given the striking difference in abundance of IFN-beta mRNA versus the other IFN-induced transcripts in DM skin (data not shown). One weakness of this approach is that it assumes that IFN transcript level faithfully reflects the level of active IFN protein in the skin biopsies—however, this assumption would only serve to weaken any positive correlation, and thus the high correlation coefficients we observed are likely of significance.

The fact that many biopsies have high levels of other type I IFN transcripts (which share the same receptor as IFN-beta) in the absence of an IFN signature (Fig. 6C) suggests that other considerations are critical for the strong induction of IFN-induced genes seen in the skin of DM patients—these may include translation of IFN transcripts, localization of IFN production and/or presence of a responder cell population that is sensitive signaling via the IFN receptor. Thus, our data do not rule out an essential role for other type I or II IFNs in the pathogenesis of DM skin disease. They also point out the important fact that elevation of a particular IFN transcript does not provide proof of its activity *in vivo*.

One limitation of our study is that our data are derived from whole skin biopsies, and thus it is unclear what cell(s) constitute the source of IFN, as well as what cell(s) are responsible for producing such high levels of IFN-induced mRNA transcripts. Previous data suggest that keratinocytes as well as inflammatory cells are included in the latter "responding" population in DM skin [16]. However, it is clear that the pattern of expression of IFN-inducible proteins depends on the protein examined [15,16,33]. In addition, it will be important to detect the source of different IFN transcripts and proteins in DM skin, which can be technically demanding. Without detailed understanding of these issues, the role of IFN in DM skin disease will remain unclear.

Another potential weakness of our study is that many of our analyses compared data generated by different investigators, using different methodologies, across different microarray platforms. We attempted to mitigate this problem by only using datasets in which a control group was included, so that all data could be expressed relative to healthy patient skin. In addition, where possible, we used identical methodologies for normalizing array data. Despite this, we realize that this can always be a concern when analyzing microarray data, and thus we were more interested in the patterns of gene expression rather than absolute levels of selected genes. We believe our methodology had internal validation in that, for a given disease, independent patient samples run by independent investigators across disparate microarray platforms showed astonishingly similar patterns of gene expression over the gene modules that we were interested in studying (see Figure 3).

Our study defines patterns of gene expression that readily distinguish normal from DM skin. Many of these genes may prove to be useful as specific molecular markers that correlate with disease progression and prognosis. Our analysis provides further insight into the underlying pathogenesis of DM, including characterization of a specific IFN response in DM that may provide more effective targets for therapy.

Methods

Ethics Statement

The Stanford Panel on Medical Human Subjects approved human subjects involvement in this research project (last renewal on 04/18/2011). All subjects entered in this study signed an Informed Consent document before donating tissue.

Patients

All patients were seen in the adult Stanford Dermatology Clinics between August 2004 and March 2006 and agreed to sign an Informed Consent before participating in the study. All patients were diagnosed with DM based upon diagnostic cutaneous findings suggested previously [35] and all patients had a skin biopsy consistent with DM. Exclusion criteria included: (1) age less than 18 years old, and/or (2) evidence of medication-induced DM or mixed-connective tissue disease or other overlap syndromes. There were no restrictions on concomitant medications. We analyzed skin biopsies from 23 DM patients (16 active and 7 inactive) and 10 healthy controls (Table S1). All biopsies were taken from an area that was considered to be representative of active disease. In patients considered to have inactive skin disease (but active myositis), biopsies were taken from areas of telangiectasia and/or pigmentary alteration consistent with prior active DM skin disease. Because skin disease localization in DM patients can be variable, many of these biopsies are from different anatomic sites, although the majority of biopsies were from the arm or neck/upper back (Table S1). 23 DM patients provided a total of 25 biopsies, with 9 technical replicates for a total of 34 samples. 10 healthy controls provided a total of 15 biopsies, with 3 technical replicates, for a total of 18 samples. The DM patients were significantly older than the healthy control patients (mean age 53.1 vs 38.2, $p = .019$) and had a mean disease duration of 6.0 years. Four of the patients (17%) had cancer-associated DM. 8 of the patients (35%) had skin predominant disease–5 of them with a past history of myositis, and 3 never experiencing myositis (amyopathic). We also included skin biopsies from 4 patients with cutaneous lupus erythematosus (2 with acute cutaneous lupus and 2 with discoid lupus lesions).

Skin biopsy Processing and Microarray Analysis

Poly-adenylated RNA was extracted from snap-frozen skin biopsy specimens (DM and lupus) using a two step method. First, total RNA was extracted with phenol-guanidine thiocyaniate extraction (RNAbee, Tel-Test, Friendswood TX). Next, poly-adenylated RNA was purified using RNeasy Kit (Quiagen, Chatsworth, CA) according to the manufacturer's instructions. Sample RNA and reference mRNA (Stratagene) were amplified using an Amino Allyl MessageAmp II aRNA kit (Ambion, Austin, TX). Amplified skin RNA (labeled with Cy5) and amplified Human Universal Reference RNA (labeled with Cy3) (Stratagene, La Jolla, CA) were competitively hybridized to HEEBO (human exon evidence based oligonucleotide) microarrays as described (http://www.microarray.org/sfgf/heebo.do).

Array data were filtered based on fluorescent hybridization signal ≥1.5-fold over local background in either the Cy5 or the Cy3 channel and if the data were technically adequate in ≥80% of experiments. Array data underwent LOWESS normalization, and the data were displayed as a $\log_2$ ratio of LOWESS-normalized Cy5/Cy3 ratio (span parameter = 0.4). These array data are publicly available at Gene Expression Omnibus (GEO), accession number GSE32245.

For experiments assessing the platform independence of our DM array findings (Fig. 3) and for quantifying IFN expression in DM skin (Fig. 6), several independent DM ($n = 39$) and healthy control ($n = 18$) biopsies were obtained in the exact manner as described above. These biopsies were processed and hybridized to Affymetrix Human Genome U133 Plus 2.0 GeneChip arrays as described [32]. These array data were normalized using Robust Multichip Averaging (RMA) using Genespring (www.agilent.com/chem/genespring).

For all datasets, after filtering and normalization, expression data of each sample for all probes mapping to the same UnigeneID were averaged in linear space before any analysis was performed. Genes which showed significantly different expression between DM and controls were identified using Significance Analysis of Microarrays, with a false discovery rate (FDR)<0.043 and a minimum average expression of 2-fold greater or less than controls.

Average linkage hierarchical clustering was performed using GeneCluster ver3.0 software (http://bonsai.ims.u-tokyo.ac.jp/~mdehoon/software/cluster/software.htm). Clustered trees and gene expression heat maps were viewed using Java TreeView Software (http://jtreeview.sourceforge.net/).

Module Maps

Gene module map was done as described with the program Genomica (http://genomica.weizmann.ac.il/) using gene sets derived from Gene Ontology and KEGG Pathway annotations and the gene expression profiles of skin from patients with dermatomyositis and normal controls.

Briefly, given this collection of precompiled gene sets and this compendium of expression arrays, the method identifies the gene sets that are induced or repressed significantly in the set of arrays ($p \leq 0.05$, hypergeometric distribution).

Comparisons with publicly available microarray data

Publicly available gene expression data was obtained for psoriasis (GSE13355, GSE14905), atopic dermatitis (GSE5667, GSE6012), acne vulgaris (GSE6475), allergic contact dermatitis (GSE6281), HSV-2 infection (GSE18527), systemic sclerosis and morphea (GSE9285), DM muscle (GSE1551, GSE5370), DM blood (courtesy S. Greenberg, Brigham and Women's Hospital), and systemic lupus (GSE8650). The following array platforms were used for these studies: Affymetrix U133A (GSE5667, GSE6012, GSE1551, GSE5370, GSE8650) Affymetrix U133A 2.0 (GSE6475, 5667); Affymetrix U133 plus 2.0 (GSE6281, GSE13355, GSE14905); Agilent Whole Human Genome Oligo Microarray G4112A (GSE9285); Illumina humanref-8 v. 2.0 (GSE18527). Only scleroderma samples that classified as "inflammatory subgroup" were used for comparisons [36], given that we wished to enrich these data for samples that might express an IFN signature. For Affymetrix data, all array data was normalized using Robust Multichip Averaging (RMA) using Genespring (www.agilent.com/chem/genespring).

In order to compare data from different experiments, all expression data were first mapped to a common EntrezGene number. A set of 7783 unique EntrezGene IDs that were common to all platforms was used in these comparisons ("comparison matrix"). Probes that matched to multiple genes were not used. For instances in which multiple probes mapped to the same EntrezGene, these data were averaged by calculating the mean value in linear space to give a single value for each EntrezGene ID. Next, data for each gene in a given disease sample were normalized to the mean expression value of all control samples for that gene. Control samples were always skin biopsies from healthy donors, with the exception of the data from the HSV-2 patients (GSE18527), as the only control data available were derived from patient skin from uninvolved sites. Thus, each experiment was normalized to its own internal control samples, in order to facilitate comparison across experiment sets.

RT PCR analysis of individual transcripts

The expression level of several microarray target genes was assessed in patient tissue using Taqman quantitative one-step RT-

PCR (Applied Biosystems, Foster City, California, United States). Fifty nanograms of total RNA was used in each assay. Assay on demand primers for fatty acid desaturase 1 (Assay ID: Hs00203685_m1), IFN-b1 (Assay ID: Hs00277188_s1), 3-hydroxy-3-methylglutaryl-Coenzyme A synthase 1 (Assay ID: Hs00266810_m1), IFN α 2 (Assay ID: Hs02621172_s1), IFN-a1 (Assay ID: Hs00256882_s1), IFN-induced protein with tetratricopeptide repeats 3 (Assay ID: Hs00155468_m1) and IFN-alpha-inducible protein 6 (Assay ID: Hs00242571_m1) were normalized to GAPDH (Assay ID: Hs99999905_m1) levels and relative abundance was calculated using delta-delta threshold analysis. All assays were conducted on a Stratagene MX3000P thermocycler (La Jolla, CA). RT-PCR analysis of IFN mRNA transcripts was performed as described previously [32].

Mapping the DM module across disease states

Due to differences across array platforms, we first determined that 490 of the 946 genes from the DM module were present across all samples in the "comparison matrix" (defined above). One-way hierarchical clustering was performed (genes only) and the data were viewed as described above, with 5 representative examples from each inflammatory disease used for comparison.

Method for defining genes comprising core IFN signature

We reasoned that the skin has keratinocytes, fibroblasts, endothelial cells, and leukocytes, among other cells that could potentially respond differently to IFN. Thus we generated our list of IFN-stimulated genes from all publicly available expression data pertaining to in vitro stimulation with either IFN-gamma, -alpha, -beta, or other IFN preparations—these included data derived from the use of keratinocytes, lung epithelial cells, macrophages, endothelial cells, and fibroblasts as responder cells. These specific datasets used had the following GEO identifiers: GSE1132, GSE7216, GSE5542, GSE3920, GSE1925, GSE1740. The time of stimulation and concentration of IFN varied between studies. For each study, pre- and post-stimulation data were placed in $\log_2$ space and mean-centered for each gene. All data were then combined and evaluated using Statistical Analysis of Microarrays using a two-class analysis (pre vs post-treatment). From this analysis, 749 genes were identified as significantly regulated by IFN. From this set, we selected only genes that were regulated by an average of two-fold or greater, leaving a final set of 161 genes. Of these 161 genes, 117 were contained in the set of 7783 comprised in the "comparison matrix" gene list discussed above, and thus this set was used as the final "core IFN signature" (Table S4).

Correlation matrices and principal components analysis

Spearman's rank correlations were calculated between individual arrays for various disease/specimen sources and various *in vitro* stimulations with IFN-alpha or IFN-gamma on different responding cell types using the DM module gene set (490 genes) as well as the IFN signature (as described above). The same expression data of the 117 core IFN signature were further utilized to calculate principal components analysis (PCA). Both the correlations and PCA were conducted using the R statistical computing environment (http://r-project.org). The missing values in the data matrix were imputed by the method *svdImpute* (from the R package "pcaMethods") and the principal components were calculated with the function *prcomp*.

Supporting Information

Figure S1 Inactive DM skin samples cluster with healthy controls and not active DM skin samples. Shown is a hierarchical clustering dendrogram using two-dimensional clustering of gene expression data from active DM skin (gold branches), skin from patients with inactive skin disease (green branches), and healthy controls (light blue branches). The 946 gene "DM module" was used to cluster the skin samples. The red bar to the right of the dendrogram indicates the cluster of IFN-induced genes.

Figure S2 Detailed view of heat map of expression of DM module across skin samples. Two-dimensional hierarchical clustering was performed on gene expression data from active DM skin lesions and skin from healthy controls. A set of 946 genes whose average expression significantly differed between DM and healthy controls (the "DM module) was used to group sample expression data and is shown on the thumbnail diagram at the left. Major clusters of genes are shown with the colored bars and labeled with letters A-G. Shown at the panel on the right are enlarged details of expression data for the labeled clusters, with selected groups of genes labeled at the right. Clusters of genes are: A—epidermal activation; B—leukocyte function; C-IFN signature; D-epidermal differentiation; E—immunoglobulin expression; G—lipid metabolism.

Figure S3 DM skin module map (detailed). Module map of the Gene Ontology (GO), Kyoto Encyclopedia of Genes and Genomes (KEGG), and selected other Biological Processes differentially expressed among the active DM samples is shown. Each column represents a single microarray (e.g. patient) and each row represents a single biological process. Only modules that were significantly enriched (minimum 2-fold change, $p = 0.05$) on at least 4 micoarrays are shown. The average expression of the gene hits from each enriched gene set is displayed here. Only gene sets that show significant differences after multiple hypothesis testing were included. Selected GO or KEGG biological processes are shown. The entire figure with all biological processes can be viewed in Supplementary Figure S3.

Figure S4 Spearman's rank coefficient matrix using the DM module across different inflammatory disease tissues. Correlation correlation similarity matrix for 16 cohorts of disease/specimen source groups with 4–5 replicates per each cohort using the 490 genes in the DM module. DM (HEEBO) and DM (Affy) represent data from independent DM skin biopsies run on either HEEBO or Affymetrix arrays, respectively. The remaining datasets were obtained from publicly available GEO omnibus data (see Methods). All data are derived from skin biopsies with the exception of the three diseases on the rightmost region of the x-axis, as indicated. The color legend at the bottom indicates the range of Spearman p values, with general degrees of correlation indicated at each threshold (e.g. low, no (no correlation), mod (moderate), high, or identity). This figure represents the individual array comparisons from the data presented in Figure 3.

Figure S5 Spearman's rank coefficient matrix using 117 IFN inducible genes both *in vitro* and *in vivo* across diseases. Correlation correlation similarity matrix for 16 cohorts of disease/specimen source groups as well as various *in vitro* stimulations with IFN-alpha or IFN-gamma on different responding cell types with 2–7 replicates per each cohort using 117 IFN inducible genes. Similar to the information presented in Figure 4A, the leftmost columns on the x-axis shows the correlation patterns of this IFN signature following various *in vitro* stimulations with

IFN-alpha or IFN-gamma on different responding cell types, as indicated. The rightmost columns on the x-axis show the expression patterns of the IFN signature across multiple disease states. The data from the disease states were derived from publicly available data as described in Figure 3 and Methods. The color legend at the bottom indicates the range of Spearman p values, with general degrees of correlation indicated at each threshold (e.g. low, no (no correlation), mod (moderate), high, or identity). This figure represents the individual array comparisons from the data presented in Figure 4A.

Table S1 Patients in this study. [1]Limited to immunomodulatory medications. [2]Skin disease graded as active or inactive. Active disease considered based on erythema, induration and/or pruritus. Inactive disease based on absence of erythema with pigmentary alteration and/or telangiectasia. [3]Defined if any of the following were found: proximal muscle weakness, eleveated muscle enzymes (CPK, aldolase), EMG findings consistent with inflammatory myopathy, muscle biopsy consistent with DM. Abbreviations. DM = DM; NT = not tested; Pred = prednisone (daily dose in mg); MTX = methotrexate; AZA = azathioprine; CSA = cyclosporine; MMF = mycophenolate moefitil; HCQ = hydroxychloroquine; Doxy = doxycycline; homo = homogeneous; unk = unknown; Ca = cancer; ILD = interstitial lung disease.

Table S2 List of genes significantly dysregulated in DM skin. Genes significantly dysregulated in DM skin (compared to skin from healthy donors) were determined using SAM analysis as described in Methods. "Average fold change" refers to the ratio of the mean of the average expression in DM samples divided by the mean of the average expression in control (healthy) samples.

Table S3 Top 25 upregulated genes in DM skin. The top 25 upregulated genes from Table S2 are ordered (highest to lowest expression values relative to healthy controls). Genes previously identified to be induced by IFN are bolded.

Table S4 Core IFN gene list. The 117 genes comprising the "core IFN gene list" are listed (highest to lowest expression values relative to unstimulated cells). The list was derived as described in Methods.

Author Contributions

Conceived and designed the experiments: DW BK DF. Performed the experiments: DW BK RP BH WZ DF. Analyzed the data: DW BK BH YY PB DF. Contributed reagents/materials/analysis tools: DW BK WZ YY PB DF. Wrote the paper: DW BK DF.

References

1. Mammen AL (2010) Dermatomyositis and polymyositis: Clinical presentation, autoantibodies, and pathogenesis. Ann N Y Acad Sci 1184: 134–153.
2. O'Hanlon TP, Miller FW (2009) Genetic risk and protective factors for the idiopathic inflammatory myopathies. Curr Rheumatol Rep 11: 287–294.
3. Greenberg SA, Amato AA (2004) Uncertainties in the pathogenesis of adult dermatomyositis. Curr Opin Neurol 17: 359–364.
4. Arahata K, Engel AG (1984) Monoclonal antibody analysis of mononuclear cells in myopathies. I: Quantitation of subsets according to diagnosis and sites of accumulation and demonstration and counts of muscle fibers invaded by T cells. Ann Neurol 16: 193–208.
5. Page G, Chevrel G, Miossec P (2004) Anatomic localization of immature and mature dendritic cell subsets in dermatomyositis and polymyositis: Interaction with chemokines and Th1 cytokine-producing cells. Arthritis Rheum 50: 199–208.
6. De Paepe B, Creus KK, De Bleecker JL (2009) Role of cytokines and chemokines in idiopathic inflammatory myopathies. Curr Opin Rheumatol 21: 610–616.
7. Greenberg SA (2010) Dermatomyositis and type 1 interferons. Curr Rheumatol Rep 12: 198–203.
8. Niewold TB, Kariuki SN, Morgan GA, Shrestha S, Pachman LM (2009) Elevated serum interferon-alpha activity in juvenile dermatomyositis: associations with disease activity at diagnosis and after thirty-six months of therapy. Arthritis Rheum 60: 1815–1824.
9. Baechler EC, Bauer JW, Slattery CA, Ortmann WA, Espe KJ, et al. (2007) An interferon signature in the peripheral blood of dermatomyositis patients is associated with disease activity. Mol Med 13: 59–68.
10. Walsh RJ, Kong SW, Yao Y, Jallal B, Kiener PA, et al. (2007) Type I interferon-inducible gene expression in blood is present and reflects disease activity in dermatomyositis and polymyositis. Arthritis Rheum 56: 3784–3792.
11. Krathen MS, Fiorentino D, Werth VP (2008) Dermatomyositis. Curr Dir Autoimmun 10: 313–332.
12. Crowson AN, Magro CM (1996) The role of microvascular injury in the pathogenesis of cutaneous lesions of dermatomyositis. Hum Pathol 27: 15–19.
13. Mascaro JM, Jr., Hausmann G, Herrero C, Grau JM, Cid MC, et al. (1995) Membrane attack complex deposits in cutaneous lesions of dermatomyositis. Arch Dermatol 131: 1386–1392.
14. Magro CM, Crowson AN (1997) The immunofluorescent profile of dermatomyositis: a comparative study with lupus erythematosus. J Cutan Pathol 24: 543–552.
15. Wenzel J, Scheler M, Bieber T, Tuting T (2005) Evidence for a role of type I interferons in the pathogenesis of dermatomyositis. Br J Dermatol 153: 462–463; author reply 463–464.
16. Wenzel J, Schmidt R, Proelss J, Zahn S, Bieber T, et al. (2006) Type I interferon-associated skin recruitment of CXCR3+ lymphocytes in dermatomyositis. Clin Exp Dermatol 31: 576–582.
17. Shrestha S, Wershil B, Sarwark JF, Niewold TB, Philipp T, et al. (2010) Lesional and nonlesional skin from patients with untreated juvenile dermatomyositis displays increased numbers of mast cells and mature plasmacytoid dendritic cells. Arthritis Rheum 62: 2813–2822.
18. McNiff JM, Kaplan DH (2008) Plasmacytoid dendritic cells are present in cutaneous dermatomyositis lesions in a pattern distinct from lupus erythematosus. J Cutan Pathol 35: 452–456.
19. Greenberg SA, Fiorentino D (2009) Similar topology of injury to keratinocytes and myofibres in dermatomyositis skin and muscle. Br J Dermatol 160: 464–465.
20. Callen JP, Wortmann RL (2006) Dermatomyositis. Clin Dermatol 24: 363–373.
21. Caproni M, Torchia D, Cardinali C, Volpi W, Del Bianco E, et al. (2004) Infiltrating cells, related cytokines and chemokine receptors in lesional skin of patients with dermatomyositis. Br J Dermatol 151: 784–791.
22. Saaf AM, Tengvall-Linder M, Chang HY, Adler AS, Wahlgren CF, et al. (2008) Global expression profiling in atopic eczema reveals reciprocal expression of inflammatory and lipid genes. PLoS One 3: e4017.
23. Gudjonsson JE, Ding J, Johnston A, Tejasvi T, Guzman AM, et al. (2010) Assessment of the psoriatic transcriptome in a large sample: additional regulated genes and comparisons with in vitro models. J Invest Dermatol 130: 1829–1840.
24. Der SD, Zhou A, Williams BR, Silverman RH (1998) Identification of genes differentially regulated by interferon alpha, beta, or gamma using oligonucleotide arrays. Proc Natl Acad Sci U S A 95: 15623–15628.
25. Sanda C, Weitzel P, Tsukahara T, Schaley J, Edenberg HJ, et al. (2006) Differential gene induction by type I and type II interferons and their combination. J Interferon Cytokine Res 26: 462–472.
26. Indraccolo S, Pfeffer U, Minuzzo S, Esposito G, Roni V, et al. (2007) Identification of genes selectively regulated by IFNs in endothelial cells. J Immunol 178: 1122–1135.
27. Gudjonsson JE, Ding J, Li X, Nair RP, Tejasvi T, et al. (2009) Global gene expression analysis reveals evidence for decreased lipid biosynthesis and increased innate immunity in uninvolved psoriatic skin. J Invest Dermatol 129: 2795–2804.
28. Yao Y, Richman L, Higgs BW, Morehouse CA, de los Reyes M, et al. (2009) Neutralization of interferon-alpha/beta-inducible genes and downstream effect in a phase I trial of an anti-interferon-alpha monoclonal antibody in systemic lupus erythematosus. Arthritis Rheum 60: 1785–1796.
29. Plager DA, Leontovich AA, Henke SA, Davis MD, McEvoy MT, et al. (2007) Early cutaneous gene transcription changes in adult atopic dermatitis and potential clinical implications. Exp Dermatol 16: 28–36.
30. Greenberg SA, Pinkus JL, Pinkus GS, Burleson T, Sanoudou D, et al. (2005) Interferon-alpha/beta-mediated innate immune mechanisms in dermatomyositis. Ann Neurol 57: 664–678.
31. Tezak Z, Hoffman EP, Lutz JL, Fedczyna TO, Stephan D, et al. (2002) Gene expression profiling in DQA1*0501+ children with untreated dermatomyositis: a novel model of pathogenesis. J Immunol 168: 4154–4163.
32. Yao Y, Richman L, Morehouse C, de los Reyes M, Higgs BW, et al. (2008) Type I interferon: potential therapeutic target for psoriasis? PLoS One 3: e2737.
33. Wenzel J, Tuting T (2008) An IFN-associated cytotoxic cellular immune response against viral, self-, or tumor antigens is a common pathogenetic feature in "interface dermatitis". J Invest Dermatol 128: 2392–2402.

5

Chronic Stress Suppresses the Expression of Cutaneous Hypothalamic–Pituitary–Adrenocortical Axis Elements and Melanogenesis

Silin Pang[1,2], Huali Wu[1,2], Qian Wang[1,2], Minxuan Cai[1,2], Weimin Shi[3], Jing Shang[1,2]*

1 New Drug Screening Center, China Pharmaceutical University, Nanjing, China, **2** State Key Laboratory of Natural Medicines, China Pharmaceutical University, Nanjing, China, **3** Shanghai First People Hospital, Shanghai, China

Abstract

Chronic stress can affect skin function, and some skin diseases might be triggered or aggravated by stress. Stress can activate the central hypothalamic–pituitary–adrenocortical (HPA) axis, which causes glucocorticoid levels to increase. The skin has HPA axis elements that react to environmental stressors to regulate skin functions, such as melanogenesis. This study explores the mechanism whereby chronic stress affects skin pigmentation, focusing on the HPA axis, and investigates the role of glucocorticoids in this pathway. We exposed C57BL/6 male mice to two types of chronic stress, chronic restraint stress (CRS) and chronic unpredictable mild stress (CUMS). Mice subjected to either stress condition showed reduced melanogenesis. Interestingly, CRS and CUMS triggered reductions in the mRNA expression levels of key factors involved in the HPA axis in the skin. In mice administered corticosterone, decreased melanin synthesis and reduced expression of HPA axis elements were observed. The reduced expression of HPA axis elements and melanogenesis in the skin of stressed mice were reversed by RU486 (a glucocorticoid receptor antagonist) treatment. Glucocorticoids had no significant inhibitory effect on melanogenesis in vitro. These results suggest that, high levels of serum corticosterone induced by chronic stress can reduce the expression of elements of the skin HPA axis by glucocorticoid-dependent negative feedback. These activities can eventually result in decreased skin pigmentation. Our findings raise the possibility that chronic stress could be a risk factor for depigmentation by disrupting the cutaneous HPA axis and should prompt dermatologists to exercise more caution when using glucocorticoids for treatment.

Editor: Andrzej T Slominski, University of Tennessee, United States of America

Funding: This work was supported by 2012–2014 National Science and Technology Infrastructure Program (2012BAI30B001), PI 2011–2013 Mega-projects of Science Research for the 12th Five-Year Plan of China (2011ZX09401-007), PI. The funders had no role in study design, data collection and analysis, decision to publish, or preparation of the manuscript.

Competing Interests: The authors have declared that no competing interests exist.

* E-mail: shangjing21cn@163.com

Introduction

Substantial evidence suggests that chronic stress can affect the function of multiple physiological systems, including skin function [1–4]. Stress has been associated with the onset and aggravation of many skin disorders, such as psoriasis, alopecia, atopic dermatitis, and vitiligo [5–10]. The "brain–skin connection" may underlie skin diseases triggered or aggravated by stress [3,4,7,11].

During exposure to stressful events, the central hypothalamic–pituitary–adrenocortical (HPA) axis is activated. In brief, during stress, corticotropin-releasing hormone (CRH) is synthesized and released, which increases pro-opiomelanocortin (POMC) expression. POMC is converted into adrenocorticotropic hormone (ACTH) and other melanocortin peptides, such as α-MSH. ACTH then binds to the melanocortin type 2 receptor (MC2R) of the adrenal cortex and stimulates glucocorticoid synthesis and secretion into systemic circulation to exert various physiological effects. In the adrenal cortex, P450scc (Gene symbol: CYP11A1) acts as a key enzyme in glucocorticoid synthesis. Glucocorticoid binding to glucocorticoid receptors (GRs) in hypophysiotropic neurons and the anterior pituitary gland can inhibit the release of CRH and ACTH to allow for negative feedback regulation of the HPA axis [12–15].

The skin is the largest organ in the human body and can be regulated by the immune and neuroendocrine systems [3,16–18]. Skin reacts to environmental stressors, such as ultraviolet radiation (UVR), in a strikingly similar manner to the activities of the central HPA axis [3,19,20]. The skin and its major appendages express key molecules, including CRH or urocortin (UCN1), POMC, and P450scc, along the classical HPA axis. CRH or UCN1 can interact with CRH receptor type 1 (CRHR1) to produce POMC-derived peptides, with the latter stimulating the local production of glucocorticoids [21–28]. After exposure to UVR, the gene expression levels of CRH or UCN1, POMC, and CYP11A1 in the skin increase [19,29]. Simultaneously, the skin is also the target organ of CRH and the related urocortin peptide, POMC-derived peptides, and glucocorticoids [3,4,22,23,26,27,30]. Treating melanocytes with CRH has been shown to induce melanogenesis [22,26,31]. POMC, ACTH, and α-MSH also increase melanogenesis in melanocytes [31–33]. Thus, skin pigmentation has a close relationship with cutaneous HPA axis activation.

Because of the evolutionary conservation of HPA-like networks at the central and cutaneous levels, interactions may exist between these systems, and such interactions could affect the functions of each systerm [4,34]. For example, UVR of the skin results in excitation of the central nervous system [3,35], and skin disorder is associated with higher central HPA axis activity [36]. The possibility of communication between the cutaneous and systemic HPA axes poses an interesting question for research [3]. However, to our knowledge, very few studies have investigated the influence of the higher central HPA axis on the skin. Thus, this study aimed to explore the effects of chronic stress on skin function and to test whether the cutaneous HPA axis is involved. Here, C57BL/6 male mice were subjected to two types of chronic stress, and the effects of these stresses on skin were observed. Because high levels of serum corticosterone were observed in stressed mice, normal mice were administered corticosterone and stressed mice were administered a glucocorticoid receptor antagonist to explore the role of glucocorticoids in the effects of stress on the skin.

Materials and Methods

Animals

Male C57BL/6 mice (5 weeks old, 20.6±2.1 g) were obtained from the Laboratory Animal Services Center of the Yangzhou University. Animals were maintained on a 12-h light/dark cycle at a regulated temperature (22±2°C), humidity (50±10%) and fed a standard diet and water ad libitum. Animals were acclimatized for 7 days. This study was carried out in strict accordance with the guidelines of the "Principles of Laboratory Animal Care" (NIH Publication No. 80–23, revised in 1996). This study was specifically approved by the Animal Experimentation Ethics Committee of the Chinese Pharmaceutical University (Approval ID: SCXK - (Su) 2011–0003). All efforts were made to minimize suffering.

Chronic stress application

Mice were randomly divided into the following three groups: (1) control group, (2) chronic restraint stress (CRS) group, and (3) chronic unpredictable mild stress (CUMS) group. The CRS procedure was performed as described before [37]. The CUMS procedure was performed as described before with adjustments [38]. In brief, CUMS consisted of a variety of unpredictable stressors, namely, 14-h food deprivation, 14-h water deprivation, 3-min swimming, 1-min tail pinch, 0.5 h cage shock, 24-h soiled cage, and overnight illumination. One of these stressors was given every day for 21 days.

Drugs

Corticosterone was purchased from Sigma-Aldrich (MO, USA). Mice were randomly divided into control and corticosterone (CORT) groups. Mice received corticosterone injections (20 mg/kg, subcutaneously), once per day for 21 days.

RU486 (a glucocorticoid receptor antagonist) was purchased from Sigma-Aldrich. Mice were randomly divided into the following three groups: (1) control group, (2) CUMS group with no drug injection and the application of CUMS, and (3) CUMS+RU486 group with the application of CUMS concomitant with 100 mg/kg/day of RU486 injected subcutaneously for 21 days.

Depilation and tissue sample collection

On day 9, all mice received epilation with rosin and paraffin (1:1, w:w) to induce anagen of the hair cycle (Fig. 1) [39]. Mice were maintained under intraperitoneal anesthesia with chloral hydrate (300 mg/kg) during epilation. On day 22, mice were sacrificed after taking blood samples from eyes under anesthesia between 09:00 am and 10:00 am. Blood was incubated at room temperature for 1 h to allow clotting to occur, and serum was then separated by centrifugation and stored at −70°C until use. The back skin of mice was collected and stored in liquid nitrogen until use.

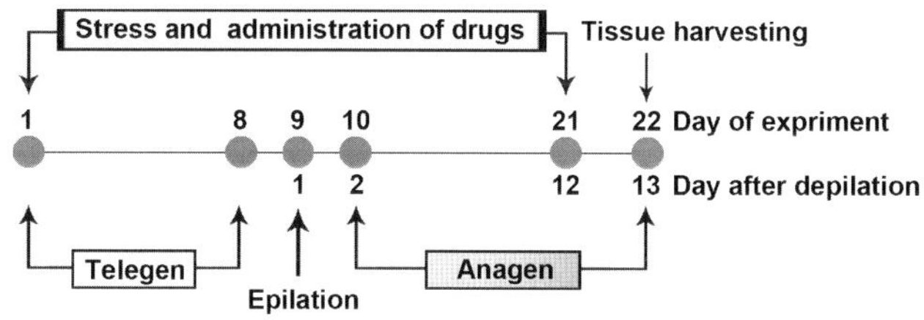

Figure 1. Time table of the experiments. CRS or CUMS was administered beginning on day 1 and continued for 21 days. Drugs were also administered from day 1 for 21 days. All mice received epilation to induce anagen of the hair cycle at day 9. Mice were photographed on days 10 and 22, which were 2 and 13 days post-depilation. Tissue samples were collected on day 22.

Cell culture

The B16F10 murine melanoma cells were purchased from the Cell Bank of the Chinese Academy of Sciences. Cell culture was performed as described before [40]. α-MSH and dexamethasone (DEX) were purchased from Sigma-Aldrich (MO, USA). To detect the effects of DEX and α MSH on melanogenesis, cells were incubated with 1 μM DEX or 50 nM α-MSH. B16F10 cells at passage numbers between 5 and 7 were used for the experiments.

Normal human epidermal melanocytes were derived from young male adult foreskins (ethnic Han/aged 18–22 years) obtained at circumcision following standard protocols [41]. Melanocytes were incubated with MCDB153 medium (Sigma-Aldrich, USA) containing 1 nM choleratoxin (Sigma-Aldrich, USA), 0.1 mM 3-isobutyl-1-methylxanthine (Sigma-Aldrich, USA), 1.6 nM phorbolesters (Sigma-Aldrich, USA), 5 μg/mL insulin (Sigma-Aldrich, USA) and incubated at 37°C in a humidified atmosphere containing 5% CO_2. To detect the effects of DEX and α-MSH on melanogenesis, cells were incubated with 1 μM DEX or 50 nM α-MSH. Melanocytes at passage numbers between 3 and 6 were used for the experiments. The studies on human material were approved by Nanjing Drum Tower Hospital, Medical Ethics Committee. All participants provided their written informed consent to participate in this study. This consent procedure was approved by the Nanjing Drum Tower Hospital, Medical Ethics Committee.

Measurement of body weight and corticosterone analysis

The body weight of all mice were recorded on days 3, 6, 9, 12, 15, 18, and 21. Serum corticosterone concentrations were measured using the IBL-AMERICA Corticosterone rat/mouse ELISA kit (IBL, USA) according to the manufacturer's instructions. Serum samples were incubated at room temperature and then directly used for detection. The lowest detectable concentration of corticosterone that could be distinguished from the "zero calibrator" was 4.1 ng/mL.

Assessment of skin pigmentary response

All mice were photographed with a digital camera (Canon, Japan) once every day after depilation. The grayscale (0–255) of specific area in the photographs (the region from neck to tail) were analyzed by Image J software and presented as ratios (grayscale/255).

Table 1. Primer sequences.

Genes	Species	Forward (F) and Reverse (R) primer sequences		Product size (bp)
MITF	mouse	F	TGCTCGCCTGATCTGGTGAAT	152
		R	GTGCCGAGGTTGTTGGTAAAGG	
TYR	mouse	F	GATGGAACACCTGAGGGACCACTAT	150
		R	GCTGAAATTGGCAGTTCTATCCATT	
Hsd11b1	mouse	F	CTCCTCCCGATCCTGGTGCTCT	132
		R	TGCCATTTCTCTTCCAATCCCTTT	
Hsd11b2	mouse	F	GTTAACAACGCTGGCCTCAATA	160
		R	CAACGGTCACAATACGTCCCCT	
Nr3c1	mouse	F	GGATGACCAAATGACCCTTCTACAG	112
		R	ATCAGGAGCAAAGCATAGCAGGTT	
CRHR1	mouse	F	CTCACGTACTCCACCGACCG	130
		R	TGCCAAACCAGCACTTTTCA	
CRHR2	mouse	F	CCCTGTGGACACTTTTGGAGC	183
		R	GGGTCGTGTTGTACTTGATGCC	
MC1R	mouse	F	GGCTGTCGTGGGCATCTGGA	204
		R	ATGGACCGCCGCCTTTTGTG	
MC2R	mouse	F	ACCATCATCACCCTAACAAT	136
		R	GACACAGGATAAAAACCAGC	
UCN1	mouse	F	CACTGTCCATCGACCTCACCTTC	117
		R	ACTTGCCCACCGAATCGAATA	
POMC	mouse	F	TTGCTGAGAACGAGTCGGC	86
		R	GACCTGCTCCAAGCCTAATGG	
CYP11A1	mouse	F	AGATGCCTGGAAGAAAGACCGAA	199
		R	GATGGACTCAAAGGAAAAGCGGA	
Actb	Mouse	F	CAGGTCATCACTATTGGCAACGAG	87
		R	GATGCCACAGGATTCCATACCC	
MITF	Human	F	ACGAGAACAGCAACGCGCAAA	145
		R	GCAGAGACCCGTGGATGGAATA	
TYR	Human	F	GTTGCGGTGGGAACAAGAAATC	164
		R	AGAAGAATGATGCTGGGCTGAGTAA	
GAPDH	Human	F	CGCTGAGTACGTCGTGGAGTC	172
		R	GCTGATGATCTTGAGGCTGTTGTC	

Measurement of melanin contents

Cells were incubated with compounds for 72 hours. After they were washed twice with ice-cold phosphate-buffered saline (PBS), cells were lysed by incubation in cell lysis buffer [20 mM Tris PH 7.5, 150 mMNaCl, 1% TritonX-100, 2.5 mM sodium pyrophosphate, 1 mM EDTA, 1%Na3VO4, 0.5 μg/ml leupeptin, 1 mM phenylmethanesulfonyl fluoride (PMSF)] (Biyuntian, China) at 4°C for 10 min, then the lysates were centrifuged at 14,000 rpm for 15 min. The supernatant containing protein was removed and conserved. Protein concentrations were determined by BCA Protein Assay kit (Biyuntian, China) with bovine serum albumin (BSA) (Sigma-Aldrich, USA) as a standard. The precipitate containing total melanin was dissolved in 100 μL of 1N NaOH/10%DMSO for 2 h at 80°C. Total melanin content was estimated by absorbance at 405 nm and comparison made with total protein concentration, then calculated as a percent of the control.

Western blotting

The protein suspension of skin tissues was obtained using a Total Protein Extraction Kit (APPLYGEN, China) and the protein concentrations were detected by BCA Protein Assay kit with BSA as a standard. The same amount of total protein was assayed for each Western blot. Proteins were separated by SDS-PAGE and transferred to nitrocellulose membranes. The membranes were incubated with primary antibodies: POMC (1:200, Santa Cruz Biotechnology Inc, USA) and β-Actin (1:4000, Sigma-Aldrich, USA) for 1.5 h at room temperature then washed with Tris-buffered saline, including 0.1% Tween-20, exposed to peroxidase-conjugated secondary antibodies (1:4000, Sigma-Aldrich, USA) for 1 h at room temperature, washed. Proteins were visualized using an enhanced chemiluminescence detection system. Densitometric analysis was performed by using Quantity One (Bio-Rad, USA). Three animals were used for each data point. Western blot assay results reported here are representative

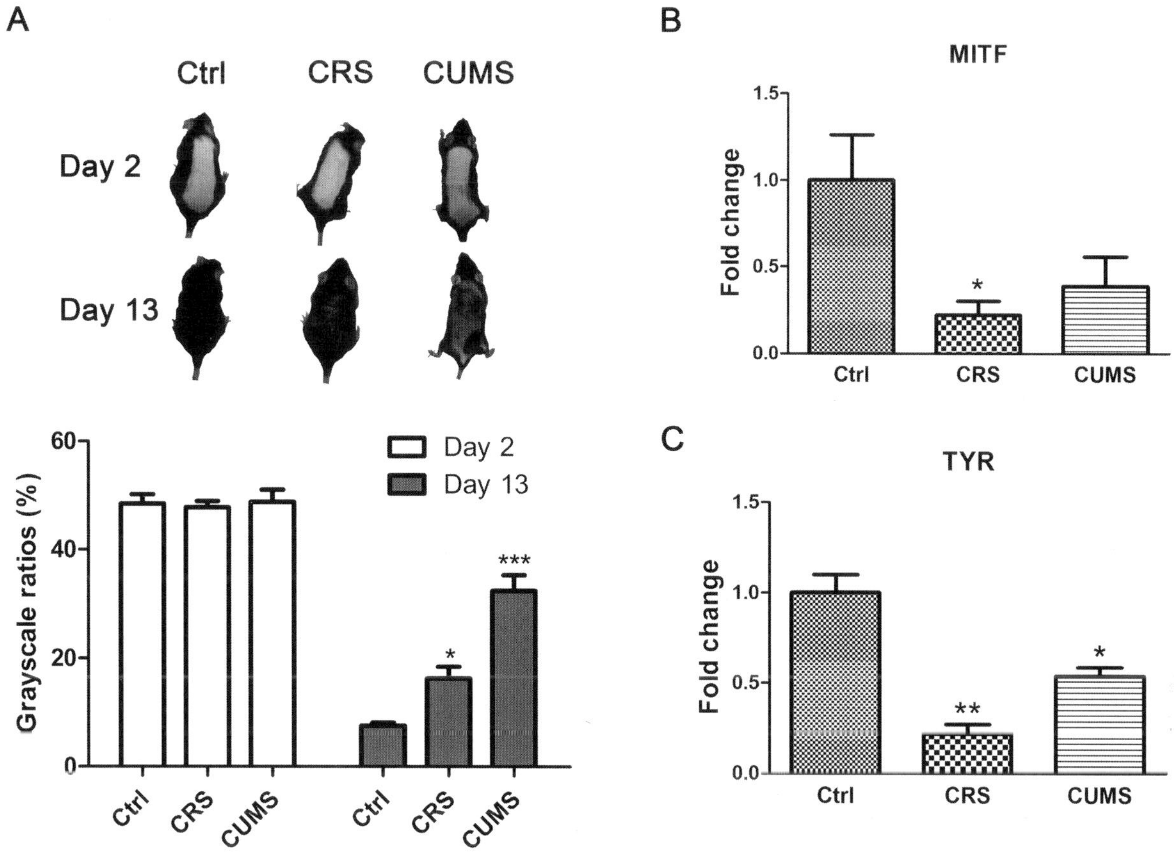

Figure 2. Chronic stress causing reduction of melanogenesis in mice dorsal skin. A: Photographs of mice back skin on day 2 and day 13 after epilation showing the reduction of melanin in the skin of CRS and CUMS group mice on day 13. **B**: The mRNA expression levels of microphthalmia-associated transcription factor (MITF) in mouse skin. **C**: The mRNA expression levels of tyrosinase (TYR) in mouse skin. The expression levels of each gene were normalized against β-Actin then calculated as fold change using the comparative $2^{-\Delta\Delta}$CT method. Data are showed in mean ± SEM, n = 8, and the data were analyzed by one-way ANOVA with Tukey's post hoc test. * *P<0.05*, ** *P<0.01*, *** *P<0.001*, compared with control.

of three independent experiments. The related protein bands, cut and displayed in the same figure, are from the same membrane.

Quantitative real-time PCR

Total RNA was extracted from cells or mouse dorsal skin using TRIZOL reagent (Gibco-BRL, USA) and total RNA concentration was quantified spectrophotometrically. First strand cDNA was synthesized with PrimeScript RT Master Mix (Takara, Japan) according to the manufacturer's instructions. The quantitative real-time PCR was performed on an iQ5 multicolor real-time PCR detection system (Bio-Rad, USA) by using SYBR Premix Ex TaqTM2 (Takara, Japan) according to the manufacturer's instructions. Primer sequences are shown in Table 1. Real-time PCR conditions were: 1 cycle of 2 min at 50°C, 95°C for 10 min, followed by 40 cycles of 95°C cDNA denaturation for 20 s, 60°C primer annealing for 30 s and 72°C extension for 30 s. Melting curve analyses were performed to confirm absence of nonspecific bands. The expression levels of each gene were normalized against β-Actin (Gene symbol: Actb) or GAPDH, then calculated as fold change using the comparative $2^{-\Delta\Delta CT}$ method and the results were from at least three independent experiments according to the manufacturer's protocols [42].

Statistical analysis

Statistical analysis was performed using GraphPadPrismVersion 5.0c (GraphPad Software). Data were analyzed by unpaired, two-tailed Student's t test or by one-way ANOVA with Tukey's post hoc test, as appropriate. P<0.05 was regarded as significant. Results are presented as mean ± SEM.

Results

Effects of chronic stress on the mouse dorsal skin melanogenesis

Mice were photographed after epilation. Upon visual examination, all groups of mice had a similar skin color on the second day after epilation. However, on the thirteenth day, the skin color showed visible differences, and stressed mice showed lighter skin color than control mice (Fig. 2A).

Experiments were performed to detect any changes in microphthalmia-associated transcription factor (MITF) or tyrosinase (TYR) mRNA expression levels in the dorsal skin. MITF is a key transcription factor for melanogenesis that effectively transactivates the TYR genes by binding to an M-box motif in the TYR promoter [43]. Tyrosinase is the rate-limiting enzyme in two critical steps in melanogenesis [44]. The CRS mice showed reduced mRNA expression levels of MITF (P<0.05) and TYR (P<0.01) (Fig. 2B, C). The CUMS mice showed reduced mRNA expression levels of TYR (P<0.05) (Fig. 2C).

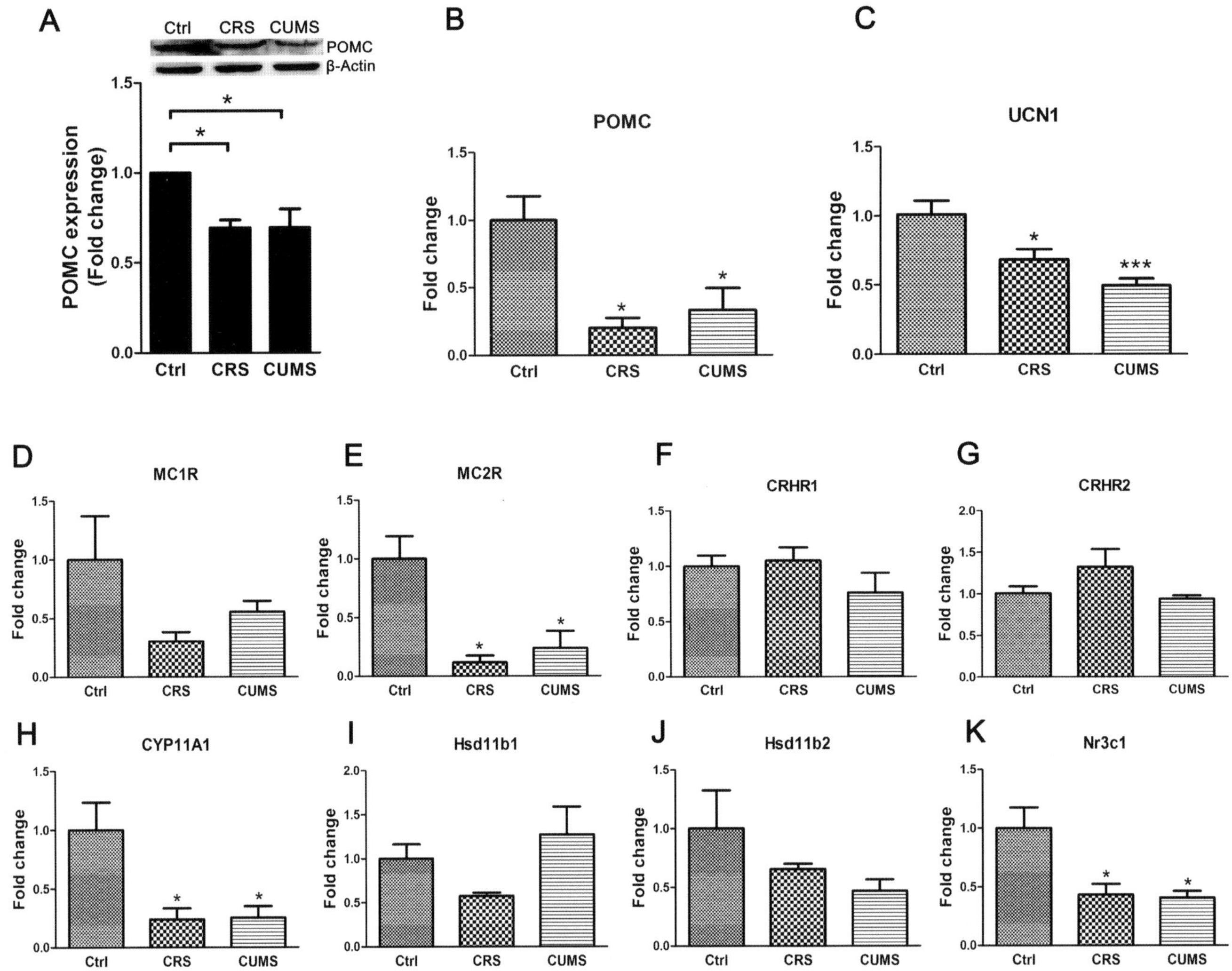

Figure 3. Chronic stress causing disrupted expressions of cutaneous HPA axis elements. A: POMC expression was analyzed by immunoblotting. β-Actin expression was indicated as a loading control. Western blot assay are representative of three experiments. Densitometric scanning of band intensities obtained from three separate experiments was used to quantify change of proteins expression. Three animals were used for each data point. Data are showed in mean ± SEM. **B–K**: The mRNA expression levels of POMC, UCN1, MC1R, MC2R, CRHR1, CRHR2, CYP11A1, Hsd11b1, Hsd11b2, and Nr3c1 in mouse skin. The expression levels of each gene were normalized against β-Actin then calculated as fold change using the comparative $2^{-\Delta\Delta CT}$ method. Data are showed in mean ± SEM, n = 8. Data were analyzed by one-way ANOVA with Tukey's post hoc test. * *P<0.05*, ** *P<0.01*, compared with control.

Effects of chronic stress on the cutaneous HPA axis

The expression of POMC was examined in mouse skin. POMC expression levels were reduced by both CRS (P<0.05) and CUMS (P<0.05) (Fig. 3A). Similarly, the mRNA expression levels of POMC in mouse skin were also reduced by CRS (P<0.05) and CUMS (P<0.05) (Fig. 3B). The mRNA expression levels of POMC cleavage product receptors were also measured, and chronic stress reduced MC2R mRNA expression levels (Fig. 3E). Although there were decreased mRNA expression levels of MC1R in the skin of stressed mice, the changes were not significantly different from the levels in control mice (Fig. 3D).

Alterations of POMC expression in the skin of stressed mice may be caused by changes in UCN1 expression, thereby affecting the cutaneous HPA axis, and may lead to changes in the expression of CYP11A1. To test this possibility, experiments were performed to measure mRNA expression of UCN1 and CYP11A1, and both genes were found to be reduced in the skin of stressed mice (Fig. 3C, H). UCN1 exerts biological effects by binding to its receptors [28,45,46]. The mRNA expression levels of CRHR1 and CRHR2 did not significantly change in the skin of stressed mice (Fig. 3F, G). 11β-hydroxysteroid dehydrogenase type 1 (11β-HSD1, Gene symbol: HSD11b1), 11β-hydroxysteroid dehydrogenase type 2 (11β-HSD2, Gene symbol: HSD11b2), and glucocorticoid receptor (GR) play key roles in the regulation of glucocorticoid activities [47–50]. The expression of the genes that encode 11β-HSD1 (Hsd11b1) and 11β-HSD2 (Hsd11b2) showed no significant changes in the skin of stressed mice, whereas the expression of the gene that encodes GR (Gene symbol: Nc3r1) was reduced (Fig. 3I–K).

Effects of chronic stress on body weight and serum corticosterone levels

Our data indicated that CRS and CUMS did not significantly inhibit mouse body weight gain compared to the control group (Fig. 4A).

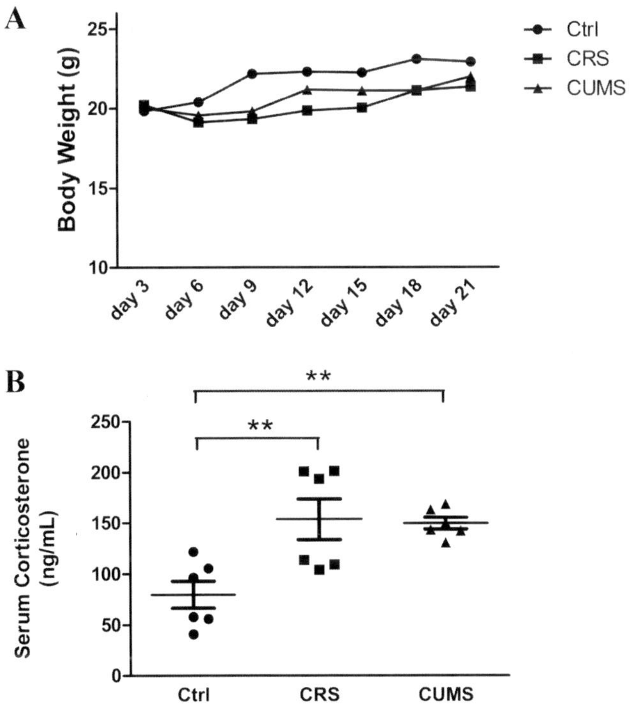

Figure 4. Effects of chronic stress on mice body weight gain and serum corticosterone levels. A: On days 3, 6, 9, 12, 15, 18, and 21, CRS and CUMS did not inhibit mice body weight gain significantly compared with control. **B**: The serum corticosterone levels in mice of different group. Serum for corticosterone measurement was collected on day 22, one day after the final stressor. Data are showed in mean ± SEM, n = 6, and the data were analyzed by one-way ANOVA with Tukey's post hoc test. ** *P<0.01*, compared with control.

Sustained activation of the central HPA axis by chronic stress can lead to elevated glucocorticoid levels [51]. Compared to controls (Ctrl, 79.72±12.08 ng/mL), chronic stress caused a significant elevation of serum corticosterone levels (CRS, 153.83±18.36 ng/mL; CUMS, 149.75±5.31 ng/mL) (Fig. 4B).

Effects of corticosterone on the dorsal skin of mice

Considering that chronic stress caused a marked elevation of serum corticosterone levels, further studies were conducted to investigate whether corticosterone affects the dorsal skin of mice in vivo. On the thirteenth day after epilation, mice that received corticosterone injections had a significantly lighter observable skin color than controls (Fig. 5A). In the CORT group, mice had significantly lower MITF expression (Fig. 5B). These results suggest that corticosterone reduces skin melanogenesis.

The expression levels of key factors along the HPA axis were evaluated in the dorsal skin of mice that received chronic corticosterone injections. POMC expression was reduced after corticosterone injections (Fig. 5C). Corticosterone also significantly suppressed mRNA expression levels of UCN1, POMC, CYP11A1, MC2R, CRHR1, CRHR2 and Nr3c1 (Fig. 5D).

Effects of RU486 on the dorsal skin of stressed mice

Because chronic stress caused a marked elevation of serum corticosterone levels, further studies were conducted to test whether RU486 (a glucocorticoid receptor antagonist) could reverse the effects of CUMS on the dorsal skin of mice in vivo. On the thirteenth day after epilation, mice that received RU486 injections had a significantly darker observable skin color than CUMS mice (Fig. 6A). The CUMS mice showed reduced expression of MITF and TYR, but RU486 reversed this effect (Fig. 6B, C). Additionally, administration of RU486 significantly ameliorated the CUMS-induced reduction of POMC expression (Fig. 6D). Furthermore, RU486 also normalized the CUMS-induced reduction of mRNA expression levels of UCN1, POMC, and CYP11A1 (Fig. 6E). These results suggested that stress-induced alterations of these mediators might be mediated by glucocorticoids.

Effects of HPA axis-related hormones on melanin synthesis in vitro

To determine whether corticosterone could directly inhibit melanogenesis, NHEMs or B16F10 cells were incubated with α-MSH or DEX, a synthetic corticosteroid. In NHEMs, both α-MSH and DEX significantly increased melanin content, and α-MSH showed a stronger effect than DEX (Fig. 7A). Next, we used RT-PCR to examine the effects of these hormones on the expression of genes associated with melanogenesis. Both α-MSH and DEX increased mRNA expression levels of MITF and TYR, and again α-MSH showed a stronger effect than DEX (Fig. 7B, C). In B16F10 cells, α-MSH significantly increased the melanin content, whereas DEX showed no significant effect (Fig. 7D). We found that α-MSH increased the mRNA expression levels of MITF and TYR, whereas DEX showed no significant effect (Fig. 7E, F). These results suggested that glucocorticoids showed no inhibitory effects on melanogenesis in B16F10 cells and that glucocorticoids promoted melanogenesis in NHEMs.

Discussion

Our data demonstrate that chronic stress can suppress cutaneous melanogenesis and the expression levels of cutaneous HPA axis elements. Moreover, chronic stress can cause the elevation of serum corticosterone levels, suggesting that increased corticosterone levels may contribute to the suppression of chronic stress. Consistent with this possibility, mice that received subcutaneous injections of corticosterone showed reduced expression of cutaneous HPA axis elements and decreased pigmentation. Additionally, the glucocorticoid receptor antagonist increased the CUMS-induced reductions of melanogenesis and cutaneous HPA axis element expression levels. These findings suggest that stress can suppress the activation of the cutaneous HPA axis through glucocorticoids and thereby cause reduced melanogenesis.

In a study of human hair follicles in vitro, the glucocorticoid receptor agonist hydrocortisone could reduce follicular CRH expression [22]. The skin of DEX-treated mice shows attenuated production of POMC mRNA [52]. These data, along with our observations that subcutaneous injections of corticosterone can reduce the expression of HPA axis hormones in the skin of mice, suggest that the skin has HPA axis-like regulatory feedback systems that are mediated by glucocorticoids. Stress is the main factor that drives increased central HPA axis activation [1]. Both CRS and CUMS cause sustained responsiveness of the central HPA axis [53,54] and caused high levels of serum glucocorticoids in our study. These results imply that stress may attenuate the activation of the cutaneous HPA axis. Some researchers have reported that 2 h restraint stress treatment could suppress cutaneous POMC mRNA expression levels [55]. Together with the inhibitory effect of chronic stress on the cutaneous HPA axis, it is possible that this phenomenon is caused by glucocorticoid-dependent negative feedback.

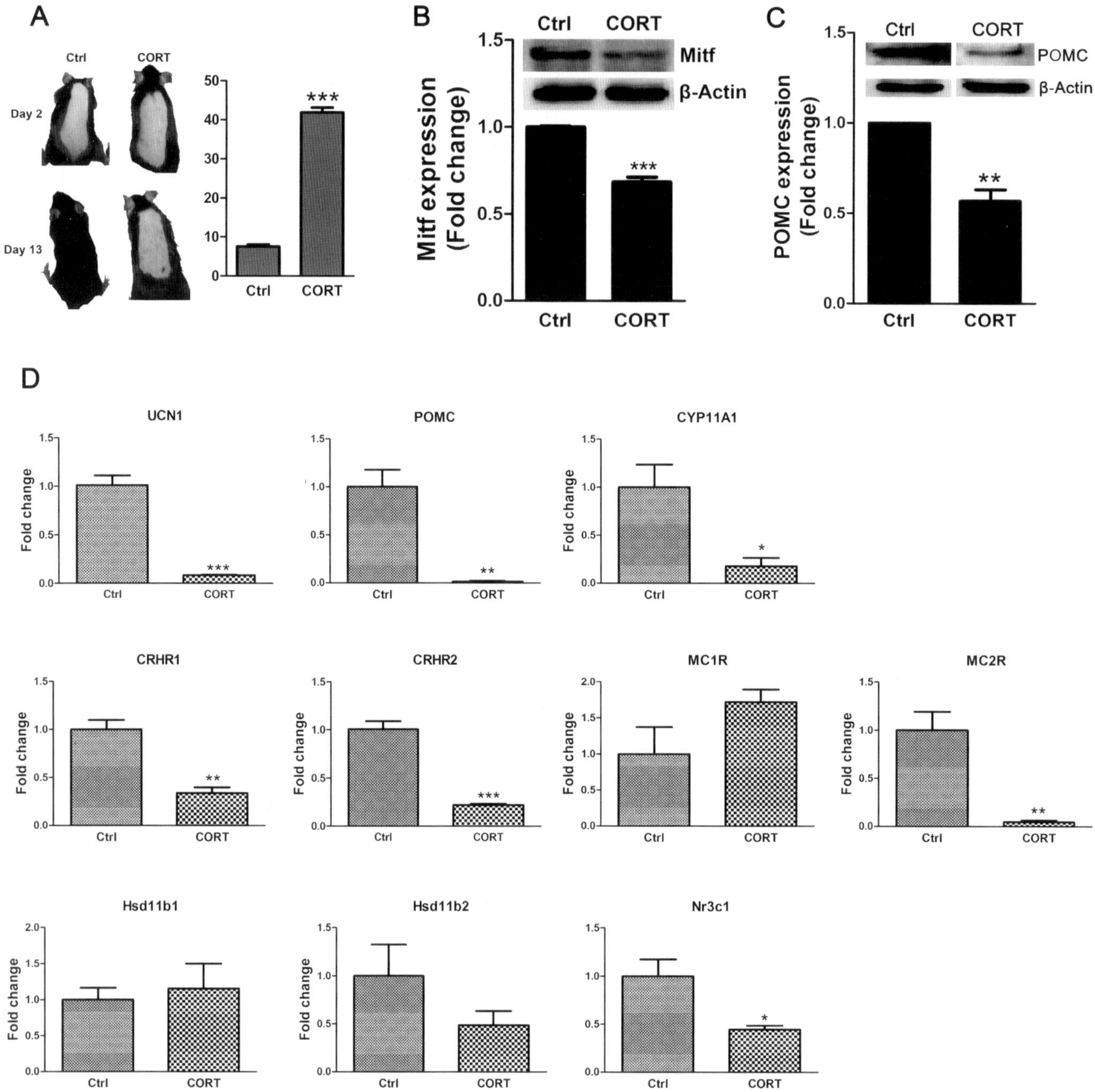

Figure 5. Corticosterone causing reduction of melanogenesis and disrupted expressions of cutaneous HPA axis elements. A: Photographs of mice back skin on day 2 and day 13 after epilation showing the reduction of melanin in corticosterone treated mice on day 13. **B**: MITF expression was analyzed by immunoblotting. **C**: POMC expression was analyzed by immunoblotting. β-Actin expression was indicated as a loading control. Western blot assay are representative of three experiments. Densitometric scanning of band intensities obtained from three separate experiments was used to quantify change of proteins expression. Three animals were used for each data point. Data are showed in mean ± SEM. **D**: The mRNA expression levels of UCN1, POMC, CYP11A1, CRHR1, CRHR2, MC1R, MC2R, Hsd11b1, Hsd11b2, and Nr3c1 in mouse skin. The expression levels of each gene were normalized against β-Actin then calculated as fold change using the comparative $2^{-\Delta\Delta CT}$ method. Data are showed in mean ± SEM, n = 8. Data were analyzed by Student's t test. * *P<0.05*, ** *P<0.01*, *** *P<0.001*, compared with control.

In addition to the decreased expression of hormones along the cutaneous HPA axis in situ, chronic stress also leads to changes in the expression of cognate receptors for these hormones. Mice that experienced chronic stress or long-term corticosterone injections exhibited reduced MC2R mRNA expression levels in skin. ACTH binds to MC2R to promote glucocorticoid synthesis [56]. Reduced expression of MC2R and POMC may cause a reduction in glucocorticoid synthesis, which is consistent with the reduced expression of CYP11A1 observed in our experiments. CRHR1 and CRHR2 are important receptors of the HPA axis. Hypothalamic CRHR1 gene transcription in mice has been shown to be inhibited by glucocorticoid administration [56]. Corticosterone-treated mice had decreased cutaneous expression levels of CRHR1 and CRHR2, whereas stressed mice showed no

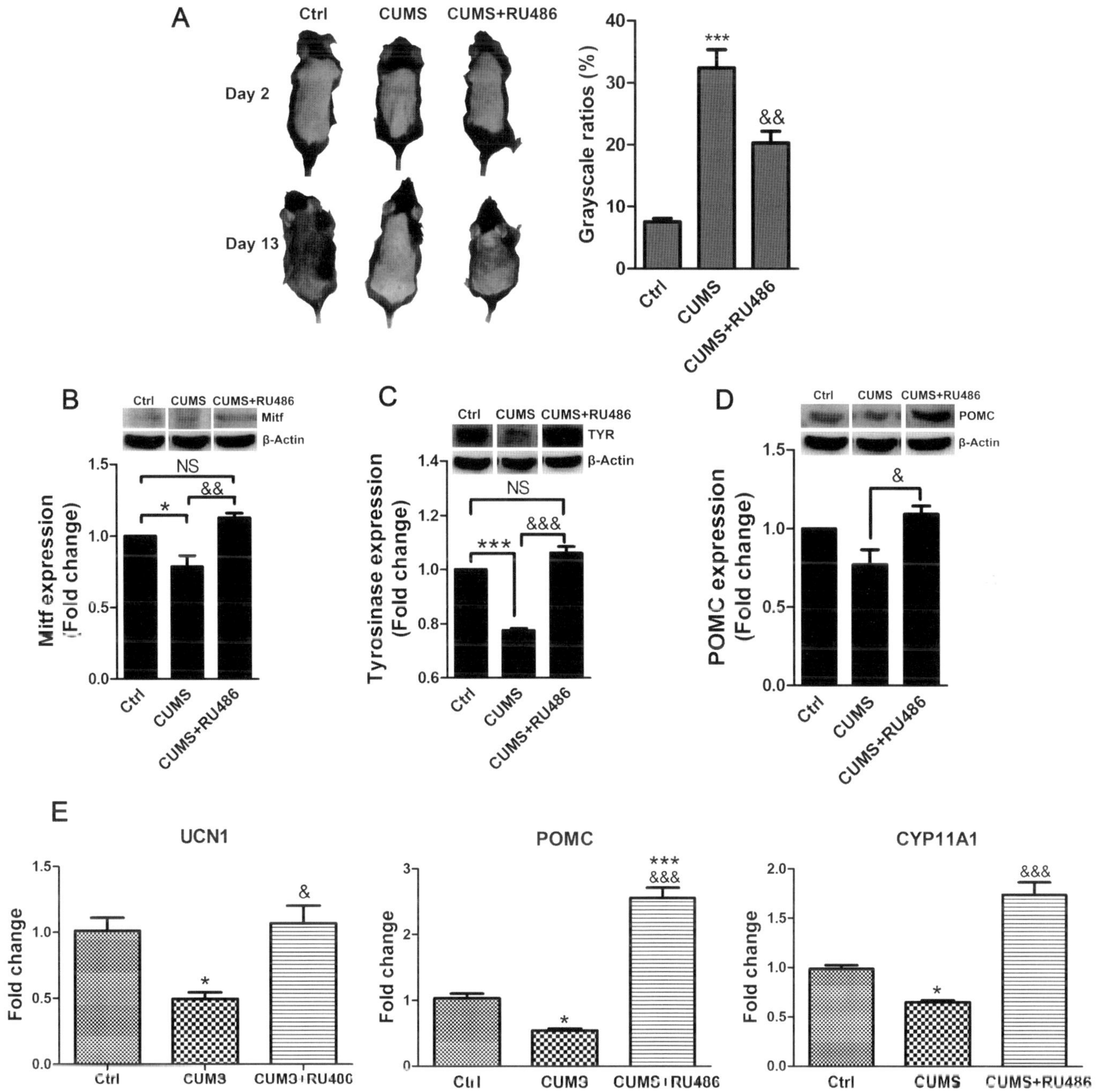

Figure 6. Effects of RU486 on the dorsal skin of stressed mice. A: Photographs of mice back skin on day 2 and day 13 after epilation showing that the mice received RU486 injection had a significantly darker observable skin color than CUMS mice. **B**: MITF expression was analyzed by immunoblotting. **C**: TYR expression was analyzed by immunoblotting. **D**: POMC expression was analyzed by immunoblotting. β-Actin expression was indicated as a loading control. Western blot assay are representative of three experiments. Densitometric scanning of band intensities obtained from three separate experiments was used to quantify change of proteins expression. Three animals were used for each data point. Data are showed in mean ± SEM. **E**: The mRNA expression levels of UCN1, POMC, and CYP11A1 in mouse skin. The expression levels of each gene were normalized against β Actin then calculated as fold change using the comparative $2^{-\Delta\Delta CT}$ method. Data are showed in mean ± SEM, n = 8. The data were analyzed by one-way ANOVA with Tukey's post hoc test. * *P*<0.05, *** *P*<0.001, compared with control; $^{\&}$*P*<0.05, $^{\&\&}$*P*<0.01, $^{\&\&\&}$*P*<0.001, compared with CUMS.

significant differences. Substance P can increase the expression of CRHR1 in mast cells in human skin [57]. There is increased Substance P protein expression in cutaneous peripheral nerve fibers in chronically stressed mice [58]. The involvement of other factors that increase in response to stress in skin might underlie the differential expression of CRHR1 and CRHR2 in chronically stressed and corticosterone-treated mice.

Based on our findings, glucocorticoids play an important role in the regulation of chronic stress. In humans, two key enzymes that regulate local cortisol availability are 11β-HSD1 and 11β-HSD2, which induce intracellular conversion of cortisol, and, together with GR, play a key role in regulating glucocorticoid activities [47–50]. Expression of 11β-HSD1, 11β-HSD2, and GR has been detected in human skin [59,60]. We found that the mRNA

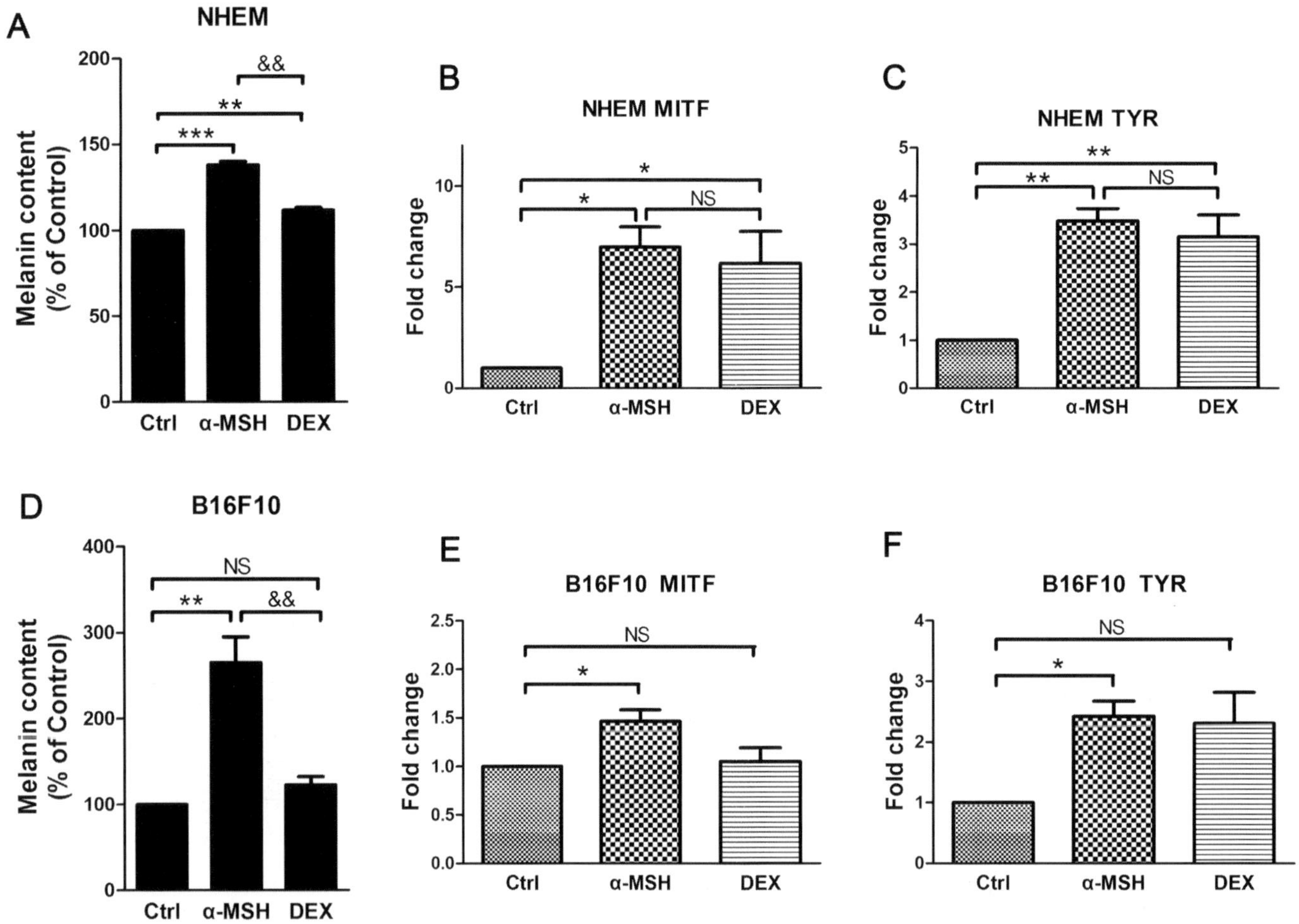

Figure 7. Effects of HPA axis-related hormones on melanin synthesis in vitro. A: Measurement of melanin contents in normal human epidermal melanocytes (NHEMs) after treatment with 50 nM α-MSH or 1 μM DEX for 72 h. **D**: Measurement of melanin contents in B16F10 cells after treatment with 50 nM α-MSH or 1 μM DEX for 72 h. **B–C**: The mRNA expression levels of MITF and TYR in NHEMs after treatment with 50 nM α-MSH or 1 μM DEX for 24 h. **E–F**: The mRNA expression levels of MITF and TYR in B16F10 cells after treatment with 50 nM α-MSH or 1 μM DEX for 24 h. The expression levels of each gene were normalized against β-Actin or GAPDH then calculated as fold change using the comparative $2^{-\Delta\Delta CT}$ method. Data are combined from three separate experiments and showed in mean ± SEM, and the data were analyzed by one-way ANOVA with Tukey's post hoc test. * *P<0.05*, ** *P<0.01*, *** *P<0.001*, compared with control; $^{\&\&}$*P<0.01*, compared with α-MSH.

expression levels of HSD11b1 and HSD11b2 could be detected in the skin of mice and that the expression level of these genes was not affected by chronic stress or corticosterone injections. Recent studies have shown that chronic stress can reduce GR expression in the brain, and this effect may be mediated by elevated glucocorticoid levels [61,62]. We found that both chronically stressed and corticosterone-treated mice showed reduced mRNA expression of Nr3c1. This phenomenon may be caused by desensitization of skin exposed to high glucocorticoid concentrations.

human skin expresses mRNAs for three obligatory enzymes of steroid synthesis including cytochromes P450scc, P450c17 and P450c21 [63]. P450scc also shows pleiotropic effects in cutaneous secosteroidal system [3,64,65]. Since chronic stress and corticosterone treatment suppressed mRNA expression levels of CYP11A1, we propose that chronic stress and glucocorticoids treatment may affect steroidogenesis and secosteroidogenesis in the skin.

Clinically, glucocorticoids are used to treat many skin diseases [66–68]. Although the precise role of the cutaneous HPA axis in skin function remains to be determined, the multiple functions of HPA axis-derived hormones on the skin adds further evidence to the role of the cutaneous HPA axis in maintaining homeostasis in the skin microenvironment [11,20,69]. In addition to some direct effects of glucocorticoids on skin [68,70,71], local glucocorticoid treatment may affect skin function by restraining the activation of the cutaneous HPA axis. Moreover, skin disorder is accompanied by psychological pressure, which can lead to elevated cortisol levels [2]. Based on our data, we speculate that these patients could have attenuated expression of cutaneous HPA axis elements. Our findings should prompt dermatologists to be more cautious when using glucocorticoids for treatment.

Melanogenesis is an important function of the skin that protects the body against radiation and helps maintain homeostasis of the skin microenvironment [33,72,73]. Melanogenesis is closely related to activation of the skin HPA axis. In patients with depigmentation, decreased epidermal POMC processing and α-MSH levels have been previously reported [74]. In this study, we found no significant inhibitory effect of glucocorticoids on melanogenesis in B16F10 cells. In NHEMs, glucocorticoids could promote melanogenesis, however this effect was weaker than α-MSH treatment. However, administering corticosterone to mice resulted in reduced melanin synthesis, which is consistent with a previous report that the application of DEX to the skin of mice decreased tyrosinase protein concentration [52]. The inhibitory effect of corticosterone and chronic stress on melanogenesis in vivo appears to be indirect. The reduced pigmentation may be caused by the repressed expression of skin HPA axis elements, which are caused by glucocorticoids. Taking into account that glucocorticoids promotes melanin synthesis and that glucocorticoids exert their biological effects by binding to their receptor, the reduced expression of glucocorticoid receptor in chronically stressed and corticosterone-treated mice may have also caused the reduced pigmentation.

In summary, our data demonstrate that chronic stress can suppress the expression of skin HPA axis-related genes and proteins. This restriction of the cutaneous HPA axis may be caused by negative feedback control via high glucocorticoid concentrations induced by stress. Additionally, the suppressed expression of elements of the cutaneous HPA axis is accompanied by reduced pigmentation, emphasizing that chronic stress may be a risk factor for the development of skin problems.

Acknowledgments

We thank Feng Wang, Liangliang Zhou and Jinpeng Lv for expert technical assistance.

Author Contributions

Conceived and designed the experiments: SP JS. Performed the experiments: SP HW QW MC. Analyzed the data: SP HW. Contributed reagents/materials/analysis tools: JS WS. Wrote the paper: SP.

References

1. McEwen BS (2008) Central effects of stress hormones in health and disease: Understanding the protective and damaging effects of stress and stress mediators. Eur J Pharmacol 583: 174–185.
2. Schut C, Weik U, Tews N, Gieler U, Deinzer R, et al. (2013) Psychophysiological effects of stress management in patients with atopic dermatitis: a randomized controlled trial. Acta Derm Venereol 93: 57–61.
3. Slominski AT, Zmijewski MA, Skobowiat C, Zbytek B, Slominski RM, et al. (2012) Sensing the environment: regulation of local and global homeostasis by the skin's neuroendocrine system. Adv Anat Embryol Cell Biol. 212: v, vii, 1–115.
4. Slominski AT, Zmijewski MA, Zbytek B, Tobin DJ, Theoharides TC, et al. (2013) Key Role of CRF in the Skin Stress Response System. Endocr Rev 34: 827–884
5. Evers AW, Verhoeven EW, Kraaimaat FW, de Jong EM, de Brouwer SJ, et al. (2010) How stress gets under the skin: cortisol and stress reactivity in psoriasis. Br J Dermatol 163: 986–991.
6. Hadshiew IM, Foitzik K, Arck PC, Paus R (2004) Burden of hair loss: stress and the underestimated psychosocial impact of telogen effluvium and androgenetic alopecia. J Invest Dermatol 123: 455–457.
7. Hall JM, Cruser D, Podawiltz A, Mummert DI, Jones H, et al. (2012) Psychological Stress and the Cutaneous Immune Response: Roles of the HPA Axis and the Sympathetic Nervous System in Atopic Dermatitis and Psoriasis. Dermatol Res Pract 2012: 403908.
8. Hunter HJ, Griffiths CE, Kleyn CE (2013) Does psychosocial stress play a role in the exacerbation of psoriasis? Br J Dermatol 169: 965–974.
9. Lonne-Rahm SB, Rickberg H, El-Nour H, Marin P, Azmitia EC, et al. (2008) Neuroimmune mechanisms in patients with atopic dermatitis during chronic stress. J Eur Acad Dermatol Venereol 22: 11–18.
10. Manolache L, Benea V (2007) Stress in patients with alopecia areata and vitiligo. J Eur Acad Dermatol Venereol 21: 921–928.
11. Arck PC, Slominski A, Theoharides TC, Peters EM, Paus R (2006) Neuroimmunology of stress: skin takes center stage. J Invest Dermatol 126: 1697–1704.
12. Vale W, Spiess J, Rivier C, Rivier J (1981) Characterization of a 41-residue ovine hypothalamic peptide that stimulates secretion of corticotropin and beta-endorphin. Science 213: 1394–1397.
13. Rivier C, Vale W (1983) Modulation of stress-induced ACTH release by corticotropin-releasing factor, catecholamines and vasopressin. Nature 305: 325–327.
14. Munck A, Guyre PM, Holbrook NJ (1984) Physiological functions of glucocorticoids in stress and their relation to pharmacological actions. Endocr Rev 5: 25–44.
15. Bamberger CM, Schulte HM, Chrousos GP (1996) Molecular determinants of glucocorticoid receptor function and tissue sensitivity to glucocorticoids. Endocr Rev 17: 245–261.
16. Tanida M, Katsuyama M, Sakatani K (2007) Relation between mental stress-induced prefrontal cortex activity and skin conditions: a near infrared spectroscopy study. Brain Res 1184: 210–216.
17. Dhabhar FS (2013) Psychological stress and immunoprotection versus immunopathology in the skin. Clin Dermatol 31: 18–30.
18. Slominski A, Wortsman J (2000) Neuroendocrinology of the skin. Endocr Rev 21: 457–487.
19. Skobowiat C, Dowdy JC, Sayre RM, Tuckey RC, Slominski A (2011) Cutaneous hypothalamic-pituitary-adrenal axis homolog: regulation by ultraviolet radiation. Am J Physiol Endocrinol Metab 301: E484–493.
20. Slominski A, Mihm MC (1996) Potential mechanism of skin response to stress. Int J Dermatol 35: 849–851.
21. Slominski A, Zbytek B, Nikolakis G, Manna PR, Skobowiat C, et al. (2013) Steroidogenesis in the skin: Implications for local immune functions. J Steroid Biochem Mol Biol 137: 107–123
22. Ito N, Ito T, Kromminga A, Bettermann A, Takigawa M, et al. (2005) Human hair follicles display a functional equivalent of the hypothalamic-pituitary-adrenal axis and synthesize cortisol. FASEB J 19: 1332–1334.
23. Slominski A, Zbytek B, Szczesniewski A, Semak I, Kaminski J, et al. (2005) CRH stimulation of corticosteroids production in melanocytes is mediated by ACTH. Am J Physiol Endocrinol Metab 288: E701–706.
24. Slominski A, Zjawiony J, Wortsman J, Semak I, Stewart J, et al. (2004) A novel pathway for sequential transformation of 7-dehydrocholesterol and expression of the P450scc system in mammalian skin. Eur J Biochem 271: 4178–4188.
25. Slominski A, Pisarchik A, Tobin DJ, Mazurkiewicz JE, Wortsman J (2004) Differential expression of a cutaneous corticotropin-releasing hormone system. Endocrinology 145: 941–950.
26. Slominski A, Wortsman J, Luger T, Paus R, Solomon S (2000) Corticotropin releasing hormone and proopiomelanocortin involvement in the cutaneous response to stress. Physiol Rev 80: 979–1020.
27. Slominski A, Wortsman J, Pisarchik A, Zbytek B, Linton EA, et al. (2001) Cutaneous expression of corticotropin-releasing hormone (CRH), urocortin, and CRH receptors. FASEB J 15: 1678–1693.
28. Slominski A, Zbytek B, Zmijewski M, Slominski RM, Kauser S, et al. (2006) Corticotropin releasing hormone and the skin. Front Biosci 11: 2230–2248.
29. Skobowiat C, Nejati R, Lu L, Williams RW, Slominski AT (2013) Genetic variation of the cutaneous HPA axis: An analysis of UVB-induced differential responses. Gene 530: 1–7
30. Talaber G, Jondal M, Okret S (2013) Extra-adrenal glucocorticoid synthesis: Immune regulation and aspects on local organ homeostasis. Mol Cell Endocrinol 380: 89–98
31. Kauser S, Slominski A, Wei ET, Tobin DJ (2006) Modulation of the human hair follicle pigmentary unit by corticotropin-releasing hormone and urocortin peptides. FASEB J 20: 882–895.
32. Rousseau K, Kauser S, Pritchard LE, Warhurst A, Oliver RL, et al. (2007) Proopiomelanocortin (POMC), the ACTH/melanocortin precursor, is secreted by human epidermal keratinocytes and melanocytes and stimulates melanogenesis. FASEB J 21: 1844–1856.
33. Slominski A, Tobin DJ, Shibahara S, Wortsman J (2004) Melanin pigmentation in mammalian skin and its hormonal regulation. Physiol Rev 84: 1155–1228.
34. Slominski A (2007) A nervous breakdown in the skin: stress and the epidermal barrier. J Clin Invest 117: 3166–3169.
35. Kourosh AS, Harrington CR, Adinoff B (2010) Tanning as a behavioral addiction. Am J Drug Alcohol Abuse 36: 284–290.
36. Zhang X, Yu M, Yu W, Weinberg J, Shapiro J, et al. (2009) Development of alopecia areata is associated with higher central and peripheral hypothalamic-pituitary-adrenal tone in the skin graft induced C3H/HeJ mouse model. J Invest Dermatol 129: 1527–1538.
37. Zhao X, Seese RR, Yun K, Peng T, Wang Z (2013) The role of galanin system in modulating depression, anxiety, and addiction-like behaviors after chronic restraint stress. Neuroscience 246: 82–93.
38. Willner P, Towell A, Sampson D, Sophokleous S, Muscat R (1987) Reduction of sucrose preference by chronic unpredictable mild stress, and its restoration by a tricyclic antidepressant. Psychopharmacology (Berl) 93: 358–364.
39. Muller-Rover S, Handjiski B, van der Veen C, Eichmuller S, Foitzik K, et al. (2001) A comprehensive guide for the accurate classification of murine hair follicles in distinct hair cycle stages. J Invest Dermatol 117: 3–15.
40. Ping F, Shang J, Zhou J, Song J, Zhang L (2012) Activation of neurokinin-1 receptor by substance P inhibits melanogenesis in B16-F10 melanoma cells. Int J Biochem Cell Biol 44: 2342–2348.
41. Kim NS, Cho JH, Kang WH (2000) Behavioral differences between donor site-matched adult and neonatal melanocytes in culture. Arch Dermatol Res 292: 233–239.
42. Bustin SA, Benes V, Garson JA, Hellemans J, Huggett J, et al. (2009) The MIQE guidelines: minimum information for publication of quantitative real-time PCR experiments. Clin Chem 55: 611–622.

43. Yasumoto K, Yokoyama K, Shibata K, Tomita Y, Shibahara S (1995) Microphthalmia-associated transcription factor as a regulator for melanocyte-specific transcription of the human tyrosinase gene. Mol Cell Biol 15: 1833.
44. Sulaimon SS, Kitchell BE (2003) The biology of melanocytes. Vet Dermatol 14: 57–65.
45. Perrin MH, Vale WW (1999) Corticotropin releasing factor receptors and their ligand family. Ann N Y Acad Sci 885: 312–328.
46. Krause K, Schnitger A, Fimmel S, Glass E, Zouboulis CC (2007) Corticotropin-releasing hormone skin signaling is receptor-mediated and is predominant in the sebaceous glands. Horm Metab Res 39: 166–170.
47. Bujalska I, Shimojo M, Howie A, Stewart PM (1997) Human 11 beta-hydroxysteroid dehydrogenase: studies on the stably transfected isoforms and localization of the type 2 isozyme within renal tissue. Steroids 62: 77–82.
48. Bujalska IJ, Walker EA, Hewison M, Stewart PM (2002) A switch in dehydrogenase to reductase activity of 11β-hydroxysteroid dehydrogenase type 1 upon differentiation of human omental adipose stromal cells. Journal of Clinical Endocrinology & Metabolism 87: 1205–1210.
49. Draper N, Stewart PM (2005) 11beta-hydroxysteroid dehydrogenase and the pre-receptor regulation of corticosteroid hormone action. J Endocrinol 186: 251–271.
50. Tomlinson JW, Walker EA, Bujalska IJ, Draper N, Lavery GG, et al. (2004) 11beta-hydroxysteroid dehydrogenase type 1: a tissue-specific regulator of glucocorticoid response. Endocr Rev 25: 831–866.
51. Raone A, Cassanelli A, Scheggi S, Rauggi R, Danielli B, et al. (2007) Hypothalamus-pituitary-adrenal modifications consequent to chronic stress exposure in an experimental model of depression in rats. Neuroscience 146: 1734–1742.
52. Ermak G, Slominski A (1997) Production of POMC, CRH-R1, MC1, and MC2 receptor mRNA and expression of tyrosinase gene in relation to hair cycle and dexamethasone treatment in the C57BL/6 mouse skin. J Invest Dermatol 108: 160–165.
53. Aguilera G, Kiss A, Lu A, Camacho C (1996) Regulation of adrenal steroidogenesis during chronic stress. Endocr Res 22: 433–443.
54. Joels M, Karst H, Alfarez D, Heine VM, Qin Y, et al. (2004) Effects of chronic stress on structure and cell function in rat hippocampus and hypothalamus. Stress 7: 221–231.
55. Flint MS, Morgan JB, Shreve SN, Tinkle SS (2003) Restraint stress and corticotropin releasing hormone modulation of murine cutaneous POMC mRNA. Stress 6: 59–62.
56. Chen A, Perrin M, Brar B, Li C, Jamieson P, et al. (2005) Mouse corticotropin-releasing factor receptor type 2alpha gene: isolation, distribution, pharmacological characterization and regulation by stress and glucocorticoids. Mol Endocrinol 19: 441–458.
57. Asadi S, Alysandratos KD, Angelidou A, Miniati A, Sismanopoulos N, et al. (2012) Substance P (SP) induces expression of functional corticotropin-releasing hormone receptor-1 (CRHR-1) in human mast cells. J Invest Dermatol 132: 324–329.
58. Liu N, Wang LH, Guo LL, Wang GQ, Zhou XP, et al. (2013) Chronic restraint stress inhibits hair growth via substance P mediated by reactive oxygen species in mice. PLoS One 8: e61574.
59. Tiganescu A, Walker EA, Hardy RS, Mayes AE, Stewart PM (2011) Localization, age- and site-dependent expression, and regulation of 11beta-hydroxysteroid dehydrogenase type 1 in skin. J Invest Dermatol 131: 30–36.
60. Skobowiat C, Sayre RM, Dowdy JC, Slominski AT (2013) Ultraviolet radiation regulates cortisol activity in a waveband-dependent manner in human skin ex vivo. Br J Dermatol 168: 595–601.
61. Chiba S, Numakawa T, Ninomiya M, Richards MC, Wakabayashi C, et al. (2012) Chronic restraint stress causes anxiety- and depression-like behaviors, downregulates glucocorticoid receptor expression, and attenuates glutamate release induced by brain-derived neurotrophic factor in the prefrontal cortex. Prog Neuropsychopharmacol Biol Psychiatry 39: 112–119.
62. Meyer U, van Kampen M, Isovich E, Flugge G, Fuchs E (2001) Chronic psychosocial stress regulates the expression of both GR and MR mRNA in the hippocampal formation of tree shrews. Hippocampus 11: 329–336.
63. Slominski A, Ermak G, Mihm M (1996) ACTH receptor, CYP11A1, CYP17 and CYP21A2 genes are expressed in skin. J Clin Endocrinol Metab 81: 2746–2749.
64. Slominski AT, Kim TK, Chen J, Nguyen MN, Li W, et al. (2012) Cytochrome P450scc-dependent metabolism of 7-dehydrocholesterol in placenta and epidermal keratinocytes. Int J Biochem Cell Biol 44: 2003–2018.
65. Slominski AT, Kim T-K, Shehabi HZ, Semak I, Tang EK, et al. (2012) In vivo evidence for a novel pathway of vitamin D3 metabolism initiated by P450scc and modified by CYP27B1. The FASEB Journal 26: 3901–3915.
66. Luger T, Loske KD, Elsner P, Kapp A, Kerscher M, et al. (2004) [Topical skin therapy with glucocorticoids—therapeutic index]. J Dtsch Dermatol Ges 2: 629–634.
67. Schafer-Korting M, Kleuser B, Ahmed M, Holtje HD, Korting HC (2005) Glucocorticoids for human skin: new aspects of the mechanism of action. Skin Pharmacol Physiol 18: 103–114.
68. Werth VP (2013) The safe and appropriate use of systemic glucocorticoids in treating dermatologic disease. J Am Acad Dermatol 68: 177–178.
69. Slominski A, Wortsman J, Tuckey RC, Paus R (2007) Differential expression of HPA axis homolog in the skin. Mol Cell Endocrinol 265–266: 143–149.
70. Kao JS, Fluhr JW, Man MQ, Fowler AJ, Hachem JP, et al. (2003) Short-term glucocorticoid treatment compromises both permeability barrier homeostasis and stratum corneum integrity: inhibition of epidermal lipid synthesis accounts for functional abnormalities. J Invest Dermatol 120: 456–464.
71. Zoller NN, Kippenberger S, Thaci D, Mewes K, Spiegel M, et al. (2008) Evaluation of beneficial and adverse effects of glucocorticoids on a newly developed full-thickness skin model. Toxicol In Vitro 22: 747–759.
72. Agar N, Young AR (2005) Melanogenesis: a photoprotective response to DNA damage? Mutat Res 571: 121–132.
73. Slominski A, Wortsman J, Plonka PM, Schallreuter KU, Paus R, et al. (2005) Hair follicle pigmentation. J Invest Dermatol 124: 13–21.
74. Spencer JD, Gibbons NC, Rokos H, Peters EM, Wood JM, et al. (2007) Oxidative stress via hydrogen peroxide affects proopiomelanocortin peptides directly in the epidermis of patients with vitiligo. J Invest Dermatol 127: 411–420.

6

Sociodemographic and Disease Correlates of Body Image Distress among Patients with Systemic Sclerosis

Lisa R. Jewett[1,5], Marie Hudson[3,5,6], Vanessa L. Malcarne[8], Murray Baron[3,5,6], Brett D. Thombs[1,2,3,4,5,6,7]*, Canadian Scleroderma Research Group[¶]

1 Department of Psychiatry, McGill University, Montréal, Québec, Canada, **2** Department of Epidemiology, Biostatistics, and Occupational Health, McGill University, Montréal, Québec, Canada, **3** Department of Medicine, McGill University, Montréal, Québec, Canada, **4** School of Nursing, McGill University, Montréal, Québec, Canada, **5** Lady Davis Institute for Medical Research, Jewish General Hospital, Montréal, Québec, Canada, **6** Division of Rheumatology, Jewish General Hospital, Montréal, Québec, Canada, **7** Department of Psychiatry, Jewish General Hospital, Montréal, Québec, Canada, **8** Department of Psychology, San Diego State University, San Diego, California, United States of America

Abstract

Background: Body image concerns are infrequently studied in systemic sclerosis (SSc), even though significant visible disfigurement is common. The objective of this study was to identify sociodemographic and disease-related correlates of dissatisfaction with appearance and social discomfort among people with SSc.

Methods: SSc patients came from the 15-center Canadian Scleroderma Research Group Registry. Sociodemographic information was based on patient self-report. Disease characteristics were obtained via physician examinations. The Brief-SWAP was used to assess dissatisfaction with appearance and social discomfort. Structural equation models were conducted with MPlus to determine the relationship of dissatisfaction with appearance and social discomfort with age, sex, education, marital status, race/ethnicity, disease duration, skin involvement, telangiectasias, skin pigmentation changes, and hand contractures.

Results: A total of 489 SSc patients (432 female, 57 male) were included. Extent of skin involvement was significantly associated with both dissatisfaction with appearance and social discomfort (standardized regression coefficients = 0.02, p = 0.001; 0.02, p = 0.020, respectively), as was skin involvement in the face (0.18, p = 0.016; 0.23, p = 0.006, respectively). Greater social discomfort was robustly associated with younger age (−0.017, p<0.001) and upper-body telangiectasias (0.32, p = 0.021). Dissatisfaction with appearance was associated with hand contractures (0.07, p = 0.036).

Conclusion: This study found that dissatisfaction with appearance and social discomfort were associated with numerous disfiguring characteristics of SSc, in addition to age. These results underline that there are multiple factors contributing to body image distress in SSc, as well as the need to attend to both disease and social contexts in understanding the impact of disfigurement among patients.

Editor: Richard Fielding, The University of Hong Kong, Hong Kong

Funding: LJ was supported by a Canadian Scleroderma Research Group Studentship (Canadian Institutes of Health Research [CIHR] Strategic Training Initiative in Health Research Grant, #SKI 83345), a Frederick Banting and Charles Best Canadian Graduate Scholarship – Master's Award from the CIHR, and a Bourses de Formation – Formation de Maîtrise from the Fonds de recherche santé Québec. MB is the director of the Canadian Scleroderma Research Group, which has received grant funding from the CIHR; the Scleroderma Society of Canada and its provincial chapters, Scleroderma Society of Ontario, Sclérodermie Québec, and the Ontario Arthritis Society; and educational grants from Actelion Pharmaceuticals and Pfizer Inc. BT and MH were supported by New Investigator Awards from the Canadian Institutes of Health Research and Établissement de Jeunes Chercheurs awards from the Fonds de Recherche santé Québec. The funders had no role in study design, data collection and analysis, decision to publish, or preparation of the manuscript.

Competing Interests: MB is the director of the Canadian Scleroderma Research Group, which received educational grants from Actelion Pharmaceuticals and Pfizer Inc. This does not alter the authors' adherence to all the PLoS ONE policies on sharing data and materials.

* E-mail: brett.thombs@mcgill.ca

¶ Membership of the Canadian Scleroderma Research Group is provided in the Acknowledgments

Introduction

Systemic sclerosis (SSc), or scleroderma, is a multi-system, chronic autoimmune connective tissue disease characterized by vascular injury, immune dysfunction, and abnormal fibrotic processes. SSc affects the skin, as well as internal organs such as the lungs, heart, and gastrointestinal tract [1]. The rate of disease onset is highest between 30–50 years of age, and 80% of people affected are female [2,3]. Median survival time from diagnosis is approximately 11 years, with patients 3.7 times more likely to die within 10 years of diagnosis (44.9% mortality) than age, sex, and race-matched individuals without the disease (12.0% mortality) [2]. The name *scleroderma* is derived from the Greek words *scleros*, meaning hard, and *derma* meaning skin. This is because a central feature of SSc is the excessive production of collagen, which manifests itself in thickening and hardening of the skin, and commonly leads to significant visible disfigurements to various body parts, including the face, mouth, and hands [1].

Disfiguring injury or illness often results in difficulty maintaining a healthy body image and decreased comfort in social interactions, both of which can lead to anxiety and other forms of distress [4,5]. Research among patients with physical disfigurements has highlighted that characteristics of the disfigurement, including severity, visibility, and location of appearance changes, may influence body image dissatisfaction and related problems [6]. There has been relatively little research on body image distress in SSc. Nonetheless, existing studies have shown that more severe disease manifestations, such as significant skin changes in the hands, are associated with greater body image dissatisfaction, increased depressive symptoms, and reduced overall psychosocial functioning, including appearance-related anxiety and social avoidance [7–9]. One recent study of 171 SSc patients examined the impact of facial changes, and reported that patients rated facial disfigurement as the most worrying aspect of the condition [10], and another study of 129 SSc patients reported that greater objective disfigurement was linked to more distress, worry, and perceptions of noticeability by patients [9].

Research from non-disfigured populations has suggested that women are less satisfied with their appearance than men [6,11], and generally, studies of body image, broadly defined, report that women tend to have poorer body image appraisals [12]. Furthermore, in the context of social interactions, particularly for establishing intimate relationships, appearance is highly relevant. Thus, appearance concerns are sometimes more salient for unattached persons compared to those in stable marriages or intimate relationships [6]. Similarly, concerns with appearance and its importance for meeting new people and making social connections is often more pronounced earlier in life, and the broader literature on people with changes to their appearance due to illness and injury has reported that older age is generally associated with less distress related to body image [13].

Patients with SSc may experience significant emotional distress due to negative self-appraisals or dissatisfaction with their appearance, discomfort in social situations due to changes in appearance, or both. Dissatisfaction with appearance and social discomfort are related, but distinct constructs [14]. The Brief-Satisfaction with Appearance Scale (Brief-SWAP) [14] was designed to evaluate both dissatisfaction with appearance and social discomfort related to disfigurement from SSc. The Dissatisfaction with Appearance subscale assesses self-reported dissatisfaction with specific body parts commonly affected by SSc (face, hands, and arms). The Social Discomfort subscale assesses the impact of body image concerns on social interactions (e.g., comfort with strangers, feelings of unattractiveness to others) [14].

The objective of this study was to identify sociodemographic (age, sex, marital status, race/ethnicity, and education) and disease factors (skin involvement, telangiectasias, hand contractures and disfigurement, and changes in skin pigmentation) associated with (1) dissatisfaction with appearance and (2) social discomfort among patients with SSc. We hypothesized that sociodemographic variables, including age, sex, and marital status, as well as SSc disease factors, including skin involvement, telangiectasias, hand contractures, and changes in skin pigmentation would be potentially associated with dissatisfaction with appearance and social discomfort.

Methods

Ethics Statement

This study consisted of an analysis of data from within the Canadian Scleroderma Research Group's (CSRG) pan-Canadian Registry. Ethics approval for the Registry and this study was provided by the research ethics committee of McGill University. In addition, the research ethics committees of each of the 15 CSRG centres approved data collection for inclusion in the Registry. All patients provided written informed consent.

Participants and Procedure

The sample consisted of patients who completed annual visits as part of the CSRG Registry between 2008, when the Brief-SWAP was first included in the Registry, and 2010. To be eligible for the Registry, patients must have a diagnosis of SSc made by a Registry rheumatologist, be ≥18 years of age, and be fluent in English or French. Registry patients undergo physician evaluations at their initial visit and at subsequent yearly visits. Patients were included in the study if they had complete data for the Brief-SWAP and all other variables included in analyses. Some patients completed the Brief-SWAP at more than one visit, but only data from the first administration were analyzed in this study.

Measures

Dissatisfaction with appearance and social discomfort were measured by the Brief-SWAP [14]. Sociodemographic variables included in analyses were assessed by patient self-report and consisted of age, sex, marital status (married or living as married versus single, divorced, or widowed), race/ethnicity (white versus other race/ethnicity), and education (high school or less versus higher education). Disease-related variables included in analyses were measured via clinical histories and examinations by study physicians and consisted of disease duration; total body skin involvement (modified Rodnan skin score, mRss), as well as body area-specific skin involvement scores; upper-body telangiectasias; skin pigmentation changes (hyper-and/or hypo-pigmentation); and fingertip-to-palm distance to assess hand contractures. In addition, disease subtype was recorded, but it was not entered into the analyses because of the high degree of overlap with mRss. Although over 1,000 variables are collected at each CSRG visit, only the variables described here were considered for inclusion in analyses.

The Brief-Satisfaction with Appearance Scale (Brief-SWAP). The 6-item Brief-SWAP [14] assesses dissatisfaction with appearance and social discomfort related to disfigurement in SSc. It was adapted from the original 14-item Satisfaction with Appearance Scale (SWAP) [15] that was designed to measure non-weight related body image dissatisfaction among burn survivors. The Brief-SWAP includes two subscales: Dissatisfaction with Appearance, reflecting dissatisfaction with the appearance of specific body parts relevant to patients with SSc (face, hands, arms), and Social Discomfort, reflecting social discomfort relative to disfigurement from SSc. Respondents to the Brief-SWAP rate the degree to which they feel each item reflects their thoughts and feelings about their appearance on a 7-point scale ranging from 0 (*strongly disagree*) to 6 (*strongly agree*). Item scores can be summed to calculate total subscale scores with higher scores indicating greater dissatisfaction or social discomfort. The range of possible scores is 0–18 for each subscale. Each subscale of the Brief-SWAP is comprised of three items. Items from the Dissatisfaction with Appearance subscale are: (1) I am satisfied with the appearance of my face, (2) I am satisfied with the appearance of my hands, and (3) I am satisfied with the appearance of my arms. Items from the Social Discomfort subscale are (1) Because of changes in my appearance caused by my scleroderma, I am uncomfortable in the presence of strangers, (2) I feel that my scleroderma is unattractive to others, and (3) I don't think people would want to touch me. In a previous study of 654 SSc patients from the CSRG Registry, the internal consistency reliability was good for both the

Dissatisfaction with Appearance ($\alpha = 0.81$) and Social Discomfort ($\alpha = 0.81$) subscales. The Brief-SWAP total score was highly correlated with the full 14-item SWAP total score ($r = 0.95$), and all correlations of the Brief-SWAP total score and full SWAP total score with measures of convergent validity were substantively equal with no statistically significant differences [14]. The raw sum scores of the Dissatisfaction with Appearance subscale and Social Discomfort subscale were only moderately correlated at $r = 0.46$ (correlation of latent factors = 0.56) [14], thus, in the current study, subscale scores, rather than a total score, were used.

Disease-Related Variables. SSc disease duration was defined as the time from onset of the first non-Raynaud's disease symptoms based on clinical history established by study physicians. Limited/diffuse status was recorded and defined as per LeRoy's definition. Limited disease was defined as skin involvement distal to the elbows and knees with or without face involvement and diffuse disease as skin involvement proximal to the elbows and knees and/or involving the trunk [16]. Total body skin involvement was assessed using the mRss, a previously validated method that has been used in other SSc samples [17–21]. Skin involvement is an important component of disease severity in SSc [17,18]. For each of 17 body areas, physicians rate the skin from 0 (*normal*) to 3 (*hidebound*), summing to obtain the mRss; scores can range in severity from 0 to 51. In addition, to determine the most salient body areas of potential concern, area-specific scores were derived for six body regions, including (1) the face, (2) hands/fingers, (3) arms, (4) chest/abdomen, (5) thighs, and (6) legs and feet. The area-specific scores were defined by the maximum severity score for each area (possible maximum score 0–3). For instance, the arms comprised four individual parts (i.e., right upper arm, right lower arm, left upper arm, left lower arm), and we defined the variable "arms" as the highest score from any of those parts. Telangiectasias were defined as including either macular or dot telangiectasias, or both; these involve the visible dilatation of superficial cutaneous blood vessels that collapse upon pressure and fill slowly when pressure is released, and exclude normal sun exposure-related telangiectasias. This definition is based on an adapted definition from Medsger et al. [17], as there is no uniform, validated definition of telangiectasias. Telangiectasias were coded separately for the upper body and lower body as present or absent. However, we used only upper-body telangiectasias because very few patients had lower-body, but not upper-body telangiectasias (4 of 390 with any telangiectasias in the current sample, 1.0%). Hyper- and/or hypo-pigmentation of the skin were each scored by physicians as present or absent. For analyses, we coded patients as having any pigmentation change versus none due to the high degree of overlap between occurrences of hyper- and hypo-pigmentation. In the current sample, only 23 of 119 patients with hypo-pigmentation did not have hyper-pigmentation as well (19.3%). To determine the presence of possible disfigurement because of hand contractures, fingertip-to-palm distances of both hands were measured by asking patients to make a fist, and the distance from the tip of the finger pad of the third finger to the distal palmar crease in full flexion was recorded in centimetres. This is a consistently used surrogate marker of contractures that is based on established methods [17,18]. In this study, the greater fingertip-to-palm distance of the right and left hand was used.

Data Analysis

To simultaneously assess correlates of dissatisfaction with appearance and social discomfort, we used the software MPlus [22] and replicated the two-factor confirmatory factor analysis model that was previously reported for the Brief-SWAP (Dissatisfaction with Appearance and Social Discomfort) [14]. Item responses for the Brief-SWAP are ordinal Likert data, so the weighted least squares estimator with a diagonal weight matrix, robust standard errors, and a mean-and variance-adjusted chi-square statistic was used with delta parameterization [22]. A chi-square goodness-of-fit test and three fit indices were used to assess model fit, including the Tucker-Lewis Index (TLI) [23]; the comparative fit index (CFI) [24]; and the root mean square error of approximation (RMSEA) [25]. Since the chi-square test is highly sensitive to sample size and can lead to the rejection of well-fitting models, practical fit indices were emphasized [26]. Guidelines proposed by Hu and Bentler [27] suggest that models with TLI and CFI close to .95 or higher and the RMSEA close to .06 or lower are representative of good fitting models. A CFI of .90 or above [28] and a RMSEA of .08 or less [29] may also be considered to represent reasonably acceptable model fit.

In an initial model, we regressed the Dissatisfaction with Appearance and Social Discomfort latent factors on *a priori* specified sociodemographic (age, sex, education, marital status, and race/ethnicity) and disease-related variables (disease duration, mRss, upper-body telangiectasias, hyper- and/or hypo-pigmentation, and fingertip-to-palm distance). We removed sociodemographic and disease-related variables from the model if they were not associated with the Dissatisfaction with Appearance or Social Discomfort subscales ($p > 0.25$), if their inclusion worsened overall model fit, and if their removal did not substantively or significantly influence links between other sociodemographic or disease variables and the Brief-SWAP latent factors.

Due to the significant association between mRss and the Dissatisfaction with Appearance and Social Discomfort subscales, in order to determine the body areas where skin involvement was most closely linked to these body image factors, in a second model, we replaced the mRss with body area-specific scores for the (1) face, (2) hands/fingers, (3) arms, (4) chest/abdomen, (5) thighs, and (6) legs and feet. We did this by initially entering the area-specific scores individually in separate models then including the body area with the most robust association with each factor. Subsequently, we kept that body area in the model and added other areas that were significant, starting with largest associations first.

Results

Sample Characteristics

A total of 489 patients were included in the study. Sociodemographic and disease characteristics are presented in Table 1, as well as Pearson bivariate correlations between sociodemographic and disease variables and Brief-SWAP subscales. The mean age of the sample was 57.1 years (SD = 11.7, range = 21–84 years), 88% of patients were female, and 91% were White. The mean time since onset of the first non-Raynaud's disease symptoms was 10.4 years (SD = 8.7), and the mean mRss was 9.0 (SD = 8.7; internal consistency $\alpha = 0.94$). Mean mRss was significantly higher in diffuse (mean = 19.2, SD = 9.8) compared to limited disease patients (mean = 5.9, SD = 4.2; $p < 0.001$). The Pearson correlation between limited/diffuse status and mRss was 0.65 ($p < 0.001$). As shown in Table 2, Pearson correlations between body area-specific scores ranged from 0.32 to 0.66. The mean Dissatisfaction with Appearance subscale score was 8.4 (SD = 5.2), and the mean Social Discomfort subscale score was 5.1 (SD = 5.1). Both subscales had good internal consistency reliability (Dissatisfaction with Appearance $\alpha = 0.82$, Social Discomfort $\alpha = 0.83$).

Table 1. Sociodemographic Variables, Disease Characteristics for SSc Patients, and Pearson Correlations with Brief-SWAP Subscales (N = 489).

Sociodemographic Variables:		**Correlation with Dissatisfaction with Appearance**	**Correlation with Social Discomfort**
Age *(mean years, SD)*	57.1 (11.7)	−0.04 (p = 0.400)	−0.20 (p<0.001)
Female sex *(n, %)*	432 (88.3)	−0.01 (p = 0.818)	0.06 (p = 0.220)
White *(n, %)*	447 (91.4)	−0.03 (p = 0.516)	−0.06 (p = 0.167)
Married *(n, %)*	344 (70.3)	−0.05 (p = 0.306)	−0.06 (p = 0.205)
Above high school education *(n, %)*	227 (46.4)	0.05 (p = 0.232)	0.01 (p = 0.839)
Disease Characteristics:			
Disease duration *(mean years, SD)*	10.4 (8.7)	0.001 (p = 0.977)	0.01 (p = 0.877)
Limited SSc *(n, %)*	323 (71.0)	0.16 (p = 0.001)	0.21 (p<0.001)
Modified Rodnan Skin Score (0–51) *(mean, SD)*	9.0 (8.7)	0.24 (p<0.001)	0.23 (p<0.001)
Maximum Skin Scores for Specific Body Areas:			
Face (0–3) *(mean, SD)*	0.6 (0.8)	0.18 (p<0.001)	0.21 (p<0.001)
Right/left hands and right/left fingers (0–3) *(mean, SD)*	1.7 (1.0)	0.18 (p<0.001)	0.17 (p<0.001)
Right/left upper arms and right/left forearms (0–3) *(mean, SD)*	0.5 (0.8)	0.20 (p<0.001)	0.20 (p<0.001)
Chest and abdomen (0–3) *(mean, SD)*	0.2 (0.6)	0.17 (p<0.001)	0.22 (p<0.001)
Right/left thighs (0–3) *(mean, SD)*	0.4 (1.1)	0.18 (p<0.001)	0.17 (p<0.001)
Right/left lower leg and right/left feet (0–3) *(mean, SD)*	0.6 (0.9)	0.16 (p<0.001)	0.11 (p = 0.013)
Upper-body telangiectasias	386 (78.9)	0.08 (p = 0.080)	0.11 (p = 0.020)
Hyper- and/or hypo-pigmentation	210 (42.9)	0.14 (p = 0.002)	0.18 (p<0.001)
Fingertip-to-palm distance (greater of right and left hands) *(mean cm, SD)*	1.0 (1.7)	0.18 (p<0.001)	0.16 (p = 0.001)
Body Image:			
Brief-SWAP *(mean,* SD)	13.5 (8.8)	------	------
Brief-SWAP Dissatisfaction with Appearance Subscale	8.4 (5.2)	------	0.59 (p<0.001)
Brief-SWAP Social Discomfort Subscale	5.1 (5.1)	0.59 (p<0.001)	------

Correlates of Dissatisfaction with Appearance and Social Discomfort

In the initial model, mRss was significantly associated with both greater Dissatisfaction with Appearance (standardized regression coefficient = 0.02, p = 0.001) and greater Social Discomfort (0.02, p = 0.020). When we replaced the mRss in the model with body-specific areas, each was significantly associated with Dissatisfaction with Appearance and Social Discomfort latent factors (p<0.05) with face being the most robust. In the final model (see Figure 1), face skin involvement was significantly associated with both factors (Dissatisfaction with Appearance, 0.18, p = 0.016, Social Discomfort, 0.23, p = 0.006). Once scores for the face were included in the model, no other area-specific scores were statistically significant when added. Model fit was good ($\chi^2(30) = 84$, CFI = 0.99, TLI = 0.98, RMSEA = 0.06), and all item factor loadings were ≥0.79 for the Dissatisfaction with Appearance factor and ≥0.67 for the Social Discomfort factor. The correlation between the Dissatisfaction with Appearance and Social Discomfort factors was 0.59. The model accounted for 13% of the variance in the Social

Table 2. Pearson Correlations between Body Area-Specific Scores[1].

	Face	Hands and Fingers	Arms	Chest and Abdomen	Thighs	Legs and Feet
Face	1.00	0.47	0.48	0.43	0.33	0.32
Hands and Fingers		1.00	0.49	0.36	0.35	0.35
Arms			1.00	0.63	0.65	0.44
Chest and Abdomen				1.00	0.66	0.38
Thighs					1.00	0.51
Legs and Feet						1.00

[1]All correlations p<0.01.

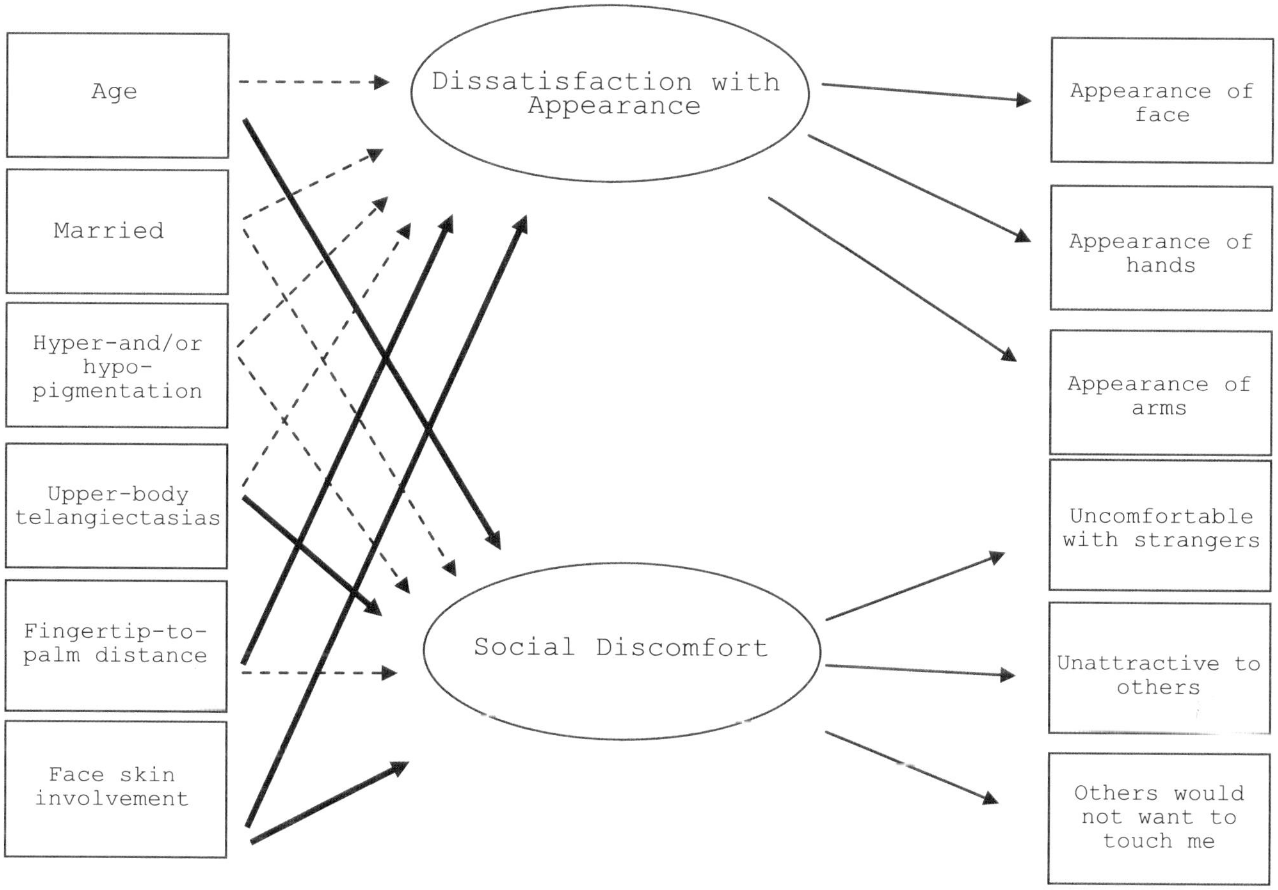

Figure 1. Structural equation model of relationships with sociodemographic and disease variables.

Discomfort latent factor and 6% of the variance in the Dissatisfaction with Appearance latent factor. Model parameters are shown in Table 3. Fingertip-to-palm distance, the measure of hand contractures, was significantly related to greater Dissatisfaction with Appearance (0.07, $p = 0.036$). Social Discomfort was significantly associated with presence of upper-body telangiectasias (0.32, $p = 0.021$) as well as younger age (per year) (−0.017, $p < 0.001$). Skin pigmentation changes were not significantly associated with either factor, but there was some suggestion of an association (Dissatisfaction with Appearance, 0.15, $p = 0.161$; Social Discomfort, 0.22, $p = 0.068$). Education, race/ethnicity, and sex were not associated with either Dissatisfaction with Appearance or Social Discomfort at $p < 0.25$, and their inclusion reduced model fit, so they were not included in the model.

Discussion

This study found that, in multivariate analyses, both disease factors and age were related to Dissatisfaction with Appearance and Social Discomfort among people with SSc. The findings

Table 3. Brief-SWAP Structural Equation Model of Relationships with Sociodemographic and Disease Variables.

Variables	Dissatisfaction with Appearance		Social Discomfort	
	Standardized Regression Coefficients	p value	Standardized Regression Coefficients	p value
Age	−0.001	0.863	−0.017	<0.001
Married	−0.16	0.138	−0.19	0.104
Upper-body telangiectasias	0.04	0.774	0.32	0.021
Face skin involvement	0.18	0.016	0.23	0.006
Fingertip-to-palm distance	0.07	0.036	0.05	0.199
Hyper- and/or hypo-pigmentation change	0.15	0.161	0.22	0.068
Correlation of Dissatisfaction with Appearance and Social Discomfort Factors	0.59			

highlighted the multifaceted nature of these two body image factors, as they were related to various disfiguring aspects of SSc, including skin involvement, upper-body telangiectasias, and disfigurement from hand contractures. Younger patients were more socially uncomfortable than older patients; however, age was not strongly related to Dissatisfaction with Appearance.

The associations of disfiguring physical changes with Dissatisfaction with Appearance and Social Discomfort are not surprising. For instance, relationships among extensive skin involvement, decreased appearance self-esteem, and heightened dissatisfaction with appearance have been documented previously in SSc [4,30,31] and in other types of acquired disfigurements [32]. A previous study, for instance, found that skin thickening was associated with lower appearance self-esteem in a sample of women with SSc [4]. Beyond SSc, previous research has documented social anxiety and avoidance behaviours among persons who have sustained visible disfigurement from a variety of sources to the face and other socially relevant body parts [33]. This is similarly reflected in the present study, as face skin involvement, upper-body telangiectasias, and hand contractures – salient physical changes that occur in visible and socially relevant body parts – were significantly related to either Dissatisfaction with Appearance or Social Discomfort. The current results also suggest that skin pigmentation changes may be important for both factors. It is of note that hands and fingers are visible and not easily hidden from others with clothing, but skin involvement to these areas was not associated with Dissatisfaction with Appearance or Social Discomfort in the multivariate model once face involvement was included. The hands and fingers variable was significant when face was not included, however, and the fact that it was not significant when added to the model after the face variable may be related to the relatively high degree of association between the variables.

Preoccupation with appearance and its importance for meeting new people, making social connections, and developing intimate relationships is often more pronounced earlier in life, which may account for the strong link in this study between age and Social Discomfort. We found that, although age did not play a role in individuals' ratings of Dissatisfaction with Appearance, it was an important factor in feelings of Social Discomfort. This finding is consistent with the broader literature on people with changes to their appearance due to illness and injury, which has found that older age is generally associated with less distress related to body image [13]. In the context of social interactions, particularly for establishing intimate relationships, appearance is highly relevant. Worry about a different or disfigured appearance can result in heightened focus on appearance itself, as well as its social consequences (e.g., thoughts of being disadvantaged in searching for a partner) [6]. Taken together, these findings suggest that younger patients may be at a greater risk of body image distress related to Social Discomfort based on physical appearance. However, the relatively small amount of variance explained by sociodemographic variables and disease factors suggest that psychological and personality variables may be important factors in determining vulnerability to body image distress in SSc.

There are interventions that may be useful to reduce distress related to this body image concern from SSc. For instance, cognitive-behavioral therapy for social anxiety [5] and social skills training programs [33,34] have been recommended as strategies to reduce social avoidance and increase self-esteem in social settings for other patient groups. Rheumatologists and other healthcare professionals may consider providing patients with informational resources as a starting point in providing support and in creating an atmosphere where body image concerns and issues can be discussed among SSc patients and healthcare providers. Changing Faces, a UK not-for-profit organization (www.changingfaces.org.uk), for instance, provides workshops, as well as a range of self-help informational resources related to body image concerns from disfigurement.

There are some limitations to consider when interpreting results from the current study. The sample consisted of a convenience sample of SSc patients enrolled in the CSRG Registry; therefore, the results may not represent the full spectrum of the SSc patient population. The present sample of patients with SSc generally had stable disease (mean disease duration 10.4 years). Patients who are not cared for by a rheumatologist and patients with very severe SSc who were too sick to participate or who died earlier in their disease course were not included in the present study. This may have resulted in an over-representation of healthier patients (survival cohort), and the results may not be generalizable to the full spectrum of SSc. Related to this, statistics on the number of patients approached versus consented are not available for all CSRG centres, but it is estimated that more than 80% of patients approached to participate in the Registry do enroll. This study also used cross-sectional data that did not allow for assessment over time. Additionally, apart from the mRss, the measures of disfiguring aspects of SSc were rough and not specifically validated. For instance, manifestations of telangiectasias can be quite extensive and might contribute significantly to body image issues; however, in the current sample, measurement of telangiectasias was based on large body regions (i.e. scores across upper body parts), scored as either present or absent, and telangiectasias to specific body regions (e.g., hands or arms) could not be assessed. Similarly, the method of measuring skin pigmentation changes was limited. Hyper- and/or hypo-pigmentation was scored as either present, absent, or unknown, which is a general scoring method, and may have limited the relationship between pigmentation changes and body image distress in our models. Additionally, the high proportion of White patients in our sample may not reflect the body image changes that can occur with pigment changes in other patients, and the high proportion of White patients in the sample, relative to other ethnicities, made it impossible to examine body image changes in other groups.

In sum, this study found that both Dissatisfaction with Appearance and Social Discomfort were associated with numerous disfiguring aspects of SSc. Furthermore, younger patients were more prone to discomfort in social settings. The results of this study underline the need to attend to both disease and social contexts in understanding the impact of disfigurement on body image distress among patients with SSc and to be aware that multiple factors may contribute to patient concerns about their appearance.

Acknowledgments

Canadian Scleroderma Research Group Recruiting Rheumatologists: M. Baron, Montreal, Quebec; J. Pope, London, Ontario; J. Markland, Saskatoon, Saskatchewan; D. A. Masetto, Sherbrooke, Quebec; E. Sutton, Halifax, Nova Scotia; N. A. Khalidi, Hamilton, Ontario; D. Robinson, Winnipeg, Manitoba; N. Jones, Edmonton, Alberta; E. Kaminska, Hamilton, Ontario; P. Docherty, Moncton, New Brunswick; C. D. Smith, Ottawa, Ontario; J.P. Mathieu, Montreal, Quebec; M. Hudson, Montreal, Quebec; S. Ligier, Montreal, Quebec; T. Grodzicky, Montreal, Quebec; S. Mittoo, Winnipeg, Manitoba; M. Fritzler, Advanced Diagnostics Laboratory, Calgary, Alberta.

Author Contributions

Conceived and designed the experiments: BT LJ MH MB. Performed the experiments: BT LJ. Analyzed the data: BT LJ VM MH. Wrote the paper: LJ BT. Interpretation of data: BT LJ MB MH VM. Revision and editing of manuscript: LJ BT MH VM MB. Final approval of the version to be published: LJ BT MH VM MB.

References

1. Seibold J, Harris ED, Budd RC, Genovese MC, Sergent JS (2005) Kelley's textbook of rheumatology. Philadelphia: Elsevier.
2. Mayes M (2008) Systemic sclerosis: A. clinical features. In: Klippel JH, Stone JH, Crafford LJ, White PH, eds. Primer on the Rheumatic Diseases. 13 ed. New York: Springer and Arthritis Foundation. pp 343–350.
3. Gayraud M (2007) Raynaud's phenomenon. Joint Bone Spine 74: e1–8.
4. Malcarne VL, Hansdottir I, Greensbergs HL, Clements PJ, Weisman MH (1999) Appearance self-esteem in systemic sclerosis. Cognitive Ther Res 23(2): 197–208.
5. Rumsey N, Harcourt D (2004) Body image and disfigurement: Issues and interventions. Body Image 1: 83–97.
6. Rumsey N, Harcourt D (2005) The psychology of appearance. New York: Open University Press.
7. van Lankveld WGJM, Vonk MC, Teunissen H, van den Hoogen FHJ (2007) Appearance self-esteem in systemic-sclerosis - subjective experience of skin deformity and its relationship with physician-assessed skin involvement, disease status and psychological variables. Rheumatology 46(5): 872–6.
8. Thombs BD, Taillefer SS, Hudson M, Baron M (2007) Depression in patients with systemic sclerosis: A systematic review of the evidence. Arthritis Rheum 57(6): 1089–1097.
9. Sivakumar B, Haloob N, Puri A, Latif A, Ghani V, et al. (2009) Systemic sclerosis as a model of chronic rejection in facial composite tissue transplantation. J Plast Reconstr Aesthet Surg 63(10): 1669–1676.
10. Amin K, Clarke A, Sivakumar B, Puri A, Fox Z, et al. (2011) The psychological impact of facial changes in scleroderma. Psychol Health Med 16(3): 304–12.
11. Cash TF, Pruzinsky T (2002) Body image: A handbook of theory, research, & clinical practice. New York: The Guilford Press.
12. Feingold A, Mazzella R (1998) Gender differences in body image are increasing. Psychol Sci 9: 190–5.
13. Fauerbach JA, Lawrence JW, Haythornthwaite J, McGuire M, Munster A (1996) Preinjury psychiatric illness and postinjury adjustment in adult burn survivors. Psychosomatics 37: 547–55.
14. Jewett LR, Hudson M, Haythornthwaite JA, Heinberg L, Wigley F, et al. (2010) Development and validation of the Brief-Satisfaction with Appearance Scale for systemic sclerosis. Arthritis Care Res 62(12): 1779–86.
15. Lawrence JW, Heinberg LJ, Roca R, Munster A, Spence R, et al. (1998) Development and validation of the satisfaction with appearance scale: Assessing body image among burn-injured patients. Psychol Assessment 10(1): 64–70.
16. LeRoy EC, Black C, Fleischmajer R, Jablonska S, Krieg T, et al. (1988) Scleroderma (systemic sclerosis): Classification, subsets and pathogenesis. J Rheumatol 15: 202–5.
17. Medsger TA, Jr., Bombardieri S, Czirjak L, Scorza R, Della Rossa A, et al. (2003) Assessment of disease severity and prognosis. Clin Exp Rheumatol 21: S42–6.
18. Medsger TA, Jr., Silman AJ, Steen VD, Black CM, Akesson A, et al. (1999) A disease severity scale for systemic sclerosis: Development and testing. J Rheumatol 26: 2159–67.
19. Clements PJ, Lachenbruch PA, Seibold JR, Zee B, Steen VD, et al. (1993) Skin thickness score in systemic sclerosis: An assessment of interobserver variability in 3 independent studies. J Rheumatol 20: 1892–6.
20. Akesson A, Fiori G, Krieg T, van den Hoogen FH, Seibold JR (2003) Assessment of skin, joint, tendon and muscle involvement. Clin Exp Rheumatol 21: S5–8.
21. Clements P, Seibold J, White B, Weiner S, Martin R (1995) Inter and intraobserver variability of total skin thickness score (modified Rodnan TSS) in systemic sclerosis. J Rheumatol 22: 1281–5.
22. Muthén LK, Muthén BO (1998–2004) Mplus user's guide version 3.11. Los Angeles: Muthén, LK & Muthén, BO.
23. Tucker LR, Lewis C (1973) A reliability coefficient for maximum likelihood factor analysis. Psychometrika 38: 1–10.
24. Bentler PM (1990) Comparative fit indexes in structural models. Psychol Bull 107: 238–46.
25. Steiger JH (1990) Structural model evaluation and modification: An interval estimation approach. Multivariate Behav Res 25: 173–80.
26. Reise SP, Widaman KF, Pugh RH (1993) Confirmatory factor analysis item response theory: Two approaches for exploring measurement invariance. Psychol Bull 114: 552–66.
27. Hu L, Bentler PM (1999) Cutoff criteria for fit indexes in covariance structure analysis: Conventional criteria versus new alternatives. Struct Equ Modeling 6: 131–52.
28. Kline RB (2005) Principles and practice of structural equation modeling. New York: Guilford Press.
29. Browne MW, Cudeck R (1993) Alternative ways of assessing fit. Newbury Park, CA: Sage.
30. Haythornthwaite JA, Heinberg LJ, McGuire L (2003) Psychologic factors in scleroderma. Rheum Dis Clin N Am 29: 427–39.
31. Benrud-Larson LM, Heinberg LJ, Boling C, Reed J, White B, et al. (2003) Body image dissatisfaction among women with scleroderma: Extent and relationship to psychosocial function. Health Psychol 22: 130–9.
32. Thombs BD, Notes LD, Lawrence JW, Magyar-Russell G, Bresnick MG, et al. (2008) From survival to socialization: A longitudinal study of body image in survivors of severe burn injury. J Psychosom Res 64: 205–12.
33. Newell R, Marks I (2000) Phobic nature of social difficulty in facially disfigured people. Brit J Psychiat 176: 177–81.
34. Newell RJ (1999) Altered body image: A fear-avoidance model of psycho-social difficulties following disfigurement. J Adv Nurs 30: 1230–8.

7

The Expression of BAFF, APRIL and TWEAK Is Altered in Eczema Skin but Not in the Circulation of Atopic and Seborrheic Eczema Patients

Yunying Chen[1*], Sara Lind Enoksson[1], Catharina Johansson[1], Maria A. Karlsson[2], Lena Lundeberg[2], Gunnar Nilsson[3], Annika Scheynius[1¶], Mikael C. I. Karlsson[1¶]

1 Clinical Allergy Research Unit, Department of Medicine Solna, Karolinska Institutet and Karolinska University Hospital Solna, Stockholm, Sweden, **2** Dermatology Unit, Department of Medicine Solna, Karolinska Institutet and Karolinska University Hospital Solna, Stockholm, Sweden, **3** Clinical Immunology and Allergy Unit, Department of Medicine Solna, Karolinska Institutet and Karolinska University Hospital Solna, Stockholm, Sweden

Abstract

The TNF family cytokines BAFF (B-cell activating factor of the TNF family) and APRIL (a proliferation-inducing ligand) are crucial survival factors for B-cell development and activation. B-cell directed treatments have been shown to improve atopic eczema (AE), suggesting the involvement of these cytokines in the pathogenesis of AE. We therefore analyzed the expression of these TNF cytokines in AE, seborrheic eczema (SE) and healthy controls (HC). The serum/plasma concentration of BAFF, APRIL and a close TNF member TWEAK (TNF-like weak inducer of apoptosis) was measured by ELISA. The expression of these cytokines and their receptors in skin was analyzed by quantitative RT-PCR and immunofluorescence. Unlike other inflammatory diseases including autoimmune diseases and asthma, the circulating levels of BAFF, APRIL and TWEAK were not elevated in AE or SE patients compared with HCs and did not correlate with the disease severity or systemic IgE levels in AE patients. Interestingly, we found that the expression of these cytokines and their receptors was altered in positive atopy patch test reactions in AE patients (APT-AE) and in lesional skin of AE and SE patients. The expression of APRIL was decreased and the expression of BAFF was increased in eczema skin of AE and SE, which could contribute to a reduced negative regulatory input on B-cells. This was found to be more pronounced in APT-AE, the initiating acute stage of AE, which may result in dysregulation of over-activated B-cells. Furthermore, the expression levels of TWEAK and its receptor positively correlated to each other in SE lesions, but inversely correlated in AE lesions. These results shed light on potential pathogenic roles of these TNF factors in AE and SE, and pinpoint a potential of tailored treatments towards these factors in AE and SE.

Editor: Silvano Sozzani, University of Brescia, Italy

Funding: This study was supported by grants from The Centre for Allergy Research, Karolinska Institutet, The Swedish Research Council, The Swedish Medical Society, The Hesselman Foundation, The Swedish International Development Agency, The Swedish Foundation for Strategic Research, Magnus Bergvall's Foundation, and through the regional agreement on medical training and clinical research (ALF) between Stockholm County Council and The Karolinska Institutet. The funders had no role in study design, data collection and analysis, decision to publish, or preparation of the manuscript.

Competing Interests: The authors have declared that no competing interests exist.

* E-mail: yunying.chen@ki.se

¶ These authors contributed equally to this work.

Introduction

Atopic eczema (AE) is a chronic inflammatory skin disorder and known to be caused by a combination of multiple factors, including genetic predisposition, skin barrier dysfunction, immunological deviation and environmental allergens [1]. Most AE patients have elevated concentration of total and allergen-specific serum IgE [2]. Some patients also have IgE against self-antigens, such as manganese superoxide dismutase (MnSOD) [2,3]. The lipophilic yeast *Malassezia* belongs to the commensal skin microflora, however, it can induce specific IgE and T-cell reactivity in AE patients [2,3]. Seborrheic eczema (SE) is another chronic inflammatory skin disorder associated with *Malassezia* reactivity but without IgE production [4].

Although the exact role of B-cells in AE is not fully understood, the contribution of B-cells to AE etiopathogenesis has become evident by studies showing that B-cell-depleting treatment with anti-CD20 Ab improved AE skin lesions with reduced mRNA expression of IL-5 and IL-13 and decreased infiltration of T and B-cells in skin, whereas total and allergen-specific IgE levels were not reduced, suggesting other functions than Ab production of B-cells in the disease mechanisms [5]. It has recently become appreciated that aberrant regulation and activation of B-cells result in chronic inflammatory and autoimmune-mediated disorders. They contribute to the disease pathogenesis not only by being the Ab producers, but also as APCs (antigen-presenting cells) and cytokine/chemokine producers [6,7]. Accordingly, B-cell directed therapy, including Abs against B-cell specific markers and inhibitors of survival and signalling factors for B-cells, is currently introduced for the treatment of inflammatory and autoimmune diseases [6,7].

The TNF ligand members BAFF (B-cell activating factor of the TNF family) and APRIL (a proliferation-inducing ligand) are two crucial survival factors for peripheral B-cells [8]. They can promote Ab class switching independently of the CD40/CD40L pathway [8]. BAFF and APRIL are expressed mainly by innate immune cells, to a less extent by T-cells and activated B-cells, as well as non-haematopoietic tissue resident cells [8]. BAFF and APRIL share the receptors TACI (transmembrane activator and calcium-modulator and cyclophilin ligand interactor) and BCMA (B-cell maturation antigen). In addition, BAFF binds to BAFFR and APRIL interacts with heparan sulphate proteoglycans [8]. BAFF is expressed as both surface-bound and soluble factors, whereas APRIL is processed inside the cell and released as a soluble protein [8]. However, APRIL can be attached to the cell surface by being a natural fusion protein with TWEAK (TNF-like weak inducer of apoptosis), called TWE-PRIL, sharing receptors with APRIL [9]. Thus, these factors form a network of mediators interacting with an overlapping set of receptors.

In humans, increased levels of BAFF and/or APRIL in serum or target tissues have been described in a number of autoimmune conditions and often correlated to disease progression [8]. In allergic diseases, so far, an elevated serum level of BAFF has been suggested as a diagnostic parameter for asthma [10]. In AE, an increased serum BAFF level in children has been reported [11]. However, another group has published data in adult AE patients having an elevated serum level of APRIL, but not BAFF [12].

When not fused to APRIL, full length TWEAK is a multifunctional cytokine, regulating cell proliferation, migration, differentiation, apoptosis, angiogenesis and inflammation [13], playing either beneficial or detrimental biological effects in mouse models, depending on the tissue injury or disease model that is used [14]. Its receptor Fn14 (Fibroblast growth factor-inducible 14) is expressed by many cell types, but absent on lymphocytes [13]. The expression of TWEAK and Fn14 is relatively low in normal tissues and up-regulated by tissue injury or disease [13]. It has recently been reported that TWEAK and TNF-α can cooperate in the induction of keratinocyte apoptosis, suggesting a role of TWEAK in eczema formation of AE [15] . Apart from this, TWEAK/Fn14 interaction in human keratinocytes has also been shown to induce the production of the chemokine RANTES, suggesting the potential involvement of TWEAK/Fn14 in the pathophysiology of inflammatory skin disorders [16].

To define the role of BAFF, APRIL and TWEAK in inflammatory skin disease, we characterized their expression in the circulation and the skin in AE, SE and HC. To get a more complete picture of the dynamic regulation of these factors, positive atopy patch test reactions in AE patients (APT-AE) was included, which mimics the early stage of AE lesions [17,18]. Our results demonstrate that unlike other inflammatory diseases, the levels of BAFF, APRIL and TWEAK are not elevated in the circulation and do not correlate with the severity of AE. Instead, the levels and expression patterns of these cytokines are changed in eczema skin of both AE and SE compared to skin of HC, showing an altered balance in the eczema skin for these TNF members.

Results

Circulating levels of BAFF, APRIL and TWEAK are not elevated in AE or SE patients

First, we measured plasma/serum levels of BAFF, APRIL and TWEAK by ELISA. We found that these cytokines were not elevated in AE or SE patients compared to HC (Fig. 1A–C). When investigating subgroups of AE patients (Fig. 1D–F), the plasma levels of BAFF were found to be decreased in patients with severe AE (Fig. 1D), as well as in the subgroup with elevated total IgE (Fig. 1E). However, the plasma/serum levels of these cytokines did not correlate with the SCORAD index or with the plasma levels of total IgE or *Malassezia*-specific IgE in AE patients (Table 1). Since the circulating levels of these factors have been found to be increased in autoimmune disease [8,13], we analyzed a subgroup of AE patients to elucidate whether their specific IgE levels to human MnSOD (n = 5) [19] correlated with the circulating levels of these cytokines, however, no correlation was found (data not shown).

The mRNA expression of BAFF is increased in SE and APT-AE, but not in AE lesions

To analyze the expression of BAFF, APRIL and TWEAK in eczema lesions, skin biopsies from AE and SE patients as well as HC were randomly selected from the respective groups in table 2

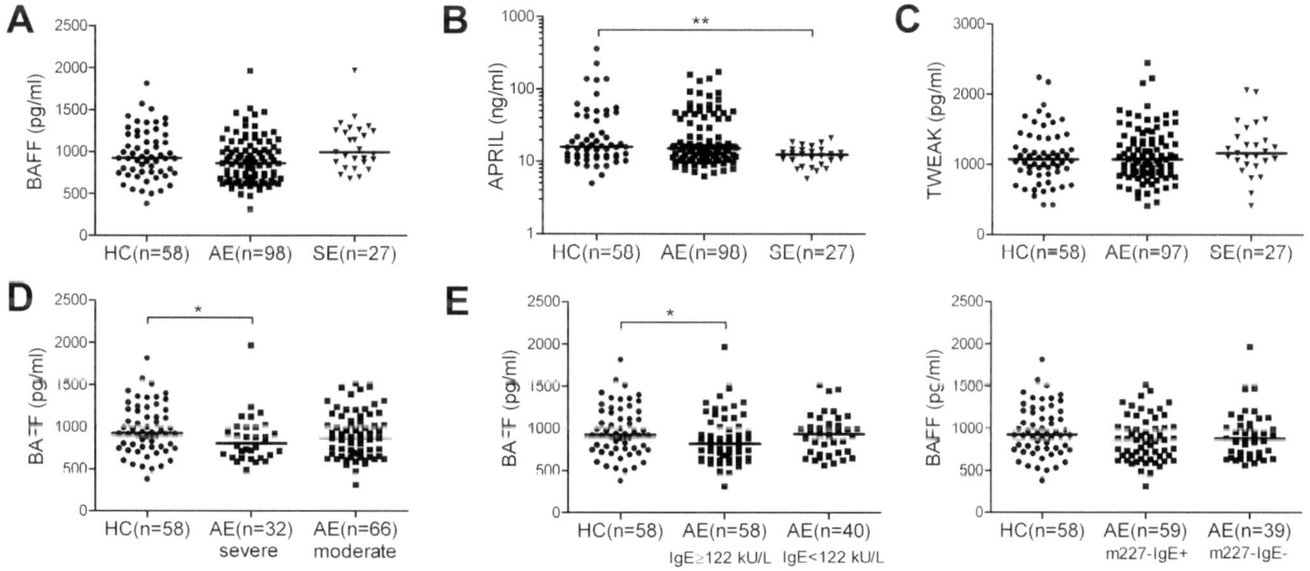

Figure 1. Plasma/serum levels of BAFF, APRIL and TWEAK in HC and patients with AE or SE. (A) BAFF, (B) APRIL and (C) TWEAK measured by ELISA in HC and patients with AE or SE. (D–F) Plasma levels of BAFF in subgroups of AE patients with (D) severe or moderate AE, (E) with/without increased total plasma IgE and (F) with/without *Malassezia* (m227)-specific plasma IgE. Data shown as individual patients or healthy controls, horizontal bar indicates the median, *$p<0.05$, **$p<0.01$ by Mann-Whitney test.

Table 1. Correlations between the serum/plasma levels of BAFF, APRIL, TWEAK and SCORAD, plasma levels of total-IgE or *Malassezia*-IgE in patients with AE, respectively.

Correlation	R value	P value
BAFF and SCORAD	−0.114	0.263
BAFF and total IgE	−0.179	0.078
BAFF and *Malassezia*-IgE	−0.120	0.240
APRIL and SCORAD	0.063	0.539
APRIL and total IgE	0.130	0.202
APRIL and *Malassezia*-IgE	0.094	0.360
TWEAK and SCORAD	0.018	0.861
TWEAK and total IgE	−0.078	0.449
TWEAK and *Malassezia*-IgE	−0.099	0.337

Correlations were assessed with the Spearman's rank correlation (n = 97–98).

(Table S1). The samples were analyzed by quantitative RT-PCR and verified for protein expression by immunofluorescence.

We found that mRNA expression of BAFF was about 10 times higher in APT-AE and about 7 times higher in SE lesions compared to HC (Fig. 2A). The mRNA levels of BAFFR and TACI were decreased in all the inflammatory conditions (Fig. 2B). Since these two receptors are known to be mainly expressed by B-cells [8], we normalized the mRNA levels of BAFFR and TACI to the mRNA levels of a B-cell specific marker CD19, the relative mRNA expression of these two receptors appeared similar in all groups (data not shown). We next verified the protein expression pattern of BAFF in skin. Immunostaining indicated that the cellular origins of BAFF in healthy skin were keratinocytes and cells in dermis co-stained with anti-CD68 mAb (Fig. 2C). The expression of BAFF by keratinocytes in healthy skin was confirmed by immunostaining of human keratinocytes (Fig. 2D). However, immunostaining for BAFFR and TACI expression on skin sections and on cultured keratinocytes revealed that these two receptors were not expressed by keratinocytes (data not shown). In lesional skin of AE, APT-AE and SE, besides the keratinocytes, subpopulations of the infiltrating CD3$^+$ T cells and CD68$^+$ macrophages also expressed BAFF, as shown by double-immunostaining on skin sections (Fig. 2E).

Table 2. Characterization of patients with AE or SE and healthy controls.

	Healthy controls	AE patients	SE patients
Total number of participants	58	99	27
Gender (female/male)	36/22	51/48	5/22
Age (years)	37 (18–64)[a]	28 (18–65)[a]	39 (22–63)[a]
SCORAD	-	35 (15–69)[a]	-
Mild AE/moderate AE/severe AE[b]	-	(0/66/33)	-
Plasma total IgE (kU/L)	20 (3.2–140)[a]	280 (2–15100)[a]	17 (2–390)[a]
Plasma *Malassezia*-IgE	0%	60%	0%
Phadiatop® positive	0%	80%	22%
Asthma and/or rhinitis	0%	74%	22%

[a]) Median (range);
[b]) Defined according to the objective SCORAD index (range 0–83; mild <15, moderate = 15–40, severe >40) [37].

The mRNA expression of APRIL is decreased in lesional skin of AE, APT-AE and SE

In contrast to BAFF, the relative mRNA levels of APRIL were decreased in lesional skin of AE, APT-AE and SE, compared to HC (Fig. 3A). Similarly, "TWE-PRIL", the cell surface bound form of APRIL, showed a tendency of lower expression in lesional skin (Fig. 3A). In healthy skin, APRIL was expressed by keratinocytes and by cells in dermis co-stained with anti-CD3 (Fig. 3B) or anti-CD68 mAb (data not shown). We confirmed the expression of APRIL in healthy keratinocytes by immunostaining of cultured human keratinocytes, which showed a similar intracellular expression pattern as found in HC skin (Fig. 3C) and was different from the cell membrane associated staining pattern of BAFF seen in figure 2. The expression of APRIL by keratinocytes in lesional skin of AE and APT-AE was decreased and among the infiltrating CD3$^+$ T-cells in APT-AE, only a small subpopulation was found to express APRIL (Fig. 3B), which was in line with the decreased mRNA expression of APRIL observed in these inflammatory skin lesions.

The mRNA expression of Fn14 is increased in AE and APT-AE skin lesions

Local expression of TWEAK and its receptor Fn14 have been shown to be increased in target tissues of several diseases [13]. Here, we found a decreased mRNA expression of TWEAK in lesional skin of AE, APT-AE and SE (Fig. 4A), whereas the mRNA expression of Fn14 showed having an increased tendency in lesional skin of AE, SE and APT-AE (Fig. 4A). Interestingly, the mRNA levels of Fn14 and TWEAK positively correlated to each other in SE, while these factors correlated inversely in AE (Fig. 4B). Furthermore, the mRNA levels of Fn14 in APT-AE correlated inversely with the APT scores (Fig. 4C). The protein expression pattern of TWEAK in skin specimens from all groups was similar, where TWEAK was expressed by keratinocytes and cells in dermis (Fig. 4D). The expression of Fn14 was in the dermal-epidermal basement membrane zone in both healthy skin of HC (Fig. 4D) and skin of AE, SE and APT-AE. Primary keratinocytes in culture did not stain with anti-TWEAK mAb and anti-Fn14 mAb (data not shown), which suggest that the local environment is important for their expression.

The mRNA expression of BAFF in cultured keratinocytes is regulated by IFN-γ and IL-27 and is correlated with that of IL-18 in lesional AE skin

The correlation between the protein levels of BAFF, APRIL and TWEAK in the circulation and mRNA levels in the skin was analyzed, however, no correlation was found (data not shown), suggesting that the systemic expression of these cytokines is not connected to the levels in the local environment in eczema skin. We and others have previously shown that the plasma level of IL-18, a product of activation of the inflammasome, is increased in AE patients [20,21,22]. In addition, the expression of IL-18 has been found to be increased in inflamed skin [23]. Thus, as a measure of local inflammation for means of correlation, we investigated the expression of IL-18 in lesional skin of AE and SE. IL-18 was found to be expressed at the level of the single basal layer of keratinocytes in HC, whereas expression in the suprabasal layers of keratinocytes was observed in lesional skin of AE, and particularly in APT-AE and SE (Fig. 5A). The mRNA level of IL-

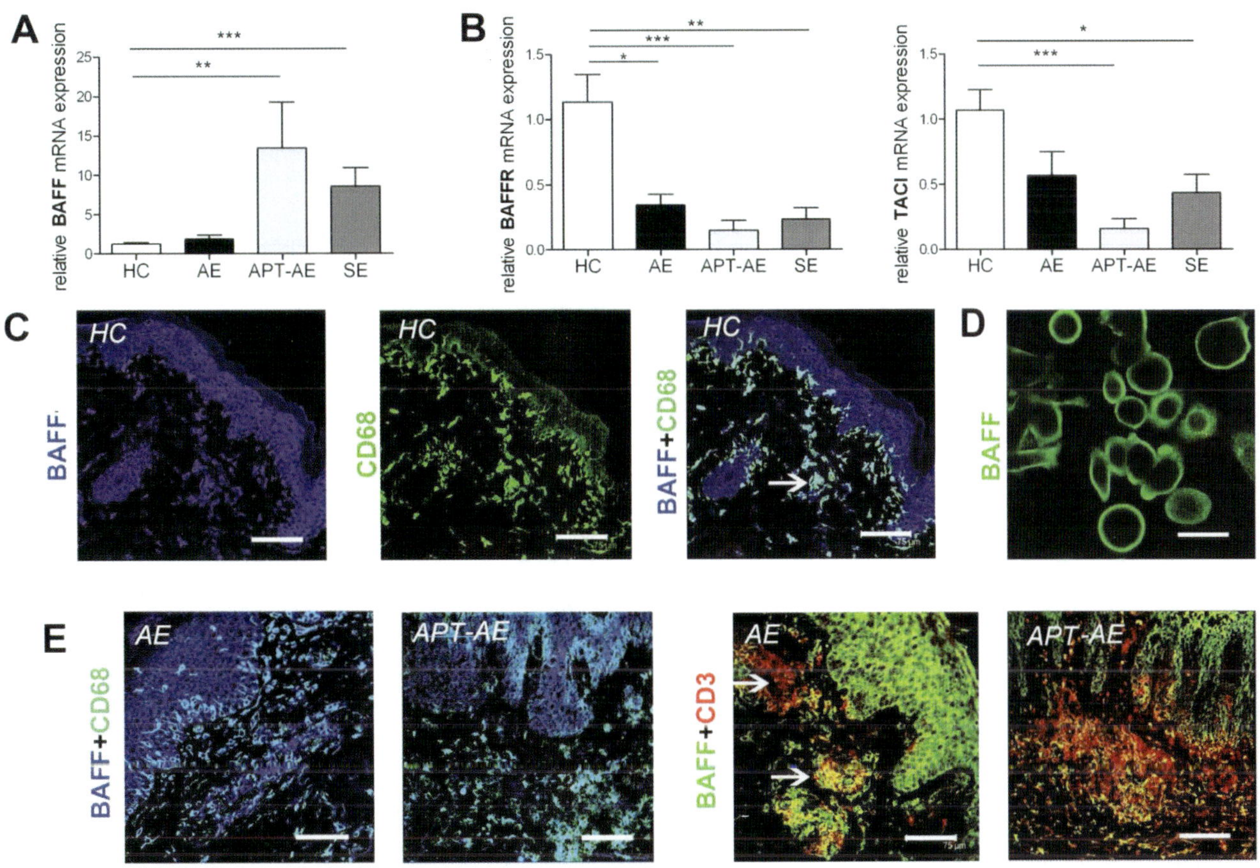

Figure 2. Expression of BAFF in skin of HC and lesional skin of AE and SE determined by quantitative RT-PCR and immunofluorescence. (A–B) Relative mRNA expression of BAFF, BAFFR and TACI in skin of HC (n = 9), lesional skin of AE (n = 9), APT-AE (n = 6) and SE (n = 6). Data shown as mean ± SEM, $^{*}p<0.05$, $^{**}p<0.01$, $^{***}p<0.001$ by Mann-Whitney test. (C) Representative picture of double-immunostaining with anti-BAFF and anti-CD68 mAb on sections of skin biopsies from HC (bar = 75 µm). The arrow indicates representative cells double positive for anti-BAFF and anti-CD68 staining. (D) Immunostaining with anti-BAFF mAb on cultured human keratinocytes (bar = 30 µm). (E) Representative pictures of double-immunostaining with anti-BAFF and anti-CD68/anti-CD3 mAb on sections of lesional AE skin and APT-AE skin specimens (bar = 75 µm). The upper arrow indicates the red cells stained with only anti-CD3 mAb. The lower arrow indicates the yellow cells stained with both anti-CD3 and anti-BAFF mAb.

18 was found to correlate with BAFF and APRIL in lesional skin of AE and APT-AE (Fig. 5B, C), but not in HC and SE lesions (data not shown). No correlation between IL-18 and TWEAK was found (data not shown). Since we found expression of BAFF and APRIL in healthy keratinocytes (Fig. 2D and Fig. 3C), we wanted to investigate if this expression could be regulated by IL-18, as well as other stimuli involved in the pathogenesis of AE. We found that IFN-γ and IL-27 dramatically increased the mRNA level of BAFF but not that of APRIL, TWEAK and Fn14 in keratinocytes stimulated for 24 hours (Fig. 5D). The other stimuli tested, *M. sympodialis* extract, LPS, LTA (Lipoteichoic acid), TNF-α, IL-4, IL-18 and IL-31, did not influence the mRNA levels analyzed (Fig. 5D).

Discussion

The role of B-cells in the pathology of allergy is undisputable, and their contribution beyond IgE production has recently started to be appreciated [6]. However, the factors influencing B-cell activation and homeostasis in allergic diseases, in both systemic and target tissue environments, need to be characterized. Here, we sought to define the role for BAFF, APRIL and TWEAK in inflammatory skin disease by comparing the systemic levels and skin expression in AE and SE patients as well as HCs.

Unlike other inflammatory diseases including autoimmune diseases and asthma [8,10], we found that the circulating levels of BAFF and APRIL were not elevated in patients with AE and they did not correlate with AE severity and plasma levels of total IgE or *Malassezia*-specific IgE. Notably, a recent publication has shown that the serum levels of BAFF were increased in children with AE [11], but this was not the case in adult patients [12], in agreement with our results. These findings suggest that BAFF might play a role at an early stage of AE but not at a later adult stage. Indeed, this seems to be the case in the local skin environment, where the mRNA expression of BAFF is found to be dramatically increased in APT-AE, which mimics the acute lesion.

Matsushita *et al* reported an increased level of APRIL in AE patients compared to HCs [12], which is not found in the cohort of patients investigated here. The reason for this is unclear, but might suggest that larger cohorts and multiple studies are needed to settle if levels of these factors are really altered in AE patients. On the other hand, our results show that AE and SE, two different chronic inflammatory skin diseases, can be distinguished by the systemic

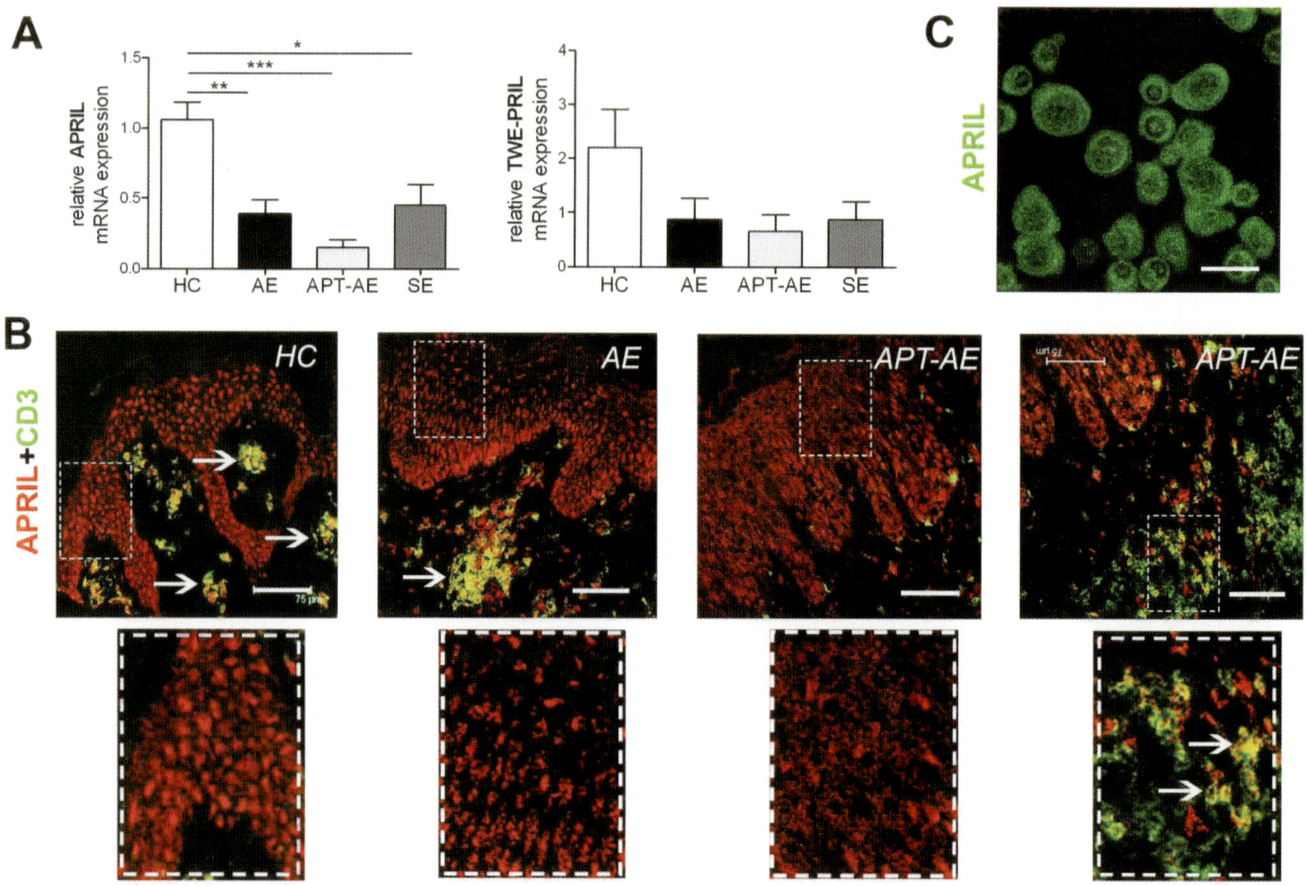

Figure 3. Expression of APRIL in skin of HC and lesional skin of AE and SE determined by quantitative RT-PCR and immunofluorescence. (A) Relative mRNA expression of APRIL and TWE-PRIL in skin of HC (n = 9), lesional skin of AE (n = 9), APT-AE (n = 6) and SE (n = 6). Data shown as mean ± SEM, *p<0.05, **p<0.01 by Mann-Whitney test. (B) Representative pictures of double-immunostaining with anti-APRIL and anti-CD3 mAb on sections of skin biopsies from HC, lesional AE skin and APT-AE skin specimens (bar = 75 μm). The arrows indicate representative yellow cells double positive for anti-CD3 and anti-APRIL staining. (C) Cultured human keratinocytes immunostained with anti-APRIL mAb (bar = 30 μm).

APRIL levels. Patients with SE displayed lower systemic APRIL concentration compared to HCs. The pathological role of the decreased serum APRIL level in SE remains to be determined.

The keratinocytes in skin, besides the barrier function, can also secrete numerous cytokines, chemokines and some of the growth factors in an autocrine manner regulating barrier homeostasis, and this ability of keratinocytes has been shown to be dysregulated in AE lesional skin [24]. It is known that BAFF and APRIL can be expressed by resident cells in several kinds of tissues [8]. We report here that healthy keratinocytes can also synthesize and express BAFF and APRIL, both *in vivo* and *ex vivo*, and in lesional skin of AE, APT-AE and SE the keratinocytes have impaired APRIL expression compared to HCs. Different from other TNF ligands, APRIL only functions as a soluble protein. By immunohistological analysis, we confirmed the intracellular expression pattern of APRIL in keratinocytes both *in vivo* and *ex vivo*, which is different from the cell membrane associated expression pattern of BAFF. We then studied the regulation of BAFF and APRIL *in vitro* in keratinocytes using some factors involved in the pathogenesis of eczema and we found that the BAFF mRNA level was dramatically increased by IFN-γ and IL-27. IL-27 is a member of the IL-12 family, produced by activated APCs [25]. The increased expression of IFN-γ and IL-27 in chronic eczema skin lesions has been demonstrated before [1,25], and both IFN-γ and IL-27 have been shown to greatly induce the production of CXCL 9–11 in normal human keratinocytes [26,27], the chemokines known to attract Th1 cells, triggering and sustaining skin inflammation [26,27]. Here we suggest that IFN-γ and IL-27 can amplify the skin inflammation not only through the regulation of the chemokine production in keratinocytes, but also through the regulation of BAFF expression in these cells.

By immunostaining we did not found the expression of TACI or BAFFR by keratinocytes both *in vivo* and *ex vivo*, indicating that the expression of BAFF and APRIL by keratinocytes is not regulated by feedback autocrine mechanism. BAFF and APRIL thus presumably have no regulatory role for the homeostasis of keratinocytes. TACI and BAFFR are mainly expressed by B-cells [8] and the presence of B-cells in normal skin and the infiltration of B-cells in AE eczema skin have been demonstrated by Simon *et al* [5]. We could detect the expression of these two receptors in skin, however, the mRNA level of these two receptors in inflamed skin of APT-AE, AE and SE was not found to be increased. The reason for this could be the dilute effect by the influx of a large number of T-cells and macrophages in inflammatory skin lesions. Indeed, when the mRNA levels of these two receptors were normalized to the expression level of a B-cells maker CD19, the relative mRNA expression of TACI and BAFFR appeared similar in all groups.

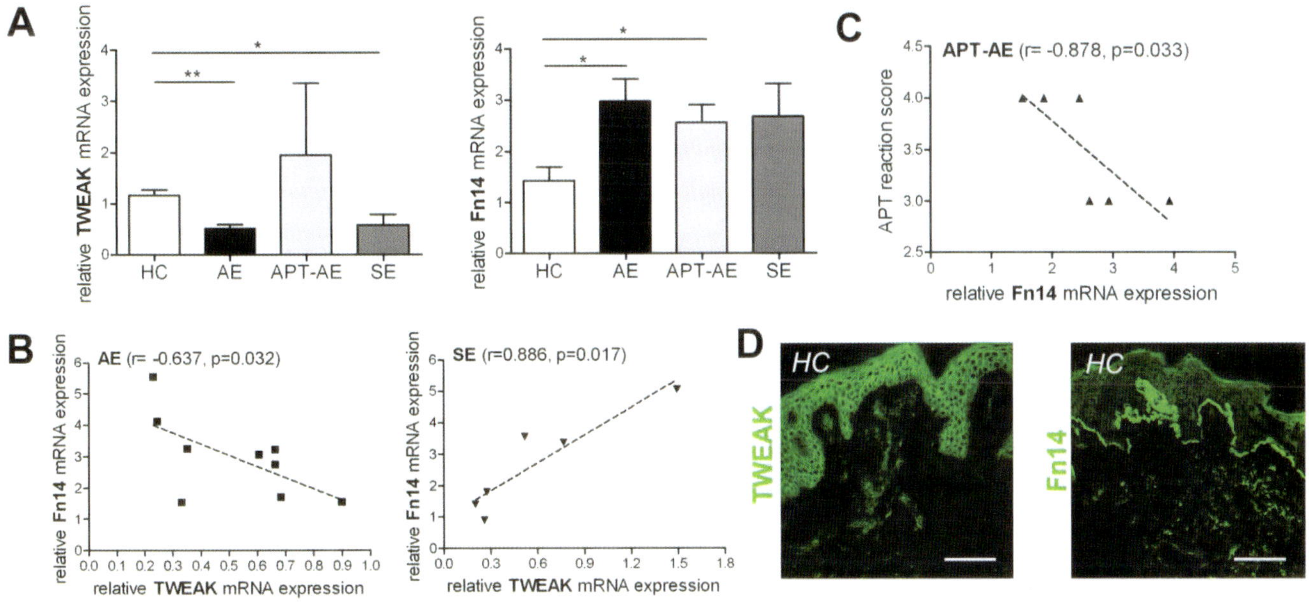

Figure 4. Expression of TWEAK in skin of HC and lesional skin of AE and SE determined by quantitative RT-PCR and immunofluorescence. (A) Relative mRNA expression of TWEAK and Fn14 in skin of HC (n = 9), lesional skin of AE (n = 9), APT-AE (n = 6) and SE (n = 6). Data shown as mean ± SEM, *$p<0.05$, **$p<0.01$ by Mann-Whitney test. (B) Correlation of relative mRNA levels of TWEAK and Fn14 in AE (n = 9) and SE (n = 6) skin specimens. (C) Correlation of relative mRNA levels of Fn14 and APT reaction scores in APT-AE (n = 6) skin specimens. The correlations were analyzed using Spearman's rank correlation. (D) Representative picture of immunostaining with anti-TWEAK or anti-Fn14 mAb on sections of skin specimens from HC (bar = 75 μm).

APRIL is a close homologue to BAFF and they share many functions and receptors. Here we demonstrate that opposite to BAFF, the expression of APRIL, as well as the cell surface APRIL hybrid TWE-PRIL, is down-regulated in the skin lesions of APT-AE, AE and SE. It has been shown that APRIL binding to TACI delivers a negative signal to B-cells [28]. Since APRIL does not bind to BAFFR, it does not deliver a BAFFR mediated positive signal to B-cells. Therefore, the decreased expression of APRIL and TWE-PRIL together with the increased BAFF expression in eczema skin could contribute to a reduced negative regulatory input on B-cells, which is more pronounced in the initiating acute stage of AE, resulting in dysregulation of over-activated B-cells in lesional skin of AE and SE. Our data of the down-regulation of APRIL and the up-regulation of BAFF in the eczema skin of AE and SE is also important for guiding potential clinical treatment. When targeting BAFF and APRIL in the therapy for AE and SE, the agents neutralizing only BAFF but having no effect on APRIL might be more suitable than those targeting both BAFF and APRIL.

The up-regulation of IL-18 in suprabasal keratinocytes in skin lesions has been described in psoriasis [29]. Here we report that this phenomenon is also present in APT-AE, AE and SE. Indeed, IL-18 has been shown to play a harmful effect to enhance inflammation in several autoimmune and inflammatory diseases [30]. Since B-cells are known to lack the expression of the IL-18 receptor, the effect of IL-18 on B-cell related activation has not been well studied. We suggest that there might be a direct or indirect interplay between IL-18 and BAFF/APRIL in AE, since the mRNA level of BAFF/APRIL correlates with that of IL-18 in lesional skin of AE and APT-AE. A connection between these factors is supported by a mouse model where daily i.p. injections of IL-18 for 10 days induce production of both IgE [31,32] and BAFF (our own unpublished observation). Furthermore, we demonstrated that although IL-18 itself had no direct effect on the regulation of BAFF and APRIL production in cultured keratinocytes, IFN-γ dramatically increased the BAFF mRNA level in these cells. Since IL-18 is known to be a powerful stimulator of IFN-γ production [33], we therefore suggest that IL-18 could be produced locally by inflammatory cells and indirectly regulate the production of BAFF and APRIL in keratinocytes through IFN-γ.

Elevated serum levels of TWEAK have been found in patients with chronic inflammatory diseases and been suggested to be playing either a protective or harmful role [14]. For example, in systemic sclerosis where TWEAK is associated with a low frequency of pulmonary fibrosis [34] and in rheumatoid arthritis where the levels of TWEAK reflect disease activity [35]. In our patient cohort, we found no difference in the serum level of TWEAK in patients with AE or SE compared with HCs. This is in agreement with a recent study, where the serum level of TWEAK was reported to be similar among patients with AE or psoriasis and HCs [15]. Thus, unlike other chronic inflammatory diseases, increased level of TWEAK is not a candidate for a systemic role in the pathogenesis of AE and SE. Zimmermann *et al* also found that the TWEAK mRNA expression in healthy keratinocytes was not influenced by various eczema related stimuli [15] in agreement with our results. However, although the authors found similar mRNA expression of TWEAK between lesional and non-lesional skin from patients with AE, they found that the protein expression of TWEAK was only present in the epidermis of lesional, but absent in non-lesional skin by means of immunofluorescence [15]. In the biopsy specimens used in our study we could detect TWEAK expression not only in lesional AE skin, but also in healthy skin by immunofluorescence and we also found altered mRNA levels of TWEAK and Fn14 in AE lesions compared with HC. These differences between our study and the study by Zimmermann *et al* [15] could besides different immuno-staining protocols and source of anti-TWEAK and anti-Fn14 mAb possibly

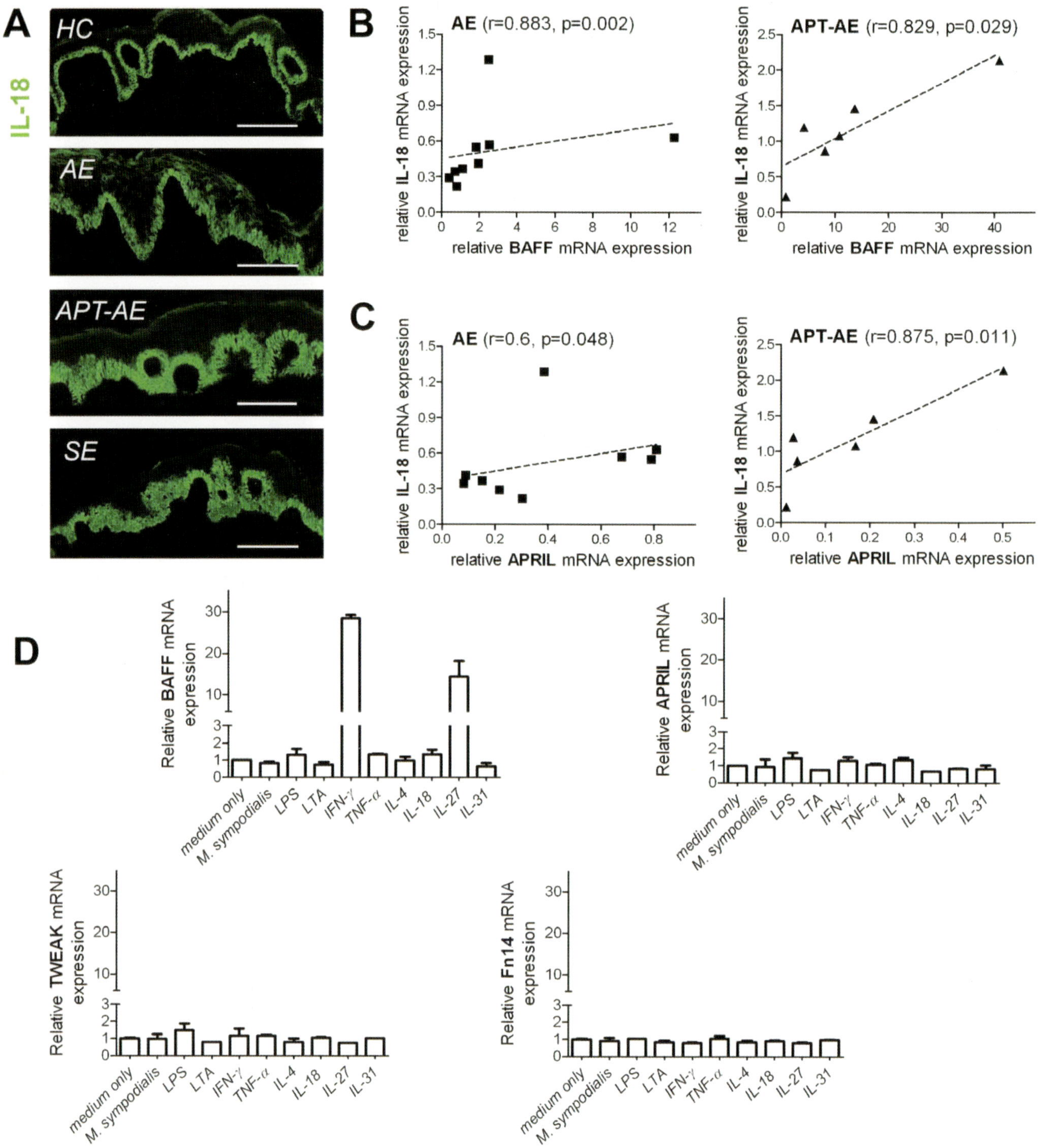

Figure 5. Expression of IL-18 in AE, SE and HC skin determined by immunofluorescence and the regulation of mRNA expression of BAFF, APRIL, TWEAK and Fn14 in healthy keratinocytes by IL-18 and other eczema related stimuli. (A) Representative pictures of immunostaining with anti-IL-18 mAb on sections of skin biopsies from HC, lesional skin of AE, APT-AE and SE (bar = 150 μm). (B) Correlation of relative mRNA levels of BAFF and IL-18 in AE (n = 9) and APT-AE (n = 6) skin specimens. (C) Correlation of relative mRNA levels of APRIL and IL-18 in AE (n = 9) and APT-AE (n = 6) skin specimens. The correlations were analyzed using Spearman's rank correlation. (D) Relative mRNA expression of BAFF, APRIL, TWEAK and Fn14 in healthy keratinocytes cultured for 24 h with indicated stimuli. Data are shown as mean ± SEM (n = 3) from two separate experiments.

be due to the source of healthy skin; they used non-lesional skin from the buttock area of patients with AE or psoriasis, whereas we used skin biopsy specimens from healthy individuals. Furthermore, the source of the primary healthy keratinocytes was from adults in their study [15] and from young individuals in ours, which might lead to the different observations on the Fn14 expression in cultured keratinocytes by immunofluorescence. Another study also reported the protein expression of Fn14 on primary keratinocytes by FACS analysis [16], but the culture system in this study is different from what we used in this study; the extra supplements in their culture media could contribute to the induction of Fn14 expression in keratinocytes *ex vivo*. Further studies are needed to verify these possibilities.

It is known that the expression of Fn14 is inducible by tissues injury and that Fn14 signalling can occur in a TWEAK-dependent or -independent manner, contributing to tissue repair or a pathological effect depending on different disease or injury setting [14]. Indeed, we found that Fn14 was expressed at a low level in healthy skin and its expression level was significantly induced in the skin of AE and APT-AE. Importantly, we report here that in AE lesions the mRNA level of Fn14 correlates inversely with that of TWEAK, suggesting a compensatory mechanism that regulates TWEAK and Fn14 expression in AE lesions, where TWEAK-independent Fn14 signalling might be more dominate. Meanwhile, our data suggest that TWEAK-independent Fn14 signalling is not at work in SE lesions, where the TWEAK-dependent signalling could be more important in this setting, since the expression levels of TWEAK and Fn14 positively correlate to each other. Thus, we suggest that the persistent activation of Fn14 signalling in skin lesions of AE and SE could result in harmful and pathological effects to perpetuate the diseases. Therefore blocking TWEAK-independent and -dependent Fn14 signalling could be a therapeutic strategy for AE and SE, respectively. Whereas we also show here that blocking Fn14 signalling might not be suitable for the acute phase of AE, since the expression level of Fn14 correlates inversely with the APT score, suggesting a protective role of Fn14 signalling in acute AE. This suggestion is also supported by the current hypothesis that TWEAK-Fn14 axis normally plays a beneficial role in tissue repair following acute injury [14].

In conclusion, our data suggests that elevated levels of BAFF, APRIL or TWEAK in the circulation are not a part of the pathogenesis of AE and SE. However, the expression of these cytokines is altered in the local inflammatory environment in lesional skin of AE and SE. Furthermore, the expression pattern in AE lesions can be distinguished from that of SE lesions, as well as from that in the acute phase of AE lesions. Therefore, we propose that BAFF, APRIL and TWEAK can be considered as potential targets for the development of different therapeutic strategies in these inflammatory skin disorders.

Materials and Methods

Subjects and Ethics

Adult patients with AE or SE and HCs were recruited in the Stockholm area (Table 2). The inclusion and exclusion criteria for the AE patients were as previously described [36]. AE disease severity was assessed by the objective SCORAD index [37]. The SE patients had no history of additional skin disease. The HC had no clinical symptoms or history of allergy or skin disease. All participants gave their written informed consent. The study was approved by the Swedish regional ethics committee.

Atopy patch test and skin biopsy specimens

APT with an in house extract from *M. sympodialis* (ATCC strain 42132) [38] was performed on non-lesional skin of AE patients as previously described [36]. The APT reaction was evaluated 48 h later and scored from 0 to 5+ on a scale proposed by European Task Force on Atopic Dermatitis [39]. Four mm punch skin biopsy specimens were taken under local anaesthesia from positive APT reactions (APT-AE), lesional skin from AE or SE patients and normal looking skin from HC. The specimens were snap-frozen and stored at −80°C until analysis.

Serology

The concentrations of BAFF (R&D Systems, Minneapolis, MN) and APRIL (Bender Medsystems, Vienna, Austria) in plasma and TWEAK (Bender MedSystems) in sera were measured by ELISA according to the manufacturer's instruction. Total IgE (reference range 1.6–122 kU/L), *Malassezia*-specific IgE (m227, mixture of *M. sympodialis*, *M. globosa* and *M. restricta*, positive≥0.35 kU/L) and specific IgE to any of 11 common aeroallergens (Phadiatop®, positive≥0.35 kU/L) were measured in plasma using ImmunoCAP™ (Phadia AB, Uppsala, Sweden).

Keratinocyte culture

Human keratinocytes originally isolated from skin of healthy young boys in connection with a routine surgical operation on the foreskin [40] were cultured in Keratinocyte-SFM® containing 5 µg/L human recombinant epidermal growth factor (EGF 1–53) and 50 mg/L bovine pituitary extract (BPE) (GIBCO® Invitrogen Cell Culture, Auckland, New Zealand) and 1% penicillin at 37°C in humidified atmosphere plus 5% CO_2. The third- or fourth-passage keratinocytes were added to sterile microscope slides (Novakemi AB, Stockholm, Sweden) and incubated overnight to let the cells attach on the slides. The slides were then washed with PBS, air-dried and stored at −80°C until analysis. In addition, the keratinocytes were cultured in duplicates in 24-well plates (Becton Dickinson, Franklin lakes, NJ) for 24 h in 700 µl culture medium alone or stimulated with 10 µg/ml extract from *M. sympodialis* (ATCC strain 42132) [38], 10 µg/ml LPS (strain O111:B4, Sigma, St Louise, MO), 10 µg/ml Lipoteichoic acid (LTA, from *Staphylococcus aureus*, Sigma), 10 ng/ml rhIFN-γ (Sigma), 10 ng/ml rhTNF-α (R&D Systems, Minneapolis, MN), 10 ng/ml rhIL-4 (Invitrogen, Camarillo, CA), 100 ng/ml rhIL-18 (MBL International Corporation, Woburn, MA), 100 ng/ml rhIL-27 and 100 ng/ml rhIL-31 (R&D Systems). Total RNA of the keratinocytes was then isolated for quantitative QT-PCR analysis (see below).

Quantitative RT-PCR

Total RNA from cultured keratinocytes or snap-frozen skin biopsies randomly selected from the participants (Table S1) was isolated by the TRIzol method (Invitrogen, Carlbad, CA). Isolated RNA was reversely transcribed by iScript TM cDNA synthesis kit (Bio-Rad, Hercules, CA). The cDNA was quantified in duplicates by means of real-time PCR with iQTM SYBR Green Supermix in the iCycler iQTM Multicolor real-time detection system (Bio-Rad). The primer sets for genes of interest were designed by Primer-BLAST program at NCBI databases. For each primer set (Table S2), non-template controls and melting curve were performed to control the specificity of the amplification. Relative expression level of a certain gene to the housekeeping gene GAPDH was calculated with the Pfaffl-formula [41].

Immunofluorescence

Six-µm cryosections of skin biopsies and keratinocytes attached to slides were fixed in acetone. After blocking with goat serum, sections were incubated with primary mAb, followed by several washes in PBS and incubation with fluorescently-labelled secondary Abs. The following Abs were used: anti-BAFF (Buffy-2, rat IgM) and anti-APRIL (Aprily-8, mouse IgG_1) (Axxora, Lausen, Switzerland); anti-TWEAK (CARL-1, mouse IgG_3), anti-BAFFR (11c1, mouse IgG_1), biotin conjugated anti-TACI (1A1, rat IgG_{2a})

and anti-Fn14 (ITEM-1, mouse IgG_1) (Biolegend, San Diego, CA); anti-IL-18 (25-2G, mouse IgG_1; Medical & Biological Laboratories, Naka-ku Nagoya, Japan); Alexa-488 or 546-conjugated $F(ab')_2$ of goat anti-mouse IgG and Alexa-488 or 647-conjugated goat anti-rat IgG (Invitrogen, Eugene, OR). In double-stainings, FITC or PE-conjugated anti-CD3 (SK7, mouse IgG_1; BD biosciences, San Jose, CA) or Alexa-488-conjugated anti-CD68 (KP1, mouse IgG_1; Santa Cruz Biotechnology, Heidelberg, Germany) were used. Stainings with isotype controls were performed to confirm the specificity of the immunostainings. Images were acquired using a confocal laser scanning microscope (TCS SP2; Leica Microsystems, Mannheim, Germany).

Statistical analysis

Mann-Whitney test was used to test the difference between two groups. Correlation was assessed by Spearman's rank correlation. All calculations were performed by GraphPad Prism 5 software (GraphPad Software Inc., La Jolla, CA). $p<0.05$ was considered significant.

Supporting Information

Table S1 Characterization of the patients with AE or SE and HC included in analysis of skin specimens.

Table S2 Genes of interest and primer sequences.

Acknowledgments

We thank Ylva Kaiser, Agnetha Beinhoff, Dr. Fredrik Wermeling, and Emilie Domange Jordö, (Karolinska Institutet) for important input and helpful discussions.

Author Contributions

Conceived and designed the experiments: AS MCIK YC. Performed the experiments: YC SLE CJ. Analyzed the data: YC SLE CJ. Contributed reagents/materials/analysis tools: MAK LL GN AS MCIK. Wrote the paper: YC AS MCIK.

References

1. Bieber T (2008) Atopic dermatitis. N Engl J Med 358: 1483–1494.
2. Akdis CA, Akdis M, Bieber T, Bindslev-Jensen C, Boguniewicz M, et al. (2006) Diagnosis and treatment of atopic dermatitis in children and adults: European Academy of Allergology and Clinical Immunology/American Academy of Allergy, Asthma and Immunology/PRACTALL Consensus Report. Allergy 61: 969–987.
3. Scheynius A, Crameri C (2010) *Malassezia* in atopic eczema/dermatitis. In: Boekhout T, Guého-Kellerman E, Mayser P, Velegraki A, eds. *Malassezia* and the skin, Springer Verlag Heidelberg, New York. pp 212–228.
4. Naldi L, Rebora A (2009) Clinical practice. Seborrheic dermatitis. N Engl J Med 360: 387–396.
5. Simon D, Hosli S, Kostylina G, Yawalkar N, Simon HU (2008) Anti-CD20 (rituximab) treatment improves atopic eczema. J Allergy Clin Immunol 121: 122–128.
6. Nagel A, Hertl M, Eming R (2009) B-cell-directed therapy for inflammatory skin diseases. J Invest Dermatol 129: 289–301.
7. Daridon C, Burmester GR, Dorner T (2009) Anticytokine therapy impacting on B cells in autoimmune diseases. Curr Opin Rheumatol 21: 205–210.
8. Mackay F, Schneider P (2009) Cracking the BAFF code. Nat Rev Immunol 9: 491–502.
9. Daridon C, Youinou P, Pers JO (2008) BAFF, APRIL, TWE-PRIL: who's who? Autoimmun Rev 7: 267–271.
10. Kang JS, Yoon YD, Ahn JH, Kim SC, Kim KH, et al. (2006) B cell-activating factor is a novel diagnosis parameter for asthma. Int Arch Allergy Immunol 141: 181–188.
11. Jee HM, Kim KW, Hong JY, Sohn MH, Kim KE (2009) Increased serum B cell-activating factor level in children with atopic dermatitis. Clin Exp Dermatol 53: 795–800.
12. Matsushita T, Fujimoto M, Echigo T, Matsushita Y, Shimada Y, et al. (2008) Elevated serum levels of APRIL, but not BAFF, in patients with atopic dermatitis. Exp Dermatol 17: 197–202.
13. Burkly LC, Michaelson JS, Hahm K, Jakubowski A, Zheng TS (2007) TWEAKing tissue remodeling by a multifunctional cytokine: role of TWEAK/Fn14 pathway in health and disease. Cytokine 40: 1–16.
14. Winkles JA (2008) The TWEAK-Fn14 cytokine-receptor axis: discovery, biology and therapeutic targeting. Nat Rev Drug Discov 7: 411–425.
15. Zimmermann M, Koreck A, Meyer N, Basinski T, Meiler F, et al. (2011) TNF-like weak inducer of apoptosis (TWEAK) and TNF-alpha cooperate in the induction of keratinocyte apoptosis. J Allergy Clin Immunol 127: 200–207, 207. e201-210.
16. Jin L, Nakao A, Nakayama M, Yamaguchi N, Kojima Y, et al. (2004) Induction of RANTES by TWEAK/Fn14 interaction in human keratinocytes. J Invest Dermatol 122: 1175–1179.
17. Mitchell EB, Crow J, Chapman MD, Jouhal SS, Pope FM, et al. (1982) Basophils in allergen-induced patch test sites in atopic dermatitis. Lancet 1: 127–130.
18. Johansson C, Eshaghi H, Linder MT, Jakobson E, Scheynius A (2002) Positive atopy patch test reaction to Malassezia furfur in atopic dermatitis correlates with a T helper 2-like peripheral blood mononuclear cells response. J Invest Dermatol 118: 1044–1051.
19. Vilhelmsson M, Glaser AG, Martinez DB, Schmidt M, Johansson C, et al. (2008) Mutational analysis of amino acid residues involved in IgE-binding to the Malassezia sympodialis allergen Mala s 11. Mol Immunol 46: 294–303.
20. Tanaka T, Tsutsui H, Yoshimoto T, Kotani M, Matsumoto M, et al. (2001) Interleukin-18 is elevated in the sera from patients with atopic dermatitis and from atopic dermatitis model mice, NC/Nga. Int Arch Allergy Immunol 125: 236–240.
21. Lind SM, Kuylenstierna C, Moll M, E DJ, Winqvist O, et al. (2009) IL-18 skews the invariant NKT-cell population via autoreactive activation in atopic eczema. Eur J Immunol 39: 2293–2301.
22. Shaker OG, El-Komy M, Tawfic SO, Zeidan N, Tomaireek RH (2009) Possible role of nerve growth factor and interleukin-18 in pathogenesis of eczematous lesions of atopic dermatitis. J Dermatol Sci 53: 153–154.
23. Wittmann M, Macdonald A, Renne J (2009) IL-18 and skin inflammation. Autoimmun Rev 9: 45–48.
24. Pastore S, Mascia F, Girolomoni G (2006) The contribution of keratinocytes to the pathogenesis of atopic dermatitis. Eur J Dermatol 16: 125–131.
25. Wittmann M, Zeitvogel J, Wang D, Werfel T (2009) IL-27 is expressed in chronic human eczematous skin lesions and stimulates human keratinocytes. J Allergy Clin Immunol 124: 81–89.
26. Kanda N, Shimizu T, Tada Y, Watanabe S (2007) IL-18 enhances IFN-gamma-induced production of CXCL9, CXCL10, and CXCL11 in human keratinocytes. Eur J Immunol 37: 338–350.
27. Shibata S, Tada Y, Kanda N, Nashiro K, Kamata M, et al. (2010) Possible roles of IL-27 in the pathogenesis of psoriasis. J Invest Dermatol 130: 1034–1039.
28. Seshasayee D, Valdez P, Yan M, Dixit VM, Tumas D, et al. (2003) Loss of TACI causes fatal lymphoproliferation and autoimmunity, establishing TACI as an inhibitory BLyS receptor. Immunity 18: 279–288.
29. Ohta Y, Hamada Y, Katsuoka K (2001) Expression of IL-18 in psoriasis. Arch Dermatol Res 293: 334–342.
30. Sims JE, Smith DE (2010) The IL-1 family: regulators of immunity. Nat Rev Immunol 10: 89–102.
31. Yoshimoto T, Mizutani H, Tsutsui H, Noben-Trauth N, Yamanaka K, et al. (2000) IL-18 induction of IgE: dependence on CD4+ T cells, IL-4 and STAT6. Nat Immunol 1: 132–137.
32. Hoshino T, Yagita H, Ortaldo JR, Wiltrout RH, Young HA (2000) In vivo administration of IL-18 can induce IgE production through Th2 cytokine induction and up-regulation of CD40 ligand (CD154) expression on CD4+ T cells. Eur J Immunol 30: 1998–2006.
33. Okamura H, Tsutsi H, Komatsu T, Yutsudo M, Hakura A, et al. (1995) Cloning of a new cytokine that induces IFN-gamma production by T cells. Nature 378: 88–91.
34. Yanaba K, Yoshizaki A, Muroi E, Hara T, Ogawa F, et al. (2009) Elevated Circulating TWEAK Levels in Systemic Sclerosis: Association with Lower Frequency of Pulmonary Fibrosis. J Rheumatol 36: 1657–1662.
35. Park MC, Chung SJ, Park YB, Lee SK (2008) Relationship of serum TWEAK level to cytokine level, disease activity, and response to anti-TNF treatment in patients with rheumatoid arthritis. Scand J Rheumatol 37: 173–178.
36. Johansson C, Ahlborg N, Andersson A, Lundeberg L, Karlsson MA, et al. (2009) Elevated peripheral allergen-specific T cell response is crucial for a positive atopy patch test reaction. Int Arch Allergy Immunol 150: 51–58.
37. Kunz B, Oranje AP, Labreze L, Stalder JF, Ring J, et al. (1997) Clinical validation and guidelines for the SCORAD index: consensus report of the European Task Force on Atopic Dermatitis. Dermatology 195: 10–19.
38. Zargari A, Midgley G, Back O, Johansson SG, Scheynius A (2003) IgE-reactivity to seven Malassezia species. Allergy 58: 306–311.

8

B-RAF Mutant Alleles Associated with Langerhans Cell Histiocytosis, a Granulomatous Pediatric Disease

Takeshi Satoh[1,9], Alexander Smith[2,9], Aurelien Sarde[1,9], Hui-chun Lu[3], Sophie Mian[2], Celine Trouillet[1], Ghulam Mufti[2], Jean-Francois Emile[4], Franca Fraternali[3], Jean Donadieu[5], Frederic Geissmann[1]*

1 School of Medicine, Centre for Molecular and Cellular Biology of Inflammation (CMCBI), King's College London, London, United Kingdom, **2** Haematology Department, King's College London, London, United Kingdom, **3** Randall Division of Molecular Biophysics, King's College London, London, United Kingdom, **4** Hopital Ambroise-Pare, Pathology department, AP-HP, Paris, France, **5** Centre de Référence de l'Histiocytose, Hopital d'Enfants Armand Trousseau, Pediatric Hematology Unit, AP-HP, Paris, France

Abstract

Background: Langerhans cell histiocytosis (LCH) features inflammatory granuloma characterised by the presence of CD1a+ dendritic cells or 'LCH cells'. Badalian-Very et al. recently reported the presence of a canonical ^{V600E}B-RAF mutation in 57% of paraffin-embedded biopsies from LCH granuloma. Here we confirm their findings and report the identification of two novel B-RAF mutations detected in LCH patients.

Methods and Results: Mutations of B-RAF were observed in granuloma samples from 11 out of 16 patients using 'next generation' pyrosequencing. In 9 cases the mutation identified was ^{V600E}B-RAF. In 2 cases novel polymorphisms were identified. A somatic ^{600DLAT}B-RAF insertion mimicked the structural and functional consequences of the ^{V600E}B-RAF mutant. It destabilized the inactive conformation of the B-RAF kinase and resulted in increased ERK activation in 293 T cells. The ^{600DLAT}B-RAF and ^{V600E}B-RAF mutations were found enriched in DNA and mRNA from the CD1a+ fraction of granuloma. They were absent from the blood and monocytes of 58 LCH patients, with a lower threshold of sequencing sensitivity of 1% 2% relative mutation abundance. A novel germ line ^{T599A}B-RAF mutant allele was detected in one patient, at a relative mutation abundance close to 50% in the LCH granuloma, blood monocytes and lymphocytes. However, ^{T599A}B-RAF did not destabilize the inactive conformation of the B-RAF kinase, and did not induce increased ERK phosphorylation or C-RAF transactivation.

Conclusions: Our data confirmed presence of the ^{V600E}B-RAF mutation in LCH granuloma of some patients, and identify two novel B-RAF mutations. They indicate that ^{V600E}B-RAF and ^{600DLAT}B-RAF mutations are somatic mutants enriched in LCH CD1a^{+} cells and absent from the patient blood. Further studies are needed to assess the functional consequences of the germ-line ^{T599A}B-RAF allele.

Editor: Alice Y. W. Chang, Kaohsiung Chang Gung Memorial Hospital, Taiwan

Funding: TS is a fellow of the Japan Society for the Promotion of Science (JSPS) and FG is the Arthritis Research UK Chair of Inflammation Biology, at King's College London. This study was also funded by grants from the Histiocytosis Research Trust (HRT) and MRC G0900867 from the Medical Research Council (UK) to FG. The funders had no role in study design, data collection and analysis, decision to publish, or preparation of the manuscript.

Competing Interests: The authors have declared that no competing interests exist.

* E-mail: frederic.geissmann@kcl.ac.uk

9 These authors contributed equally to this work.

Introduction

Langerhans cell histiocytosis (LCH) is a pediatric granulomatous disease with an incidence of four to eight cases per million children [1,2,3]. The clinical spectrum of LCH is remarkably broad, ranging from isolated skin or bone lesions to a disseminated disease that may require aggressive chemotherapy [1,4,5]. LCH can lead to severe dental and periodontal lesions [6]. LCH also frequently leads to diabetes insipidus [1,2,3]. Apart from diabetes insipidus, central nervous system involvement in Langerhans cell histiocytosis (LCH) is rare but represent a serious complication with neurological deterioration, including progressive cerebellar ataxia [7].

LCH lesions feature granulomatous collections of immature CD1a+ langerin/CD207+ DC ('LCH cells') presumed to be pathologic [8,9,10], admixed with abundant eosinophils [11], polyclonal T cells including abundant FoxP3^{+} CD4^{+} T cells [12], activated macrophages and osteoclast-like multinucleated giant cells [13]. These granuloma are therefore heterogeneous in cellular composition as well as anatomical distribution. The pathophysiology of LCH is largely unknown [10,14], although a genetic component is suggested by a higher concordance rate between monozygotic twins compared with dizygotic twins [15]. The tropism of skin lesions to flexures also suggests that external stimuli may trigger inflammation [16]. However, the nature of the initiating event(s), and the mechanisms of local tissue destruction by LCH and other inflammatory cells are still largely unknown.

Clonality of LCH granulomas has been reported in 1994 [17,18]. Its significance remained controversial, since specific genetic abnormalities were not consistently observed [19], until recently. Progress came from the identification by Badalian-Very et al., of a ^{V600E}B-RAF mutation by pyrosequencing of formalin-fixed, paraffin-embedded material, from 35 out of 61 archived specimens (57%) [20]. This ^{V600E}B-RAF mutation is likely to be somatic, because a germ-line activating ^{V600E}B-RAF allele is embryonic lethal in mice [21]. B-RAF is a protein kinase activated by ras-coupled receptor tyrosine kinases (RTK) that is central to signaling via the Mitogen Activated Kinase (MAPK) and phosphorylates its downstream target MEK and ERK kinases [22]. The RAS-RAF-MAPK pathway coordinates a large variety of cellular responses involved in development, cell cycle regulation, cell proliferation and differentiation, cell survival and apoptosis, and many other physiological processes, by transmitting extracellular signals to various nuclear, cytoplasmic and membrane-bound targets [22].

Data obtained from murine model using Cre-mediated activation of a conditionnal B-RAF allele indicate that ^{V600E}B-RAF can contribute to tumour initiation [23]. For example, ^{V600E}B-RAF induces high levels of cyclin D1-mediated cell proliferation. However, ^{V600E}B-RAF also induces oncogene-induced senescence (OIS) that may restrain further development of the tumour [23,24]. In human, somatic ^{V600E}B-RAF mutation have been found in a number of benign and malignant tumors including non-malignant naevi [25], melanoma [26], colon and thyroid tumors [21,22,24,26]. Thus ^{V600E}B-RAF may represent a first step toward the development of a malignant tumor, although the presence of a ^{V600E}B-RAF mutation is not synonymous with cancer.

Of note, the clinical features of LCH are not typical of cancer [10,14] and LCH lesions frequently regress, either spontaneously or after local treatment [1,4,5]. In addition, LCH CD1a+ cells, which are presumed to be pathologic, very slowly proliferate in most patients [12], while the expansion of a monocyte or dendritic cell compartment, which represent candidate precursors for these CD1a+ cells of the granuloma, was not consistently observed in the blood of LCH patients [12,27].

Identification of dysregulation of the RAS-RAF-MAPK pathway in LCH is nevertheless an important step towards a molecular understanding of the pathophysiology of this pediatric granuloma. It suggests possible novel therapeutic approaches, e.g. the use of B-RAF or MEK inhibitors. Moreover, if ^{V600E}B-RAF was detectable in the patient's blood, this could be of use for diagnostic, monitoring of treatment efficacy, and potentially prognostic purposes.

We therefore sought firstly to confirm the finding of Badalian-Very using another methodology i.e. analyzing flow sorted CD1a+ cells from fresh LCH granuloma tissue instead of paraffin embedded biopsies. We then aimed to compare relative mutation abundance of V600E B-RAF mutations between CD1a+ and CD1a− cells from LCH granuloma, and whether mutations can be detected in the peripheral blood of patients. Finally we investigated whether additional B-RAF mutations can be found in LCH patients, to further reinforce the link between LCH and the RAS-RAF pathway.

Results

B-RAF polymorphisms associated with LCH

We investigated the presence of B-RAF mutations by 'next generation' pyrosequencing (Roche GS FLX 454) in a series of 16 granuloma samples obtained at diagnosis from 16 patients with LCH from a cohort followed in the French LCH Registry (Tables 1 & 2). Among granuloma samples 11/16 carried B-RAF mutations as detected by pyrosequencing of granuloma genomic DNA (gDNA) and cDNA (Table 1). In 9/11 cases (patients #1–9) we found a g1799 T>A transition resulting in the previously described ^{V600E}B-RAF mutation [20] (Figure 1 A). In one patient (patient #10) we found a novel in-frame insertion of 12 nucleotides, leading to the insertion of 4 amino acids (Asp-Leu-Ala-Thr, or DLAT) (Figure 1 A). In one other patient we observed an A>G transversion, producing a ^{T599A}B-RAF allele (Table 2, Figure 1 A). The ^{T599A}B-RAF and ^{600DLAT}B-RAF alleles were not previously reported in the literature, dbSNP (v131), or in data from 1000 genomes project (Nov 10 release).

Somatic B-RAF mutations

The ^{V600E}B-RAF and ^{600DLAT}B-RAF, mutations were detected in granuloma from patients 1–10 with a high relative mutation abundance (RMA) (Table 2) We therefore investigated whether these alleles were germ-line or somatic mutants, and which cellular fraction of the granuloma was bearing the mutation. In 4 cases of ^{V600E}B-RAF mutation (Patients 4, 5, 8, 9) and in the sample carrying the ^{600DLAT}B-RAF mutation (patient #10) (Table 2), CD1a+ cells were enriched from fresh granuloma tissue using antibody-coupled beads [8]. The CD1a-depleted fractions (Effluent, Table 2) were also collected in 4 cases (Patients 5, 8, 9, 10, Table 2). Genomic DNA and cDNA were extracted from all samples and analysed by next generation sequencing. In all cases B-RAF mutated alleles were enriched in the CD1a+ fraction at the genomic DNA and cDNA level, in comparison with the CD1a-depleted fractions, with a relative mutation abundance of up to 48% (Table 2), suggesting that the CD1a+ 'LCH cells' carry a heterozygous B-RAF mutant allele, though we did not assess heterozygosity at the single cell level. We then investigated whether ^{V600E}B-RAF or ^{600DLAT}B-RAF mutations could be found in the patients circulating myeloid or lymphoid cells, either because of a germ-line mutation, or because of a mosaicism in bone marrow progenitors. Analysis by pyrosequencing of whole blood and of purified monocytes (CD14+) and lymphocytes (CD14−) from patient 1 indicated the absence of detectable B-RAF mutations, with a lower threshold of sequencing sensitivity of 1%–2% relative mutation abundance. Analysis of whole blood from patient 2 with the same method also failed to detect a ^{V600E}B-RAF mutation. Blood samples were not available for the 8 other patients with a ^{V600E}B-RAF or ^{600DLAT}B-RAF mutation.

We therefore investigated the presence of B-RAF mutations in peripheral blood mononuclear cells of an additional series of LCH patients for whom blood samples were available either at diagnosis or relapse (n = 22) (Table 3), or under treatment (n = 32). Neither ^{V600E}B-RAF or ^{600DLAT}B-RAF were detectable by pyrosequencing in these 56 peripheral blood mononuclear cell samples (Tables 2 & 3, and data not shown). Unfortunately granuloma samples were not availables for these patients, however based on the frequency of B-RAF mutation in LCH granuloma, 57% in the Badalian-Very study, and 11/16 (68%) in the present study, it is likely that several of the 56 patients had a B-RAF mutation in their granuloma.

In aggregate, these data indicate that ^{V600E}B-RAF and ^{600DLAT}B-RAF mutations are detectable in granuloma but not in the blood, and thus strongly suggest they are somatic events. In addition, lack of detection of B-RAF mutations in the blood from patients 1 and 2 and from the 22 others patients for whom blood samples were available at diagnosis or relapse suggests that detection of potential circulating B-RAF mutated cells will require a threshold of sensitivity below 1%.

Germline B-RAF polymorphisms

In contrast, the ^{T599A}B-RAF mutation was detected in both the granuloma and the whole blood of patient #16. ^{T599A}B-RAF was

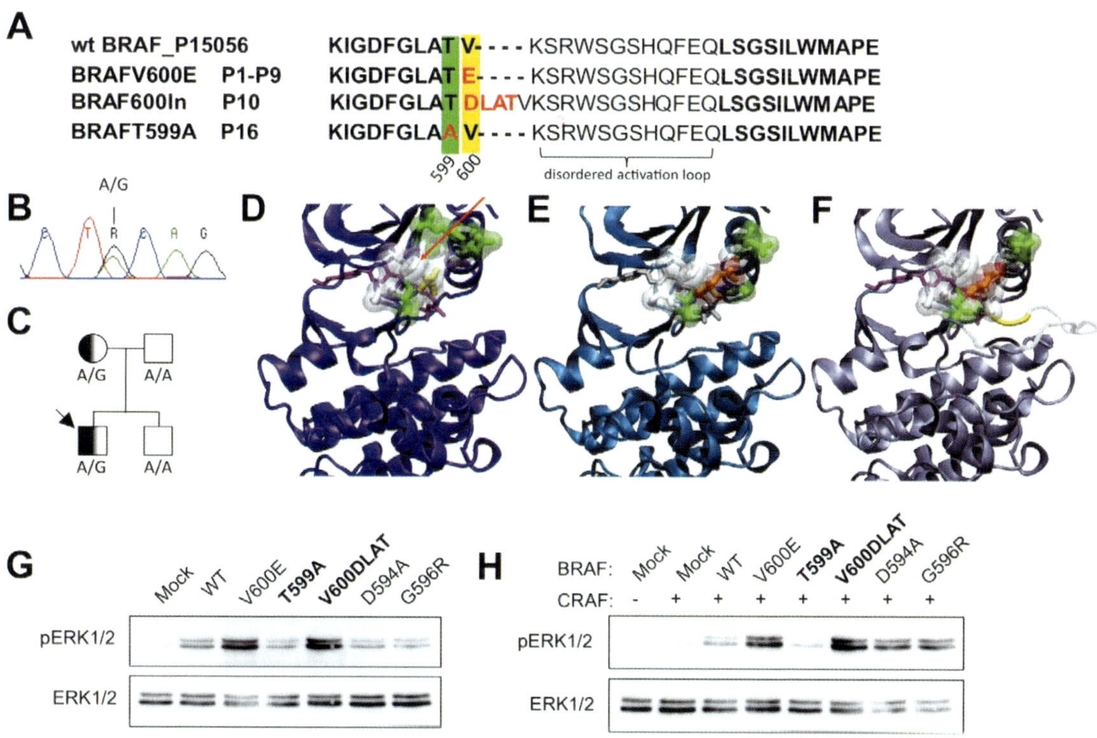

Figure 1. Analysis of B-RAF mutant. A. Sequence alignment, results from 454 pyrosequencing of granuloma cells from patients 1–10 and 16. **B.** 'Sanger' sequencing of patient 16 blood; A/G transition at nucleotide 1795. **C.** Pedigree of patient 16. Both the patient and his mother carry a ^{T599A}B-RAF allele, while his father is ^{wt}B-RAF. **D–E.** Comparison between ^{wt}B-RAF 5P_15056 (D, purple), ^{V600E}B-RAF structure (E, cyan) and the modeled mutant ^{600DLAT}B-RAF (F, grey). In D, Val600 (yellow) forms a hydrophobic contact with Phe468 (red arrow). In E and F charged residues Asp and Glu (in orange) disrupt the hydrophobic network of interactions, stabilising the active conformation of the P-loop. In F, insertion Asp-Leu-Ala-Thr shifted Val600 and disrupt the hydrophobic cluster. **G, H.** MEK phosphorylation in 293 T cells. 293 T cells were transiently transfected with with mock or B-RAF mutant expressing vectors (WT, V600E, T599A, 600DLAT, D594A, G596R), and with (H) or without (G) wtC-RAF. Twenty-four hours after transfection, the medium was changed to serum-free DMEM, followed by further 18 hours culture. Total cell lysates were immunoblotted with the indicated antibodies.

Table 1. Age, sex, and clinical characteristics of patients 1 to 16.

Patient#	NUP	age at diagnosis (y)	sex	clinical features
#1	1506614	7.9	F	bone
#2	1506751	9	M	bone
#3	2106401	0.26	M	skin, lung, lymph node
#4	2106143	0.5	M	LETTERER SIWE hematological dysfunction, bone, liver, spleen
#5	1406259	8.4	F	bone
#6	1506706	19	M	Skin
#7	2106169	0.438	F	LETTERER SIWE hematological dysfunction, bone, liver, spleen, pituitary
#8	1406253	8.6	F	bone
#9	1406254	7.6	M	bone
#10	1406015	0	F	LETTERER SIWE hematological dysfunction, bone, liver, spleen, pituitary, lung, lymph nodes
#11	1406210	10	M	bone
#12	1506008	0.97	F	LETTERER SIWE hematological dysfunction, bone, lung, liver, spleen
#13	1406215	5.3	M	bone
#14	1406247	7.59	F	bone, lymph node
#15	1506766	11.79	F	bone
#16	1506646	1	M	skin, bone

Table 2. Presence and relative abundance of B-RAF mutant clones identified in granuloma and blood from patients with LCH.

		granuloma							
		total	gDNA		cDNA		blood, gDNA		
Patient#	NUP	gDNA	CD1a+	effluent	CD1a+	effluent	whole blood	CD14+	CD14−
#1	1506614	V600E 13,5%					wt	wt	wt
#2	1506751	V600E 29,4%					wt		
#3	2106401	V600E 16%							
#4	2106143		V600E 35%		V600E 40%				
#5	1406259		V600E 38%	V600E 22%	V600E 46%	V600E 24%			
#6	1506706	V600E 8%							
#7	2106169	V600E 9%							
#8	1406253		V600E 21%	V600E 8%	V600E 48%	V600E 6%			
#9	1406254		V600E 35%	V600E 23%	V600E 47%	V600E 35%			
#10	1406015		600DLAT 11%	600DLAT 5%	600DLAT 28%	600DLAT 11%			
#11	1406210	wt							
#12	1506008	wt							
#13	1406215	wt							
#14	1406247	wt							
#15	1506766	wt						wt	wt
#16	1506646	T599A 44%					T599A 37%	T599A 37%	T599A 45%

detected in the monocytic (CD14+) and lymphoid fractions (CD14−), at a high frequency of 37 to 45% relative mutation abundance, respectively, similar to its abundance in the granuloma (Table 2). This pattern suggested a germ-line mutation. Conventional 'Sanger' sequencing of peripheral blood mononuclear cells from the patient and from the patient's mother with an Applied Biosystem Genetic analyzer 3730xl confirmed the presence of an allelic mutation (Figure 1 B). Therefore the ^{T599A}B-RAF mutation was present in the peripheral blood of the patient and his mother, indicating a germ-line transmitted allele (Figure 1 C).

Altogether, these data indicate that ^{V600E}B-RAF and ^{600DLAT}B-RAF are somatic events while ^{T599A}B-RAF is a germ-line polymorphism.

B-RAF 600DLAT is an activating B-RAF mutant

Substitution of Val600 with Glu (^{V600E}B-RAF) strongly activates B-RAF [28,29]. ^{600DLAT}B-RAF is an in-frame insertion of 12 nucleotides leading to the insertion of 4 amino acids (Asp-Leu-Ala-Thr, or DLAT) starting from position 600 (Figure 1 A). This insertion, in the structural alignment superimposed to the V600 position, therefore effectively results in a B-RAFV600D substitution, leaving the insertion constituted only by a LATV segment. We have examined the residues surrounding D600 in the structure within a cut-off range of 6 Å. As reported by Wan et al. [29] the V600 residue is in a cluster of hydrophobic residues with Phe468, therefore the presence of a negative charge (residue D) will disrupt this cluster, resulting in destabilization of the inactive conformation of ^{600DLAT}B-RAF, exactly as for the V600E mutant (Figure 1 D–F). As expected from our structural modelisation study, ^{600DLAT}B-RAF resulted in increased MEK and ERK activation upon transient transfection in 293 T cells in comparison to wild-type B-RAF, similar to what is observed for ^{V600E}B-RAF [29] (Figure 1). However, we could not investigate the role of ^{V600E}B-RAF and ^{600DLAT}B-RAF in myeloid cells, since, when transfected in U937 and THP1 myeloid cell lines both ^{V600E}B-RAF and ^{600DLAT}B-RAF resulted in growth arrest and cell death (data not shown).

B-RAF T599A is a dead-kinase B-RAF mutant that does not transactivate C-RAF

Thr599 is a major phosphorylation site in the B-RAF activation domain [28], and substitution of Thr599 with alanine was shown in vitro to suppress B-RAF activity. Indeed, in contrast to ^{V600E}B-RAF and ^{600DLAT}B-RAF, ^{T599A}B-RAF substitutes a polar uncharged residue with a hydrophobic residue, causing the loss of short-ranged interactions with residues D576 and D594 (Figure 1 A, B). This does not predict a destabilization of the inactive conformation of B-RAF. Indeed transfection of ^{T599A}B-RAF in 293 T cells did not increase MEK and ERK phosphorylation, in comparison to wt control (Figure 1 G). Co-transfection of C-RAF did not increase MEK and ERK phosphorylation in the presence of ^{T599A}B-RAF (Figure 1 H). To further investigate the function of ^{T599A}B-RAF in myeloid cells, we retrovirally transfected ^{wt}B-RAF and ^{T599A}B-RAF in THP1 myeloid cells. As shown in Figure 2 C and 2 D ^{T599A}B-RAF did not induce MEK and ERK phosphorylation in THP1 cells above control (Figure 2 C). Thus ^{T599A}B-RAF may represent a mutant devoid of intrinsic kinase activity.

However, some B-RAF mutants found in cancer such as ^{D594A}B-RAF, albeit devoid of intrinsic B-RAF kinase activity, can transactivate C-RAF and the MEK/ERK pathway [30,31]. We thus compared the activity of ^{T599A}B-RAF with that of ^{wt}B-RAF and ^{D594A}B-RAF after retroviral transfection into U937 cells. Results indicated that unlike ^{D594A}B-RAF, ^{T599A}B-RAF did not induce MEK/ERK phosphorylation (Figure 2 D, E) or IL-8 production (Figure 2 F) by U937 cells.

Table 3. Age, sex, clinical features, and molecular findings in 22 patients with available blood samples at the time of diagnosis or relapse.

patient #	NUP	Clinical features	status at the time of blood sample	BRAF		
				whole blood	CD14+	CD14−
#17	1406220	bone skin, ENT, pituitary, neuro	active/progressive disease	na	wt	wt
#18	1506752	skin	active/progressive disease	wt	na	na
#19	1506604	Bone, skin, hematological dysfunction	active/progressive disease	wt	na	na
#20	1506648	Bone, skin, ENT, lung, liver, hematological dysfunction	active/progressive disease	wt	na	na
#21	1506882	Skin, ENT	active/progressive disease	wt	na	na
#22	1506863	Bone, skin, ENT, lung, liver, hematological dysfunction	active/progressive disease	wt	na	na
#23	1506009	Bone, skin, ENT, nodes, pituitary, lung, liver, spleen, hematological dysfunction	active/progressive disease	wt	na	na
#24	1507109	skin, ENT, pituitary	active/progressive disease	wt	na	na
#25	2106005	Bone, skin, ENT, CNS mass lesion	active/progressive disease	wt	na	na
#26	1509003	bone	at diagnosis, before treatment	wt	na	na
#27	1506819	bone	at diagnosis, before treatment	wt	na	na
#28	1507093	bone	at diagnosis, before treatment	wt	wt	na
#29	1506957	lung	at diagnosis, before treatment	wt	na	na
#30	1506973	bone, pituitary	at diagnosis, before treatment	wt	na	na
#31	1507062	Skin	at diagnosis, before treatment	wt	wt	wt
#32	1506869	bone	1 MONTH DIAGNOSIS	wt	na	na
#33	1507096	bone	<2 MONTH DIAGNOSIS	na	wt	wt
#34	1506754	skin	2 MONTHS DIAGNOSIS	wt	na	na
#35	1506865	bone	2 MONTH DIAGNOSIS	wt	na	na
#36	1507084	skin	2 MONTH DIAGNOSIS	wt	wt	wt
#37	1506932	bone	3 MONTH DIAGNOSIS	wt	wt	na
#38	1506984	skin	3 MONTH DIAGNOSIS	wt	na	na

Clinical features of patients with B-RAF mutations

^{V600E}B-RAF mutations were found both in children with granuloma of bones or isolated skin disease, and in infants with early-onset multi-organ disease (Table 1). Among the 16 studied patients, we compared the proportion of patients with or without B-RAF mutations according to the extension of the disease by Fisher exact test and according to the age of diagnosis by Kruskall Wallis Test. No significant difference was observed as the p value was above 0.05 for all tests. However the sample size was small and may not be representative of a population based sample of patients. The patient with a ^{600DLAT}B-RAF insertion presented with early-onset multi-organ disease, but responded well to treatment (Patient #10, Table 1). The patient with a germ-line ^{T599A}B-RAF allele (Patient #16, Table 1) presented at the age of 10 months with persistent swelling of the left parietal bone. Two months after, clinical examination revealed 10 small skin nodules. Biopsy of one skin element demonstrated the histological diagnosis of LCH with the presence of CD1a+ cells. Patient #16 received therapy by vinblastine and steroid, as per the LCH III protocol, for a total duration of one year. No reactivation of the disease or sequellae was observed during a 7-year follow-up. His mother, who carried the same allelic mutation, is in good health and did not report a personal history of LCH.

Discussion

In this study we confirm the findings by Badalian-Very et al. [20], that ^{V600E}B-RAF mutations are detected in LCH granuloma, and identify two additional mutations ^{600DLAT}B-RAF and ^{T599A}B-RAF in two LCH patients. The ^{600DLAT}B-RAF mutants mimics ^{V600E}B-RAF at the structural and functional level. Our results also indicate that ^{V600E}B-RAF and ^{600DLAT}B-RAF mutations are enriched in CD1a+ 'LCH' granuloma cells and absent from the blood of 58 patients, suggesting the presence of somatic mutations in CD1a+ cells, and arguing against a mosaicism in the myeloid lineage or a bone marrow clonal disease, within the sensitivity limits of our deep sequencing assay. We also identified a novel germ-line ^{T599A}B-RAF polymorphism in a patient with LCH, although it remains unclear whether ^{T599A}B-RAF is involved in the pathophysiology of LCH in this patient. The data presented here strengthen the association between B-RAF mutation and a dysregulation of the RAS-RAF-MEK pathway in CD1a+ LCH cells from LCH granuloma.

Both the study by Badalian-Very [20] and our present report fail to show a correlation between the presence of B-RAF mutations in LCH granuloma and the patient's age, clinical presentation, or outcome. However, the total number of cases analysed reported (77 in total) is still too small to allow a powerful

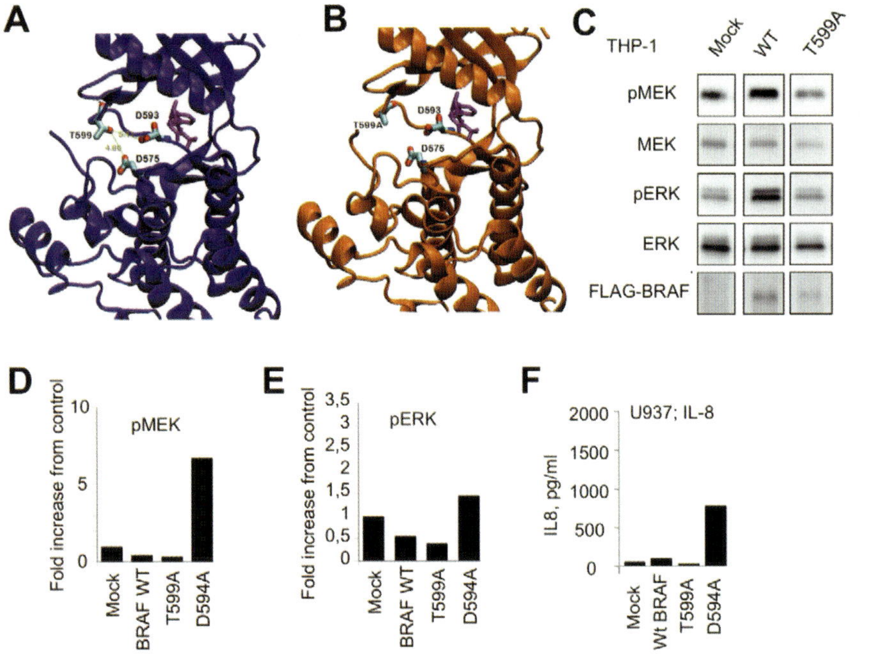

Figure 2. Analysis of ^{T599A}B-RAF. (**A, B**) Comparison between models of ^{WT}B-RAF 5P_15056 (A, violet) and ^{T599A}B-RAF (B, gold). ^{T599A}B-RAF substitutes a polar uncharged residue with a hydrophobic residue, causing the loss of short-ranged interactions with residues D576 and D594. **C.** Analysis of MEK and ERK phosphorylation in THP1 cell lines stably transfected with ^{WT}B-RAF-FLAG and ^{T599A}B-RAF-FLAG. Experiment was repeated twice with similar results. (**D–F**) Analysis of MEK and ERK phosphorylation and IL-8 production in U937 cell lines stably transfected with ^{WT}B-RAF, ^{T599A}B-RAF, and ^{D594A}B-RAF. Experiment was repeated twice with similar results.

statistical analysis, given the marked clinical heterogeneity of the disease [1,4,5]. A statistical study of the possible association or lack of association of B-RAF somatic mutations with subgroups of LCH patients or with the natural history of the disease remains to be done, in a population based approach.

Our results indicate that both ^{600DLAT}B-RAF and ^{V600E}B-RAF mutations are somatic events which are not detected in the blood of patients. LCH granulomas may thus arise from a local process within affected tissues, rather than from the continuous recruitment of putative precursors, such as monocytes or dendritic cells carrying activating B-RAFV600E or B-RAF600DLAT alleles. Nevertheless, given the threshold sensitivity of 1%–2% of our deep-sequencing method, we cannot exclude the contribution of a minor myeloid-restricted clone in the bone marrow of patients, or of a subset of patients, and a prospective investigation is required to further investigate whether detection of rare circulating or bone marrow B-RAF mutated cells may be useful to monitor residual disease.

While substitution of Val600 with Glu (^{V600E}B-RAF) strongly activates B-RAF, substitution of Thr599 with Ala (^{T599A}B-RAF) impairs B-RAF kinase activity [28,29] given that Thr599 is the major phosphorylation site in the B-RAF activation domain [28]. Other mutations that affect intrinsic B-RAF kinase activity such as ^{D594A}B-RAF can also transactivate C-RAF and the MEK/ERK pathway, albeit less strongly [30,31]. However we have shown here that ^{T599A}B-RAF was both impaired in its intrinsic B-RAF kinase activity and unable to transactivate C-RAF. At this time, we do not have a molecular explanation for this observation. Further studies will therefore be needed to potentially unveil the functional consequences of the ^{T599A}B-RAF allele on cell activation. The patient's mother born in 1977 carried the same B-RAFT599A allele while in good health, and without a personal history of LCH. Therefore, although the ^{T599A}B-RAF allele is not a common polymorphism, there is no evidence that ^{T599A}B-RAF is involved in the pathophysiology of LCH in our patient. However the clinical spectrum of LCH is remarkably broad, and the age of onset highly variable [1,4,5], preventing us to definitely conclude to the absence of LCH in the mother of the patient. For instance, in one previously reported case of familial LCH, a monostotic lesion was diagnosed in a 20-year-old woman and then also in her daughter when aged 30 months [32].

Finally, ^{V600E}B-RAF mutations are observed in a number of benign and tumoral diseases (e.g. naevi and melanoma [25,26]). In itself this mutation thus do not characterize a malignant disease. It is posssible that the effects of activating B-RAF mutations such as ^{V600E}B-RAF and ^{600DLAT}B-RAF are different whenever they occur in stem cells or and differentiated cells, and depending on the lineage of the mutated cells, i.e. epithelial or myeloid. Therefore, more work is needed to understand the consequences of ^{V600E}B-RAF and ^{600DLAT}B-RAF in myeloid cells. We observed that retroviral transduction of either ^{V600E}B-RAF or ^{600DLAT}B-RAF in U937 and THP1 myeloid cell lines resulted in growth arrest and cell death. This suggests that an in vivo approach may be preferable, since an appropriate cellular environment could be required to support cell growth of ^{V600E}B-RAF or ^{600DLAT}B-RAF expressing myeloid cells. In this regard, mouse models of conditional expression of B-RAF mutant alleles in different cell lineages [23], should prove extremely useful.

Materials and Methods

Patients

Patients were registered in the National French Registry for Langerhans Cell Histiocytosis. LCH diagnosis was established on the basis of the patients' clinical history, histological examination and the mandatory presence of CD1a+ histiocytes in clinical biopsy specimens, and reviewed by a national panel of pathologists. Patient's parents gave written informed consent for the study. The Study was approved by the Institutional Review Board of the University Hospital of Nantes, France. Characteristic of patients 1–16 are summarized in Table 1. Biopsies samples and/or blood were obtained at diagnosis from 15 patients with various clinical forms of the disease, isolated involvement of bone (n = 9), early-onset multisystem disease (n = 4), isolated skin (n = 1) and skin and lung disease (n = 1) (Table 1). Purified CD1a+ cells were isolated from biopsies from patients with eosinophilic granuloma of bone (n = 3) and early-onset multisystem disease (n = 3). Blood was obtain from patient 16 and his parents, and epithelial cells from patient 16, his parents and brother.

Preparation of DNA from granuloma samples, whole blood, and purified cellular fractions

Samples from CD1a+ LCH cells were obtained as previously described [8]. In brief, after frozen section examination, sterile tissue from eosinophilic granuloma was harvested in RPMI 1640 supplemented with 2 mM L-glutamine, 100 U/mL penicillin, 100 µg/mL streptomycin, and 10% heat-inactivated fetal calf serum (FCS) myoclone (all from GIBCO BRL, Gaithersburg, MD), referred to below as complete medium. Tissues were immediately gently dissociated through a nylon mesh. The cell suspension was washed 3 times and incubated with human IgG to block Fc receptor, and anti-CD1a antibody (BLG; Immunotech, Marseille, France). The cells were washed twice, incubated with antimouse microbeads (MACS; Miltenyi Biotec, Bergisch Gladbach, Germany) for 15 minutes at 4°C. Cells were washed again, and then CD1a+ LCH cells were separated by positive immunomagnetic selection by using a magnetic cell separator (MACS) according to the manufacturer's instructions. Between 2.105 and 6.105 CD1a+ cells were recovered from each sample. Purity of CD1a+ and CD1alow/neg sorted fraction was 80% or greater and mortality 10% or less. Genomic DNA and RNA from frozen granuloma cells, sorted CD1a+ cells and effluent fractions lysed and stored in Trizol were extracted using chloroform, the organic phase was transferred to a fresh tube to extract genomic DNA, and RNA was extracted using the RNA microkit from Qiagen. cDNA was obtained using the Superscript III Reverse-transcriptase kit (Invitrogen) according to the manufacturer's procedure. Genomic DNA extraction from paraffin sections (Patient 16) was performed as per Qiagen protocol for this material. Genomic DNA extraction from whole Blood was performed using the GenElute Blood genomic DNA kit mini prep from Sigma Aldrich according to the manufacturer procedure. Peripheral blood mononuclear cells (PBMCs) were obtained by the standard Ficoll-Hypaque method. CD14+ and CD14− fraction were separated by negative magnetic depletion by using hapten-conjugated CD3, CD7, CD19, CD45RA, CD56, and anti-IgE antibodies (MACS; Miltenyi Biotec) and a MACS according to the manufacturer's instructions. gDNA and RNA were extracted from CD14+ and CD14− MACS purificated monocytes fractions using the RNA/DNA AllPrep QIAgen Minikit (Quiagen).

B-RAF mutation detection

Pyrosequencing assay was performed using with 454 sequencing (Roche GS FLX platform). Primers sets were designed to amplify B-RAF exons 11 and 15 from both genomic DNA and cDNA, which incorporated a universal forward and reverse sequence tag. A second round of PCR was also performed utilizing the universal tags, to incorporate a sample specific 10 bp "barcode" sequence as well as additional tags utilized in the sequencing process (Roche GS FLX Titanium). Sequencing was performed to yield a 'depth' in excess of 500 clonal reads (500×) per exonic amplicon, per patient sample in most cases. This allowed detection of mutant clones down to around 1–2% relative mutation abundance, defined as the proportion of sequence reads that contain the mutation. Independent PCR and GS FLX sequencing experiments were carried out to confirm mutations and to reduce sampling error for calculations of mutation abundance. Somatic mutation in patient #16, his parents and his sibling were confirmed using a Applied Biosystem Genetic analyzer 3730xl (primers available on request).

B-RAF mutation modeling

The B-RAF patient mutations ^{600DLAT}B-RAF and ^{T599A}B-RAF have been modeled starting from the structure of the B-RAF kinase domain [29] using the Modeller 9v8 program [33]. The sequence alignment on this domain with the observed patient mutations was performed with the program Praline [34]. The structural alignment of the mutated sequences with the chosen template (pdb code 1WUH) was performed with the program T-coffee [35]. For each mutant, 200 structures have been generated and the ones with the best DOPE score have been selected for further investigations. The VMD program [36] has been used for graphical representations and for structural analyses.

Transfection of B-RAF alleles in 293 T cells

293 T (Lenti-X 293 T) was purchased from Clontech, and maintained in DMEM supplemented with 10% FBS, 100 units/ml Penicillin, and 100 mg/ml Streptomycin. cDNA fragments of human B-RAF (Genbank accession number: NM_004333) and C-RAF (Genbank accession number: NM_002880) were amplified by RT-PCR from human PBMC cDNA and cloned into pMXs-puro vector. V600E, T599A, D594A, and G596R B-RAF mutants construct were obtained by site-direct mutagenesis (Agilent Technologies). DLAT insertion B-RAF mutant construct was generated by PCR. The constructs were FLAG-tagged and cloned into pMXs-puro and pMXs-IRES-GFP vectors. The mutations were confirmed by DNA sequencing.

293 T was transiently transfected with pMXs-puro, FLAG-B-RAF WT, V600E, T599A, 600DLAT, D564A, G596R, or FLAG-CRAFvectors as indicated in the figure. Transfection was carried out with jetPEI according to the manufacture's instructions (Polyplus transfections, Inc.).

Generation of stable B-RAF transfectants using retroviral vector

Retrovirus packaging cell line, Plat-A was purchased from Cell Biolabs, Inc., and maintained in DMEM supplemented with 10% FBS, 100 units/ml Penicillin, and 100 mg/ml Streptomycin. U937 was kindly donated by Dr. Taams. THP-1 was kindly donated by Dr. Neil. These cell lines were maintained in RPMI supplemented with 10% FBS, 100 units/ml Penicillin, and 100 mg/ml Streptomycin (complete medium). Plat-A was transiently transfected with pMXs-IRES-GFP, FLAG-B-RAF WT, V600E, T599A, 600DLAT, D594A, and G596R vectors using jetPEI. Twenty-four hours after transfection, the medium was changed to fresh DMEM, and the cells were cultured for further 24 hours. The virus supernatants were collected and the debris was removed by centrifuge. The supernatants were mixed with DOTAP Liposomal Transfection Reagent (Roche) and added to U937 or THP-1 culture, followed by centrifuge at 30°C at 1100×g for 2 hours. Forty-eight hours after infection, GFP positive cells were sorted using BD FACSAria (BD Biosciences) and maintained in complete medium.

Western-Blot analysis

Twenty-four hours after transfection to 293 T cells, culture medium was changed to serum-free DMEM and cells starved for 18 hours. Cells were lysed with RIPA buffer (20 mM Tris-HCl (pH7.4), 150 mM NaCl, 2 mM EDTA, 1% Nonidet-P 40, 0.1% Sodium dodecyl sulfate, 0.1% Sodium deoxycolate, 50 mM Sodium fluoride, 1 mM b-Glycerophosphate, 1 mM Sodium orthovanadate, 1 mM Phenylmethylsulfonyl fluoride, and Protease inhibitor cocktail (Sigma-Aldrich)). For the experiment using THP-1 transfectant, 1×10^6 of growing cells were colllected by centrifuge and lysed in RIPA buffer. The cell lysates were separated on 10% SDS-PAGE gel and transferred onto nitrocellulose membranes (Bio-Rad). The membrane were blotted with anti-phospho-MEK1/2 mAb (41G9), anti-MEK1/2 mAb (L38C12), anti-phospho-ERK1/2 (D13.14.4E), anti-ERK1/2 mAb (L34F12) all from Cell Signaling Technology, Inc., and anti-FLAG M2 (Sigma Aldrich). Horseradish peroxidase-coupled secondary antibodies were used to detect the primary antibodies. Signal was revealed by enhanced chemiluminescence (SuperSignal West Pico Chemiluminescent Substrate, Pierce) using a molecular imager Chemidoc™ XRS+, Biorad. Band intensity was quantified by ImageLab™ Analysis Software.

Quantification of pMEK, pERK, and IL-8 from U937 transfectant by Bio-Plex

For the measurement of IL-8 secretion, 1×104 of U937 transfectants ware laid in a 96 well plate in 100 microL. After 24 hours, the plate were centrifuged and supernatants were collected. For pMEK and pERK, 1×104 of U937 were lysed using Bio-Plex Cell Lysis kit. The samples were analyzed according to manufactures instructions.

Statistics

Unsupervised students t-test on single comparisons was compared to analyse significance. A P value$<$0.05 was considered significant.

Acknowledgments

The authors thank patients and their families for participating to the study, Dempsey and his family, and the association Histiocytose france for constant support. We thank Dr Elisa Gomez-Perdigero and Dr Brigitte Senechal for helpful discussions.

Author Contributions

Conceived and designed the experiments: FG JD TS. Performed the experiments: A. Smith A. Sarde H-CL SM CT. Analyzed the data: FG FF JD. Contributed reagents/materials/analysis tools: GM JFE. Wrote the paper: FG.

References

1. Guyot-Goubin A, Donadieu J, Barkaoui M, Bellec S, Thomas C, et al. (2008) Descriptive epidemiology of childhood Langerhans cell histiocytosis in France, 2000–2004. Pediatr Blood Cancer 51: 71–75.
2. Salotti JA, Nanduri V, Pearce MS, Parker L, Lynn R, et al. (2009) Incidence and clinical features of Langerhans cell histiocytosis in the UK and Ireland. Arch Dis Child 94: 376–380.
3. Stalemark H, Laurencikas E, Karis J, Gavhed D, Fadeel B, et al. (2008) Incidence of Langerhans cell histiocytosis in children: a population-based study. Pediatr Blood Cancer 51: 76–81.
4. Group TFLCHS (1996) A multicentre retrospective survey of Langerhans' cell histiocytosis: 348 cases observed between 1983 and 1993. Arch Dis Child 75: 17–24.
5. Ceci A, de Terlizzi M, Colella R, Loiacono G, Balducci D, et al. (1993) Langerhans cell histiocytosis in childhood: results from the Italian Cooperative AIEOP-CNR-H.X '83 study. Med Pediatr Oncol 21: 259–264.
6. Madrigal-Martinez-Pereda C, Guerrero-Rodriguez V, Guisado-Moya B, Meniz-Garcia C (2009) Langerhans cell histiocytosis: literature review and descriptive analysis of oral manifestations. Med Oral Patol Oral Cir Bucal 14: E222–228.
7. Grois N, Prayer D, Prosch H, Lassmann H (2005) Neuropathology of CNS disease in Langerhans cell histiocytosis. Brain 128: 829–838.
8. Geissmann F, Lepelletier Y, Fraitag S, Valladeau J, Bodemer C, et al. (2001) Differentiation of Langerhans cells in Langerhans cell histiocytosis. Blood 97: 1241–1248.
9. Allen CE, Li L, Peters TL, Leung HC, Yu A, et al. (2010) Cell-specific gene expression in Langerhans cell histiocytosis lesions reveals a distinct profile compared with epidermal Langerhans cells. J Immunol 184: 4557–4567.
10. Egeler RM, van Halteren AG, Hogendoorn PC, Laman JD, Leenen PJ (2010) Langerhans cell histiocytosis: fascinating dynamics of the dendritic cell-macrophage lineage. Immunol Rev 234: 213–232.
11. Annels NE, Da Costa CE, Prins FA, Willemze A, Hogendoorn PC, et al. (2003) Aberrant chemokine receptor expression and chemokine production by Langerhans cells underlies the pathogenesis of Langerhans cell histiocytosis. J Exp Med 197: 1385–1390.
12. Senechal B, Elain G, Jeziorski E, Grondin V, Patey-Mariaud de Serre N, et al. (2007) Expansion of regulatory T cells in patients with Langerhans cell histiocytosis. PLoS Med 4: e253.
13. da Costa CE, Annels NE, Faaij CM, Forsyth RG, Hogendoorn PC, et al. (2005) Presence of osteoclast-like multinucleated giant cells in the bone and nonostotic lesions of Langerhans cell histiocytosis. J Exp Med 201: 687–693.
14. Gasent Blesa JM, Alberola Candel V, Solano Vercet C, Laforga Canales J, Semler C, et al. (2008) Langerhans cell histiocytosis. Clin Transl Oncol 10: 688–696.
15. Arico M, Nichols K, Whitlock JA, Arceci R, Haupt R, et al. (1999) Familial clustering of Langerhans cell histiocytosis. Br J Haematol 107: 883–888.
16. Weitzman S, Egeler RM (2008) Langerhans cell histiocytosis: update for the pediatrician. Curr Opin Pediatr 20: 23–29.
17. Willman CL, Busque L, Griffith BB, Favara BE, McClain KL, et al. (1994) Langerhans'-cell histiocytosis (histiocytosis X)–a clonal proliferative disease. N Engl J Med 331: 154–160.
18. Yu RC, Chu C, Buluwela L, Chu AC (1994) Clonal proliferation of Langerhans cells in Langerhans cell histiocytosis. Lancet 343: 767–768.
19. da Costa CE, Szuhai K, van Eijk R, Hoogeboom M, Sciot R, et al. (2009) No genomic aberrations in Langerhans cell histiocytosis as assessed by diverse molecular technologies. Genes Chromosomes Cancer 48: 239–249.
20. Badalian-Very G, Vergilio JA, Degar BA, Macconaill LE, Brandner B, et al. (2010) Recurrent BRAF mutations in Langerhans cell histiocytosis. Blood.
21. Mercer K, Giblett S, Green S, Lloyd D, DaRocha Dias S, et al. (2005) Expression of endogenous oncogenic V600EB-raf induces proliferation and developmental defects in mice and transformation of primary fibroblasts. Cancer Res 65: 11493–11500.
22. Wellbrock C, Karasarides M, Marais R (2004) The RAF proteins take centre stage. Nat Rev Mol Cell Biol 5: 875–885.
23. Pritchard C, Carragher L, Aldridge V, Giblett S, Jin H, et al. (2007) Mouse models for BRAF-induced cancers. Biochem Soc Trans 35: 1329–1333.
24. Dhomen N, Reis-Filho JS, da Rocha Dias S, Hayward R, Savage K, et al. (2009) Oncogenic Braf induces melanocyte senescence and melanoma in mice. Cancer Cell 15: 294–303.
25. Pollock PM, Harper UL, Hansen KS, Yudt LM, Stark M, et al. (2003) High frequency of BRAF mutations in nevi. Nat Genet 33: 19–20.
26. Dankort D, Curley DP, Cartlidge RA, Nelson B, Karnezis AN, et al. (2009) Braf(V600E) cooperates with Pten loss to induce metastatic melanoma. Nat Genet 41: 544–552.
27. Rolland A, Guyon L, Gill M, Cai YH, Banchereau J, et al. (2005) Increased blood myeloid dendritic cells and dendritic cell-poietins in Langerhans cell histiocytosis. J Immunol 174: 3067–3071.
28. Zhang BH, Guan KL (2000) Activation of B-Raf kinase requires phosphorylation of the conserved residues Thr598 and Ser601. Embo J 19: 5429–5439.
29. Wan PT, Garnett MJ, Roe SM, Lee S, Niculescu-Duvaz D, et al. (2004) Mechanism of activation of the RAF-ERK signaling pathway by oncogenic mutations of B-RAF. Cell 116: 855–867.
30. Kamata T, Hussain J, Giblett S, Hayward R, Marais R, et al. (2010) BRAF inactivation drives aneuploidy by deregulating CRAF. Cancer Res 70: 8475–8486.
31. Heidorn SJ, Milagre C, Whittaker S, Nourry A, Niculescu-Duvas I, et al. (2010) Kinase-dead BRAF and oncogenic RAS cooperate to drive tumor progression through CRAF. Cell 140: 209–221.
32. de Chadarevian JP, Pawel BR (1998) Hereditary Langerhans cell histiocytosis: instances of apparent vertical transmission. Med Pediatr Oncol 31: 559.
33. Eswar N, Eramian D, Webb B, Shen MY, Sali A (2008) Protein structure modeling with MODELLER. Methods Mol Biol 426: 145–159.
34. Simossis VA, Heringa J (2005) PRALINE: a multiple sequence alignment toolbox that integrates homology-extended and secondary structure information. Nucleic Acids Res 33: W289–294.

Actinic Skin Damage and Mortality - the First National Health and Nutrition Examination Survey Epidemiologic Follow-up Study

Wei He[1], Fei Zhu[1], Xiaoguang Ma[2,3], Xinyu Zhao[1], Min Zheng[4], Zhao Chen[5], Steven B. Heymsfield[6], Shankuan Zhu[1,2]*

1 Injury Control Research Center, Obesity and Body Composition Research Center, School of Public Health, Zhejiang University, Hangzhou, China, **2** Injury Research Center, Medical College of Wisconsin, Milwaukee, Wisconsin, United States of America, **3** Department of Epidemiology and Biostatistics, Arnold School of Public Health, University of South Carolina, Columbia, South Carolina, United States of America, **4** Department of Dermatology, Second Affiliated Hospital, Zhejiang University, Hangzhou, China, **5** Division of Epidemiology and Biostatistics, Mel and Enid Zuckerman College of Public Health, University of Arizona, Tucson, Arizona, United States of America, **6** Pennington Biomedical Research Center, Baton Rouge, Louisiana, United States of America

Abstract

Background: Exposure to sunlight may decrease the risk of several diseases through the synthesis of vitamin D, whereas solar radiation is the main cause of some skin and eye diseases. However, to the best of our knowledge, the association of sun-induced skin damage with mortality remains unknown.

Methodology/Principal Findings: Subjects were 8472 white participants aged 25–74 years in the First National Health and Nutrition Examination Survey Epidemiologic Follow-up Study. Cardiovascular disease mortality, cancer mortality, and all-cause mortality were obtained by either a death certificate or a proxy interview, or both. Actinic skin damage was examined and recorded by the presence and severity (absent, minimal, moderate, or severe) of overall actinic skin damage and its components (i.e., fine telangiectasia, solar elastosis, and actinic keratoses). Cox regression and Kaplan-Meier methods were applied to explore the associations. A total of 672 cancer deaths, 1500 cardiovascular disease deaths, and 2969 deaths from all causes were documented through the follow-up between 1971 and 1992. After controlling for potential confounding variables, severe overall actinic skin damage was associated with a 45% higher risk for all-cause mortality (95% CI: 1.22, 1.72; $P<0.001$), moderate overall skin damage with a 20% higher risk (95% CI: 1.08., 1.32; $P<0.001$), and minimal overall skin damage with no significant mortality difference, when compared to those with no skin damage. Similar results were obtained for all-cause mortality with fine telangiectasia, solar elastosis, and actinic keratoses. The results were similar for cancer and cardiovascular disease mortality.

Conclusions: The present study gives an indication of an association of actinic skin damage with cardiovascular disease, cancer and all-cause mortality in white subjects. Given the lack of support in the scientific literature and potential unmeasured confounding factors, this finding should be interpreted with caution. More independent studies are needed before any practical recommendations can be made.

Editor: An-Wen Chan, Women's College Research Institute, University of Toronto, Canada

Funding: This study was supported in part by the "985" development initiative from Zhejiang University, Hangzhou, China. The funders had no role in study design, data collection and analysis, decision to publish, or preparation of the manuscript.

Competing Interests: The authors have declared that no competing interests exist.

* E-mail: zsk@zju.edu.cn

Introduction

Exposure to sunlight can provide people with a sense of wellbeing and a tanned body is viewed as a sign of good health. [1,2] Humans get vitamin D from exposure to sunlight, which may play a role not only in the maintenance of healthy bones, but also in reducing the risk of some illnesses, including autoimmune, infectious, and cardiovascular diseases, and colon, prostate, and breast cancers.[3] In addition, artificial ultraviolet (UV) radiation is used to treat several diseases under medical supervision, including rickets, psoriasis and eczema. [4]

However, overexposure to the sun also carries potential risks to human health. UV radiation is a known carcinogen and excessive exposure increases the risk of lip, skin basal cell and squamous cell carcinomas and cutaneous melanoma, particularly in fair-skinned population. [5] There is also evidence that solar UV radiation increases the risk of several eye diseases, including cortical cataract, some conjunctive neoplasms, and possibly ocular melanoma. [5]

Chronic repeated sunlight exposure can also induce degenerative changes in skin cells, fibrous tissue, and blood vessels, leading to visible signs of actinic skin damage, [4] which is partially characterized by telangiectasia, solar elastosis, and actinic keratoses. [6,7,8,9] Epidemiologic studies have found that people with accelerated aging looking have an increased mortality risk, [10,11] and the skin damage caused by overexposure to sunlight is an important environmental factor for increased facial "aging". [12] However, we are not aware of any study designed to investigate the relation between sun-induced skin damage and mortality.

The present study aims to examine the associations of actinic skin damage with cardiovascular disease mortality, cancer mortality, and all-cause mortality in whites based on the data from the First National Health and Nutrition Examination Survey (NHANES I) Epidemiologic Follow-up Study (NHEFS), which is characterized by a large sample size and an average of a 16-year follow-up.

Methods

Ethics statement

The primary NHANES I and NHEFS were approved by the National Center for Health Statistics (NCHS) Institutional Review Board.[13] The present study was approved by the Ethics Committee of Zhejiang University School of Public Health.

Participants

The First National Health and Nutrition Examination Survey (NHANES I) was conducted between 1971 and 1975 by the National Center for Health Statistics based on a probability sample of the civilian noninstitutionalized population of the United States. [14,15,16] The NHANES I Epidemiologic Follow-up Study (NHEFS) is a longitudinal follow-up of participants in NHANES I who were aged 25 to 74 years at the time of survey. [17] Detailed information on NHANES I and NHEFS are provided elsewhere. [14,15,16,17]

Of the 12, 053 white subjects followed in the NHEFS, we excluded 2760 NHANES I Augmentation Survey participants who were not administered a dermatologic examination[16]; 83 subjects who were pregnant at the time of the baseline examination, and 487 subjects whose demographic, socioeconomic, or other covariates were missing. Among the remaining participants, 251 were lost during the follow-up period, leaving 8472 participants (men, 40.5%; women, 59.5%) who contributed 139,802 person-years of follow-up to the final analyses.

Outcome definitions

Based on interviews, health care facility medical records, and death certificates, NHEFS follow-up data were collected in 4 waves: 1982 to 1984, 1986, 1987, and 1992. [17] Death was ascertained by either a death certificate or a proxy interview, or both, and the underlying cause of death was coded according to the International Classification of Diseases, Ninth Revision (ICD-9). Deaths were analyzed for all causes, cancer (ICD-9 codes 140–208, e.g., lung cancer, colon cancer, breast cancer), and cardiovascular disease (ICD-9 codes 390–448, e.g., ischemic heart disease, cerebrovascular diseases, hypertension).

Actinic skin damage assessment

A complete clinical dermatologic examination of the skin was undertaken in NHANES I to evaluate variations in texture and color, certain manifestations of aging, and all pathologic changes. The dermatologic examinations were performed by a total of 101 dermatologists during the baseline survey. All dermatologists were trained for the dermatologic examination protocol before the commencement of the survey examinations at each location. After examining the skin covering the entire body, the dermatologist recorded an estimate of the presence and severity of overall actinic skin damage and its components, including fine telangiectasia, solar elastosis (senile elastosis), and actinic keratoses. All of these measures were graded as being either absent, minimal, moderate, or severe. [18]

Covariate definitions

Several potential confounding factors derived from the baseline interview and physical examinations were included in the regression models based on findings from previously published studies. [18,19,20] These included age, gender, educational attainment ($<12^{th}$, 12th, $>12^{th}$ grade); family income (<$3000, $3000–$7000, $7000–$10000, $10000–$15000, ≥$15000); combined measure of occupational and recreational physical activity (low, medium, high); body mass index (underweight, normal, overweight, obese); vitamin supplement use (regular or irregular use, no); place of residence (rural, urban); region of residence (Northeast, Midwest, South, West); season of the year when the examination was taken (spring, summer, autumn, winter); eye color as a surrogate of skin type [21] (dark brown, light brown, gray-green-hazel, dark blue, light blue, other); frequency of alcohol consumption (less than once a month or never, once a month to several times a week, almost daily or daily). Menopause was defined by the answer "yes" for the question, "have the cycles entirely stopped?". Occupation was coded according to the 1970 census of population Alphabetical Index of Industries and Occupations [22]: professional, manager, sales worker, clerical and kindred workers, craftsmen and kindred workers, operatives, laborer, farmer, service works, and unemployment variables for retired, keeping house, and others (disabled, student, looking for work, missing). Smoking was coded as current, past, or never. Past smokers were defined as those who reported that they had smoked ≥100 cigarettes during their lifetimes but did not currently smoke cigarettes. Retrospective smoking data collected during the follow-up were used for persons with missing baseline information. Retrospective information on smoking agreed reasonably well with data collected in NHANES I. [23] Baseline diseases were defined as self-reported history of having cardiovascular diseases, cancer, diabetes, hypertension, ulcer, kidney diseases or hepatitis.

Statistical methods

Characteristics of the participants at baseline were presented as the mean or percentage stratified by severity of overall actinic skin damage. The level of statistical significance of differences were examined by using ANOVA (continuous variables) and the χ^2 test (categorical variables), with Bonferroni adjustment for multiple comparisons.

Cox proportional hazards regression models [24] were used separately to examine the associations of overall actinic skin damage and its components with all cause, cancer, and cardiovascular disease (CVD) mortality. [25] Age was used as the time scale in all time-to-event analyses, and all analyses were stratified by birth cohort using 10-year interval to control for calendar period and cohort effect. [26] Trend tests for the adjusted hazard ratios (HRs) were performed by assigning the integers of 0, 1, 2, 3 to the degrees of severity of actinic skin damage and its components, and treating the resulting score variables as continuous in the models. The Schoenfeld residual [27] test was used to check the proportional hazards assumption. In addition, we also performed the Cox regression model with time-on-study as the time-scale and baseline age as a covariate.

To assess the effect of the complex survey design on the results, Cox proportional hazard regression analyses were performed to incorporate the sample weights, the stratification and clustering in the analysis. The weighted and unweighted models yielded consistent results. Therefore, only unweighted results were presented here. To explore whether the results will be affected by skin cancer, we also performed the analyses excluding those who died from skin cancer during the follow-up period (n = 8) in all three models. Subgroup analyses by age (25–44, 45–65, 65–74 years old) were conducted to assess the robustness of our findings. Cox regressions were also performed excluding subjects with cardiovascular disease, diabetes, or cancer at baseline, and were repeated when including pregnant women. All Cox models were adjusted for the above-mentioned potential confounding factors. In addition, men and women were combined in the regression analysis as no interactions were detected between gender and actinic skin damage.

Cumulative mortality curves were plotted according to overall actinic skin damage severity using the Kaplan-Meier method. [28] The assessment of cumulative mortality rates was limited to subjects who were 40–85 years of age during the follow-up period. Because the calculation of cumulative mortality rates is sensitive to small sample sizes, moderate and severe actinic skin damage were combined into one group. Pairwise comparisons of absent, minimal, and moderate and severe overall actinic skin damage were performed using a two-sided log-rank test [29] for all-cause (n = 8431), cancer (n = 6154) and cardiovascular disease (n = 6981) mortality, respectively. Bonferroni corrections were used to control for type I error, and a two-sided P value of 0.017 was used for each comparison. All analyses were performed using Stata software (version 11.0 for Windows; Stata Corporation, College Station, TX).

Results

The baseline characteristics of participants by overall actinic skin damage are presented in **Table 1**. Compared with women, men were more likely to have overall actinic skin damage. The severity of overall actinic skin damage increased with age and decreased with family income, education attainment, and vitamin supplement use. Subjects who lived in the South, rural or with light color eyes were more likely to suffer from severe overall actinic skin damage.

Eight thousand four hundred and seventy-two participants with 139, 802 person-years of follow-up between 1971 and 1992 were included in the analyses, and 672 cancer deaths, 1500 cardiovascular disease deaths, and 2969 deaths from all causes were documented among the subjects. HRs and 95% CIs for all-cause mortality by the severity of overall actinic skin damage and its components (i.e., fine telangiectasia, solar elastosis (senile elastosis), and actinic keratoses) were presented in **Table 2**. After adjusting for potential confounding factors, severe overall actinic skin damage was associated with a 45% higher all-cause mortality (95% CI: 1.22, 1.72; $P<0.001$), moderate overall skin damage with a 20% higher mortality (95% CI: 1.08, 1.32; $P<0.001$), and minimal overall actinic skin damage with no significant mortality difference ($p = 0.752$), when compared to having no skin damage. Similar results were obtained when exploring the associations of all-cause mortality with fine telangiectasia, solar elastosis, and actinic keratoses, respectively. Significant trends were found in all

Table 1. Baseline characteristics of 8472 NHEFS participants according to actinic skin damage*.

Variable	Actinic skin damage Absent (4419)	Minimal (2125)	Moderate (1710)	Severe (218)
Age(years), mean(SD)	43.4(14.8)	54.7(14.1)^{a}	60.4(11.6)^{b,d}	64.6(8.5)^{c,e,f}
Body mass index(Kg/m^2), mean(SD)	25.2(5.1)	25.8(4.8)^{a}	25.7(4.5)^{b}	25.4(4.7)
Men, No. (%)	1311(29.7)	878(41.3)^{a}	1083(63.3)^{b,d}	161(73.9)^{c,e,f}
High physical activity, No. (%)†	604(13.7)	294(13.8)	260(15.2)	25(11.5)
Current cigarette Smoke, No. (%)	1212(27.4)	452(21.3)^{a}	367(21.5)^{b}	45(20.6)
Regular alcohol consumption, No. (%)‡	474(10.7)	270(12.7)	294(17.2)^{b,d}	24(11.0)
More than a high school education, No.(%)	1163(26.3)	436(20.5)^{a}	290(17.0)^{b,d}	31(14.2)^{c}
Family income≥$10000, No. (%)	2057(46.6)	830(39.1)^{a}	557(32.6)^{b,d}	51(23.4)^{c,e,f}
Vitamin supplements use, No. (%)§	1564(35.4)	746(35.1)	515(30.1)^{b,d}	61(28.0)
Dark brown eyes, No. (%)	1184(26.8)	385(18.1)^{a}	239(14.0)^{b,d}	19(8.7)^{c,e}
Laborer or farmer, No. (%)	102(2.3)	53(2.5)	51(3.0)	7(3.3)
Residence in rural, No. (%)	1729(39.1)	814(38.3)	741(43.3)^{b,d}	117(53.7)^{c,e,f}
Residence in the South region, No. (%)	1037(23.5)	506(23.8)	439(25.7)	101(46.3)^{c,e,f}
Examination taken in summer, No. (%)	1192(27.0)	561(26.4)	413(24.2)	41(18.8)^{c}
Baseline disease, No. (%)**	1745(39.5)	1023(48.1)^{a}	966(56.5)^{b,d}	151 (69.3) ^{c,e,f}

*Data were given as mean ± SD or numbers (%). NHEFS indicates the First National Health and Nutrition Examination Survey Epidemiologic Follow-up Study. P was corrected by Bonferroni adjustment in multiple comparisons (p/q, q = 6, $P<0.008$).
†High physical activity was defined as both get much exercise in recreational things and very active in usual day aside from recreation.
‡Regular alcohol consumption: defined as drink everyday or just about everyday.
§Vitamin supplements use was defined as the regular or irregular use of any type of vitamin supplement.
**Baseline diseases were defined as self-reported history of having cardiovascular diseases, cancer, diabetes, hypertension, ulcer, kidney diseases or hepatitis.
[a]Statistically significant difference between the minimal and absent group.
[b]Statistically significant difference between the moderate and absent group.
[c]Statistically significant difference between the severe and absent group.
[d]Statistically significant difference between the moderate and minimal group.
[e]Statistically significant difference between the severe and minimal group.
[f]Statistically significant difference between the severe and moderate group.

Table 2. All-cause mortality hazard ratios according to actinic skin damage and its components in 8472 NHEFS participants*.

	Actinic skin damage and its components				*P* for trend
	Absent	**Minimal**	**Moderate**	**Severe**	
Actinic skin damage					
Person-years	78558	34371	24253	2621	
Number of subjects†	4419 (915)	2125 (856)	1710 (1026)	218 (172)	
HR (95% CI)					
Age- adjusted**	1.0	1.07(0.97, 1.18)	1.39^c(1.27,1.52)	1.78^c(1.51,2.10)	<0.01
Age-,gender-adjusted‡	1.0	1.01(0.92,1.11)	1.16^b(1.06,1.28)	1.42^c(1.20,1.69)	<0.001
Multivariate adjusted§	1.0	1.01(0.92,1.11)	1.20^c(1.08,1.32)	1.45^c(1.22,1.72)	<0.001
Fine Telangiectasia					
Person-years	92103	26151	18438	3111	
Number of subject†	5282 (1294)	1658 (741)	1288 (755)	244 (179)	
HR (95% CI)					
Age- adjusted**	1.0	1.06(0.97,1.16)	1.39^c(1.27,1.52)	1.64^c(1.40,1.92)	<0.001
Age-,gender-adjusted‡	1.0	0.99(0.90,1.08)	1.15^b(1.04,1.26)	1.27^b(1.08,1.49)	0.001
Multivariate adjusted§	1.0	0.98(0.89,1.07)	1.16^b(1.05,1.28)	1.27^b(1.08,1.50)	<0.001
Solar Elastosis					
Person-years	99096	20470	16831	3405	
Number of subject†	5663 (1352)	1312 (620)	1217 (775)	280 (222)	
HR (95% CI)					
Age- adjusted**	1.0	1.12^a(1.02,1.23)	1.30^c(1.18,1.42)	1.53^c(1.32,1.76)	<0.001
Age-,gender-adjusted‡	1.0	1.06(0.97,1.17)	1.11^a(1.02,1.22)	1.32^c(1.14,1.53)	<0.001
Multivariate adjusted§	1.0	1.06(0.96,1.17)	1.15^b(1.05,1.27)	1.35^c(1.16,1.58)	<0.001
Actinic Keratoses					
Person-years	119640	12948	6047	1168	
Number of subject†	7004 (2012)	918 (564)	449 (308)	101 (85)	
HR (95% CI)					
Age- adjusted**	1.0	1.23^c(1.12,1.35)	1.36^c(1.21,1.54)	1.71^c(1.38,2.13)	<0.001
Age-,gender-adjusted‡	1.0	1.11^a(1.01,1.22)	1.15^a(1.02,1.31)	1.38^b(1.11,1.72)	<0.001
Multivariate adjusted§	1.0	1.08(0.97,1.19)	1.13(1.00,1.29)	1.46^b(1.16,1.82)	0.001

*NHEFS indicates the First National Health and Nutrition Examination Survey Epidemiologic Follow-up Study; HR, hazard ratio; and CI, confidence interval.
†Number of subjects at risk for all-cause mortality (number of deaths).
**stratified by birth cohort and adjusted by age.
‡Stratified by birth cohort and adjusted by age, gender.
§Stratified by birth cohort and adjusted for age, gender, physical activity, level of education, regular alcohol consumption, current cigarette smoking, body mass index, occupation, eye colors, family income, vitamin supplement use, urban-rural residence, region of residence, season of the year when the examination was taken, baseline diseases, and menopause for women.
$^a P<0.05$.
$^b P<0.01$.
$^c P<0.001$.

of the analyses. HRs and 95% CIs for cancer and cardiovascular disease mortality according to severity of overall actinic skin damage and its components are presented in **Tables 3** and **4**, respectively. The results were similar to those of all-cause mortality shown in Table 2.

The Cox regression results from the models with time-on-study as the time scale (data not shown) were consistent with the above-mentioned results. Subgroup analyses by age provided similar results. Incorporating sample design, excluding people who died from skin cancers, excluding subjects with diseases at baseline, and including pregnant women did not change the findings. Participants with a higher level of education, family income, or physical activity had lower risk for mortality in all of the three models. Risk factors for mortality included current cigarette smoking, baseline diseases, heavy alcohol consumption, male gender, and menopause in women. Significantly higher risks were found in both obese and underweight subjects except for the obese subjects in the cancer model. In the all-cause mortality model, having dark blue eyes was a protective factor. (Data not shown).

Cumulative mortality from all causes, cancer, and cardiovascular diseases in relation to the severity of overall actinic skin damage using the Kaplan-Meier method is shown in **Figure 1**. The overall mortality curves between the minimal and no actinic skin damage groups did not differ significantly in any of the comparisons. However, participants with moderate and severe overall actinic skin damage had a significantly higher cumulative mortality rate than those with no actinic skin damage in all of the comparisons.

Table 3. Cancer mortality hazard ratios according to actinic skin damage and its components in 6175 NHEFS participants*.

	Actinic skin damage and its components				P for trend
	Absent	**Minimal**	**Moderate**	**Severe**	
Actinic skin damage					
Person-years	70666	26658	16066	1226	
Number of subjects†	3732(228)	1440(171)	924(240)	79(33)	
HR (95% CI)					
Age- adjusted**	1.0	1.01(0.82,1.23)	1.62[c](1.34,1.96)	2.36[c](1.63,3.42)	<0.001
Age-,gender-adjusted‡	1.0	0.94(0.77,1.15)	1.32[b](1.09,1.61)	1.75[b](1.20,2.55)	<0.001
Multivariate adjusted§	1.0	0.97(0.79,1.19)	1.35[b](1.10,1.66)	1.78[b](1.20,2.63)	0.001
Fine Telangiectasia					
Person-years	81151	19412	12337	1716	
Number of subject†	4307(319)	1053(136)	710(177)	105(40)	
HR (95% CI)					
Age- adjusted**	1.0	0.93(0.76,1.14)	1.61[c](1.33,1.94)	2.04[c](1.46,2.84)	<0.001
Age-,gender-adjusted‡	1.0	0.86(0.70,1.06)	1.29[a](1.06,1.57)	1.51[a](1.08,2.13)	0.004
Multivariate adjusted§	1.0	0.92(0.75,1.13)	1.33[b](1.08,1.62)	1.47[a](1.04,2.09)	0.003
Solar Elastosis					
Person-years	87502	14925	10611	1579	
Number of subject†	4643(332)	817(125)	613(171)	102(44)	
HR (95% CI)					
Age- adjusted**	1.0	1.07(0.87,1.31)	1.45[c](1.19,1.75)	1.94[c](1.40,2.67)	<0.001
Age-,gender-adjusted‡	1.0	0.99(0.81,1.23)	1.22[a](1.00,1.48)	1.54[b](1.11,2.13)	0.007
Multivariate adjusted§	1.0	1.05(0.84,1.30)	1.26[a](1.03,1.55)	1.54[a](1.09,2.16)	0.004
Actinic Keratoses					
Person-years	102541	8088	3505	482	
Number of subject†	5472(480)	460(106)	209(68)	34(18)	
HR (95% CI)					
Age- adjusted**	1.0	1.22(0.98,1.50)	1.66[c](1.28,2.14)	2.35[c](1.47,3.78)	<0.001
Age-,gender-adjusted‡	1.0	1.10(0.89,1.36)	1.36[a](1.05,1.77)	1.72[a](1.07,2.78)	0.003
Multivariate adjusted§	1.0	1.13(0.91,1.41)	1.24(0.94,1.63)	1.80[a](1.08,2.98)	0.015

*NHEFS indicates First National Health and Nutrition Examination Survey Epidemiologic Follow-up Study; HR, hazard ratio; and CI, confidence interval.
†Number of subjects at risk for cancer (number of deaths).
**stratified by birth cohort and adjusted by age.
‡Stratified by birth cohort and adjusted for age, gender.
§Stratified by birth cohort and adjusted for age, gender, physical activity, level of education, regular alcohol consumption, current cigarette smoking, body mass index, occupation, eye colors, family income, vitamin supplement use, urban-rural residence, region of residence, season of the year when the examination was taken, baseline diseases, and menopause for women.
[a] $P<0.05$.
[b] $P<0.01$.
[c] $P<0.001$.

Discussion

The present study in participants from white populations indicated that the risk of death from cancer, cardiovascular disease and all causes were higher for subjects with moderate to severe actinic skin damage than those with no skin damage. Subgroup analyses by age, sensitivity analyses by excluding subjects with diseases at baseline, or incorporating complex survey design did not change our results.

Potential mechanisms

There are several possible mechanisms by which actinic skin damage may influence all-cause and cause-specific mortality. The free radical theory states that the appropriate and inappropriate production of oxidants is intricately connected to aging and lifespan [30,31] Many environmental stimuli, including ultraviolet (UV) radiation, can generate high levels of reactive oxygen species (ROS). [30] Plasma antioxidants are decreased in people with actinic keratosis, probably due to their long exposure to UV radiation. [32] ROS plays a role in the pathology of sun-induced skin damage, [33,34] and thus may potentially be involved in mechanisms responsible for an increased risk of mortality in people with moderate to severe actinic skin damage reported in this study. Recent experimental and clinical data support the hypothesis that cigarette smoke exposure increases oxidative stress as a potential mechanism for initiating cardiovascular dysfunction,

Table 4. Cardiovascular disease mortality hazard ratios according to actinic skin damage and its components in 7003 NHEFS participants*.

	Actinic skin damage and its components				*P* for trend
	Absent	Minimal	Moderate	Severe	
Actinic skin damage					
Person-years	73035	30110	18732	1748	
Number of subjects†	3934(430)	1739(470)	1194(510)	136(90)	
HR (95% CI)					
Age- adjusted**	1.0	1.15^a(1.01,1.32)	1.43^c(1.26,1.63)	2.16^c(1.72,2.72)	<0.001
Age-,gender-adjusted‡	1.0	1.08(0.95,1.24)	1.17^a(1.02,1.34)	1.64^c(1.29,2.07)	<0.001
Multivariate adjusted§	1.0	1.09(0.95,1.25)	1.24^b(1.07,1.42)	1.64^c(1.29,2.10)	<0.001
Fine Telangiectasia					
Person-years	84792	22380	14339	2113	
Number of subject†	4630(642)	1322(405)	896(363)	155(90)	
HR (95% CI)					
Age- adjusted**	1.0	1.10(0.97,1.25)	1.38^c(1.21,1.57)	1.86^c(1.49,2.32)	<0.001
Age-,gender-adjusted‡	1.0	1.02(0.90,1.15)	1.10(0.96,1.25)	1.35^b(1.08,1.70)	0.023
Multivariate adjusted§	1.0	1.01(0.88,1.15)	1.13(0.98,1.30)	1.34^a(1.06,1.70)	0.013
Solar Elastosis					
Person-years	91394	17223	12790	2219	
Number of subject†	4969(658)	1020(328)	847(405)	167(109)	
HR (95% CI)					
Age- adjusted**	1.0	1.17^a(1.02,1.34)	1.37^c(1.21,1.56)	1.63^c(1.33,2.00)	<0.001
Age-,gender-adjusted‡	1.0	1.12(0.98,1.28)	1.16^a(1.02,1.32)	1.39^b(1.13,1.71)	0.001
Multivariate adjusted§	1.0	1.13(0.98,1.29)	1.23^b(1.08,1.42)	1.43^b(1.15,1.78)	<0.001
Actinic Keratoses					
Person-years	108515	10054	4296	761	
Number of subject†	6001(1009)	653(299)	288(147)	61(45)	
HR (95% CI)					
Age- adjusted**	1.0	1.26^c(1.11,1.44)	1.38^c(1.16,1.65)	1.93^c(1.43,2.60)	<0.001
Age-,gender-adjusted‡	1.0	1.13(0.99,1.29)	1.14(0.96,1.36)	1.44^a(1.06,1.95)	0.006
Multivariate adjusted§	1.0	1.10(0.96,1.27)	1.14(0.94,1.36)	1.44^a(1.05,1.98)	0.013

*NHEFS indicates First National Health and Nutrition Examination Survey Epidemiologic Follow-up Study; HR, hazard ratio; and CI, confidence interval.
†Number of subjects at risk for cardiovascular disease (number of deaths).
**stratified by birth cohort and adjusted by age.
‡Stratified by birth cohort and adjusted for age, gender.
§Stratified by birth cohort and adjusted for age, gender, physical activity, level of education, regular alcohol consumption, current cigarette smoking, body mass index, occupation, eye colors, family income, vitamin supplement use, urban-rural residence, region of residence, season of the year when the examination was taken, baseline diseases, and menopause for women.
$^a P<0.05$.
$^b P<0.01$.
$^c P<0.001$.

[35] and histologic analysis of "smoker's skin" reveals elastic fiber thickening and fragmentation, similar to that found in sun damaged skin. [36] Thus smoking and sun-related actinic skin damage may share some common mechanisms resulting in cardiovascular disease. Furthermore, repeated UV radiation can cause DNA damage and apoptosis on human peripheral blood mononuclear cells, which indicate that sunlight exposure may cause internal diseases by affecting blood components. [37,38] In addition, UV radiation is known to activate multiple signaling cascades, leading to inflammatory reactions. [39] Despite all of these possible pathways, the mechanisms of the association between actinic skin damage and mortality remain unclear. Further study is needed to elucidate this association.

Study implications

Previous studies have found that optimal vitamin D status may not only be important for bone health but also may protect people from some cancers and other chronic diseases. [3] It has been estimated that approximately one billion people worldwide have vitamin D deficiency or insufficiency.[3] In the United States, at the end of the winter, 42% of 15-49 year-old black girls and women had a 25-hydroxyvitamin D level below 20 ng/mL. [3,40] Exposure to sunlight is the main source of vitamin D for most people. [41] For all of these reasons, although the American Academy of Dermatology (AAD) recommends that an adequate amount of vitamin D should be obtained from a healthy diet and/or vitamin D supplement,[42] people are

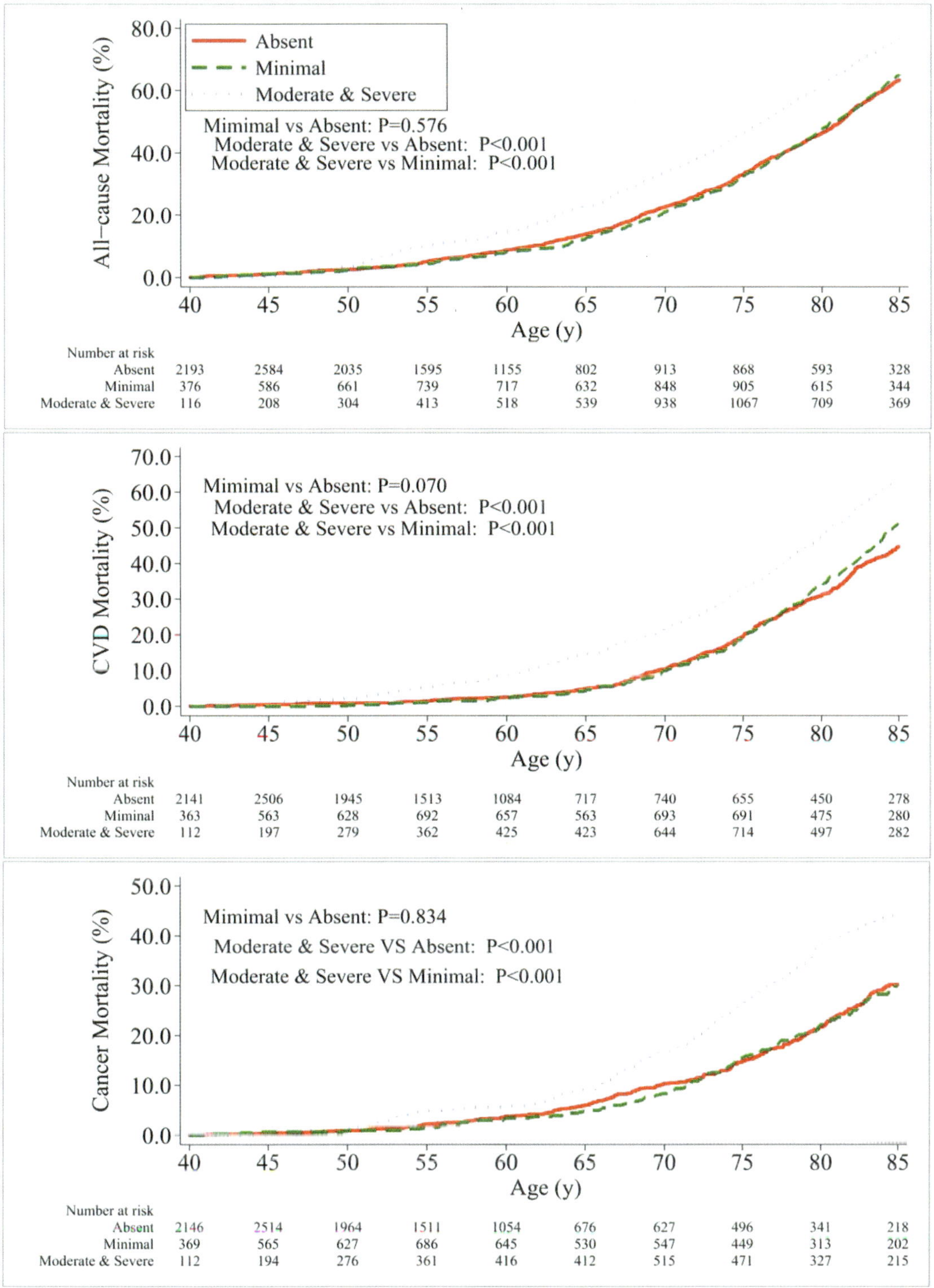

Figure 1. Cumulative mortality from all-cause, cardiovascular disease or cancer according to severity of overall actinic skin damage in NHEFS. Overall actinic skin damage was defined as absent, minimal, or moderate & severe. NHEFS, the First National Health and Nutrition Examination Survey Epidemiology Follow-up Study. P values were corrected by Bonferroni adjustment in multiple comparisons (p/q, $q = 3$, $P < 0.017$).

encouraged to increase their sun exposure to prevent vitamin D deficiency by many studies, [3,43,44] and the WHO is now addressing the issue of whether current sun protection messages are too strong. [45] However, the prevalence of hypovitaminosis D was only 4.2% for white women of reproductive age, [40]. Hence to better understand the risk and benefit of sun exposure to human health is needed. It is well known that over exposure to sun increase risk for skin cancer and skin damage. If the finding from our research about the positive association between skin damage and mortality can be confirmed by other studies, an evaluation on the sun protective message should be warranted.

Children are at high-risk for sun-induced skin damage. An estimated 50% to 80% of the skin's lifetime sun damage is thought to occur in childhood and adolescence. [46] Among youths aged 11 to 18 years in the United States, 72% reported having had at least one summer sunburn, 30% reported at least 3, and 12% reported at least 5 sunburns. [47] Sunbathers are another group at high risk for actinic skin damage. [47] In a national survey, 59% of white adults reported sunbathing during the past year, and 25% reported frequent sunbathing. Of the subsample who reported sunbathing during the month before the interview, only 47% routinely used sunscreen. [48] Other high risk populations include tourists, outdoor workers, and fair skinned people living in lower latitudes. [4]

Skin damage caused by over exposure to sunlight is preventable. By running programs such as education, provision of shade in open spaces, rescheduling of work and sports activities, removal of sales taxes from approved sunscreens, and provision of cheap sunscreens, there have been substantial changes in knowledge, attitudes, and beliefs about sunlight and suntans, as well as an increase in sun protection behavior in Australia. [49]

Sunlight exposure plays an important role in both vitamin D synthesis and actinic skin damage pathology, which means that whether increased sun exposure is a protective or risk factor for chronic disease may depend on the balance between the UV induced production of vitamin D and UV induced skin damage. Throughout the United States, the estimated daily solar exposure to maintain a serum 25(OH)D level of 30 ng/mL is 15 minutes in early fall or later spring, from 11:00 AM to 2:00 PM under clear skies, assuming exposure of arms, shoulders, and back. [50,51] Ultraviolet exposure beyond the minimal erythemal dose does not increase vitamin D production further. [51] The concentration of previtamin D in the skin reaches an equilibrium in white skin within 20 min of ultraviolet exposure. [51] However, the optimal amount of sunlight exposure a person should receive is not known but is likely to depend on many factors related to skin type, latitude, and sunscreen application. [4]

Study limitations

A major limitation of this study is that the measurements of actinic skin damage were subject to errors of classification. [18,52] Although the 101 examiners received training, the written instructions for this component of the examination were limited, and there were no diagnostic criteria employed in the definition of actinic skin damage severity. [52] In addition, the actinic skin damage severity evaluation was done subjectively by dermatologists. [18] However, the impact of any particular dermatologist's judgments on the overall results was minimized by the large number of examiners used in the survey. [18] In addition, the follow-up survey did not specifically collect dermatologic data [17] and we thus had to assume that the subjects' actinic skin damage did not vary over time, a factor that might result in biased hazard ratios. Another study limitation is the lack of information in potentially important characteristics such as skin type, outdoor/indoor workers or sun seeking behavior. In the present study, we used other surrogates, such as eye color, occupation and family income, to minimize these affects. Furthermore, baseline actinic skin damage data were collected almost 40 years ago, hence the study findings may not be generalizable to the current US population.

Despite these limitations, our study used a large population-based cohort with an average of 16 years of follow-up, focusing on whites only. The fact that follow-up information was available for more than 97% of the study participants and that an extensive number of covariates were available for the NHANES I subjects further enhanced the validity of our findings. Moreover, to the best our knowledge, this is the first study to investigate the relation between sun-induced skin damage and mortality.

Age could be the most important confounder in this study, because age has a very strong relationship with both actinic skin damage and all-cause mortality. [20] To adjust adequately for chronological age, we used age as the time scale and all analyses were stratified by birth cohort to control for calendar period and cohort effector. [26] Furthermore, subgroup analyses by age provided similar results. After further controlling for potential confounding factors such as smoking, occupation, region of residency, season and social-economic status, the association of over-all actinic skin damage and its components with all-cause mortality persisted, and the results remained similar when we used cancer and cardiovascular disease as the outcome.

Conclusions

In conclusion, our study detected an association of actinic skin damage with cardiovascular disease, cancer and all-cause mortality in whites. However, this result should be interpreted with caution since unmeasured or incompletely measured confounding factors cannot be ruled out in this study and since mechanisms for these associations are lacking. More independent studies are needed before any practical recommendations can be made.

Author Contributions

Conceived and designed the experiments: SZ WH. Performed the experiments: WH SZ. Analyzed the data: WH FZ XM XZ MZ ZC SBH SZ. Contributed reagents/materials/analysis tools: SZ. Wrote the paper: WH SZ SBH FZ XM XZ MZ ZC. Study supervision: SZ.

References

1. Arthey S, Clarke VA (1995) Suntanning and sun protection: a review of the psychological literature. Soc Sci Med 40: 265–274.
2. Ness AR, Frankel SJ, Gunnell DJ, Smith GD (1999) Are we really dying for a tan? Br Med J 319: 114–116.
3. Holick MF (2007) Vitamin D deficiency. N Engl J Med 357: 266–281.
4. World Health Organization (2003) INTERSUN. The global UV project: a guide and compendium. Geneva: WHO.
5. Gallagher RP, Lee TK (2006) Adverse effects of ultraviolet radiation: A brief review. Prog Biophys Mol Biol 92: 119–131.
6. Matts PJ, Fink B (2010) Chronic sun damage and the perception of age, health and attractiveness. Photochem Photobiol Sci 9: 421–431.
7. Calderone DC, Fenske NA (1995) The clinical spectrum of actinic elastosis. J Am Acad Dermatol 32: 1016–1024.
8. Salasche SJ (2000) Epidemiology of actinic keratoses and squamous cell carcinoma. J Am Acad Dermatol 42: S4–S7.
9. Wulf HC, Sandby-Moller J, Kobayasi T, Gniadecki R (2004) Skin aging and natural photoprotection. Micron 35: 185–191.
10. Christensen K, Iachina M, Rexbye H, Tomassini C, Frederiksen H, et al. (2004) "Looking old for your age": Genetics and mortality. Epidemiology 15: 251–252.
11. Purba MB, Kouris-Blazos A, Wattanapenpaiboon N, Lukito W, Rothenberg E, et al. (2001) Can skin wrinkling in a site that has received limited sun exposure be used as a marker of health status and biological age? Age Ageing 30: 227–234.
12. Rexbye H, Petersen I, Johansens M, Klitkou L, Jeune B, et al. (2006) Influence of environmental factors on facial ageing. Age Ageing 35: 110–115.
13. NCHS Research Ethics Review Board (ERB)Approval. http://www.cdc.gov/nchs/nhanes/irba98.htm Accessed August 26, 2010.
14. Miller HW (1973) Plan and operation of the health and nutrition examination survey. United states 1971-1973. Vital Health Stat 1: 1–46.
15. (1973) Plan and operation of the health and nutrition examination survey: United States-1971-1973. Vital Health Stat 1: 1–77.
16. Engel A, Murphy RS, Maurer K, Collins E (1978) Plan and operation of the HANES I augmentation survey of adults 25-74 years United States, 1974-1975. Vital Health Stat 1: 1–110.

17. Cox CS, Mussolino ME, Rothwell ST, Lane MA, Golden CD, et al. (1997) Plan and operation of the NHANES I Epidemiologic Followup Study, 1992. Vital Health Stat 1: 1–231.
18. Engel A, Johnson ML, Haynes SG (1988) Health-effects of sunlight exposure in the United-States - results from the 1st National Health and Nutrition Examination Survy, 1971-1974. Arch Dermatol 124: 72–79.
19. Brown TT, Quain RD, Troxel AB, Gelfand JM (2006) The epidemiology of sunburn in the US population in 2003. J Am Acad Dermatol 55: 577–583.
20. Holman CDJ, Evans PR, Lumsden GJ, Armstrong BK (1984) The determinants of actinic skin damage - problems of confounding among environmental and constitutional variables. Am J Epidemiol 120: 414–422.
21. Fitzpatrick TB (1988) The validity and practicality of sun-reactive skin type-I through type-VI. Arch Dermatol 124: 869–871.
22. US Bureau of the Census (1971) 1970 Census of the population: Alphabetical index of industries and occupation. Washington: US Government Printing Office.
23. Machlin SR, Kleinman JC, Madans JH (1989) Validity of mortality analysis based on retrospective smoking information. Stat Med 8: 997–1009.
24. Cox DR (1972) Regression models and life - tables. J R Stat Soc Series B Stat Methodol 34: 187–&.
25. Ingram DD, Makuc DM (1994) Statistical issues in analyzing the NHANES I Epidemiologic Followup Study. Series 2: Data evaluation and methods research. Vital Health Stat 2: 1–30.
26. Korn EL, Graubard BI, Midthune D (1997) Time-to-event analysis of longitudinal follow-up of a survey: Choice of the time-scale. Am J Epidemiol 145: 72–80.
27. Grambsch PM, Therneau TM (1994) Proportional hazards tests and diagnostics based on weighted residuals. Biometrika 81: 515–526.
28. Kaplan EL, Meier P (1958) Nonparametric-estimation from incomplete observations. J Am Stat Assoc 53: 457–481.
29. Mantel N (1966) Evaluation of survival data and two new rank order statistics arising in its consideration. Cancer Chemother Rep 50: 163–170.
30. Finkel T, Holbrook NJ (2000) Oxidants, oxidative stress and the biology of ageing. Nature 408: 239–247.
31. Beckman KB, Ames BN (1998) The free radical theory of aging matures. Physiol Rev 78: 547–581.
32. Vural P, Canbaz M, Selcuki D (1999) Plasma antioxidant defense in actinic keratosis and basal cell carcinoma. J Eur Acad Dermatol Venereol 13: 96–101.
33. Yaar M, Gilchrest BA (2007) Photoageing: mechanism, prevention and therapy. Br J Dermatol 157: 874–887.
34. Fisher GJ, Kang SW, Varani J, Bata-Csorgo Z, Wan YS, et al. (2002) Mechanisms of photoaging and chronological skin aging. Arch Dermatol 138: 1462–1470.
35. Ambrose JA, Barua RS (2004) The pathophysiology of cigarette smoking and cardiovascular disease - An update. J Am Coll Cardiol 43: 1731–1737.
36. Frances C, Boisnic S, Hartmann DJ, Dautzenberg B, Branchet MC, et al. (1991) Changes in the elastic tissue of the non-sun-exposed skin of cigarette smokers. Br J Dermatol 125: 43–47.
37. Narbutt J, Cebula B, Lesiak A, Sysa-Jedrzejowska A, Norval M, et al. (2009) The Effect of Repeated Exposures to Low-Dose UV Radiation on the Apoptosis of Peripheral Blood Mononuclear Cells. Arch Dermatol 145: 133–138.
38. Moller P, Wallin H, Holst E, Knudsen LE (2002) Sunlight-induced DNA damage in human mononuclear cells. FASEB J 16: 45–53.
39. Muthusamy V, Piva TJ (2010) The UV response of the skin: a review of the MAPK, NF kappa B and TNF alpha signal transduction pathways. Arch Dermatol Res 302: 5–17.
40. Nesby-O'Dell S, Scanlon KS, Cogswell ME, Gillespie C, Hollis BW, et al. (2002) Hypovitaminosis D prevalence and determinants among African American and white women of reproductive age: third National Health and Nutrition Examination Survey, 1988-1994. Am J Clin Nutr 76: 187–192.
41. Holick MF (2004) Sunlight and vitamin D for bone health and prevention of autoimmune diseases, cancers, and cardiovascular disease. Am J Clin Nutr 80: 1678S–1688S.
42. American Academy of dermatology (2009) American Academy of Dermatology Issues Updated Position Statement on Vitamin D. http://www.aad.org/Forms/Policies/Uploads/PS/PS-Vitamin%20D.pdf. Accessed December 27, 2010.
43. Holick MF (2008) Sunlight, UV-radiation, vitamin D and skin cancer: How much sunlight do we need? Sunlight, Vitamin D and Skin Cancer. pp 1–15.
44. Gillie O (2006) A new government policy is needed for sunlight and vitamin D. Br J Dermatol 154: 1052–1061.
45. Lucas RM, Repacholi MH, McMichael AJ (2006) Is the current public health message on UV exposure correct? Bull World Health Organ 84: 485–491.
46. Robinson JK, Rigel DS, Amonette RA (2000) Summertime sun protection used by adults for their children. J Am Acad Dermatol 42: 746–753.
47. Davis KJ, Cokkinides VE, Weinstock MA, O'Connell MC, Wingo PA (2002) Summer sunburn and sun exposure among US youths ages 11 to 18: National prevalence and associated factors. Pediatrics 110: 27–35.
48. Koh HK, Bak SM, Geller AC, Mangione TW, Hingson RW, et al. (1997) Sunbathing habits and sunscreen use among White adults: Results of a national survey. Am J Public Health 87: 1214–1217.
49. Marks R (1994) Melanoma prevention: is it possible to change a population's behavior in the sun? Pigment Cell Res 7: 104–106.
50. Garland CF, Garland FC, Gorham ED, Lipkin M, Newmark H, et al. (2006) The role of vitamin D in cancer prevention. Am J Public Health 96: 252–261.
51. Vieth R (1999) Vitamin D supplementation, 25-hydroxyvitamin D concentrations, and safety. Am J Clin Nutr 69: 842–856.
52. Safavi K (1994) Data resources for epidemiology of skin diseases. J Invest Dermatol 102: S51–S53.

High Prevalence of Skin Diseases and Need for Treatment in a Middle-Aged Population. A Northern Finland Birth Cohort 1966 Study

Suvi-Päivikki Sinikumpu[1]*, Laura Huilaja[1], Jari Jokelainen[2,3], Markku Koiranen[2], Juha Auvinen[2], Päivi M. Hägg[1], Erika Wikström[1], Markku Timonen[2], Kaisa Tasanen[1]

1 Department of Dermatology, Medical Research Center, University of Oulu and Oulu University Hospital, Oulu, Finland, **2** Institute of Health Sciences, Faculty of Medicine University of Oulu, Oulu, Finland, **3** Unit of General Practice, Oulu University Hospital, Oulu, Finland

Abstract

To determine the overall prevalence of skin diseases a whole-body skin examination was performed for 1,932 members (46-years of age) of the Northern Finland Birth Cohort (NFBC 1966), which is a comprehensive longitudinal research program (N = 12,058). A high prevalence of all skin diseases needing treatment was found (N = 1,158). Half of the cases of skin findings were evaluated to be serious enough to require diagnostic evaluation, treatment or follow-up either in a general health care, occupational health care or a secondary care setting. The remaining half were thought to be slight and self-treatment was advised. Males (70%) had more skin diseases needing treatment than females (52%) (P<0.001). The most common skin finding was a benign skin tumor, which was found in every cohort member. Skin infections (44%), eczemas (27%) and sebaceous gland diseases (27%) were the most common skin diseases in the cohort. Moreover, skin infections and eczemas were more commonly seen in the group with low education compared to those with high education (P< 0.005). The results strengthen the postulate that skin diseases are common in an adult population.

Editor: Katariina Laine, Oslo University Hospital, Ullevål, Norway

Funding: The authors are grateful to Oulu University Hospital, the Northern Finland Cancer Association, the Academy of Finland and the University of Oulu for their support. The funders had no role in study design, data collection and analysis, decision to publish, or preparation of the manuscript.

Competing Interests: The authors have declared that no competing interests exist.

* E-mail: suvi-paivikki.sinikumpu@oulu.fi

Introduction

Skin diseases are common and they are found in more than half of adult population [1]. The most common skin diagnoses are benign tumors, eczemas, viral warts, sebaceous gland diseases and fungal infections [1], [2], [3]. About one in every three of all patients at general practitioner suffers from a skin disorder [2], [4]. Most dermatologic diseases are chronic in nature and decrease the daily quality of life [2], [5].

Despite the high morbidity and substantial load for primary health care, epidemiological studies addressing the overall prevalence of skin diseases at population level (among a healthy population) are sparse and controversial [1], [3], [6], [7]. In a pioneering study by Rea and co-workers over one-fifth out of 614 study cases had a moderate or severe skin lesion, and age, sex, and social class trends in prevalence were found in certain groups of skin disease [1]. There was a slight (61% versus 48%) female predominance in the prevalence of skin diseases [1]. Another large epidemiologic study by Johnson and Roberts was also conducted as early as in the 1970s [1], [3]. In this diverse Health and Nutrition Examination Survey nearly one-third of persons 1–74 years of age had at least one skin condition that required an evaluation by a physician and the prevalence of skin diseases increased rapidly with age [3]. In a recent German study the prevalence of skin diseases and the need of treatment were investigated by means of a wide cross-sectional analysis of 90,880 employed study cases [6]. Need of treatment was higher in males (31% versus 22%) compared with females [6]. Another recent analysis of 1457 randomly selected adults in Australia revealed following prevalences of skin diseases: eczemas 31.6%, psoriasis 6.6% and acne 12.8%, but the association between skin diseases and socioeconomic classes was not addressed [7].

Due to the scarce epidemiological-level evidence of the prevalences of skin diseases we decided to study the overall prevalence of all skin disorders among an unselected middle-aged population in a developed country, which was the primary aim of the study. Furthermore, the association between skin disorders and sex or socioeconomic status is poorly understood. Consequently, another aim was to investigate the possible sex differences in skin diseases and finally, the association between skin diseases and socioeconomic status.

Materials and Methods

Study population

We performed a comprehensive birth-cohort study to find out cross-sectional point prevalence of skin diseases in a middle-aged population. The study population is part of the Northern Finland Birth Cohort 1966 study (NFBC 1966), which is a longitudinal research program in the two northernmost provinces in Finland. NFBC 1966 included initially all 12,058 children whose expected time of delivery was in the year 1966. The whole NFBC 1966 cohort has been evaluated regularly since birth by means of health questionnaires and clinical examinations.

In connection with a 46-year follow-up survey, altogether 3,181 persons currently living in a given geographical area (in the city of Oulu and within 100 km of it, including rural areas) were asked to the clinical examination; 1,932 of them were reached (60.7%) to form the skin study population, which is here called the cohort. Cohort members were 45–47 years of age at this stage.

Ethics Statement

The Ethical Committee of the Northern Ostrobothnia Hospital District approved the study (§94/2011), which was performed according to the Helsinki Declaration of 1983. Written consent for scientific purposes was received from all participants.

Clinical examination

Between April 2012 and May 2013, all 1,932 study cases were evaluated by multidisciplinary examination including body index, blood pressure, heart echo recording, dental status and several other health measurements. For the purpose of this study, full dermatologic status was comprehensively determined at an out-hospital visit. This examination began with visual observation of the whole skin and was performed by a specialist in dermatology or an experienced resident. Skin tumors were further investigated by a dermatoscope. Bacterial, viral and fungal skin infections were diagnosed on the basis of clinical picture without laboratory investigations. This group of diseases includes virus warts, folliculitis, onychomycosis and tinea pedis. Inflammatory skin diseases like atopic eczema were classified by an international eczema area and severity index (EASI-index, 0–72 points) consisting of assessment of redness, thickness, scratching and lichenification of eczema in four different body region, as was psoriasis using a psoriasis area and severity index (PASI-index, 0–72 points) which combines the severity and percentage of the affected skin area [8], [9]. International classification of disease characteristics was used for rosacea, acne vulgaris and androgenetic alopecia [10], [11], [12], [13]. Location and duration of all skin symptoms and their severity were recognized.

Registering of findings and the definition of need of treatment

All cutaneous findings were documented in a computerized database. For additional analysis, the cohort members were classified into four subgroups according to their need of further interventions: I) Subjects with no further care needed, II) those who would recover with self-treatment, III) those to whom a visit at general practitioner was recommended and IV) cases that required further treatment by a dermatologist. This classification was based on a clinical whole body examination. It was decided for every study case whether any follow-up or treatment was required; the chosen treatment was based on cutaneous findings and an expert opinion concerning the accepted clinical practice in dermatology. The group *"no further care needed"* included for example benign tumors, androgenetic alopecia and erytematoteleangiectatic rosacea. The study cases suspected of presenting any skin malignancy or premalignant finding were referred to the Department of Dermatology, University Hospital of Oulu, for biopsy or other further examination and treatment. All other skin diseases requiring treatment, diagnostic investigations or follow-up were referred to primary health care units. The study cases with multiple pigmented nevi were advised to follow their nevi and to protect their skin against sun radiation.

The classification of education level

The association of the socioeconomic status with the prevalence of skin diseases was investigated by analyzing the relationship between the level of education and the cutaneous findings and diseases. The cohort members were classified in three subgroups of education: basic, secondary and tertiary education (Table 1). The information about education level was obtained from National Education Register [14] and was supplemented with self-reported questionnaires.

Statistical analysis

The overall prevalence of all common skin diseases as well as the prevalence of each dermatologic diagnosis was calculated. The Chi Square test, and Fisher's exact test when appropriate, was used to test difference in categorical variables. The modified Poisson regression model with a robust error variance was used to estimate crude and adjusted prevalence ratios and their 95% confidence intervals [15]. The adjusted model included both sex and educational level variables. Interactions for sex and the educational levels were also tested. All statistical analyses were performed with SAS 9.3 for Windows (The SAS Institute, Cary, NC, USA). All significance tests were two-tailed, and values of $P < 0.05$ were considered statistically significant.

Results

Characteristics of the study population

A slight majority of the cohort members were females (53.7%, N = 1,036). Of them, 77% were married or cohabitant. The corresponding figure for males was 80%. Almost 60% of the study population had secondary level education, 38.7% had completed tertiary level and 2.8% had basic education (Table 1).

Prevalence of skin findings and diseases

A whole-body skin examination revealed that every cohort member presented at least one pigmented naevus. Thus, benign skin tumors were the most common skin findings. About 12% of the cases showed multiple (>50) pigmented nevi. All other benign skin tumors are presented in Table 2. Androgenetic alopecia was frequent; it was found in 69% of the males, 27% of the cases being severe, 32% moderate and 38% mild.

The most common skin disease was tinea pedis, found in 26.8% of all cohort members; 20% of them had also onychomycosis. Total prevalence of onychomycosis was 9.4%. Rosacea was also quite common, affecting 15.1%, while acne vulgaris was found in 7.9% of the cohort members.

The most commonly seen eczemas were hand eczema (8.9%) and seborrhoeic eczema (7.3%). The prevalence of atopic eczema was 4.8%, the mean EASI value being 4.7 (range 0.1–36), reflecting mild diseases. The prevalence of psoriasis was 2.1%, mean PASI being 3.1 (range 0.1–13.7). Approximately one in every three of all psoriatics reported joint symptoms (33.3%), and a third (30.6%) had nail deformities. The most usual autoimmune skin disease was vitiligo, found in 1.6% of study cases.

Already at the age of 46 years there were twelve (0.62%) cases of solar keratosis in the study population. Finally, seven (0.36%) basal cell carcinomas and one malignant melanoma (0.05%) were also found (Table 2).

Furthermore, there were several other skin findings that were rare or transient in nature, and because of that they have not been included in Table 2. These skin disorders were for example herpes simplex, pustulosis palmoplantaris, acanthosis nigricans and polymorphic light eruption.

Table 1. Characteristics of the study population and the classification of need of treatment according to found skin disease.

	Total N = 1930 n (%)	Male N = 894 (46.3%) n (%)	Female N = 1036 (53.7%) n (%)	*P*-value*
Marital status				0.036
Married/cohabitant	1465 (78.3)	689 (79.7)	776 (77.1)	
Single	396 (21.2)	175 (20.2)	221 (22.0)	
Widower/widow	10 (0.5)	1 (0.1)	9 (0.9)	
Educational level#				0.149
Basic (9 years)	54 (2.8)	30 (3.4)	24 (2.3)	
Secondary (10–12 years)	1130 (58.6)	535 (59.8)	595 (57.4)	
Tertiary (over 13 years)	746 (38.7)	329 (36.8)	417 (40.3)	
No. of skin diseases¤				<0.001
None	649 (33.6)	218 (24.4)	431 (41.6)	
1	688 (35.7)	328 (36.7)	360 (34.8)	
2	372 (19.3)	203 (22.7)	169 (16.3)	
3	151 (7.8)	96 (10.7)	55 (5.3)	
4 or more	70 (3.6)	49 (5.5)	21 (2.0)	
Evaluation of need of treatment				<0.001
No need of care	772 (40.0)	270 (30.3)	502 (48.5)	
Need a self-treatment	646 (33.5)	347 (38.9)	299 (28.9)	
Need care by a general practioner	472 (24.5)	256 (28.7)	216 (20.8)	
Need care in a special health care	38 (2.0)	19 (2.1)	19 (1.8)	

*Pearson's Chi-Squared test or Fisher's Exact test.
#Basic education (comprehensive schools), secondary level (upper secondary schools, vocational schools), tertiary level (universities, polytechnics).
¤Skin findings which did not require treatment are excluded (for example benign skin tumors, androgenetic alopecia and erytematoteleangiectatic rosacea).

Finally, we analyzed if some study participants had multiple skin diseases; this revealed that 39% of males and 24% of females had more than one diagnosed skin disease (Table 1).

Distribution of skin findings and diseases by sex

When compared to females, seborrhoeic eczema (RR 3.8), eczema nummulare (RR 2.4), eczema infectiosum (RR 3.4) and neurodermatitis (RR 3.4) were more common in males. Also the two most common mycoses, tinea pedis (RR 2.0) and onychomycosis (RR 2.6) predominated in males. Similarly, folliculitis (RR 3.3) and hyperhidrosis affected more males (RR 3.7) than females. In contrast, contact eczema (RR 0.1) and hand eczema (RR 0.7) were less common among males. Certain benign skin tumors, such as dermatofibromas (RR 0.7), cherry angiomas (RR 0.8), seborrheic keratosis (RR 0.9), lentigo senilis (RR 0.6) and naevus flammeus (RR 0.8), were less common among males than females. Lipoma was more common in males (RR 2.4), while rosacea predominated in females (RR 1.9). No significant difference in sex distribution was found in atopic dermatitis and psoriasis (Table 3).

Socioeconomic status and the prevalence of skin diseases

We analyzed the association of socioeconomic status, defined as education level, with the prevalence of skin diseases. When compared with tertiary education level, tinea pedis (RR 1.28), onychomycosis (RR 1.34), eczema infectiosum (RR 3.5) and folliculitis (RR 1.63) were more common among those with secondary level education ($P<0.05$). In comparison between tertiary and basic education, the corresponding values were: tinea pedis (RR 1.63), onychomycosis (RR 1.94) and eczema infectiosum (RR 10.3) ($P<0.05$).

The need of treatment

Skin diseases defined as serious enough in order to be in need of care was high being 59.9% (N = 1156). Importantly, almost half (40.8%, N = 472) were referred to a general practitioner or occupational health care, and 3.3% (N = 38) to secondary care. However, about half of the cases in need of treatment were mild and were given advice on self-care treatment (N = 646). The need for treatment was higher among males (70%) than females (52%) ($P<0.001$) as well as in lower educational class (basic education 61%, secondary level 63% and tertiary level 56%) ($P<0.05$) (Table 1).

Discussion

The novel and most important finding of our epidemiological study among nearly 2,000 subjects (aged 45–46 years) of NFBC 1966 was the high prevalence of doctor-diagnosed skin diseases (60%) serious enough to need further treatment, either by a physician or self-treatment. Thus, skin disorders are unquestionably one of the most common reasons of morbidity in an adult general population. In addition, we found that socioeconomic status and sex are associated with the prevalence of some skin diseases.

In this study, the need for treatment was higher compared to previous British and German population based studies: the prevalence of skin diseases requiring any therapy in these earlier

Table 2. Prevalences of found skin diseases and skin findings in the study population, their total numbers and distribution by sex.

	Total	Male	Female	
	% (n)	% (n)	% (n)	*P*-value*
Benign skin tumors#	1930 (100)	894 (100)	1036 (100)	
Pigmented naevus, >50 nevi	222 (11.5)	116 (13.0)	106 (10.2)	0.060
Granuloma pyogenicum	0 (0.0)	0 (0.0)	0 (0.0)	
Blue naevus	26 (1.3)	8 (0.9)	18 (1.7)	0.109
Naevus spilus	90 (4.7)	39 (4.4)	51 (4.9)	0.561
Halo naevus	16 (0.8)	7 (0.8)	9 (0.9)	0.836
Dermatofibroma	428 (22.2)	155 (17.3)	273 (26.4)	<0.001
Cherry angioma	1158 (60.0)	476 (53.2)	682 (65.9)	<0.001
Keloid	52 (2.7)	24 (2.7)	28 (2.7)	0.980
Seborrheic keratosis	855 (44.3)	366 (40.9)	489 (47.2)	0.006
Lentigo senilis	262 (13.6)	90 (10.1)	172 (16.6)	<0.001
Lipoma	61 (3.2)	41 (4.6)	20 (1.9)	<0.001
Congenital melanocytic naevus	78 (4.0)	44 (4.9)	34 (3.3)	0.068
Naevus flammeus	495 (25.6)	195 (21.8)	300 (29.0)	<0.001
Cafe au lait spot	240 (12.4)	107 (12.0)	133 (12.8)	0.564
Skin infections	840 (43.5)	483 (54.0)	357 (34.5)	<0.001
Pityriasis versicolor	38 (2.0)	19 (2.1)	19 (1.8)	0.646
Onychomycosis	181 (9.4)	126 (14.1)	55 (5.3)	<0.001
Tinea pedis	517 (26.8)	327 (36.6)	190 (18.3)	<0.001
Tinea corporis	8 (0.4)	4 (0.4)	4 (0.4)	0.834
Folliculitis	116 (6.0)	86 (9.6)	30 (2.9)	<0.001
Pyoderma	1 (0.1)	0 (0.0)	1 (0.1)	0.353
Verruca plantaris	179 (9.3)	76 (8.5)	103 (9.9)	0.277
Verruca palmaris	51 (2.6)	22 (2.5)	29 (2.8)	0.644
Sebaceus gland diseases	515 (26.7)	210 (23.5)	305 (29.4)	0.003
Acne vulgaris	152 (7.9)	66 (7.4)	86 (8.3)	0.451
Comedo acne	26 (1.3)	8 (0.9)	18 (1.7)	0.109
Papulopustular acne	130 (6.7)	64 (7.2)	66 (6.4)	0.495
Cystic acne	8 (0.4)	4 (0.4)	4 (0.4)	0.836
Acne scars	188 (9.8)	103 (11.5)	85 (8.2)	0.015
Rosacea	292 (15.1)	94 (10.5)	198 (19.1)	<0.001
Erytematoteleangiectatic	242 (12.6)	78 (8.7)	164 (15.9)	<0.001
Papulopustular	45 (2.3)	12 (1.3)	33 (3.2)	0.007
Phymatotic	3 (0.2)	3 (0.3)	0 (0.0)	0.062
Ocular	1 (0.1)	0 (0.0)	1 (0.1)	0.352
Perioraldermatitis	14 (0.7)	1 (0.1)	13 (1.3)	0.003
Eczemas and psoriasis	563 (29.2)	295 (33.0)	268 (25.9)	<0.001
Eczemas	528 (27.4)	277 (31.0)	251 (24.2)	<0.001
Atopic eczema	93 (4.8)	35 (3.9)	58 (5.6)	0.084
Hand eczema	171 (8.9)	66 (7.4)	105 (10.1)	0.033
Seborrheic eczema	141 (7.3)	108 (12.1)	33 (3.2)	<0.001
Eczema nummulare	37 (1.9)	25 (2.8)	12 (1.2)	0.009
Eczema infectiosum	28 (1.5)	21 (2.3)	7 (0.7)	0.002
Contact eczema	19 (1.0)	2 (0.2)	17 (1.6)	0.002
Eczema staticum	15 (0.8)	8 (0.9)	7 (0.7)	0.586
Neurodermatitis	35 (1.8)	26 (2.9)	9 (0.9)	<0.001
Psoriasis	40 (2.1)	23 (2.6)	17 (1.6)	0.202
Hair follicle diseases	654 (33.9)	629 (70.4)	25 (2.4)	a)<0.001
Alopecia areata	7 (0.4)	5 (0.6)	2 (0.2)	0.182

Table 2. Cont.

	Total % (n)	Male % (n)	Female % (n)	P-value*
Androgenetic alopecia	627 (32.5)	613 (68.6)	14 (1.4)	<0.001
Hyperhidrosis	42 (2.2)	32 (3.6)	10 (1.0)	<0.001
Autoimmune diseases	81 (4.2)	32 (3.6)	49 (4.7)	0.209
Lichen ruber planus	13 (0.7)	8 (0.9)	5 (0.5)	0.270
Dermatitis herpetiformis	6 (0.3)	2 (0.2)	4 (0.4)	0.523
DLE	1 (0.1)	0 (0.0)	1 (0.1)	0.353
SLE	1 (0.1)	0 (0.0)	1 (0.1)	0.353
Vitiligo	32 (1.7)	10 (1.1)	22 (2.1)	0.085
Urticaria	10 (0.5)	5 (0.6)	5 (0.5)	0.815
Malign skin tumors	12 (0.6)	7 (0.8)	5 (0.5)	0.403
Melanoma	1 (0.1)	1 (0.1)	0.0 (0)	0.353
Solar keratosis	12 (0.6)	7 (0.8)	5 (0.5)	0.403
Basal cell carcinoma	7 (0.4)	2 (0.2)	5 (0.5)	0.346

*P-value for difference of prevalence between males and females evaluated using Pearson's Chi-Squared test or Fisher's Exact test.
#All study cases had at least one pigmented naevus.

reports was 23% and 27%, respectively [1], [6]. However, in Rea and co-worker's study the population was relatively small (N = 614), part of the skin findings were diagnosed by a nurse, and some skin findings were classified as trivial, not justifying medical attention. The recent study by Augustin and co-workers (2011) included exclusively health ensured employed cases with a wide age distribution (16 years to 70 years). In contrast, a clear advantage of our study was the pure population-based study design with altogether 2,000 unselected members who were all examined by an expert. We determined "skin disease" as a condition that required follow-up or treatment, and thus for example benign tumors, androgenetic alopecia and erytematoteleangiectatic rosacea were excluded from this category. Nevertheless, we decided to recognize and report all cutaneous findings since they may have clinical importance. For example, tinea pedis may predispose to severe infections or present a primary sign of general diseases such as diabetes, but patients do not seek medical care due to the triviality of the symptoms. On the other hand, pigmented nevi, seborrheic keratosis and other benign tumors cause numerous visits to health care. In general, doctor-seeking behavior is determined not only by the severity of condition, but is also influenced by personal, financial and cultural factors.

The other remarkable finding in our study was that the need of treatment was significantly higher with low socioeconomic status. Interestingly, we found that skin infections and specific eczemas were more common in lower socioeconomic status compared to higher socioeconomic status. This is in line with the general postulate of Adler and others: the lower the socioeconomic status, the higher the risk of diseases [16]. However, the relationship between socioeconomic status and skin diseases has remained controversial: Dalstra and co-workers did not find any association between socioeconomic status and skin diseases [17]; on the other hand, the prevalences of atopic disease and skin cancer have been reported to be higher in high socioeconomic status [17], [18], [19], [20].

The majority of epidemiological studies in dermatology have focused on the prevalence of single skin diseases, the most commonly investigated ones being atopic eczema, psoriasis, acne vulgaris, rosacea, and hand eczema [21], [22], [23], [24], [25], [26], [27]. It is noteworthy that our study is the first one in Scandinavia covering widely the prevalence of cutaneous findings. In our study, psoriasis was seen in two percent of the cases, which is in line with previous studies [6], [28]. Therefore, our finding supports the existing understanding that psoriasis is not dependent on a single characteristic of any geographical region [5]. Hand eczema was seen in 8.9% in our cohort, more often in females, in line with previous reports [29], [30], [31]. In contrast, atopic eczema was clearly more common (4.8%) than previously reported (from 1.3% to 2.9%) [6], [32]. The difference is understandable because the incidence of atopic eczema varies between countries and continents [21]. Interestingly, as many as one in every six (15%) of our cohort members presented rosacea. Existing epidemiological data on rosacea is controversial, with reported prevalences varying between 2% and 22% [6], [26], [33]. An increased risk for rosacea has been connected more to female sex [10], fair-skinned population [34] and middle-aged people. The last two of these describe our cohort members and could therefore explain our high prevalence.

Our current work brings certain new considerations to the existing epidemiological literature with regard to more sparsely studied dermatological entities. In our study, over two thirds (69%) of males had some form of hair loss while nearly one third (27%, N = 171) had severe androgenetic alopecia. In comparison, in an Italian study (N = 1390), the prevalence of androgenetic alopecia consisting of frontal and vertex androgenetic alopecia (severe) was only 19% (men under 55 years, N = 52) [35]. Early androgenetic alopecia can work as a marker of insulin resistance [36]. Androgenetic alopecia has also been shown to be associated with several other diseases [37] and to decrease the quality of life [38].

An unexpected high number of middle-aged cohort members (44.3%) showed seborrheic keratosis. Albeit benign in nature, its presence may cause distress to patients due to fear of malignant tumors; even today, it is often surgically removed in vain. Multiple pigmented nevi (>50) were found in up to 11.5% of the cohort members, supporting the previous results [39], [40]. The total number of nevi has been shown to be one of the strongest risk

Table 3. The effect of male sex to the prevalence of skin findings and diseases, compared to females.

	Unadjusted RRs		Adjusted* RRs	
	RR	95% CI	aRR	95% CI
Benign skin tumor				
Dermatofibroma	0.66	0.55–0.78	0.66	0.55–0.79
Cherry angioma	0.81	0.75–0.87	0.81	0.75–0.88
Seborrheic keratosis	0.87	0.78–0.96	0.87	0.78–0.96
Lentigo senilis	0.61	0.48–0.77	0.61	0.48–0.77
Lipoma	2.38	1.40–4.02	2.40	1.42–4.06
Naevus flammeus	0.75	0.64–0.88	0.75	0.64–0.88
Skin infections	1.57	1.41–1.74	1.56	1.40–1.73
Onychomycosis	2.65	1.96–3.60	2.63	1.94–3.56
Tinea pedis	1.99	1.71–2.33	1.98	1.70–2.31
Folliculitis	3.32	2.21–4.98	3.27	2.18–4.91
Sebaceus gland diseases	0.80	0.69–0.93	0.79	0.68–0.92
Acne scars	1.40	1.07–1.84	1.39	1.06–1.83
Rosacea	0.55	0.44–0.69	0.54	0.43–0.68
Erytematoteleangiectatic	0.55	0.43–0.71	0.54	0.42 – 0.70
Papulopustular	0.42	0.22–0.81	0.42	0.22–0.81
Perioraldermatitis	0.09	0.01–0.68	0.09	0.01–0.70
Eczemas	1.28	1.11–1.48	1.28	1.10–1.48
Atopic eczema	0.70	0.46–1.05	0.70	0.47–1.06
Hand eczema	0.73	0.54–0.98	0.73	0.54–0.98
Seborrheic eczema	3.79	2.59–5.54	3.78	2.59–5.53
Eczema nummulare	2.41	1.22–4.77	2.37	1.21–4.67
Eczema infectiosum	3.47	1.48–8.13	3.36	1.43–7.86
Contact eczema	0.14	0.03–0.59	0.13	0.03–0.58
Neurodermatitis	3.34	1.58–7.10	3.36	1.59–7.10
Hair follicle diseases	29.16	19.75–43.04	29.13	19.73–43.02
Androgenetic alopecia	50.74	30.10–85.53	50.73	30.09–85.52
Hyperhidrosis	3.71	1.83–7.50	3.68	1.82–7.47

Abbrevations: RR, relative risk; aRR, adjusted relative risk; CI, confidence interval.
* Adjusted for education.

factors of melanoma [41], and the incidence of malignant melanoma has increased noticeably in recent decades [42]. Melanoma has been reported to be more common in Scandinavian countries and to have female predominance [43].

In our study, tinea pedis (26%) was more frequent than previously reported (5–15%) in other industrial countries [6], [44]. This is an important finding because it is associated with other diseases, e.g. erysipelas [45], and its treatment among diabetics is important. Tinea pedis influences people widely, being also common in athletics [46]. Our high prevalence may be explained by the fact that also minor manifestations, still fulfilling the clinical criterion of tinea pedis, were included.

The predominance of mycotic and bacterial skin infections as well as almost all eczemas in male cohort members, and specific benign skin tumors such as dermatofibromas and seborrheic keratosis in female cohort members, is in line with the findings with a German study [6]. In contrast to the study by Augustin and co-workers (2011) we found that hand eczema and rosacea affected females more often than males. Our important finding was that the overall need of treatment was much higher among males (70%) than females (52%).

The major strength of this study was the coverage of a wide general population with a relatively high (61%) participation rate, which means that our results are generalizable. We have good statistical power thanks to the large sample size. As a major difference to many previous epidemiological studies [6], [47], [48], our current work was not limited to any population subgroups (e.g. employed, children, mental health or patients with psoriasis). Another special advantage was the accurate clinical whole-body skin evaluation performed for every case by an experienced resident or specialist in dermatology instead of the self-reporting questionnaires used in some previous studies [49], [50], [51]. Finally, we were able to analyze the association of skin diseases with socioeconomic status using the level of education, which is reported to be most reliable indicator of socioeconomic status [52]. We concede as a weakness of our study that all those invited did not participate in the clinical examination. All the diagnoses were based solely on the clinical picture since medical history, histologic analysis and microbiologic culture or microscope analysis were not available due to the study setting. Furthermore, the investigators had to reach the diagnosis for the study purpose during one out-hospital visit without possibilities for therapeutical tests or repetitive visits, despite their importance in dermatology.

In conclusion, our major finding was a high prevalence of skin diseases requiring treatment. In clinical practice this means that careful skin evaluation is an important and essential part of the medical examination. Due to comprehensive birth cohort study design and a satisfactory, high participation rate (61%), we underline that our valuable results are valid and generalizable. We found that low socioeconomic status was a risk factor for certain skin diseases. The surprisingly high overall prevalence of skin diseases and the great need of treatment warrant further epidemiologic studies on the factors which are associated with skin diseases.

Author Contributions

Conceived and designed the experiments: SPS KT EW PMH JA. Performed the experiments: SPS LH EW KT. Analyzed the data: JJ MK SPS. Contributed reagents/materials/analysis tools: SPS LH EW KT. Wrote the paper: SPS LH KT MT.

References

1. Rea JN, Newhouse ML, Halil T (1976) Skin disease in Lambeth. A community study of prevalence and use of medical care. Br J Prev Soc Med 30: 107–114.
2. Julian CG (1999) Dermatology in general practice. Br J Dermatol 141: 518–520.
3. Johnson MT, Roberts J, National Center for Health Statistics (1978) Skin conditions and related need for medical care among persons 1–74 years, United States, 1971–1974. Hyattsville, Md.: U.S. Dept. of Health, Education, and Welfare, Public Health Service, Office of the Assistant Secretary for Health, National Center for Health Statistics. 72 p.
4. Lowell BA, Froelich CW, Federman DG, Kirsner RS (2001) Dermatology in primary care: Prevalence and patient disposition. J Am Acad Dermatol 45: 250–255.
5. Krueger G, Koo J, Lebwohl M, Menter A, Stern RS, et al. (2001) The impact of psoriasis on quality of life: Results of a 1998 national psoriasis foundation patient-membership survey. Arch Dermatol 137: 280–284.
6. Augustin M, Herberger K, Hintzen S, Heigel H, Franzke N, et al. (2011) Prevalence of skin lesions and need for treatment in a cohort of 90 880 workers. Br J Dermatol 165: 865–873.
7. Plunkett A, Merlin K, Gill D, Zuo Y, Jolley D, et al. (1999) The frequency of common nonmalignant skin conditions in adults in central Victoria, Australia. Int J Dermatol 38: 901–908.
8. Hanifin JM, Thurston M, Omoto M, Cherill R, Tofte SJ, et al. (2001) The eczema area and severity index (EASI): Assessment of reliability in atopic dermatitis. EASI evaluator group. Exp Dermatol 10: 11–18.
9. Schmitt J, Wozel G (2005) The psoriasis area and severity index is the adequate criterion to define severity in chronic plaque-type psoriasis. Dermatology 210: 194–199.
10. Crawford GH, Pelle MT, James WD (2004) Rosacea: I. etiology, pathogenesis, and subtype classification. J Am Acad Dermatol 51: 327–341.
11. Wilkin J, Dahl M, Detmar M, Drake L, Feinstein A, et al. (2002) Standard classification of rosacea: Report of the national rosacea society expert committee on the classification and staging of rosacea. J Am Acad Dermatol 46: 584–587.
12. White GM (1998) Recent findings in the epidemiologic evidence, classification, and subtypes of acne vulgaris. J Am Acad Dermatol 39: S34–7.
13. Norwood OT (1975) Male pattern baldness: Classification and incidence. South Med J 68: 1359–1365.
14. Isohanni I, Jarvelin MR, Rantakallio P, Jokelainen J, Jones PB, et al. (2001) Juvenile and early adulthood smoking and adult educational achievements—a 31-year follow-up of the Northern Finland 1966 birth cohort. Scand J Public Health 29: 87–95.
15. Zou G (2004) A modified poisson regression approach to prospective studies with binary data. Am J Epidemiol 159: 702–706.
16. Adler NE, Boyce WT, Chesney MA, Folkman S, Syme SL (1993) Socioeconomic inequalities in health. No easy solution. JAMA 269: 3140–3145.
17. Dalstra JA, Kunst AE, Borrell C, Breeze E, Cambois E, et al. (2005) Socioeconomic differences in the prevalence of common chronic diseases: An overview of eight European countries. Int J Epidemiol 34: 316–326.
18. Shack L, Jordan C, Thomson CS, Mak V, Moller H, et al. (2008) Variation in incidence of breast, lung and cervical cancer and malignant melanoma of skin by socioeconomic group in England. BMC Cancer 8: 271.
19. Bergmann RL, Edenharter G, Bergmann KE, Lau S, Wahn U (2000) Socioeconomic status is a risk factor for allergy in parents but not in their children. Clin Exp Allergy 30: 1740–1745.
20. Forastiere F, Agabiti N, Corbo GM, Dell'Orco V, Porta D, et al. (1997) Socioeconomic status, number of siblings, and respiratory infections in early life as determinants of atopy in children. Epidemiology 8: 566–570.
21. Williams H, Robertson C, Stewart A, Ait-Khaled N, Anabwani G, et al. (1999) Worldwide variations in the prevalence of symptoms of atopic eczema in the international study of asthma and allergies in childhood. J Allergy Clin Immunol 103: 125–138.
22. Herd RM, Tidman MJ, Prescott RJ, Hunter JA (1996) Prevalence of atopic eczema in the community: The Lothian atopic dermatitis study. Br J Dermatol 135: 18–19.
23. Remes ST, Korppi M, Kajosaari M, Koivikko A, Soininen L, et al. (1998) Prevalence of allergic rhinitis and atopic dermatitis among children in four regions of Finland. Allergy 53: 682–689.
24. Parisi R, Symmons DP, Griffiths CE, Ashcroft DM Identification and Management of Psoriasis and Associated ComorbidiTy (IMPACT) project team (2013) Global epidemiology of psoriasis: A systematic review of incidence and prevalence. J Invest Dermatol 133: 377–385.
25. Gelfand JM, Weinstein R, Porter SB, Neimann AL, Berlin JA, et al. (2005) Prevalence and treatment of psoriasis in the United Kingdom: A population-based study. Arch Dermatol 141: 1537–1541.
26. Berg M, Liden S (1989) An epidemiological study of rosacea. Acta Derm Venereol 69: 419–423.
27. Susitaival P, Husman L, Horsmanheimo M, Notkola V, Husman K (1994) Prevalence of hand dermatoses among Finnish farmers. Scand J Work Environ Health 20: 206–212.
28. Nevitt GJ, Hutchinson PE (1996) Psoriasis in the community: Prevalence, severity and patients' beliefs and attitudes towards the disease. Br J Dermatol 135: 533–537.
29. Meding B, Liden C, Burstrom B (2004) "You get what you ask for"—impact of the wording of questions on skin disease. Scand J Work Environ Health 30: 334.
30. Meding B, Swanbeck G (1990) Occupational hand eczema in an industrial city. Contact Dermatitis 22: 13–23.
31. Thyssen JP, Johansen JD, Linneberg A, Menne T (2010) The epidemiology of hand eczema in the general population—prevalence and main findings. Contact Dermatitis 62: 75–87.
32. Muto T, Hsieh SD, Sakurai Y, Yoshinaga H, Suto H, et al. (2003) Prevalence of atopic dermatitis in japanese adults. Br J Dermatol 148: 117–121.
33. Abram K, Silm H, Oona M (2010) Prevalence of rosacea in an estonian working population using a standard classification. Acta Derm Venereol 90: 269–273.
34. Gibson GE, Codd MB, Murphy GM (1997) Skin type distribution and skin disease in Ireland. Ir J Med Sci 166: 72–74.
35. Severi G, Sinclair R, Hopper JL, English DR, McCredie MR, et al. (2003) Androgenetic alopecia in men aged 40-69 years: Prevalence and risk factors. Br J Dermatol 149: 1207–1213.
36. Matilainen V, Koskela P, Keinanen-Kiukaanniemi S (2000) Early androgenetic alopecia as a marker of insulin resistance. Lancet 356: 1165–1166.
37. Yi SM, Son SW, Lee KG, Kim SH, Lee SK, et al. (2012) Gender-specific association of androgenetic alopecia with metabolic syndrome in a middle-aged korean population. Br J Dermatol 167: 306–313.
38. Cash TF (1999) The psychosocial consequences of androgenetic alopecia: A review of the research literature. Br J Dermatol 141: 398–405.
39. Karlsson P, Stenberg B, Rosdahl I (2000) Prevalence of pigmented naevi in a Swedish population living close to the Arctic Circle. Acta Derm Venereol 80: 335–339.
40. Augustsson A, Stierner U, Suurkula M, Rosdahl I (1991) Prevalence of common and dysplastic naevi in a Swedish population. Br J Dermatol 124: 152–156.
41. Swerdlow AJ, English J, MacKie RM, O'Doherty CJ, Hunter JA, et al. (1986) Benign melanocytic naevi as a risk factor for malignant melanoma. Br Med J (Clin Res Ed) 292: 1555–1559.
42. Lens MB, Dawes M (2004) Global perspectives of contemporary epidemiological trends of cutaneous malignant melanoma. Br J Dermatol 150: 179–185.
43. Osterlind A (1992) Epidemiology on malignant melanoma in Europe. Acta Oncol 31: 903–908.
44. Elewski B, Hay RJ (1995) International summit on cutaneous antifungal therapy. Boston, Massachusetts, Nov. 11–13, 1994. J Am Acad Dermatol 33: 816–822.
45. Dupuy A, Benchikhi H, Roujeau JC, Bernard P, Vaillant L, et al. (1999) Risk factors for erysipelas of the leg (cellulitis): Case-control study. BMJ 318: 1591–1594.
46. Lacroix C, Baspeyras M, de La Salmoniere P, Benderdouche M, Couprie B, et al. (2002) Tinea pedis in European marathon runners. J Eur Acad Dermatol Venereol 16: 139–142.
47. Goulden V, Stables GI, Cunliffe WJ (1999) Prevalence of facial acne in adults. J Am Acad Dermatol 41: 577–580.
48. Schultz Larsen F, Diepgen T, Svensson A (1996) The occurrence of atopic dermatitis in North Europe: An international questionnaire study. J Am Acad Dermatol 34: 760–764.
49. Wallenhammar LM, Nyfjall M, Lindberg M, Meding B (2004) Health-related quality of life and hand eczema—a comparison of two instruments, including factor analysis. J Invest Dermatol 122: 1381–1389.

50. Montnemery P, Nihlen U, Lofdahl CG, Nyberg P, Svensson A (2005) Prevalence of hand eczema in an adult Swedish population and the relationship to risk occupation and smoking. Acta Derm Venereol 85: 429–432.
51. Meding B, Jarvholm B (2004) Incidence of hand eczema-a population-based retrospective study. J Invest Dermatol 122: 873–877.
52. Winkleby MA, Jatulis DE, Frank E, Fortmann SP (1992) Socioeconomic status and health: How education, income, and occupation contribute to risk factors for cardiovascular disease. Am J Public Health 82: 816–820.

Global Activation of CD8+ Cytotoxic T Lymphocytes Correlates with an Impairment in Regulatory T Cells in Patients with Generalized Vitiligo

Yang Lili[1], Wei Yi[1], Yang Ji[1], Sun Yue[2], Shi Weimin[2], Li Ming[1]*

1 Departments of dermatology, Zhongshan Hospital, Fudan University, Shanghai, China, **2** Departments of dermatology, Shanghai First People's Hospital, Shanghai Jiaotong University, Shanghai, China

Abstract

Melanocyte-specific $CD8^+$ cytotoxic T lymphocytes (CTLs) play a pivotal role in vitiligo-induced depigmentation. Yet, the mechanisms underlying the high frequency of generalized autoimmune disorders associated with generalized vitiligo (GV) are unknown. We hypothesized that an imbalance between activated $CD8^+$ CTLs and regulatory T cells (Tregs) exists in patients with GV . Assessment of the circulating $CD8^+$ CTLs and Tregs by flow cytometric analysis revealed an obvious expansion of $CD8^+$ CTLs and a concomitant decrease in Treg cells in GV patients. The percentages of skin infiltrating $CD8^+$ CTLs and Tregs were evaluated by immunohistochemistry and revealed dramatically increased numbers of both $CD8^+$ CTLs and Tregs in the perilesional skin of GV patients. However, peripheral Tregs were impaired in their ability to suppress the proliferation and cytolytic capacity of autologous $CD8^+$ T cells, suggesting that a functional failure of Tregs and the hyper-activation of $CD8^+$ CTLs may contribute to progressive GV. Our data indicate that reduced numbers and impaired function of natural Tregs fail to control the widespread activation of $CD8^+$ CTLs, which leads to the destruction of melanocytes and contributes to the elevated frequency of various associated autoimmune diseases. This knowledge furthers our understanding of the mechanisms of immune tolerance that are impaired in GV patients and may aid in the future development of effective immunotherapy for GV patients.

Editor: Derya Unutmaz, New York University, United States of America

Funding: This work was supported by the Innovation Fund granted by Fudan University. The funders had no role in study design, data collection and analysis, decision to publish, or preparation of the manuscript.

Competing Interests: The authors have declared that no competing interests exist.

* E-mail: li.ming@zs-hospital.sh.cn

Introduction

Vitiligo is an acquired depigmentation disorder characterized by the loss of melanocytes from the epidermis. This condition affects approximately 0.5–1% of the world's population [1]. The exact etiology of vitiligo remains obscure, but autoimmune factors have been strongly implicated in the development of the disease, especially in generalized vitiligo (GV), because approximately 30% of vitiligo patients are affected with at least one additional autoimmune disorder [2].

$CD8^+$ T cell-mediated tissue damage has been demonstrated in common organ-specific autoimmune diseases, such as type I diabetes and multiple sclerosis, and a role for $CD8^+$ T cells has been postulated in the pathogenesis of GV . Previous studies have largely focused on melanocyte-specific cytotoxic T lymphocytes (CTLs) and identified their pivotal role in inducing melanocyte destruction [3–5]. The presence or activation of melanocyte-specific CTLs, however, does not explain why GV patients often present with other generalized autoimmune conditions, such as autoimmune thyroid disease, Addison's disease, systemic lupus erythematosus and pernicious anemia [2]. Several reports have shown that increases in globally activated $CD8^+$ CTLs correlate with disease activity in various autoimmune disorders [6,7]. We therefore hypothesized that the skin depigmentation of GV patients resulted from a global expansion of activated $CD8^+$ CTLs that progressively destroyed melanocytes and led to a high frequency of associated generalized autoimmune diseases. Thus far, the immune mechanisms underlying the induction and activation of autoreactive $CD8^+$ CTLs and the loss of tolerance to auto-antigens are not clear.

$CD4^+$ $CD25^+$ $CD127^-$ $Foxp3^+$ regulatory T cells (Tregs) are important in maintaining self-tolerance and regulating immune responses in both physiological and disease conditions [8]. Accumulating data indicate that a deficiency or dysfunction of Tregs is associated with impaired immune homeostasis and the development of autoimmune diseases. To date, few papers have investigated Treg numbers or function in GV patients. One report revealed a defect in Treg cell homing to the skin, based on the finding of drastically reduced Treg numbers in vitiligo skin without any systemic drop in their abundance or activity [9]. In contrast, a recent report identified increased numbers of Tregs in perilesional skin despite a functional defect of circulating Tregs in progressive vitiligo [10]. Whether the prevalence and/or function of Tregs are truly impaired in GV patients is still controversial. Moreover, studies presenting the reciprocal relationship between $CD4^+$ $CD25^+$ $CD127^-$ $Foxp3^+$ Tregs and $CD8^+$ CTLs in GV progression are lacking.

To address these issues, 50 GV patients were enrolled in this study. The frequencies of Tregs and $CD8^+$ CTLs were analyzed in serum or skin samples of GV patients with progressive or stable disease, respectively. The ability of Tregs to suppress polyclonal $CD8^+$ T cell responses was also assessed using cells from GV patients. Our results showed that $CD8^+$ CTLs that express interferon-γ (IFN-γ), Granzyme B (GrB) and Perforin exhibited a global expansion, whereas circulating $CD4^+$ $CD25^+$ $CD127^-$ Treg cells were significantly reduced among the peripheral blood mononuclear cells (PBMCs) of GV patients. Depletion of natural Tregs was related to the expansion of $CD8^+$ CTLs. Moreover, while both $CD8^+$ T and $Foxp3^+$ Tregs were increased in the perilesional skin of GV patients, we reasoned that GV patients' Tregs would exhibit a functional failure based on the observation that circulating Tregs failed to effectively suppress $CD8^+$ T cell proliferation and/or the release of cytolytic molecules. Our data indicate that the pathophysiology of GV, and its associated increase risk of autoimmune disorders, might be linked to a defect in the homeostatic control of activated $CD8^+$ CTLs and/or natural Treg cell subpopulations.

Results

Highly enriched circulating $CD8^+$ cytotoxic T lymphocytes in patients with GV

Effector $CD8^+$ CTLs play a key role in the host defense through the production of cytokines, such as IFN-γ, and the effector molecules, GrB and Perforin. $CD8^+$ CTLs can also support deleterious effects when they react against self tissues. As the actual functional molecules for killing target cells, IFN-γ, GrB and Perforin can be used as markers for effector $CD8^+$ CTLs [11]. In our study, PBMCs obtained from 38 progressive GV patients, 12 stable GV patients, and 20 normal controls were analyzed for the frequency of $CD3^+$ $CD8^+$ T cells and the expression of IFN-γ, GrB and Perforin by flow cytometry (Figure 1A). There was a significantly higher number of circulating IFN-γ^+ $CD8^+$ T among $CD3^+$ T cells in progressive GV (mean ± SD 14.80±3.56%; $P<0.01$) and stable GV (13.46±3.69%; $P<0.01$) patients compared to healthy individuals (8.66±2.59%) (Figure 1B, left). The percentage of GrB^+ $CD8^+$ T cells among circulating $CD3^+$ T cells was significantly increased in active GV (40.16±14.60%; $P<0.001$) and inactive GV (32.47±12.77%; $P<0.05$) patients compared to healthy individuals (18.59±11.73%) (Figure 1B, middle). In addition, we observed that Perforin expression in the $CD3^+$ $CD8^+$ T cell subset was significantly higher in GV patients (progressive GV, 5.64±2.08%, $P<0.001$; stable GV, 4.48±2.03%, $P<0.01$) than in normal controls (2.25±1.26%) (Figure 1B, right). Interestingly, no significant difference in the numbers of circulating IFN-γ^+ $CD8^+$ T cells, GrB^+ $CD8^+$ T cells and $Perforin^+$ $CD8^+$ T cells in $CD3^+$ T cells was observed between patients with progressive GV and stable GV (Figure 1B).

We next questioned whether the percentage of $CD8^+$ CTLs varied within the same individual in relation to disease status. To assess this, 6 individuals with progressive GV were tested longitudinally; there was a significant decrease in the percentage of $CD8^+$ CTLs after the patient's disease was stabilized by treatment with oral traditional Chinese herbs and topical steroids (Figure 1C).

Decrease of circulating $CD4^+$ $CD25^+$ $CD127^-$ Treg cells in GV patients

Natural Treg cells play a key role in peripheral immune tolerance and prevent the occurrence of autoimmune diseases. In this study, natural Treg cells were quantified by flow cytometric analysis, according to their CD4, CD25 and CD127 surface marker expression [12] (Figure 2A). The percentage of $CD4^+$ $CD25^+$ $CD127^-$ T cells was significantly decreased in the 38 patients with progressive GV (7.0%±1.8%, $P<0.001$) and the 12 patients with inactive disease (7.2%±1.4%, $P<0.01$) compared to the 20 healthy controls (10.4%±3.2%) (Figure 2C). However, the numbers of circulating Tregs did not differ significantly between progressive GV and stable patients ($P>0.05$). We compared the frequency of natural Treg cells among $CD4^+$ T cells and the frequency of IFN-γ^+ $CD8^+$, GrB^+ $CD8^+$ or $Perforin^+$ $CD8^+$ cells among $CD3^+$ T cells in progressive GV patients, revealing a strong negative correlation between these two cell populations (Spearman correlation coefficient, $r=-0.512$, $P=0.001$, $n=38$; $r=-0.524$, $P=0.001$, $n=38$; $r=-0.585$, $P<0.001$, $n=38$) (Figure 2B).

We next sought to determine whether the percentage of natural Treg cells varied within the same individual in relation to disease status. Six individuals were tested twice, once during active GV and once after their diseases were stabilized with treatment. The percentage of natural Treg cells within these patients increased significantly after treatment ($P<0.05$) (Figure 2D).

Increased frequency of $CD8^+$ T cells and Tregs in GV skin tissue samples

To visualize $CD8^+$ T cells and Treg cells in the skin of GV, we performed immunohistochemical staining for CD8 and Foxp3 expression. The number of cells staining positive for these markers were identified in skin tissue samples from normal controls or in non-lesional, perilesional and lesional skin samples from GV patients. Foxp3 is a reliable and specific marker of Tregs because it serves as the dedicated mediator of the genetic program governing Treg cell development and function [13–15]. We observed that perilesional skin samples from patients with progressive GV exhibited pathologic changes including a large number of infiltrating $CD8^+$ T and $Foxp3^+$ cells predominantly adjacent to the epidermal basal layer (Figure 3A).

$CD8^+$ T cell counts in each high-power field (400×) were significantly increased in 16 perilesional skin samples from patients with progressive GV (mean ± SD 22.96±2.29), compared to skin from 6 healthy individuals (12.79±6.89, $P<0.05$), the 2 lesional skin samples from patients with stable disease (10.83±6.53, $P<0.05$) or 8 non-lesional GV skin samples (11.19±4.4, $P<0.05$). However, no significant difference was observed between lesional skin and non-lesional skin from GV patients or healthy skin from controls ($P>0.05$) (Figure 3B). In contrast to previous studies [10], we observed that $Foxp3^+$ lymphocyte infiltration was also significantly increased in the 16 perilesional skin samples from patients with progressive GV (9.39±2.66) compared to any of the other sample types. skin samples from 6 healthy individuals (3.69±3.04, $P<0.01$), lesional skin from patients with stable disease ($n=2$; 2.49±0.6, $P<0.01$) or non-lesional GV skin ($n=8$; 3.28±2.47, $P<0.05$) (Figure 3C). No significant difference was observed between the lesional and non-lesional skin of GV patients or healthy skin from control individuals ($P>0.05$) (Figure 3C). Importantly, we observed a positive correlation between the number of $CD8^+$ T cells and $Foxp3^+$ cells in 16 perilesional skin samples from progressive GV patients (Spearman correlation coefficient, $r=0.706$, $P<0.001$) (Figure 3D). These results provide evidence that Tregs can be recruited to inflammatory sites from the circulation, and the increase in local $CD8^+$ T cells and $Foxp3^+$ cells might be involved in the GV disease process.

Analysis of Treg-mediated suppression of polyclonal $CD8^+$ T cell responses

Treg/$CD8^+$ T cell cocultures were used to evaluate the in vitro suppressive capacity of Tregs toward $CD8^+$ T cells using

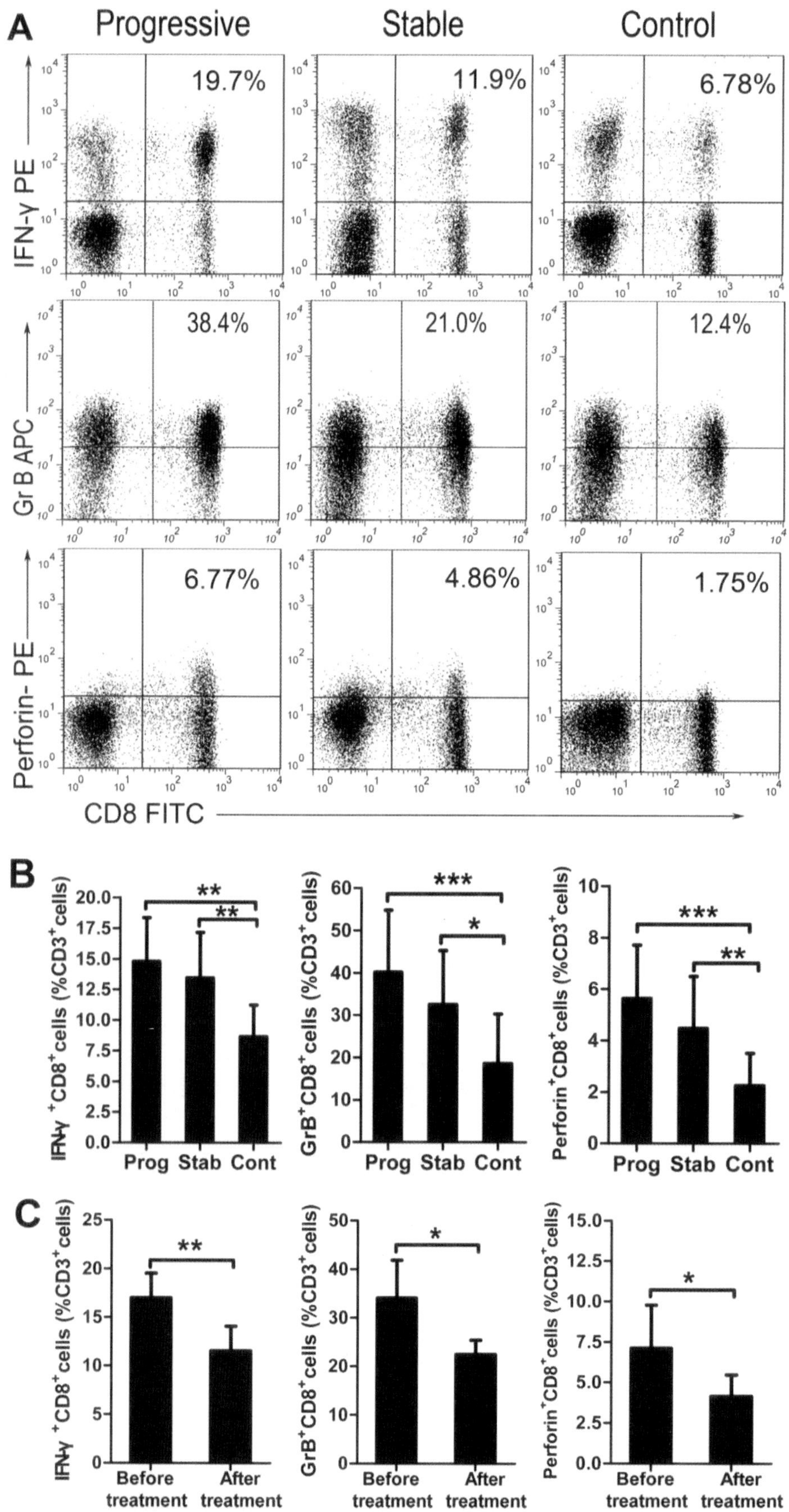

Figure 1. Circulating CD8$^+$ CTLs are increased significantly in GV patients. (A) IFN-γ, GrB and Perforin–expressing cells were detected by intracellular staining. Values are the percentage of IFN-γ^+ CD8$^+$, GrB$^+$ CD8$^+$ or Perforin$^+$ CD8$^+$ cells among CD3$^+$ T cells (Representative cases). (B) Flow cytometric analysis of IFN-γ^+ CD8$^+$, GrB$^+$ CD8$^+$ and Perforin$^+$ CD8$^+$ cells within the CD3$^+$ T cell populations from patients with progressive GV (n = 38),

stable GV (n = 12) and control subjects (n = 20). * = P<0.05, ** = P<0.01, *** = P<0.001. (C) The $CD8^+$ CTL population of 6 patients was monitored longitudinally: The percentage of IFN-γ^+ $CD8^+$ T cells, GrB^+ $CD8^+$ T cells and $Perforin^+$ $CD8^+$ T cells was measured initially during GV progression and again following stabilization after treatment. * = P<0.01, ** = P<0.001.

magnetically sorted $CD8^+$ T cells and $CD4^+$ $CD25^+$ Treg cells from either progressive GV patients (n = 6) or normal control subjects (n = 4). T cells were labeled with CFSE and cocultured in the presence of anti-CD3 and anti-CD28 antibodies (anti-CD3/CD28 Abs) at the ratio of either 1:0.1 or 1:1 (Figure 4A). By analyzing CFSE intensity by flow cytometric analysis on day 5, we detected a dose-dependent suppression of autologous $CD8^+$ T cells by $CD4^+$ $CD25^+$ Treg cells from both normal controls and GV patients. However, Tregs from GV patients showed a significantly lower suppressive capacity than that of normal controls (mean ± SD 11.97±3.08% vs. 17.92±4.15% at a ratio of 1:0.1, P<0.05; 27.76±5.71% vs. 49.03±5.80% at a ratio of 1:1, P<0.01) (Figure 4C). In addition, the $CD4^+$ $CD25^+$ T cells of normal controls and the majority of GV patients (5/6) were hyporesponsive to polyclonal TCR stimulation when cultured alone, as the majority of Tregs remained $CFSE^{high}$ (Figure 4B). These data

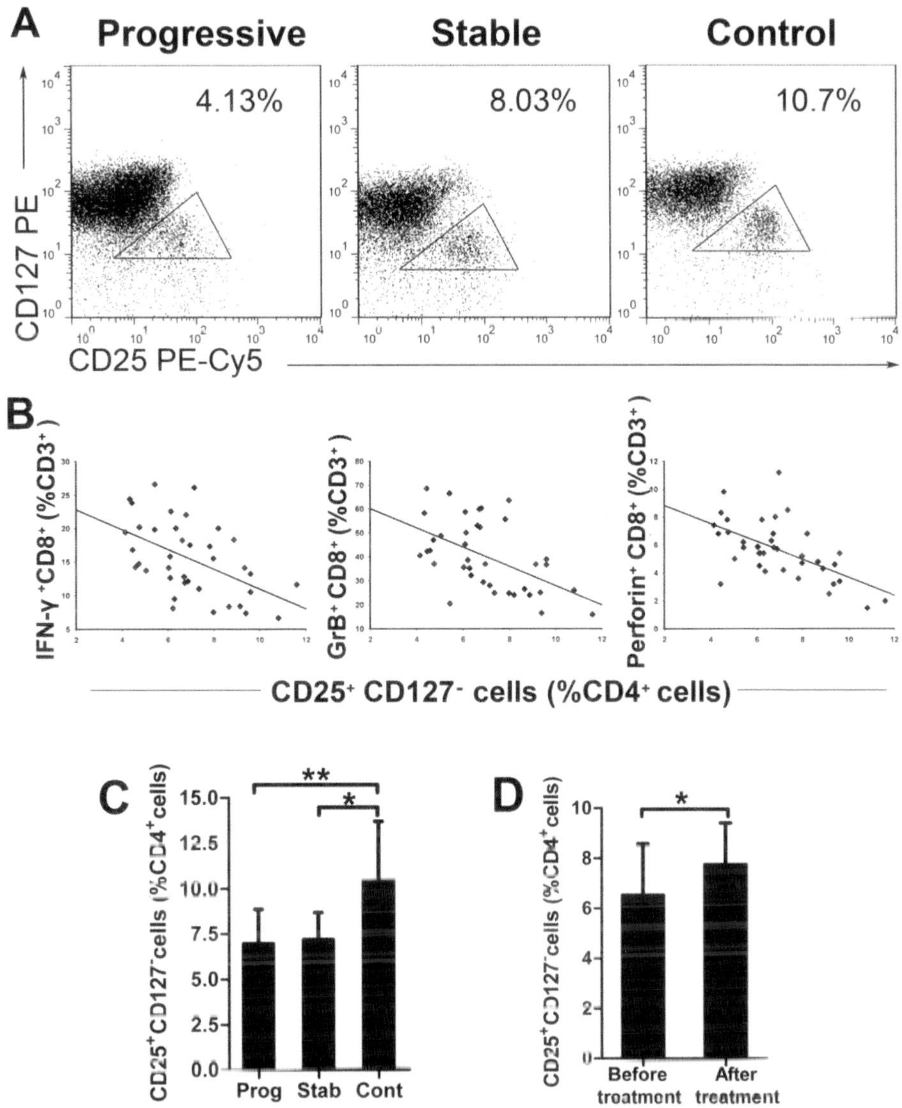

Figure 2. Circulating $CD4^+$ $CD25^+$ $CD127^-$ Tregs are decreased significantly in GV patients. (A) Human PBMCs were labeled with lymphocyte-specific antibodies (CD4, CD25 and CD127). Representative flow data showing the gating strategy and percent of natural Treg cells within the $CD4^+$ T cell population are given for one patient from each of the 3 studied groups. (B) A negative correlation was found between the frequency of $CD4^+$ natural Treg cells and the expression of IFN-γ ($r = -0.512$, P = 0.001), GrB ($r = -0.524$, P = 0.001) or Perforin ($r = -0.585$, P<0.001) from $CD3^+$ CTLs in patients with progressive GV (n = 38). (C) The results of the flow cytometric analysis of natural Treg cells in patients with progressive GV (n = 38), stable GV (n = 12) and control subjects (n = 20) are shown. * = P<0.01, ** = P<0.001. (D) Longitudinal monitoring of natural Treg cells in 6 patients. The percentage of $CD4^+$ natural Treg cells was measured twice: once during a vitiligo flare and once following resolution after treatment. * = P<0.05.

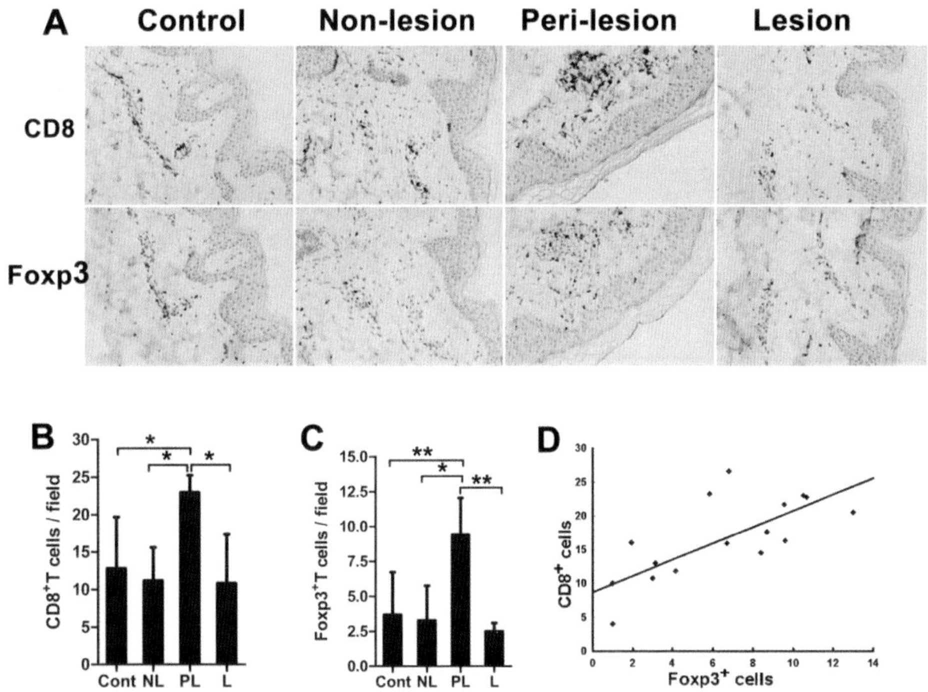

Figure 3. Skin-infiltrating CD8+ cells and Foxp3+ cells in GV patients. (A) Consecutive sections were used for immunohistochemical detection of T cells expressing CD8 or Foxp3+ in skin samples from healthy controls or GV patients (representative fields, 200×). Positive cells appear brown. Both CD8+ (B) and Foxp3+ (C) T cell numbers were increased significantly in the perilesional (PL) tissues of progressive GV patients (n = 16). In contrast, no significant differences were observed between lesional (L) (n = 2) and non-lesional GV skin (NL) (n = 8), as compared to normal skin from unaffected adults (Cont) (n = 6). * = P<0.05, ** = P<0.01. (D) The number of CD8+ and Foxp3+ T cells in perilesional GV skin samples exhibited a positive correlation (r = 0.706, P<0.001; n = 16). Values in B–C are the mean and SD.

indicate that $CD4^+$ $CD25^+$ Treg cells in progressive GV patients could not effectively suppress $CD8^+$ T cell proliferation.

Interestingly, when cocultured with autologous Tregs, $CD8^+$ T cells of GV patients had markedly enhanced levels of IFN-γ and TNF-α upon stimulation with anti-CD3/CD28 Abs compared to healthy individuals (Figure 4D and E). These findings suggest that the Tregs of GV patients may not effectively suppress the production of certain cytokines involved in $CD8^+$ T cell activation.

Discussion

A functional $CD8^+$ T cell response is an essential component of the adaptive immune response to various cancers and pathogens [16]. Upon engagement with antigen, naive $CD8^+$ T cells rapidly expand and differentiate into effector $CD8^+$ T cells, which produce cytokines, including IFN-γ, and effector molecules, such as GrB and Perforin, that mediate a local inflammatory response and effect target cell apoptosis [17,18]. Although effector cytotoxic T lymphocytes (CTLs) play a key role in host defense, they can be detrimental when they react against self tissues. $CD8^+$ T cell-mediated tissue damage has been demonstrated in many autoimmune diseases, including vitiligo [19,20]. Substantial evidence suggests that increased numbers of melanocyte antigen-reactive $CD8^+$ T cells contribute to the pathogenesis of GV [3,21,22]. However, they fail to explain why generalized autoimmune diseases are present at elevated frequencies among GV patients.

According to a large survey on the epidemiology of vitiligo and associated autoimmune diseases in 2,624 Caucasian probands, approximately 30% of vitiligo patients reported at least one associated autoimmune diseases [2]. The most frequent vitiligo-associated disorder was autoimmune thyroid disease, principally Hashimoto's thyroiditis, occurring in more than 19% of adult Caucasian vitiligo probands. Pernicious anemia, Addison's disease, systemic lupus erythematosus and inflammatory bowel disease all occurred at significantly increased frequencies in vitiligo probands. We previously performed a preliminary survey (unpublished) on associated autoimmune diseases and allergic diseases in 118 Chinese GV patients and observed that 35.59% of GV patients declared at least one associated autoimmune disease or allergic disease. The most frequent vitiligo-associated disease was thyroiditis, occurring in 14.41% of patients. Other autoimmune or allergic phenomena reported in this GV cohort were as follows: urticaria 11.02%, allergic rhinitis 11.02%, asthma 6.78%, eczema 2.54%, systemic lupus erythematosus 0.85% and psoriasis 0.85%. These results confirm previous evidence of an association between GV and other autoimmune diseases [23,24] and clarify the magnitude of these associations in Caucasian and Chinese patients.

$CD8^+$ T lymphocytes play a significant role in autoimmune disorders, as demonstrated in several reports that identify that an increase in the number of activated $CD8^+$ T lymphocytes expressing Perforin and GrB correlates with disease activity in patients with systemic lupus erythematosus [6] and multiple sclerosis [7]. These data suggest that widespread activation of $CD8^+$ CTLs might be involved in disease flare-ups. We therefore hypothesized that global activation of $CD8^+$ CTLs may correlate with GV disease activity and that this activation was responsible for the progress of depigmentation and an increased frequency of associated autoimmune disorders in GV patients. Thus, our studies were designed to delineate the ability of circulating $CD8^+$

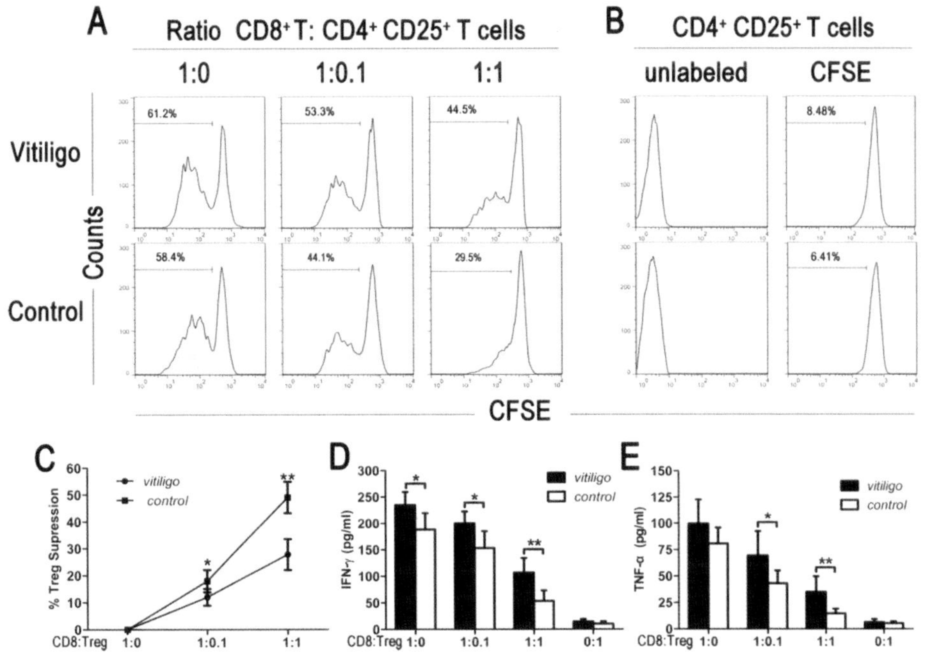

Figure 4. Tregs suppress proliferation and cytokine production of autologous CD8$^+$ T cells. (A) Detection of Treg suppression for CD8$^+$ T cells. CFSE-labeled CD8$^+$ T cells were stimulated in the presence of CD4$^+$ CD25$^+$ Treg cells at the indicated ratios for 5 days. Cellular division was measured by flow cytometric analysis based on the intensity of CFSE signal. Representative CFSE profiles from a GV patient and a normal control are shown. Values given represent the percentage of CFSE^{low} cells among CFSE$^+$ T cells. (B) Treg cells are largely unresponsive to TCR stimulation. Unlabeled and CFSE labeled CD4$^+$ CD25$^+$ T cells were cultured with anti-CD3/CD28 Abs, under the same stimulatory conditions as above, but without autologous CD8$^+$ T cells present. Values given are the percentage of CFSE^{low} cells among CFSE$^+$ Treg cells (Representative cases). (C) Dose-dependent suppression of CD8$^+$ T cell proliferation by CD4$^+$ CD25$^+$ T cells. The suppressive capacity of CD4$^+$ CD25$^+$ Tregs was compared between GV patients (n = 6) and normal control subjects (n = 4). * = P<0.05; ** = P<0.01. The production of IFN-γ (D) and TNF-α (E) was determined. CD8$^+$ T cells were cultured with Tregs at various ratios in the presence of anti-CD3/CD28 Ab stimulation for 48 hours. IFN-γ and TNF-α release into the supernatant was determined by an enzyme-linked immunosorbent assay. The data were from 6 progressive GV individuals and 4 healthy controls. * = P<0.05; ** = P<0.01.

T cells from GV patients to proliferate and/or produce cytotoxic molecules and cytokines upon stimulation with CD3/CD28 Abs.

In our study, we detected effector CD8$^+$ CTLs in the circulation of GV patients, based on their expression of IFN-γ, GrB and Perforin. These specific effector molecules are frequently used in equine research as a surrogate marker for cytotoxic cell activity [25] because studies have shown that their expression correlates well with CD8$^+$ T cell cytotoxic activity in PBMC cultures [26]. Herein, we show that patients with progressive GV exhibit an increased proportion of CD8$^+$ cells expressing IFN-γ, GrB and Perforin compared to healthy individuals (Figure 1). This demonstrates an increased prevalence of activated CD8$^+$ CTLs among PBMCs in GV patients, especially in patients with progressive disease. Furthermore, our data show that an increased proportion of CD8$^+$ T cells also accumulate in the perilesional skin of progressive GV patients, especially in areas adjacent to disappearing melanocytes. These data suggest that CD8$^+$ CTLs could migrate to sites of inflammation and participate in the destruction of melanocytes, thereby promoting vitiligo-associated depigmentation (Figure 3). Taken together, these data demonstrate that the proportion of CD8$^+$ CTLs in both circulating and perilesional skin are enhanced in the setting of progressive GV, suggesting that a global expansion of CD8$^+$ CTLs might be involved in the development of GV. In addition, we observed that the prevalence of circulating CD8$^+$ CTLs decreased significantly after efficacious treatment with oral Chinese herbs and topical steroids. Thus, the frequency of activated CTLs correlates with disease activity, whereas a normalization of this frequency may precede the clinical stabilization of GV and may be used as a predictive factor of disease outcome.

In the proliferation assay, CD8$^+$ T lymphocytes from progressive patients cultured alone showed hyper-activation and produced more IFN-γ and TNF-α upon stimulation with anti-CD3/CD28 Abs, compared with CD8$^+$ T cells from control individuals. These data suggest that the cytotoxic function of CD8$^+$ T cells may be hyperactive in progressive GV patients (Figure 4). We hypothesized that a defect in immunoregulation resulted in the global activation of effector CD8$^+$ CTLs that consequently contributed to elevated frequencies of autoimmune diseases associated with GV. Taken together, our data disclose a new and pivotal role of globally activated CD8$^+$ CTLs in GV pathogenesis.

Natural Treg cells play a key role in maintaining peripheral tolerance in vivo through the active suppression of self-reactive T cell activation and expansion [9]. A deficiency or dysfunction of Tregs has been described in several autoimmune diseases, both systemic [27,28] and organ-specific [29]. Currently, very little is known about the function of Treg cells in GV patients. In this study, we show that GV patients exhibit a decreased prevalence of circulating Tregs (Figure 2) and an increased proportion of perilesion-infiltrating Treg cells (Figure 3). Thus, regulatory T cells are likely recruited to inflamed skin lesions from the peripheral blood, despite a deficiency of circulating Tregs. These data are consistent with current findings demonstrating that circulating Tregs could migrate to sites of inflammation to balance the autoimmune response in progressive GV [10]. Our data, however, conflict with the findings reported by Klarquist et al. [9], who did not notice any deficiency in peripheral Treg cell numbers in vitiligo patients. Rather, they reported a reduced proportion of Tregs in skin samples from vitiligo patients, leading them to hypothesize that circulating Tregs are not recruited to vitiligo skin lesions. This discrepancy may be explained by the small number of patients included in their study. Nonetheless, we observed that the percentage of circulating Treg cells increased significantly after treatment-induced stabilization, suggesting that these Tregs reflected disease activity, and could therefore be a predictive factor for the stabilization of the disease.

Interestingly, the abundance of Tregs in perilesional skin could not prevent $CD8^+$ T cell-mediated cytotoxic activity toward melanocytes in progressive GV. Previous studies in some autoimmune disorders have demonstrated that defective regulatory T cell function might result in autoimmune activation [30]. This led us to evaluate the ability of circulating natural Tregs from GV patients to control $CD8^+$ T cell proliferation and activation. The suppressive effects of peripheral T regulatory cells in 6 progressive GV cases were significantly reduced, demonstrating an impairment in their ability to inhibit the proliferation and cytokine production of stimulated autologous $CD8^+$ T cells. Thus, a functional defect in Tregs might be involved in the pathogenesis of GV disease (Figure 4). For instance, a higher recruitment of functionally deficient Tregs in situ would not be able to regulate the widespread activation of self-reactive $CD8^+$ CTLs that mediate the progressive loss or destruction of melanocytes in GV patients and would also explain the elevated frequency of associated generalized autoimmunity. Our findings are consistent with a recent report from Ben Ahmed [10] in which the suppressive effects of peripheral $CD4^+$ $CD25^+$ T regulatory cells on conventional $CD4^+$ $CD25^-$ T cell proliferation were analyzed in vitiligo patients. These data revealed a functional defect in Treg cells from 7 of 15 cases. Taken together with our findings, these data indicate the presence of functional defects in Treg cells in patients with progressive GV, which would permit an active immune response against melanocytes and other self-antigens to proceed unhindered, despite the presence and recruitment of circulating peripheral Tregs in sites of diseases activity.

To demonstrate the relationship between the proportion of circulating cytotoxic $CD8^+$ T cells and natural Treg cells, we plotted the percentages of peripheral blood IFN-γ^+ $CD8^+$ T cells, GrB^+ $CD8^+$ T cells and $Perforin^+$ $CD8^+$ T cells against that of Treg cells from progressive GV patient (Figure 2C). Our data showed that these three $CD8^+$ CTL populations all correlated negatively with Tregs, suggesting a possible causal association between $CD8^+$ CTLs and Tregs in the development of GV. Although concluding whether $CD8^+$ CTL hyperactivity is a cause or a consequence of the quantitative and functional defects of Tregs requires further investigation, we hypothesize that deficiencies and dysfunction in the Treg population fail to maintain peripheral tolerance and lead to a copious expansion and activation of self-reactive $CD8^+$ CTLs, which destroys melanocytes and leads to a high frequency of generalized autoimmune diseases in GV patients.

Finally, we did not notice any significant difference in the frequency of circulating $CD8^+$ CTLs and $CD4^+$ $CD25^+$ $CD127^-$ Treg cells between patients with progressive and stable GV (Figures 1 and 2). Two reasons may account for this observation: (1) The small sample size of stable GV patients we studied may not be representative of this patient population and needs to therefore be confirmed, and (2) the classification of disease activity among our GV patients might be faulty. At present, disease activity is mainly assessed by the medical history information provided by patients themselves. However, the patients' recollection of disease activity might not be accurate. It is conceivable that minor expansions of old lesions or the appearance of new but small lesions are not always noticed by the patient, especially when these changes occur to lesions that are less conspicuous to the patient (e.g., axillae or back). Moreover, patients with extensive vitiligo involving more than 30% of the total body surface area also find it difficult to assess disease activity. Thus, it is possible that some patients with slow progressive disease were mistakenly classified as having stable vitiligo. Thus, further investigation should aim for more precise disease stage-classification standards.

In conclusion, our findings indicate that the imbalance of $CD8^+$ CTLs and natural Tregs in frequency and function might be involved in the progression of GV. The deficiency and dysfunction of natural Treg cell subpopulations lead to a global expansion and widespread activation of the $CD8^+$ CTL population, which results in the destruction of melanocytes and an elevated frequency of associated autoimmune diseases in GV patients. This knowledge furthers our understanding of the mechanisms that contribute to the autoimmune status of GV patients and provides a new avenue of investigation that may lead to the development of effective immunotherapies for patients with GV.

Methods

Patients and controls

Fifty adult patients (18 women and 32 men, mean $\pm$ SD age 38 ± 16.7 years) with a diagnosis of GV were enrolled in the study after giving informed consent. The patients were divided into two groups based on whether the existing lesions were spreading and/or new lesions had appeared within the previous 6 months: an affirmative answer to one or both of those questions led to inclusion of the patient in the progressive GV group, whereas patients with no increase in lesion size or number were included the stable GV group. Thirty-eight patients were classified with progressive GV (14 women and 24 men, age 38 ± 16 years), whereas 12 patients were included in the stable GV group (4 women and 8 men, age 38 ± 20 years). A medication-free period was required for both groups, which consisted of at least 1 month for oral drugs, and 2 weeks for topical medications or phototherapy prior to study procedures. As a control, 20 healthy individuals from Fudan University were enrolled in our study. The protocols involving human subjects were approved by the institutional review boards of Zhongshan Hospital of Fudan University. Informed consent was obtained in writing from all subjects before performing the studies.

For the 10 patients in the group of patients with active GV, we administrated oral traditional Chinese herbs and topical steroids twice a day to stop progression and improve lesions. The herbs complex is a mixture extracts of Rx. Angelicae Sinensis, Rx. Astragali, Fructus Tribuli and Caulis Spatholobi, which appears to be effective in halting disease progression and inducing repigmentation in GV. Three months later, 6 patients in 10 cases reported stabilization of their disease, and blood samples from these 6 patients were obtained again for analysis.

Four-millimeter skin biopsies were obtained from 18 patients with GV. Six healthy tissue specimens were obtained from individuals undergoing orthopedic surgery, and four healthy blood samples were obtained from age- and gender-matched volunteers for cell proliferation assays. The patients provided informed consent prior to tissue collection. The study protocol was reviewed and approved by the Zhongshan Hospital research ethics committee.

Available patient information that was relevant to this study is summarized in Table 1 and Table 2 for patients included in the

Table 1. Patient skin biopsy samples for $CD8^+$ cells and $Foxp3^+$ cells quantification by immunohistochemistry.

Patient gender	Patient age (yr)	Biopsy site	Perilesion/Lesion/Normal skin	Disease duration (yr)	Disease activity	1st degree relatives with vitiligo	Associated disease*
Female	18	Abdomen	Lesion + Normal	16	Stable	No	No
Male	45	Arm	Lesion + Normal	12	Stable	No	No
Male	34	Thorax	Perilesion + Normal	6	Progressive	No	No
Male	59	Abdomen	Perilesion + Normal	20	Progressive	No	Psoriasis
Male	20	Leg	Perilesion + Normal	1	Progressive	No	AR, Asthma
Female	36	Arm	Perilesion + Normal	24	Progressive	No	No
Male	30	Arm	Perilesion + Normal	3	Progressive	No	AR
Female	40	Abdomen	Perilesion + Normal	26	Progressive	Yes	No
Male	40	Back	Perilesion	3	Progressive	No	No
Male	62	Leg	Perilesion	6	Progressive	Yes	No
Female	69	Arm	Perilesion	30	Progressive	Yes	HT
Female	20	Arm	Perilesion	5	Progressive	No	No
Female	43	Abdomen	Perilesion	23	Progressive	No	HT
Male	30	Arm	Perilesion	10	Progressive	No	No
Female	48	Arm	Perilesion	0.5	Progressive	No	SLE
Male	77	Arm	Perilesion	1.5	Progressive	No	AA, AR
Male	46	Abdomen	Perilesion	0.2	Progressive	No	HT
Male	72	Leg	Perilesion	2	Progressive	No	No

*SLE = systemic lupus erythematosus; AA = alopecia areata; AR = allergic rhinitis; HT = Hashimoto's thyroiditis.

doi:10.1371/journal.pone.0037513.t001

Table 2. Patient PBMC samples involved in proliferation assay.

Patient gender	Patient age (yr)	Disease duration (yr)	Disease activity	Lesional Area	1st degree relatives with vitiligo	Associated disease*
Female	49	0.5	Progressive	<1%	No	No
Female	45	20	Progressive	8%	Yes	HT
Male	27	16	Progressive	1%	Yes	No
Male	16	1	Progressive	<1%	No	No
Male	48	10	Progressive	10%	No	HT
Male	18	5	Progressive	8%	Yes	AR, Asthma

*HT = Hashimoto's thyroiditis. AR = allergic rhinitis.

immunohistochemistry data set and the cell proliferation assay, respectively.

Flow cytometry

All blood samples were processed on the day of collection. Peripheral blood mononuclear cells (PBMCs) were purified on Ficoll gradients (GE Healthcare, Björkgatan, Sweden). For the detection of natural Treg cells, PBMCs were stained with fluorescein isothiocyanate (FITC)-conjugated anti-CD4, phycoerythrin-Cy5 (PE-Cy5)-conjugated anti-CD25, and PE-conjugated anti-CD127 (eBiosciences, San Diego, CA), according to the manufacturer's protocol. After staining, cells were washed twice in fluorescence-activated cell sorting solution (phosphate buffered saline [PBS] with 0.5% bovine serum albumin [BSA] and 0.02% sodium azide), fixed in PBS containing 1% paraformaldehyde, and collected the same day on a FACSCalibur system (BD Biosciences, San Jose, CA) followed by analysis using FlowJo software (Tree Star, San Carlos, CA). $CD25^+$ $CD127^-$ natural Treg cells were identified within gated $CD4^+$ T cells.

Intracellular cytokine staining

For the detection of IFN-γ, PBMCs were incubated for 4–5 hours in RPMI 1640 (containing 10% fetal bovine serum [FBS]) with 50 ng/ml phorbol myristate acetate (PMA) and 750 ng/ml ionomycin in the presence of 1.7 µg/ml monensin (Enzo Biochem, Farmingdale, New York) in a tissue culture incubator at 37°C. No incubation was performed for the detection of GrB and Perforin molecules. For intracellular staining of IFN-γ, GrB and Perforin molecules, PBMCs were first stained with PerCP-conjugated anti-CD3 and FITC-conjugated anti-CD8 antibodies and then fixed and permeabilized using FIX & PERM (Invitrogen, Carlsbad, CA), according to the manufacturer's instructions. Permeabilized cells were then stained with either PE-conjugated anti-IFN-γ or APC-conjugated anti-GrB and PE-conjugated anti-Perforin (eBioscience, San Diego, CA) for 20 minutes. Stained cells were then fixed in 1% paraformaldehyde, and 4-color flow cytometric analyses were performed using FACSCalibur and FlowJo software. For the detection of $CD8^+$ cytotoxic T cells, IFN-γ^+ $CD8^+$, GrB^+ $CD8^+$ or $Perforin^+$ $CD8^+$ T cells were analyzed among cells first included in a $CD3^+$ gate.

Immunohistochemistry

Tissues from 18 GV patients were processed and embedded in paraffin using routine methods. Tissue blocks were serially sectioned to obtain consecutive sections. Immunohistochemistry for $CD8^+$ and $Foxp3^+$ T cells was performed using the Novolink Polymer Detection System (Novocastra, Newcastle-upon-Tyne, UK) according to the manufacturer's instructions. Briefly, paraffin-embedded sections were first deparaffinized and then hydrated. After microwave antigen retrieval, endogenous peroxidase activity was blocked by the incubation of slides in 0.3% H_2O_2, whereas nonspecific binding sites were blocked with Protein Block (Novocastra). Primary monoclonal antibodies directed against CD8 (Dako, Copenhagen, Denmark) and Foxp3 (Abcam, Cambridge, UK) were used for CD8 and Foxp3 staining, respectively. Following serial incubations with primary antibodies, Primary Block, and secondary antibody treatment (Novolink polymer; Novocastra), the sections were developed in a diaminobenzidine solution and counterstained with hematoxylin. Sections incubated with PBS only served as negative controls.

For quantification of $CD8^+$ and $Foxp3^+$ cells, skin sections were examined microscopically at high power (400×). Five high-power fields of each sample were selected for digital photographs. These same five areas were counted manually by two independent observers for the number of $CD8^+$ or $Foxp3^+$ cells in each field.

Cell isolation

All blood samples were processed on the day of collection. PBMCs were purified by Ficoll-Hypaque density gradient centrifugation from heparinized blood. $CD4^+$ $CD25^+$ Tregs were isolated from PBMCs by CD4-negative selection followed by CD25-positive selection, using the $CD4^+$ $CD25^+$ T-cell isolation kit (Miltenyi Biotech, Teterow, Germany), with MidiMACS and MiniMACS separator units (both from Miltenyi Biotech), according to the manufacturer's instructions. A $CD8^+$ T-cell isolation kit (Miltenyi Biotech, Teterow, Germany) was used to isolate $CD8^+$ cells by CD8-negative selection. The purities of $CD4^+$ $CD25^+$ Tregs and $CD8^+$ T cells were 90% or greater and 98%, respectively.

$CD8^+$ T cell proliferation assay and cytokine detection

Carboxyfluorescein diacetate succinimidyl ester (CFSE) (Invitrogen Corporation, Carlsbad, CA) was used to detect the proliferation of $CD8^+$ T cells according to manufacturer's instruction. Briefly, freshly prepared CFSE stock solution was added to $CD8^+$ or $CD4^+CD25^+$ T cell suspensions at a final concentration of 4 µM and then incubated for 10 minutes at 37°C. Cells were washed and resuspended in 5 volumes of ice-cold RPMI 1640 culture medium for 5 minutes on ice to stabilize the CFSE staining. After two washes, CFSE-labeled cells were resuspended and cultured with $CD4^+$ $CD25^+$ Tregs at various ratios. In a U-bottom 96-well plate coated with 5 µg/ml anti-CD3 Abs (OKT3) (eBioscience, San Diego, CA), CFSE-labeled cells were added at 5×10^4 cells per well in RPMI 1640 (containing 10% FBS) with 2 µg/ml soluble anti-CD28 Abs (CD28.2) and incubated at 37°C and 5% CO_2. On day 3 of culture, the culture medium was replaced with fresh RPMI 1640 (containing 10% FBS) with 2 μg/ml soluble anti-CD3 and anti-CD28 Abs. Cells were harvested on day 5, and the intensity of CFSE staining of $CD8^+$ T cells or $CD4^+$ $CD25^+$ Treg populations was determined using a FACSCalibur system (BD Biosciences, San Jose, CA) and FlowJo software (Tree Star, San Carlos, CA). The suppressive capacity of Tregs toward $CD8^+$ T cells in coculture ($CD8^+$ T cell to Treg ratio of 1:0.1 or 1:1) was defined as relative inhibition based on the percentage of $CFSE^{low}$ cells used as a measure of proliferation: [100×(1-% $CFSE^{low}$ $CD8^+$ T cells in coculture/% $CFSE^{low}$ $CD8^+$ T cells alone)].

For IFN-γ and tumor necrosis factor-α (TNF-α) detection, the plate was cultured for 48 hours. Cytokine release into the supernatant was measured using the corresponding enzyme-linked immunosorbent assay kits (Bender, Vienna, Austria), according to the manufacturer's instructions.

Statistical analysis

Data analysis was performed with SPSS version 12.0 for Windows software (SPSS Inc., Chicago, IL). Quantitative data were expressed as the mean ± SD. Statistical significance was determined by an analysis of variance followed by the Bonferroni post hoc test for comparisons of multiple means or Student's t-test. Comparisons of the rates of circulating natural Treg cells, IFN-γ^+ $CD8^+$, GrB^+ $CD8^+$ and $Perforin^+$ $CD8^+$ cells during the evolution of disease were made by paired t-tests. Correlations were determined by Spearman's ranking. A P value of less than .05 was considered significant.

Acknowledgments

We thank Zeng HY for immunohistochemical slide preparation and staining, Dr. Sun SH for flow cytometry analysis, Jin JJ for technical assistance, and Dr. Xie YQ and Dr. Wu J for helpful discussions.

Author Contributions

Conceived and designed the experiments: YL LM. Performed the experiments: YL WY. Analyzed the data: YL YJ WY LM. Contributed reagents/materials/analysis tools: SY SW. Wrote the paper: YL LM.

References

1. Taieb A, Picardo M, Members V (2007) The definition and assessment of vitiligo: a consensus report of the Vitiligo European Task Force. Pigment Cell Research 20: 27–35.
2. Alkhateeb A, Fain PR, Thody A, Bennett DC, Spritz RA (2003) Epidemiology of vitiligo and associated autoimmune diseases in Caucasian probands and their families. Pigment Cell Res 16: 208–214.
3. Ogg GS, Dunbar PR, Romero P, Chen JL, Cerundolo V (1998) High frequency of skin-homing melanocyte-specific cytotoxic T lymphocytes in autoimmune vitiligo. Journal of Experimental Medicine 188: 1203–1208.
4. Palermo B, Campanelli R, Garbelli S, Mantovani S, Lantelme E, et al. (2001) Specific cytotoxic T lymphocyte responses against Melan-A/MART1, tyrosinase and Gp100 in vitiligo by the use of major histocompatibility complex/peptide tetramers: the role of cellular immunity in the etiopathogenesis of vitiligo. Journal of Investigative Dermatology 117: 326–332.
5. Lang KS, Caroli CC, Muhm A, Wernet D, Moris A, et al. (2001) HLA-A2 restricted, melanocyte-specific CD8(+) T lymphocytes detected in vitiligo patients are related to disease activity and are predominantly directed against MelanA/MART1. Journal of Investigative Dermatology 116: 891–897.
6. Blanco P, Pitard V, Viallard JF, Taupin JL, Pellegrin JL, et al. (2005) Increase in activated CD8+T lymphocytes expressing perforin and granzyme B correlates with disease activity in patients with systemic lupus erythematosus. Arthritis and Rheumatism 52: 201–211.
7. Giovanni F, Domenico P, Alessandro M, Raffaele I, Viviana N, et al. (2011) Circulating CD8(+)CD56(−)perforin(+) T cells are increased in multiple sclerosis patients. Journal of Neuroimmunology 240: 137–141.
8. Sakaguchi S (2004) Naturally arising CD4(+) regulatory T cells for immunologic self-tolerance and negative control of immune responses. Annual Review of Immunology 22: 531–562.
9. Klarquist J, Denman CJ, Hernandez C, Wainwright DA, Strickland FM, et al. (2010) Reduced skin homing by functional Treg in vitiligo. Pigment Cell Melanoma Res. England. pp 276–286.
10. Ben Ahmed M, Zaraa I, Rekik R, Elbeldi-Ferchiou A, Kourda N, et al. (2011) Functional defects of peripheral regulatory T lymphocytes in patients with progressive vitiligo. Pigment Cell Melanoma Res.
11. Wolint P, Betts MR, Koup RA, Oxenius A (2004) Immediate cytotoxicity but not degranulation distinguishes effector and memory subsets of CD8(+) T cells. Journal of Experimental Medicine 199: 925–936.
12. Liu W, Putnam AL, Xu-Yu Z, Szot GL, Lee MR, et al. (2006) CD127 expression inversely correlates with FoxP3 and suppressive function of human CD4+ T reg cells. J Exp Med 203: 1701–1711.
13. Fontenot JD, Gavin MA, Rudensky AY (2003) Foxp3 programs the development and function of CD4(+)CD25(+) regulatory T cells. Nature Immunology 4: 330–336.
14. Hori S, Nomura T, Sakaguchi S (2003) Control of regulatory T cell development by the transcription factor Foxp3. Science 299: 1057–1061.
15. Yagi H, Nomura T, Nakamura K, Yamazaki S, Kitawaki T, et al. (2004) Crucial role of FOXP3 in the development and function of human CD25(+)CD4(+) regulatory T cells. International Immunology 16: 1643–1656.
16. Kaech SM, Wherry EJ, Ahmed R (2002) Effector and memory T-cell differentiation: Implications for vaccine development. Nature Reviews Immunology 2: 251–262.
17. Trapani JA, Smyth MJ (2002) Functional significance of the perforin/granzyme cell death pathway. Nature Reviews Immunology 2: 735–747.
18. Shankaran V, Ikeda H, Bruce AT, White JM, Swanson PE, et al. (2001) IFN gamma and lymphocytes prevent primary tumour development and shape tumour immunogenicity. Nature 410: 1107–1111.
19. Walter U, Santamaria P (2005) CD8(+) T cells in autoimmunity. Current Opinion in Immunology 17: 624–631.
20. Liblau RS, Wong FS, Mars LT, Santamaria P (2002) Autoreactive CD8 T cells in organ-specific autoimmunity: Emerging targets for therapeutic intervention. Immunity 17: 1–6.
21. Oyarbide-Valencia K, van den Boorn JG, Denman CJ, Li M, Carlson JM, et al. (2006) Therapeutic implications of autoimmune vitiligo T cells. Autoimmunity Reviews 5: 486–492.
22. Wankowicz-Kalinska A, van den Wijngaard R, Tigges BJ, Westerhof W, Ogg GS, et al. (2003) Immunopolarization of CD4(+) and CD8(+) T cells to type-1-like is associated with melanocyte loss in human vitiligo. Laboratory Investigation 83: 683–695.
23. Cunliffe WJ, Hall R, Newell DJ, Stevenson CJ (1968) VITILIGO THYROID DISEASE AND AUTOIMMUNITY. British Journal of Dermatology 80: 135–&.
24. Schallreuter KU, Lemke R, Brandt O, Schwartz R, Westhofen M, et al. (1994) VITILIGO AND OTHER DISEASES - COEXISTENCE OR TRUE ASSOCIATION - HAMBURG STUDY ON 321 PATIENTS. Dermatology 188: 269–275.
25. Breathnach CC, Soboll G, Suresh M, Lunn DP (2005) Equine herpesvirus-1 infection induces IFN-gamma production by equine T lymphocyte subsets. Veterinary Immunology and Immunopathology 103: 207–215.
26. Malyguine A, Shafer-Weaver K, Derby E, Burkett M, Sayers T, et al. (2003) Granzyme B and IFN-gamma production by effector cells in cell-mediated cytotoxicity. European Cytokine Network 14: 36.
27. Antiga E, Kretz C, Klembt R, Massi D, Ruland V, et al. (2010) Characterization of regulatory T cells in patients with dermatomyositis. Journal of Autoimmunity 35: 342–350.
28. Miyara M, Amoura Z, Parizot C, Badoual C, Dorgham K, et al. (2005) Global natural regulatory T cell depletion in active systemic lupus erythematosus. Journal of Immunology 175: 8392–8400.
29. Chi LJ, Wang HB, Wang WZ (2008) Impairment of circulating CD4(+)CD25(+) regulatory T cells in patients with chronic inflammatory demyelinating polyradiculoneuropathy. Journal of the Peripheral Nervous System 13: 54–63.
30. Westerhof W, d'Ischia M (2007) Vitiligo puzzle: the pieces fall in place. Pigment Cell Research 20: 345–359.

Clinical Symptoms of Skin, Nails, and Joints Manifest Independently in Patients with Concomitant Psoriasis and Psoriatic Arthritis

Knut M. Wittkowski[1], Craig Leonardi[2], Alice Gottlieb[3], Alan Menter[4], Gerald G. Krueger[5], Paul W. Tebbey[6], Jennifer Belasco[1]*, Razieh Soltani-Arabshahi[5], John Gray[1], Liz Horn[6], James G. Krueger[1]* for the International Psoriasis Council[6]

1 The Rockefeller University, New York, New York, United States of America, **2** St. Louis University Medical School, St. Louis University, St. Louis, Missouri, United States of America, **3** Tufts Medical Center, Tufts University, Boston, Massachusetts, United States of America, **4** Baylor Institute of Research, Dermatology Research Center, Baylor University Medical Center, Baylor University, Dallas, Texas, United States of America, **5** University of Utah, Salt Lake City, Utah, United States of America, **6** International Psoriasis Council, Dallas, Texas, United States of America

Abstract

This study correlated assessment tools for evaluating the severity of skin, nail, and joint symptoms in patients with psoriasis (Pso) and psoriatic arthritis (PsA). Adults with plaque Pso (with or without PsA) were enrolled from four U.S. institutions. Patients were evaluated using a novel 10-area Linear Psoriasis Area and Severity Index (XL-PASI), Psoriatic Arthritis Assessment (PsAA), Psoriatic Arthritis Screening and Evaluation Questionnaire (PASE), Nail Assessment (NA) and Joint Assessment (JA) tools, Psoriasis Weighted Extent and Severity Index (PWESI), and Lattice Physician Global Assessment (LS-PGA). Correlations between assessment tools and individual items in the assessment tools were performed. Data from 180 patients (55 with PsA) were analyzed. Highest correlations between tools ($r = 0.77–0.88$) were between the XL-PASI, PWESI and LS-PGA. Individual items in the XL-PASI correlated with items in the PWESI for extent skin symptoms, but not for all body areas. Overall, correlations were seen between hands and feet, between face and scalp, and between buttocks, chest, and back. Only low correlation was seen between items assessing joint symptoms with items assessing skin symptoms. These data support the notion that the complex phenotype of psoriatic disease requires instruments that assess the severity of skin, nails, and joints separately.

Editor: George C. Tsokos, Harvard Medical School; Beth Israel, United States of America

Funding: This study was supported in part by a National Institutes of Health/Clinical and Translational Science Award (CTSA) grant UL1 RR024143 and an unrestricted educational grant from the International Psoriasis Council (IPC) to KMW and JGK. The project was also supported by unrestricted educational grants to the International Psoriasis Council from Abbott, Amgen/Pfizer, Astellas, Centocor, Galderma and Janssen-Cilag. The funders had no role in study design, data collection and analysis, decision to publish, or preparation of the manuscript.

Competing Interests: Alan Menter, M.D. has the following conflicts of interest in the form of compensation: Abbott, Allergen, Amgen, Astellas, Asubio, Celgene, Centocor, DUSA, Eli Lilly, GAlderma, Genentech, Novartis, Novo Nordisk, Pfizer, Promius, Stiefel, Syntrix Biosystems, Warner Chilcott and Wyeth. This compensation is not for employment. Gerald G Krueger, M.D. has received fees as a consultant or advisory board member for Abbott, Almirall, Alza, Amgen, Anacor, Astellas, Barrier Therapeutics, Boehringer Ingleheim, Bristol Myers Squibb, Centocor, CombinatoRx, Exelixis, Genentech, Genzyme, Isis, L'Oreal, Lupin Limited, Magen Biosciencs, MedaCorp, Medicis, Novartis, Nova Nordisc, Schering Plough, Somagenics, theDerm.org, Synvista, Warner Chilcot, UCB, USANA Health Sciences and ZARS. Dr. Krueger owns equities and stock options in/from ZARS. In the last 24 months Dr. Krueger has received lecture fees from Abbott, AMgen, Astellas, Boehringer Ingleheim, Centocor, Connetics, National Psoriasis Foundation, The Foundation for Better Health Care and Warner Chilcott. Dr. Krueger has received partial stipend support for a clinical research fellowship from Abbott, Amgen and Centocor. Paul Tebbey, PhD. is employed by the International Psoriasis Council to provide scientific advice. James G. Krueger, M.D., Ph.D. has the following conflicts of interest: Abbott, Centocor, Janssen-Cilag, Pfizer, Merch, Avontec and Magen. They are all lecture honoraria or consulting and all less than $10,000 a year. The other authors have no conflicts of interest to report. There are no patents, products in development or marketed products to declare. This does not alter the authors' adherence to all the PLoS ONE policies on sharing data and materials, as detailed online in the guide for authors.

* E-mail: jgk@rockefeller.edu (JGK); jbelascorockefeller.edu (JB)

Introduction

Psoriasis (Pso) is a chronic, systemic, inflammatory, multigenic disease, that manifests in the skin and has significant impact on quality of life [1]. About one quarter of patients with Pso also develop psoriatic arthritis (PsA) [2]. Nail involvement is common in patients with Pso and more so with PsA [3]. Recent studies have suggested that psoriatic skin, joint, and nail manifestations, long believed to share a common etiology, may be traits of distinct disease conditions [4–8]. This may explain why the severity and progression of skin, joint, and nail symptoms are frequently asynchronous [9], with joint disease in most patients developing up to 10 years after the initial skin presentation.

Genes within the Major Histocompatibility Complex and genes encoding cytokines have been linked to Pso and PsA [1,10–14]. Genetic evidence supports the notion that Pso and PsA are two disease conditions with comorbid association, but might have distinct genes that drive pathogenesis, progression, and severity [1,10,15]. Individual alleles for many of these genes and single nucleotide polymorphisms (SNPs) within these genes appear to be differentially associated with Pso and PsA. Recently, Nograles et al. postulated that Pso and PsA involve multiple genes with low risk effects, only some of which may be shared [16].

Biological evidence also supports a physiological differentiation. For example, selected key immune mediators of disease in the skin and joints differ. Pathologic events in the skin are mediated by autoreactive T cells [1], whereas T cells in the affected synovium of PsA patients do not exhibit the same type of autoreactivity [17]. Skin and joint symptoms frequently do not respond equally or in parallel to systemic or biologic therapeutic agents [18].

Hence, there is a need to optimize the diagnosis and recording of the appearance and progression of Pso and PsA for both clinical research purposes and clinical practice, thus optimizing treatment modalities and outcomes. The goal of this paper is to determine from existing tools the smallest number of independent scoring dimensions needed to measure the presence and severity of skin, nail and joint involvement in the broadest psoriatic patient population. Various assessment tools were then evaluated in a phase II-type clinical trial.

Methods

Study design

The clinical portion of the study was conducted from November 2007 to August 2008 in four U.S. institutions; Baylor Research Institute, Dallas; Central Dermatology, St. Louis; University of Utah, Salt Lake City; and Tufts Medical Center, Boston. The study protocol and informed consent forms were approved by all institutional review boards and all patients signed a written consent form before initiation of study-specific procedures. All statistical analyses were performed at the Rockefeller University, Center for Clinical and translational Science, New York.

Patients

Eligible patients were >18 years old and had plaque Pso (with or without PsA) with ≥5% and ≤90% body surface area (BSA) affected.

Disease assessment tools

As described below, the assessment tools comprised two categories: those that involved a physician examination and those submitted to the patient by questionnaire. Some tools were modified slightly to derive more detailed information and consequently, these are included as supplemental figures.

Psoriasis Area and Severity Index (PASI). The PASI is the most commonly used tool to assess disease severity in patients with Pso in clinical trials [19]. The PASI measures erythema, scaling, and thickness of lesions and is weighted by the area of involvement. The PASI scale ranges from 0 to 72, calculated as the extent of involvement × (score for erythema + score for scaling + score for thickness), where the extent of involvement is categorized as: 0 (0%), 1 (1–9%), 2 (10–29%), 3 (30–49%), 4 (50–69%), 5 (70–89%), or 6 (90–100%), and scores for erythema, scaling, and thickness are each rated on a scale of 0 to 4. It is seldom used in clinical practice.

Psoriatic Arthritis Assessment (PsAA). The PsAA (Fig. S1) is a composite measurement of PsA that includes questions regarding patient and family history and 6 multipart components of a physical examination. *Psoriatic Arthritis Screening and Evaluation Questionnaire (PASE).* This validated questionnaire (Fig. S2) comprises seven questions regarding symptoms and eight questions regarding function that are answered by the patient [20]. Questions are rated on a scale of 1 (strongly disagree) to 5 (strongly agree).

Nail Assessment (NA) and Joint Assessment (JA). The NA and JA (Fig. S3) evaluate nail involvement (score 0 for no involvement and score 1 for involvement by digit) and joint involvement (0/1 by digit) on the hands. The scoring is based upon physician assessment. Selected items that evaluate the type of disease for most involved nail were excluded as several assessors had included toenails; only fingernail assessments were included in this analysis.

Psoriasis Weighted Extent and Severity Index (PW-ESI). This index (Fig. S4) is used to evaluate the extent of skin disease on a scale of 0 (none) to 4 (extensive) and severity of disease on a scale of 0 (essentially clear) to (intensely inflamed) (46). Ten areas are assessed: scalp/hairline, face/neck, arms/axillae, hands/fingers/fingernails, anterior chest/abdomen, back/shoulders, genitalia/perineum/natal cleft, buttocks/thighs, knees/lower legs/ankles, and feet/toes/toenails. The physician assessment delivers a maximal composite score of 50.

Extended 10-Area Linear Psoriasis Area and Severity Index (XL-PASI). The XL-PASI (illustrated in Fig. S5) is novel assessment tool combines the PASI method [19] of scoring severity separately by erythema, thickness, and scaling with the PWESI method of dividing the body surface into ten areas. The modified PASI measure includes assessment of surface area involved, as well as dimensions for scaling, erythema, thickness and joint involvement for specific areas of psoriatic involvement. As with the PASI, severity indicators range from 0 (none) to 4 (extremely severe). As with the PWESI, body surface area was divided into ten ("X") areas. To increase the granularity of the results, each area was quantified ("Linearized") rather than categorized, i.e., the proportion of area affected was estimated numerically, rather than merely broadly categorized as in the PASI. Finally, the PASI was "eXtended" to include severity indicators for arthritis, quality of life, and sensations (pain/itching), although these additional measures were not included in this study. The scale of the XL-PASI ranges from 0 to 148.

Lattice Physician Global Assessment (LS-PGA). The LS-PGA [21] was included in the analysis of correlations between assessment tools. The results were deemed not sufficiently detailed to be included in the itemized analysis.

Data entry

Electronic versions of the instruments were generated using the Web-based Interactive Study Design, Organization, and Management (WISDOM) software, and are available for download at http://wisdom.rockefeller.edu. The meta data were extracted and automatically reformatted as screen form definitions for Research Electronic Data Capturing (REDCap) [22]. Data were entered twice by different typists and inconsistencies were resolved by an independent reviewer. One assessor entered the percentage total body area involvement as the XL-PASI proportion of involved skin, rather than percentage of body area by region. These data were analyzed as interval-censored between the highest and lowest value consistent with the input [23].

Statistical analyses

Statistical analyses were conducted using the μStat server at the Rockefeller University (http://mustat.rockefeller.edu) for computing u-scores of the binary, discrete, continuous, and interval-censored data. JMP® 7.0 software (The SAS Institute, Cary, NC) was used to generate the heatmap of the scores and Pearson correlations, equivalent to Spearman rank correlations [24]. R software (R Foundation, Vienna, Austria; http://cran.r-project.org) was used to compute odds ratios.

Results

Patients

Two hundred patients were screened for participation from the four clinical centers. Data from 180 evaluable patients that met the screening criteria were included in the analysis (Table 1). Of these, 55 (31%) patients had a diagnosis of PsA (confirmed by a rheumatologist) at baseline. The majority of patients were Caucasian (n = 154; 86%) and the remaining Asian (n = 5; 3%), Black (n = 6; 3%), Hispanic (n = 13; 7%), and Native American (n = 2; 1%).

Correlations between assessment tools

Correlations between scoring tools used to assess severity of Pso and PsA are shown in Figure 1. The highest correlation was seen between the XL-PASI and the PWESI (r = 0.88), which differ in granularity and relative weight of their components. The LS-PGA was also reasonably well correlated with the XL-PASI and PWESI (r = 0.79 and 0.77, respectively). The PsAA and the PASE also demonstrated good correlation (r = 0.655), although the self-assessment tool (PASE) discriminated less between mild and severe cases. The subsequent detailed analysis showed a surprising absence of any correlation between these two groups of tools (PsAA/PASE) and LS-PGA/XL-PASI/PWESI.

Correlations between items in the assessment tools

Correlations between individual items in the scoring tools are shown in Figure 2. The observations among fingers (or toes) were highly correlated as indicated for joint involvement (upper left corner) and nail disease (center). Individual items in the PASI score and the corresponding PWESI extent score were also highly correlated, as were the three PASI disease activity scores (erythema, thickness, and scaling) and the PWESI severity score. The extent (surface area involved per PASI) and severity (activity per PASI) of disease were highly correlated for feet, hands, genitalia/perineum/natal cleft, face, and scalp. In contrast, severity/activity of arms, knees, buttocks, chest, and back did not correlate with the extent/involvement across these body areas. The "secondary structure" of off-diagonal correlations (between severity/activity and extent/involvement within the same region) in the lower right corner of Figure 2 indicated that these items were not independent (see Figure 2 legend for details). Overall, correlations were seen between hands and feet, face and scalp, and buttocks, chest, and back.

Table 1. Patient demographics at baseline.

	Psoriasis[1] n = 182	PsA[1] n = 68	Nail Disease[1] n = 112
Sex (Female/Male)	84/98	32/36	43/69
Mean age - years (SD)	45.3 (15.0)	47.8 (13.6)	47.8 (13.8)
Minimum, maximum	18, 84	20, 72	20, 84
Mean weight - kg (SD)	204.9 (52.3)	207.5 (52.7)	209.1 (51.2)
Minimum, maximum	97, 377	97, 350	97, 377
Mean height - in (SD)	67.4 (4.3)	67.5 (3.8)	67.6 (4.2)
Minimum, maximum	50, 78	59, 76	50, 76
Patients with PsA diagnosis by a rheumatologist – n (%)	55 (30%)	53 (78%)	40 (36%)

[1]Self-reported.
Abbreviations: PsA, Psoriatic arthritis; SD, Standard deviation.

Little correlation was seen between the PASE, PsAA, and JA items describing severity of psoriatic arthritis and the PASI, PWESI, and NA. The only overlap noted among these items was individual PASE function items and extent and severity of Pso of the hands and feet. The correlations between hands/feet (XL-PASI/PWESI) and NA are likely inflated at the expense of the correlation between hands/feet and Pso of the other body areas (lower right corner) because of the design and wording of the questionnaires. Moreover, the NA items were highly correlated among each other, but had poor correlation with XL-PASI and PWESI items. Again, hands and feet were an exception, most notably for the severity by PWESI, which explicitly includes "fingernails" and "toenails" in its "hands" and "feet" categories. In particular, there were no secondary structures indicating that the joint and nail symptoms affect the same digits, an observation in contrast to the commonly believed theory.

Discussion

The results of this study do not support the hypothesis that a "least common denominator" of individual components will suffice to define the severity of the spectrum of disease along the axes of both psoriasis and psoriatic arthritis. Thus, at this time, the need for a single measurement tool that is broadly utilizable with the ability to measure the presence and severity of all clinical aspects of psoriasis remains unmet.

Our results provide evidence against an association between the severity of joint and skin involvement in patients with Pso and PsA, with the possible exception of hand symptoms. There have been few studies that have directly addressed the controversial relationship between the complexities of skin, nail and joint disease in psoriatic patients. Several small studies have reported no [25–27] or weak [9] associations between the activity of Pso and the activity, severity or functional status of the joints. However, a correlation between skin and joint severity was noted in a small group of patients who had synchronous onset of PsA and Pso [27]. All of these studies had only small sample sizes and thus low statistical power. However, in a large phase 4 clinical trial of 1122 patients, Gottlieb et al., found that baseline skin and joint disease measures were not correlated [28]. While confirming these earlier findings, the present study is limited in regard to the statistical power describing the relationship of specific psoriatic arthritis subtypes or extent of psoriatic disease. Therefore, based upon these initial unexpected observations, a more robust analysis would be necessary to better investigate the skin-joint relationship.

However, in support of previous observations regarding a qualitative association between skin and joint disease [2], and consistent with both disease conditions sharing at least some genetic risk factors, we did find a high odds ratio (19.9; $P<0.001$) for skin involvement and "any joints involved" and "any nail involved" among toes and a moderate odds ratios (2.0; $P = 0.079$) for fingers. The lack of a quantitative association requires further investigation but might involve additional genetic risk factors.

Several inconsistencies in the design of individual instruments may have affected our results. The PWESI explicitly includes nails with hands and feet, but the guidelines provided on the form do not allow even the most severe nail disease to be marked more than "noticeable" in terms of extent. The XL-PASI (like the PASI), in contrast, does not mention nails at all. The diversity of Pso manifestations on the hands and feet (palmarplantar disease) for example hyperkeratosis vs pustular or combinations thereof, further complicates the issue (Farley et al., 2009). The relatively

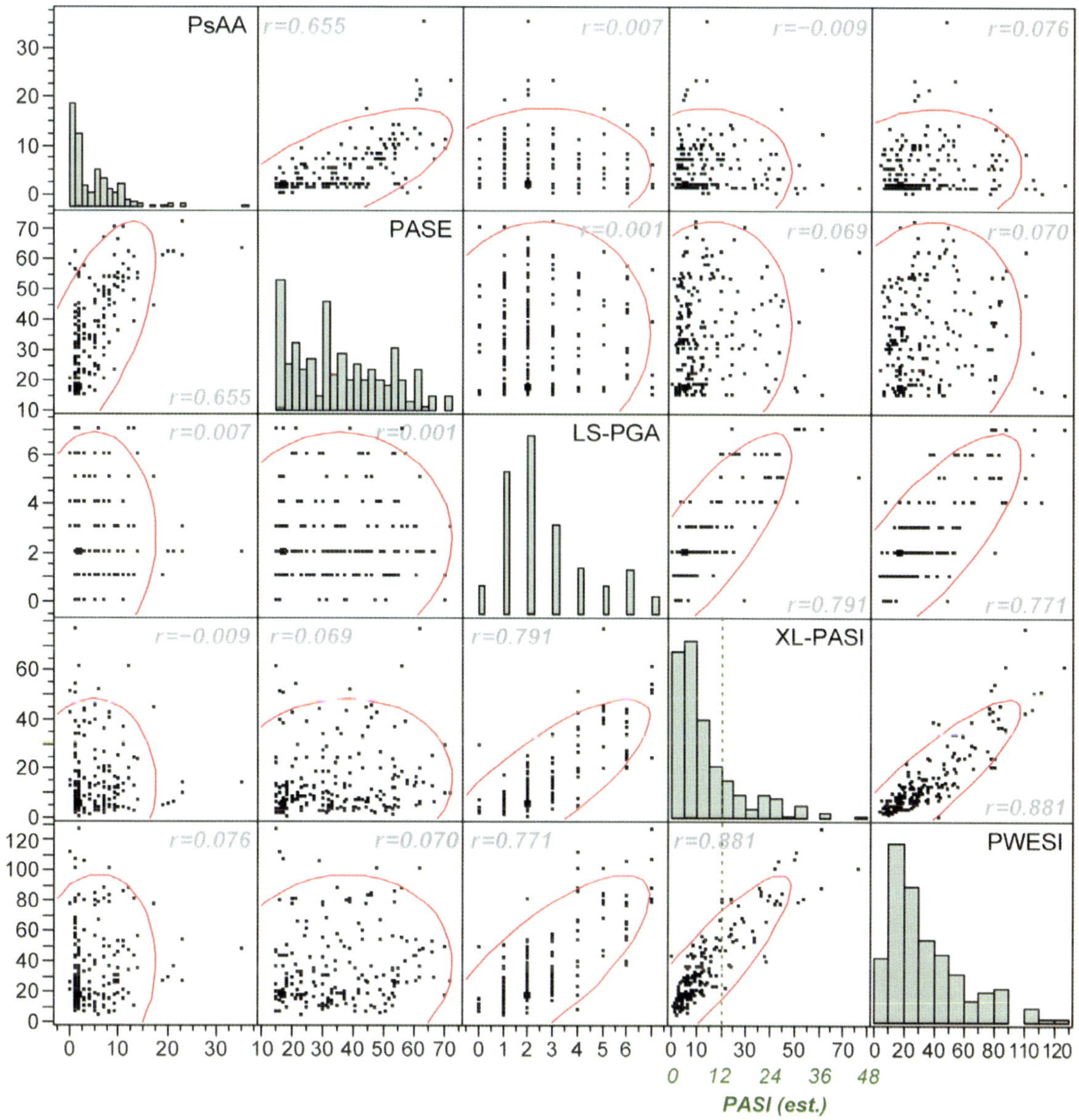

Figure 1. Correlations between tools scoring the severity of psoriasis and psoriatic arthritis and distribution of scores. x-axis and y-axis values represent the respective scores of the tools. For comparison with traditional PASI scores, the XL-PASI scores are translated into estimated PASI scores. The dotted line with an estimated PASI score of 12 separates the patients with moderate and severe disease. r: Spearman correlation.

high correlation between severity of disease and extent of disease in nails and hands/feet and the extremely low correlation between extent of disease in hands/feet and extent of disease in all other body areas may suggest that the examiners attempted to reflect severe nail disease by inflating extent and severity of skin disease of hands and feet. The XL-PASI includes a column for severity of arthritis, so that physicians were less likely to reflect joint problems by increasing the severity indicators meant to reflect skin conditions. The PWESI, by contrast, has no separate category for arthritis and, in support of this argument, had a higher correlation with severity of arthritis than the PASI.

Analysis of data to evaluate nail disease was complicated by wording of the assessment tools. The NA includes a request for a list of all involved digits (fingers and toes), but then continues with "Select the most involved fingernail and evaluate." Several completed questionnaires indicated that the examiner had included toenails in the assessment, but others may have followed the instructions literally so that the assessment could be biased to disease forms more frequently seen with hands, such as pitting. This issue highlights the importance of validating assessment tools in the appropriate clinical setting. These observations suggest that Pso of the nails might be more clearly separated from Pso of the skin if examiners were allowed to distinguish explicitly between involvement of nails and skin on both hands and feet.

The pathophysiology of nail dystrophy has been postulated to be more closely associated with joint symptoms than with skin symptoms [4]. As with the hands and feet, there is a great diversity in the clinical manifestations of nail disease, with the added problem of secondary infections (bacterial, fungal) aggravating or masking the manifestations, particularly in psoriatic toenails. PsA has been more strongly associated with nail disease than Pso alone [29]. Imaging studies have shown that the nail and the enthesis (the point at which tendons attach to bones) are linked via the distal interphalangeal joint extensor tendon [30,31]. This close

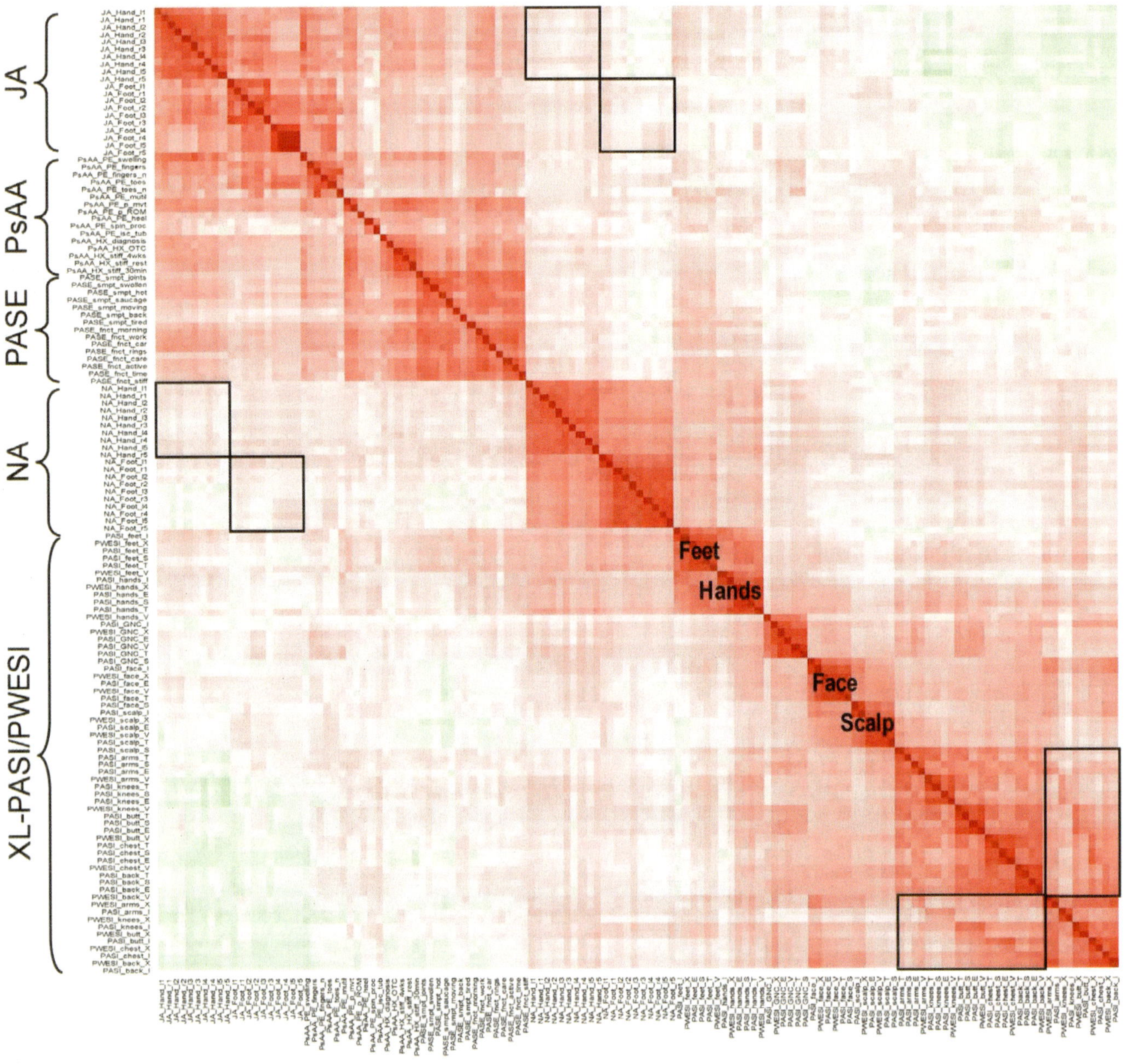

Figure 2. Correlations between individual items of psoriasis and psoriatic arthritis severity. Each cell indicates the Spearman correlation between 2 of the 52 items. Cells with dark red indicates strong positive correlation, light red indicates weak positive correlation, dark green indicates strong negative correlation, and light green indicates weak negative correlation. Boxes in the upper left portion indicate correlations between affected nails and joints on hands and feet. Boxes in the lower right corner indicate "secondary structure" (within-box diagonal) between extent/involvement and severity/activity within regions. JA: Joint Assessment; NA: Nail Assessment; PASE: Psoriatic Arthritis Screening and Evaluation Questionnaire; PsAA: Psoriatic Arthritis Assessment; XL-PASI: Extended 10-area Linear Psoriasis Area and Severity Index; PWESI: Psoriasis Weighted Extent and Severity Index.

functional relationship between the joint and the nail may explain the association between these symptoms, particularly relating to distal interphalangeal joint involvement and nail disease.

GWAS and family-based association tests for Pso as a whole have had only limited success in defining causative alleles. The results presented here, however, offer a strategy for future genetic studies with a high potential for success in elucidating genetic risk factors for Pso. More specific and statistically validated assessment instruments will allow for the clinical classification of Pso patients into specific categories based on skin, joint, and nail involvement. In addition, the identification of genetic discriminators between these categories, using novel multivariate [23], multi-locus [32], and multi-allelic [33] nonparametric methods in a well-defined subpopulation of patients with the same underlying condition, would be more accurate than studies using traditional methods for univariate, single-locus, or binary data in the more diverse population as a whole.

The clinical evidence presented herein likely signifies the existence of different psoriatic disease phenotypes, thus supporting the hypothesis that different genetic risk factors are involved in the etiology of skin, joint, and possibly nail forms of psoriatic disease. Our results suggest that the complex phenotype of psoriatic disease can only be assessed with instruments that allow the examiner to judge severity of skin, nails, and joints separately (in addition to extent of skin involvement). Moreover, the data analysis suggests that a minimum of two summary scores (one for skin and one for joints), and potentially a third for nails, are required to accurately assess severity across the full spectrum of psoriatic disease. The optimal design of such assessment tools remains the objective of this research project, with efforts continuing to identify the most meaningful contributing elements that define the full spectrum of the psoriatic disease state. Accordingly, this information is likely to be of significant benefit clinical practice as well as in the future design of clinical trials investigating developmental therapies for Pso and PsA.

Supporting Information

Figure S1 Psoriatic Arthritis Assessment (PsAA) is a composite measurement of PsA that includes questions regarding patient and family history and 6 multipart components of a physical examination.

Figure S2 Psoriatic Arthritis Screening and Evaluation (PASE) is a validated patient questionnaire that comprises questions on symptoms and functions.

Figure S3 Nail Assessment (NA) and Joint Assessment (JA) evaluates nail involvement (score 0 for no involvement and score 1 for involvement by digit) and joint involvement (0/1 by digit) on the hands, as determined by physician assessment.

Figure S4 Psoriasis Weighted Extent and Severity Index (PWESI) is used to evaluate the extent and severity of skin disease across multiple areas of the body. The extent of skin disease is measured on a scale of 0 (none) to 4 (extensive) and severity of disease on a scale of 0 (essentially clear) to (intensely inflamed). Ten areas are assessed: scalp/hairline, face/neck, arms/axillae, hands/fingers/fingernails, anterior chest/abdomen, back/shoulders, genitalia/perineum/natal cleft, buttocks/thighs, knees/lower legs/ankles, and feet/toes/toenails. This physician assessment delivers a maximal composite score of 50.

Figure S5 Extended 10-area Linear Psoriasis Area and Severity Index (XL-PASI) combines the PASI and PWESI scoring methods. This measure includes assessment of surface area involved, as well as dimensions for scaling, erythema, thickness and joint involvement for specific areas of psoriatic involvement. As with the PASI, severity indicators range from 0 (none) to 4 (extremely severe). As with the PWESI, body surface area is divided into ten ("X") areas and each area is quantified. The scale of the XL-PASI ranges from 0 to 148.

Acknowledgments

In addition to authors J. Krueger, Wittkowski, Leonardi, Gottlieb, Menter, G. Krueger, and Horn, participants in the International Psoriasis Council conference to evaluate current and predominant assessment tools in routine use for psoriatic disease and their individual components included Robert Chalmers, Dermatology Centre, University of Manchester UK; Charles Ellis, University of Michigan Dept. of Dermatology Ann Arbor, MI; Andrew Finlay, Wales College of Medicine, Cardiff University, Wales; Ron Gottschalk, Galderma Laboratories Fort Worth, TX; Stacey Hirata, Amgen, New York, NY; and Luigi Naldi, Clinica Dermatologica Bergamo, Italia.

We wish to thank Claudia Peissert for her work on the WISDOM-REDCap link, and Pradeep Mutalik for hosting REDCap. We also thank Julia R. Gage, PhD for editorial assistance.

Author Contributions

Conceived and designed the experiments: KMW CL AG GGK LH JGK. Performed the experiments: CL AG AM GGK RS-A JG. Analyzed the data: KMW CL AG AM GGK PWT JB JG LH JGK. Contributed reagents/materials/analysis tools: KMW. Wrote the paper: KMW CL AG AM GGK PWT JB RS-A JG LH JGK.

References

1. Nestle FO, Kaplan DH, Barker J (2009) Psoriasis. N Engl J Med 361: 496–509.
2. Gladman DD, Antoni C, Mease P, Clegg DO, Nash P (2005) Psoriatic arthritis: epidemiology, clinical features, course, and outcome. Ann Rheum Dis 64 Suppl 2: ii 14–17
3. Langley RG, Krueger GG, Griffiths CE (2005) Psoriasis: epidemiology, clinical features, and quality of life. Ann Rheum Dis 64 Suppl 2: ii 18–23.
4. McGonagle D, Benjamin M, Tan AL (2009) The pathogenesis of psoriatic arthritis and associated nail disease: not autoimmune after all? Curr Opin Rheumatol 21: 340–347.
5. Gladman DD (2009) Psoriatic arthritis. Dermatol Ther 22: 40–55.
6. Ritchlin C (2007) Psoriatic disease–from skin to bone. Nat Clin Pract Rheumatol 3: 698–706.
7. Makredes M, Robinson D, Jr., Bala M, Kimball AB (2009) The burden of autoimmune disease: a comparison of prevalence ratios in patients with psoriatic arthritis and psoriasis. J Am Acad Dermatol 61: 405–410.
8. McGonagle D, Tan AL, Benjamin M (2009) The nail as a musculoskeletal appendage–implications for an improved understanding of the link between psoriasis and arthritis. Dermatology 218: 97–102.
9. Cohen MR, Reda DJ, Clegg DO (1999) Baseline relationships between psoriasis and psoriatic arthritis: analysis of 221 patients with active psoriatic arthritis. Department of Veterans Affairs Cooperative Study Group on Seronegative Spondyloarthropathies. J Rheumatol 26: 1752–1756.
10. Duffin KC, Chandran V, Gladman DD, Krueger GG, Elder JT, et al. (2008) Genetics of psoriasis and psoriatic arthritis: update and future direction. J Rheumatol 35: 1449–1453.
11. Castelino M, Barton A (2010) Genetic susceptibility factors for psoriatic arthritis. Curr Opin Rheumatol 22: 152–156.
12. Cargill M, Schrodi SJ, Chang M, Garcia VE, Brandon R, et al. (2007) A large-scale genetic association study confirms IL12B and leads to the identification of IL23R as psoriasis-risk genes. Am J Hum Genet 80: 273–290.
13. Liu Y, Helms C, Liao W, Zaba LC, Duan S, et al. (2008) A genome-wide association study of psoriasis and psoriatic arthritis identifies new disease loci. PLoS Genet 4: e1000041.
14. Rahman P, Sun S, Peddle L, Snelgrove T, Melay W, et al. (2006) Association between the interleukin-1 family gene cluster and psoriatic arthritis. Arthritis Rheum 54: 2321–2325.
15. Strange A, Capon F, Spencer CC, Knight J, Weale ME, et al. (2010) A genome-wide association study identifies new psoriasis susceptibility loci and an interaction between HLA-C and ERAP1. Nature genetics 42: 985–990.
16. Nograles KE, Brasington RD, Bowcock AM (2009) New insights into the pathogenesis and genetics of psoriatic arthritis. Nat Clin Pract Rheumatol 5: 83–91.
17. Goldstein I, Simon AJ, Ben Horin S, Matzri S, Koltakov A, et al. (2008) Synovial VLA-1+ T cells display an oligoclonal and partly distinct repertoire in rheumatoid and psoriatic arthritis. Clin Immunol 128: 75–84.
18. Ritchlin C (2006) Newer therapeutic approaches: spondyloarthritis and uveitis. Rheum Dis Clin North Am 32: 75–90.
19. Feldman SR, Krueger GG (2005) Psoriasis assessment tools in clinical trials. Ann Rheum Dis 64: ii65–68.
20. Dominguez PL, Husni ME, Holt EW, Tyler S, Qureshi AA (2009) Validity, reliability, and sensitivity-to-change properties of the psoriatic arthritis screening and evaluation questionnaire. Arch Dermatol Res 301: 573–579.
21. Langley RG, Ellis CN (2004) Evaluating psoriasis with Psoriasis Area and Severity Index, Psoriasis Global Assessment, and Lattice System Physician's Global Assessment. J Am Acad Dermatol 51: 563–569.

22. Harris PA, Taylor R, Thielke R, Payne J, Gonzalez N, et al. (2009) Research electronic data capture (REDCap)–A metadata-driven methodology and workflow process for providing translational research informatics support. J Biomed Inform 42: 377–381.
23. Morales JF, Song T, Auerbach AD, Wittkowski KM (2008) Phenotyping genetic diseases using an extension of μ-scores for multivariate data. Stat Appl Genet Mol Biol 7: 19.
24. Spearman C (1904) The proof and measurement of association between two things. Am J Psychol 15: 72–101.
25. Jones SM, Armas JB, Cohen MG, Lovell CR, Evison G, et al. (1994) Psoriatic arthritis: outcome of disease subsets and relationship of joint disease to nail and skin disease. Br J Rheumatol 33: 834–839.
26. Jones SM, McHugh NJ (1998) The temporal relationship between joints, skin and nail disease in psoriatic arthritis: a prospective study of two years. Arthritis Rheum 41: S334.
27. Elkayam O, Ophir J, Yaron M, Caspi D (2000) Psoriatic arthritis: interrelationships between skin and joint manifestations related to onset, course and distribution. Clin Rheumatol 19: 301–305.
28. Gottlieb AB, Mease PJ, Jackson JM, Eisen D, Xia HA, et al. (2006) Clinical characteristics of psoriatic arthritis and psoriasis in dermatologists' offices. J Dermatolog Treat 17: 279–287.
29. Wilson FC, Icen M, Crowson CS, McEvoy MT, Gabriel SE, et al. (2009) Incidence and clinical predictors of psoriatic arthritis in patients with psoriasis: a population-based study. Arthritis Rheum 61: 233–239.
30. Tan AL, Grainger AJ, Tanner SF, Emery P, McGonagle D (2006) A high-resolution magnetic resonance imaging study of distal interphalangeal joint arthropathy in psoriatic arthritis and osteoarthritis: are they the same? Arthritis Rheum 54: 1328–1333.
31. Tan AL, Benjamin M, Toumi H, Grainger AJ, Tanner SF, et al. (2007) The relationship between the extensor tendon enthesis and the nail in distal interphalangeal joint disease in psoriatic arthritis–a high-resolution MRI and histological study. Rheumatology (Oxford) 46: 253–256.
32. Wittkowski KM, Haider A, Sehayek E, Suarez-Farinas M, Pellegrino M, et al. (2006) Bioinformatics tools enabling u-statistics for microarrays. Conf Proc IEEE Eng Med Biol Soc 1: 3464–3469.
33. Ramagopalan SV, McMahon R, Dyment DA, Sadovnick AD, Ebers GC, et al. (2009) An extension to a statistical approach for family based association studies provides insights into genetic risk factors for multiple sclerosis in the HLA-DRB1 gene. BMC Med Genet 10: 10.

Activation of PPARβ/δ Causes a Psoriasis-Like Skin Disease In Vivo

Malgorzata Romanowska[1]¶, Louise Reilly[1]¶, Colin N. A. Palmer[2], Mattias C. U. Gustafsson[3], John Foerster[1]*

1 Division of Experimental Medicine, University of Dundee, Dundee, United Kingdom, **2** Biomedical Research Institute, University of Dundee, Dundee, United Kingdom, **3** Department of Laboratory Medicine, Division of Medical Microbiology, Lund University, Lund, Sweden

Abstract

Background: Psoriasis is one of the most frequent skin diseases world-wide. The disease impacts enormously on affected patients and poses a huge financial burden on health care providers. Several lines of evidence suggest that the nuclear hormone receptor peroxisome proliferator activator (PPAR) β/δ, known to regulate epithelial differentiation and wound healing, contributes to psoriasis pathogenesis. It is unclear, however, whether activation of PPARβ/δ is sufficient to trigger psoriasis-like changes in vivo.

Methodology/Principal Findings: Using immunohistochemistry, we define the distribution of PPARβ/δ in the skin lesions of psoriasis. By expression profiling, we confirm that PPARβ/δ is overexpressed in the vast majority of psoriasis patients. We further establish a transgenic model allowing inducible activation of PPARβ/δ in murine epidermis mimicking its distribution in psoriasis lesions. Upon activation of PPARβ/δ, transgenic mice sustain an inflammatory skin disease strikingly similar to psoriasis, featuring hyperproliferation of keratinocytes, dendritic cell accumulation, and endothelial activation. Development of this phenotype requires the activation of the Th17 subset of T cells, shown previously to be central to psoriasis. Moreover, gene dysregulation in the transgenic mice is highly similar to that in psoriasis. Key transcriptional programs activated in psoriasis, including IL1-related signalling and cholesterol biosynthesis, are replicated in the mouse model, suggesting that PPARβ/δ regulates these transcriptional changes in psoriasis. Finally, we identify phosphorylation of STAT3 as a novel pathway activated by PPARβ/δ and show that inhibition of STAT3 phosphorylation blocks disease development.

Conclusions: Activation of PPARβ/δ in the epidermis is sufficient to trigger inflammatory changes, immune activation, and signalling, and gene dysregulation characteristic of psoriasis.

Editor: Jacques Zimmer, Centre de Recherche Public de la Santé (CRP-Santé), Luxembourg

Funding: The work presented here was in part funded by Cancer Research United Kingdom (role: fellowship for JF), the Anonymous Trust (role: provision of funds for consumables), and Tenovus Scotland (role: provision of funds for consumables). The funders had no role in study design, data collection and analysis, decision to publish, or preparation of the manuscript.

Competing Interests: The authors have declared that no competing interests exist.

* E-mail: j.foerster@dundee.ac.uk

¶ These authors contributed equally to this work.

Introduction

Psoriasis is one of the most frequent skin diseases world-wide, affecting appr. 2% in Caucasian, and 1% in African populations [1]. The disease represents a life-long affliction of affected patients. About 60% of psoriasis patients suffer from moderate to severe disease, i.e. more than 10% of the body surface area is covered by psoriatic plaques [2]. These patients are largely excluded from participation in activities involving public skin exposure due to stigmatization. Moreover, they exhibit increased rates of depression and alcohol consumption causing secondarily increased mortality [3,4]. Besides high direct treatment-related costs, absence from work-related indirect cost is enormous [5] and lack of employment is attributed to the disease in one-third of psoriasis patients [6]. Thus, psoriasis does not kill, but it impacts enormously on those affected and poses a huge financial burden on health care providers worldwide.

Among psoriasis patients, the prevalence of metabolic syndrome is increased [7] and an increased body mass index is a strong risk factor for psoriasis [8]. Although the molecular mechanisms underlying this association are unknown, it likely involves the existence of overlapping signalling pathways in psoriasis and other disorders of metabolism and chronic inflammation. The nuclear hormone receptor peroxisome proliferator activator (PPAR) β/δ has well established roles both in metabolism and in the skin. On the one hand, PPARβ/δ is a key regulator of adipogenesis and glucose metabolism [9]. On the other hand, it regulates keratinocyte differentiation [10]. The PPAR subfamily of nuclear hormone receptors also includes PPARα (target of fibrate class lipid lowering drugs) and PPARγ (target of the rosiglitazone-family of anti-diabetes drugs), all of which form heterodimers with the RXRα subunit of retinoid receptors and require binding of ligands in order to bind cognate promoters and transactivate distinct set of target genes. All three isoforms have been extensively reviewed elsewhere (e.g. [11]). Table S9 lists selected information on ligands. Several lines of evidence support a role for PPARβ/δ in psoriasis. It is upregulated in psoriatic skin [12,13], induced by TNFα [14,15], stimulates proliferation and blocks apoptosis in keratinocytes [16], and induces angiogenesis [17], all of which is consistent with a disease-promoting role in psoriasis. Thus, induction of PPARβ/δ in the context of metabolic dysregulation might underlie the observed clinical association of psoriasis with metabolic disease.

PPARβ/δ represents an isoform of the peroxisome – proliferator activator receptor subfamily of nuclear hormone receptors.

The inflammatory patches of psoriasis exhibit a number of characteristic properties which are important clues to the underlying pathogenesis. Macroscopically, they are inducible by wounding or other mechanical skin trauma, indicating that challenges to the skin barrier trigger specific response pathways. Histologically, they are marked by increased keratinocyte proliferation, as well as a block in terminal differentiation. Accordingly, markers of late differentiation, including fillagrin, are decreased [18]. Besides keratinocyte biology, psoriasis is marked by complex pattern of immune system activation, including expansion of $CD11c^+$ dendritic cells [19], upregulation of interferon signalling, and influx of T cells. Specifically, the Th17 subset of T cells has recently emerged as central for the disease [20]. In addition, endothelial cells are activated, bactericidal proteins accumulate, and a variety of soluble mediators are overexpressed (reviewed in [21]). Finally, the IL12/23p40 gene, the IL23 receptor, the β-defensin locus, as well as the HLA-C region harbour genetically predisposing variants [22], suggesting that quantitative differences in immune response pathways affect disease penetrance.

The combination of proliferative changes and a distinctive immune response pattern in psoriasis has long been recognized for its similarity to the wound response. Thus, like wound response pathways, the development of inflammatory psoriasis plaques are triggered by mechanical skin trauma, as well as infection. Therefore, in many respects psoriasis represents a proliferative wound response failing to terminate, suggesting the existence of molecular feed-forward circuits fuelling a vicious circle. In this regard, too, the upregulation of PPARβ/δ is notable since it is an important regulator of the wound response [10].

We report here that PPARβ/δ activation is sufficient to trigger a skin disease replicating many elements of psoriasis. Our findings identify PPARβ/δ as a molecular link between metabolism, keratinocyte differentiation, and the epidermal immune response.

Results

Overexpression of PPARβ/δ in psoriasis

We and others have previously shown that PPARβ/δ is overexpressed in psoriasis. In order to independently confirm those results, we re-analyzed two publicly available large gene expression datasets, totalling 58 paired lesional and non-lesional skin samples, for the expression of all PPAR isotypes. As shown in figure 1a, both data sets confirm highly significant upregulation of PPARβ/δ in psoriatic skin whereas both PPARα and PPARγ are downregulated, consistent with the notion that PPARβ/δ acts antagonistically to PPARγ in psoriasis, as previously proposed [12]. Furthermore, we localized the site of maximal PPARβ/δ accumulation in the skin by immunohistochemistry. As shown in figure 1b, PPARβ/δ is found in the cytosol of the lower epidermis both in normal skin and psoriasis. By contrast, strong nuclear

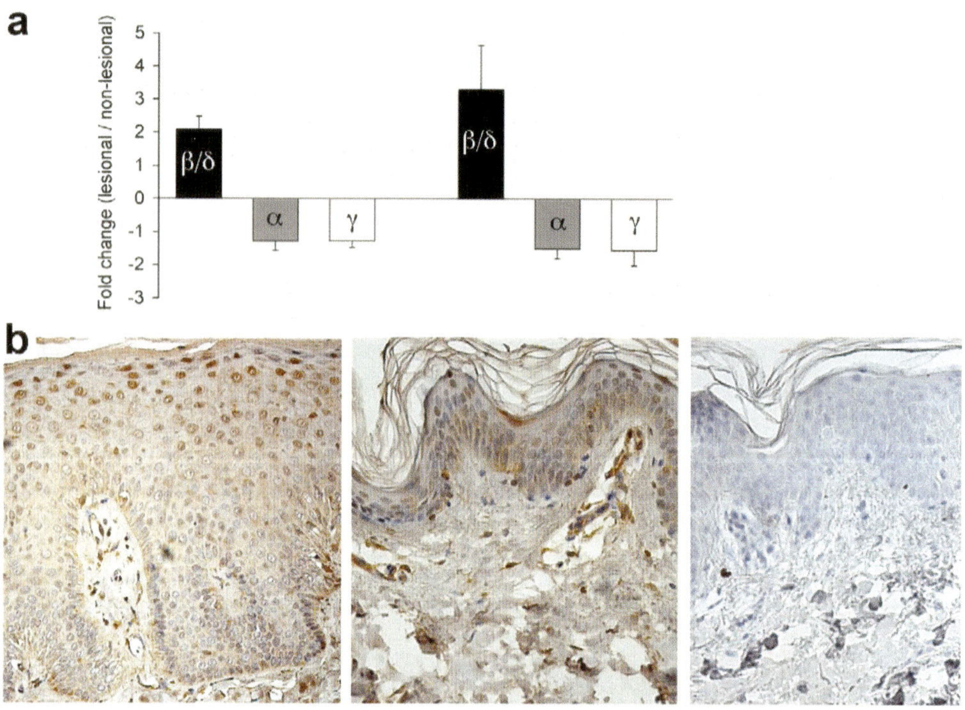

Figure 1. Overexpression of PPARβ/δ in psoriasis. A. Fold-change of mRNA expression of PPARβ/δ (black columns), PPARα (shaded), and PPARγ (white) between lesional and non-lesional skin. Data shown represent mean ± s.d. from the GAIN dataset (left, n = 30) and the GSE14905 dataset (right, n = 28). $p<10^{-3}$ for all data points shown. For each PPAR isoform, the probe yielding the highest hybridization signal was used to calculate the data shown (probesets 37152_at, 226978_at, 208510_at, respectively). **B.** Nuclear accumulation of PPARβ/δ in suprabasal epidermis in psoriasis skin lesions. Representative immunohistochemistry of paraffin-embedded lesional (left) and control (middle) skin samples stained with anti-PPARβ/δ, as well as staining control (right). Magnification 200×.

expression in the upper spinous layer was only seen in psoriasis. This pattern was highly reproducible (found in all eight lesional skin samples examined, figure S1a). These data confirm that upregulation of PPARβ/δ is a consistent feature of psoriasis and define the suprabasal epidermis as major site of its activation.

Targeting PPARβ/δ expression to suprabasal skin in mice in vivo

In mice, PPARβ/δ is not expressed in inter-follicular epidermis beyond the postnatal period [23]. To model the suprabasal expression of PPARβ/δ observed in psoriasis in humans, we initially intended to target transgenic PPARβ/δ expression using a "conventional" promoter active in suprabasal epidermis, e.g. the involucrin promoter. However, a transgenic line expressing PPARβ/δ under the control of the rat CYP1A1 promoter was already available, and turned out to afford skin-specific PPARβ/δ activation, as follows. The CYP1A1 promoter allows expression induced by the aryl hydrocarbon receptor (AhR) [24]. This promoter activity is mediated by a well-documented so-called "DXE/XRE" sequence cluster conferring responsivity to AhR [25]. In order to bind to the DXE/XRE cluster, the AhR must first be ligand-activated, which can be achieved by employing specific synthetic chemicals such as indole-3-carbinole (I3C). However, even in the absence of AhR activation and binding to the CYP1A1 promoter, a EGFP reporter gene placed under the control of the CYP1A1 promoter was found to be constitutively and strongly active in skin-associated sebaceous glands [26]. We were able to identify a G/C rich enhancer element most likely responsible for this sebaceous-specific expression, since this element had previously been shown to direct strong sebacous-gland specific expression in the keratin 5 promoter [27]. Indeed, a screen of the GEO database showed this G/C element to be highly conserved in the promoters of multiple genes belonging to the top 10% of all genes expressed in sebaceous glands (fig. 2a, bottom). Not surprisingly then, the CYP1A1 promoter also conferred high constitutive sebaceous-specific expression of PPARβ/δ in the absence of AhR activation (figure 2b). Human, rather than murine PPARβ/δ, was chosen as transgene to facilitate subsequent drug screening applications. We next observed that, unexpectedly, administration of the highly selective PPARβ/δ-agonist GW501516 to the chow of PPARβ/δ-transgenic mice induced subsequent additional expression of the PPARβ/δ-transgene in the epidermis (fig. 2c). Thus, functional activation of PPARβ/δ expressed at high level in the sebaceous glands causes secondary transgene expression in the epidermis. (RT-PCR analysis of PPARβ/δ -transgene expression revealed a borderline-detectable expression in whole skin samples, consistent with the sebaceous glands forming a small minority of all skin associated cells, Figure S8). It is known that ligand-mediated activation of PPARβ/δ in the sebaceous gland triggers sebocyte differentiation [28,29] and delivery of sebum to the skin [30], containing lipoxygenase-derived bioactive lipids that can bind and activate the AhR, such as LXA4 or 5,6-DiHETE [31,32]. Once ligand-bound, the AhR is then able to transactivate the expression of the CYP1A1-controlled PPARβ/δ transgene in the epidermis via the AhR-responsive DXE/XRE element (shown in fig. 2d). In confirmation of this proposed mechanism, the transcriptional induction of the CYP1A1-controlled PPARβ/δ transgene in the epidermis could be replicated by direct topical cream application of the AhR ligand indole-3-carbinole (I3C) to the skin (I3C, fig. 2e). Furthermore, expression of transgenic PPARβ/δ was epidermis-specific and was not detectable in dermal fibroblasts, endothelia, skin – associated T cells, or any other organ screened, including intestine, muscle, liver, spleen (Fig. S1b), confirming that activation of AhR only occurred in the skin. Taken together, use of the rat Cyp1A1-driven expression of PPARβ/δ and ligand-mediated activation by the specific PPARβ/δ agonist GW501516 promoter affords a tightly controlled epidermis-specific inducible expression of PPARβ/δ. Although we have not identified the endogenous AhR ligand(s) mediating secondary induction of the transgene in the epidermis, the net effect is a distribution and expression level of PPARβ/δ rather similar to that observed in human psoriasis (fig. 2f).

Psoriasis-like skin disease in PPARβ/δ transgenic mice

As early as seven days after initiation of PPARβ/δ - activation by GW501516 (GW), scaling, inflammation, and skin thickening was notable in all mice (figure 3a–c). Skin roughening ("hyperkeratosis") and concomitant hair loss was maximal in regions subjected to mechanical friction, such as abdomen (fig. 3b, S2), the paws (fig. 3a), or the chin (fig. S2). While psoriasis-like plaques also developed on the back in some mice (fig. 3c), changes on the dorsal skin were mostly limited to scaling (fig. S2). Thus, the overall distribution of skin changes suggest that mechanical friction contributes a trigger effect similar to that characteristic of psoriasis. Histology showed epidermal thickening (fig. 3e), dilation of dermal vessels (black arrowhead), and abundant lymphocytes (white arrowheads). Moreover, Ki67 staining demonstrated massive hyperproliferation in the basal layer of the epidermis (fig. 3g). All of these changes are highly similar to those found in psoriasis. In contrast to psoriasis, the granular layer was prominent (fig. 3f, white arrowhead), consistent with the known effect of PPARβ/δ on epidermal differentiation [33]. In order to exclude that AhR activation as such contributed to the development of skin disease, we also administered the AhR ligand I3C in the chow at a very high concentration (0.5% w/w) in the absence of GW501515 administration, which did not induce a skin phenotype. Likewise, skin disease could be effectively replicated by topical cream-based, instead of systemical, application of GW501516 + I3C to the skin, but not by I3C alone (fig. 3h), consistent with the observation that I3C induces transcription of the CYP1A1-driven PPARβ/δ transgene (fig. 2e), but does not activate it. Finally, C57Bl/6j wild type mice fed GW501516 did not exhibit skin changes. Thus, the psoriasis-like skin disease in PPARβ/δ transgenic mice is triggered solely by activation of PPARβ/δ overexpressed in the skin, but not by endogenous murine PPARβ/δ.

Immune system activation and involvement of Th17 cells in PPARβ/δ dependent skin disease

In order to further explore overlaps of the skin phenotype in PPARβ/δ transgenic mice with psoriasis, we next characterized immunological changes after disease induction. As shown in figure 4a, there was a massive influx of $CD4^+$ T cells into the dermis and, to a lesser extend, of $CD8^+$ T cells into the epidermis. CD11c+ dermal dendritic cells were abundant, while CD11c+ epidermal Langerhans cells were not found. Activation of endothelial cells was also evident by staining with CD31. All of these changes are highly consistent with those typical of psoriasis. Co-immunofluorescence studies revealed that the PPARβ/δ transgene was not found in either endothelial cells or dermal dendritic cells (fig. S3), further confirming that the skin disease in PPARβ/δ transgenic mice is driven by expression of the transgene in suprabasal epidermal keratinocytes, but not other cell types.

Th17 cells are required, but not sufficient, for phenotype development

Since the Th17-subset of T cells is of central importance in the immune activation of psoriasis, we next quantified these cells using intracellular FACS analysis. Indeed, Th17-cells, marked by

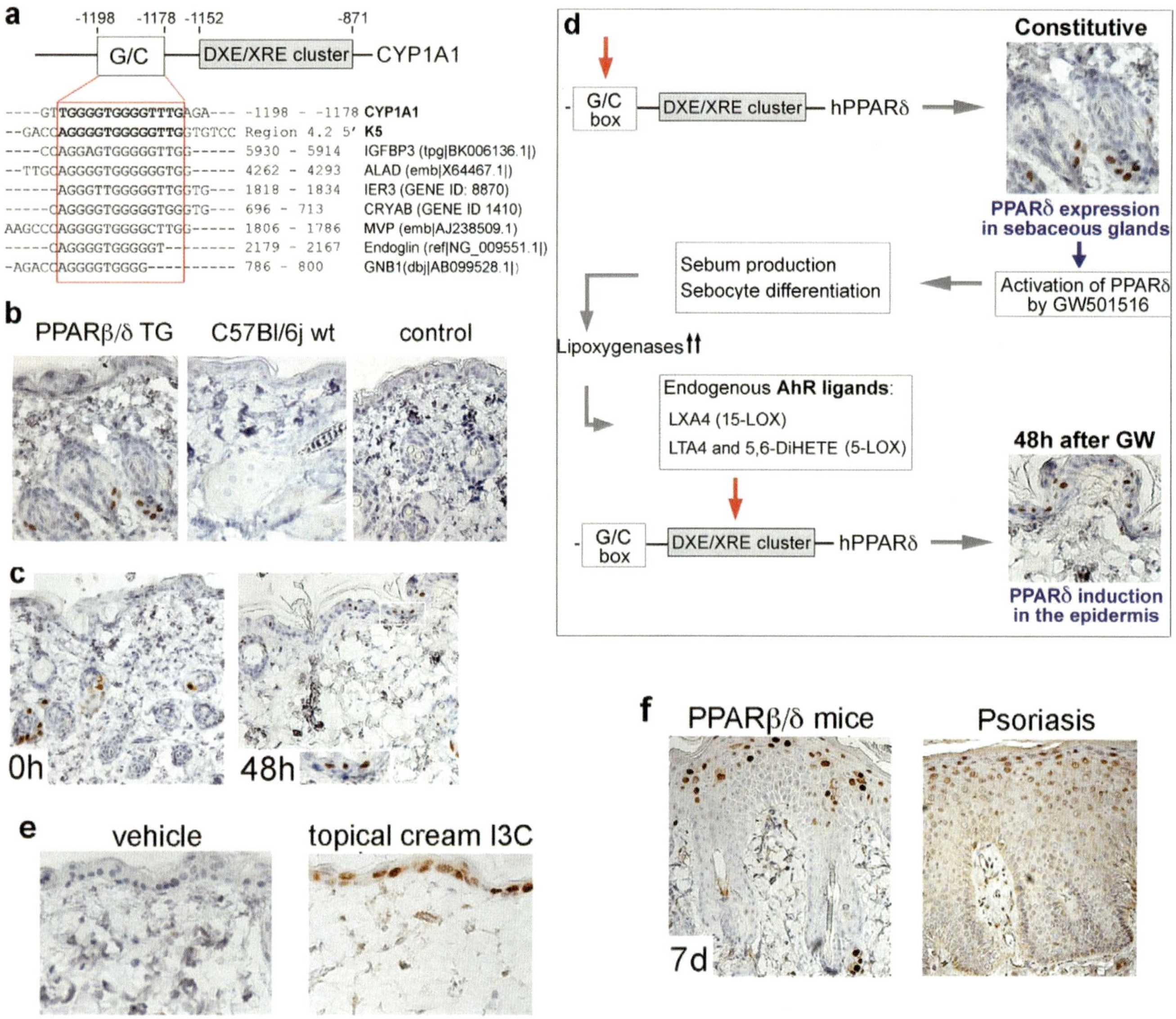

Figure 2. Inducible expression of PPARβ/δ in mouse epidermis. A. Cis-regulatory elements in the rat CYP1A1 promoter used to drive inducible expression of human PPARβ/δ. Upper panel: Map of the sebaceous – specific G/C-box element and the AHR – responsive DXE/XRE cluster in the cyp1A1 promoter as well as the human human K5 promoter. Bottom panel: ClustalW alignment of promoters identified by a BLAST search using the 20 bp G/C element of the Cyp1A1 promoter. All of the genes shown were found in the top 10% percentile of all transcripts expressed in human sebaceous glands (GDS3215 at the NCBI GEO website www.ncbi.nlm.nih.gov/geo/). **B.** Immunohistochemistry using anti-PPARβ/δ of mice transgenic for human PPARβ/δ driven by the rat CYP1A promoter (PPARβ/δ TG), as well as wild type mice. Magnification 200× **C.** Immunohistochemistry of skin samples from PPARβ/δ transgenic mice taken before, or 48 h after after initiation of PPARβ/δ activation by oral administration of the synthetic ligand GW501516 in the chow; (inset in "48 h": 400×); **d.** schematic illustrating the mechanism regulating constitutive expression of transgenic PPARβ/δ driven by the rat CYP1A1 promoter in sebaceous glands, as well as delayed PPARβ/δ expression in the epidermis after ligand-mediated activation of PPARβ/δ **e.** PPARβ/δ immunohistochemistry 48 h after topical cream application of indole-3-carbinole (I3C) to the skin of PPARβ/δ transgenic mice at 400× (right) magnification. **f.** Immunohistochemistry of PPARβ/δ in the skin of PPARβ/δ - transgenic mice after seven days of feeding of the PPARβ/δ ligand GW501516 in the chow (left) and in human psoriasis skin (right).

expression of IL17, were significantly expanded in the psoriasis-like plaques of PPARβ/δ mice, whereas the Th1 subset, marked by IFNγ^{+} expression, was not (fig. 4b,c). A small, but statistically significant expansion of IL17^{+} cells was also noted in peripheral lymphoid organs upon GW501516 stimulation (fig. S4). To assess the requirement of Th17 cells for PPARβ/δ - mediated skin disease, we depleted them *in vivo* by intraperitoneal injection of anti-IL12/23p40, analogous to the monoclonal antibody (ustekinumab) used to treat psoriasis. We extended this experiment to include the effect of injection using anti-TNFα. Blockade of TNFα is an established treatment for psoriasis. Since TNFα itself induces PPARβ/δ expression [14], blocking of TNFα- should *not* be able to completely abrogate skin phenotype development in PPARβ/δ-transgenic mice since PPARβ/δ expression is enforced downstream of TNFα in this model. As shown in fig. 4d, treatment with anti-IL12/23p40, but not with anti-TNFα, effectively suppressed expansion of Th17 cells in GW501516-treated PPARβ/δ transgenic mice, verifying that the treatment had the expected effect. Strikingly, Th17-depletion caused a significant reduction of disease severity, as shown in fig. 4e and S5. By contrast, the effect

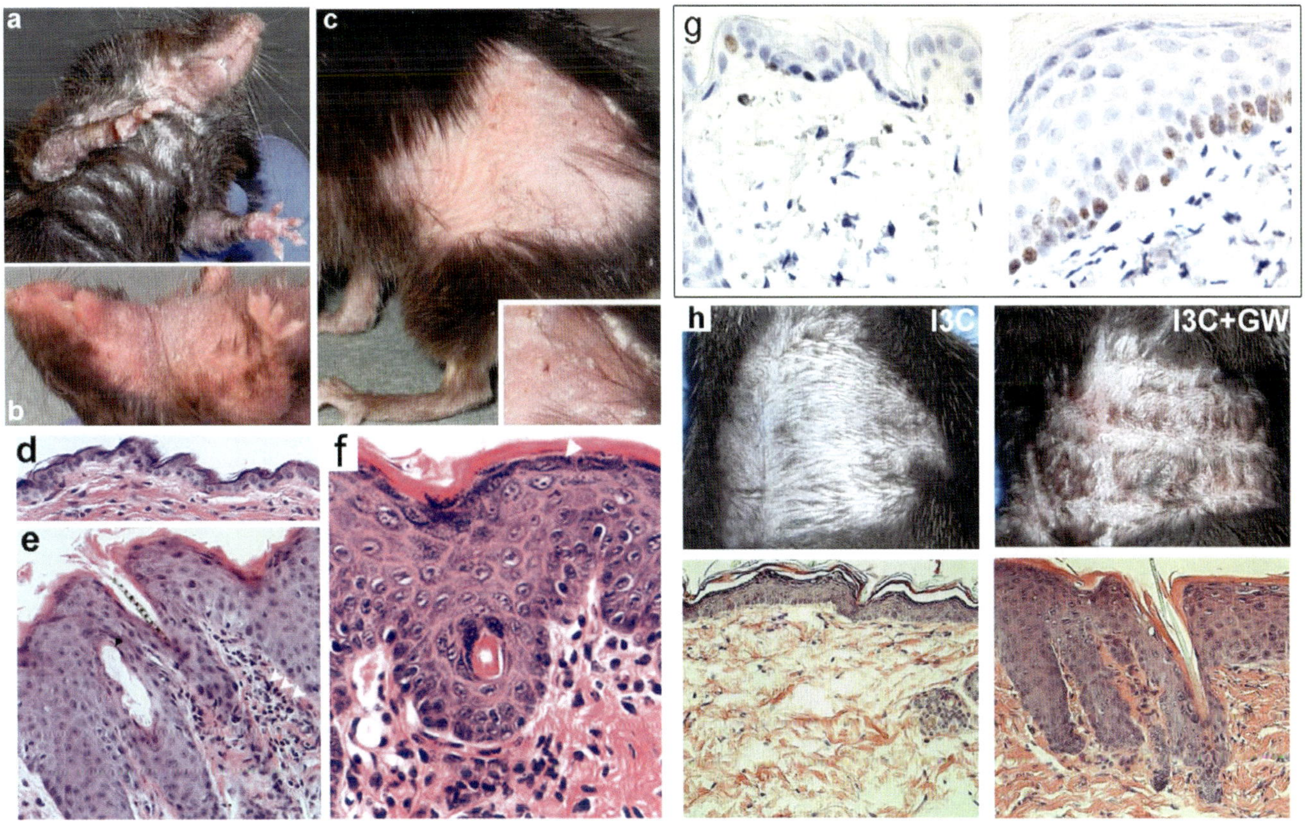

Figure 3. Skin phenotype in PPARβ/δ TG mice twenty days after GW501516 (GW) administration for twenty days. (a–c) Gross morphology, (d–e) H&E histology of control mice not treated with GW (d), or fourteen days after induction (e–g). Magnification 200× (d,e) or 400× (f). The white arrowhead in (f) denotes the granular layer. (g) Immunostaining for Ki67 of skin from PPARβ/δ TG mice maintained in the absence (left) or presence (right) of GW. Magnification 200×. (h) Induction of skin disease by topical application of either 0.3% of indole-3-carbinole (I3C, left) or I3C plus 0.3% GW501516 once daily to shaved abdominal skin. Gross macroscopic phenotype (top) and H&E histology of treated skin (bottom) was documented 10 days after beginning of treatment.

of anti-TNFα was much less pronounced, as expected. Thus, Th17 cells are required for full disease expression in PPARβ/δ transgenic mice. In order to clarify whether they are sufficient to trigger disease development, we performed adoptive transfer of splenocytes from PPARβ/δ transgenic mice with active disease to wild-type mice, which had previously been depleted of endogenous $CD4^+$ cells. This treatment failed to induce any skin phenotype even after GW501516 administration to the recipient mice. Moreover, when GW501516 was administered to naïve wild type C57Bl/6j mice, they did exhibit a modest increase of Th17 cells in peripheral organs (fig. S4), indicating that endogenous murine PPARβ/δ also stimulates Th17 cell expansion. Wild type mice did not, however, develop skin disease. Thus, Th17 cells are required, but not sufficient for development of psoriasis-like disease in PPARβ/δ transgenic mice, although we cannot rule out that their presence in the skin in high numbers might allow disease development.

Psoriasis-like gene dysregulation in PPARβ/δ transgenic mice

Although psoriasis lesions are complex, involving various cell types and a multitude of dysregulated genes, the observed changes in gene expression are remarkably reproducible between different patients. This is demonstrated by the tight correlation between two large independent expression profiling datasets (Fig. S6), thus yielding a consistent psoriasis-specific pattern of global gene dysregulation. We studied to what extent this pattern is reflected in PPARβ/δ mice. As shown in figure 5a, most of the top 50 genes upregulated in lesional skin of PPARβ/δ mice were found congruently upregulated in human psoriasis. Quantitative real-time-PCR of selected genes confirmed that the changes observed by microarray-based expression profiling were reproducible (figure S7). Indeed, 56% of all upregulated and 33% of all downregulated genes in PPARβ/δ mice were found congruently regulated in psoriasis, respectively (figure 5b, clusters I and VI). Conversely, appr. 30% of all genes dysregulated in human psoriasis were found to be regulated congruently in PPARβ/δ mice (table S3). Geneset Enrichment analysis (GSEA) independently confirmed a highly significant enrichment of those genes upregulated in psoriasis (defined as gene-set) in lesional skin of PPARβ/δ mice (figure 5c). Only two small subsets of genes (8.3% of all, clusters III and IV) displayed inverse regulation between psoriasis and PPARβ/δ mice. When analysing the functional profile of these, we observed that cluster III, containing genes *up*regulated in PPARβ/δ mice but *down*regulated in psoriasis, was enriched for markers of late epidermal differentiation (e.g. FLG, PCDH21), indicative of cells in the so-called granular layer, which is prominent in PPARβ/δ mice (fig. 3f) but absent in psoriasis. Cluster IV, containing genes *up*regulated in psoriasis but *down*regulated in PPARβ/δ mice, was highly enriched for interferon-signalling (fig. 5b, table S3), where we were able to identify the mechanism underlying this discrepancy (see below). Taken together, expression profiling

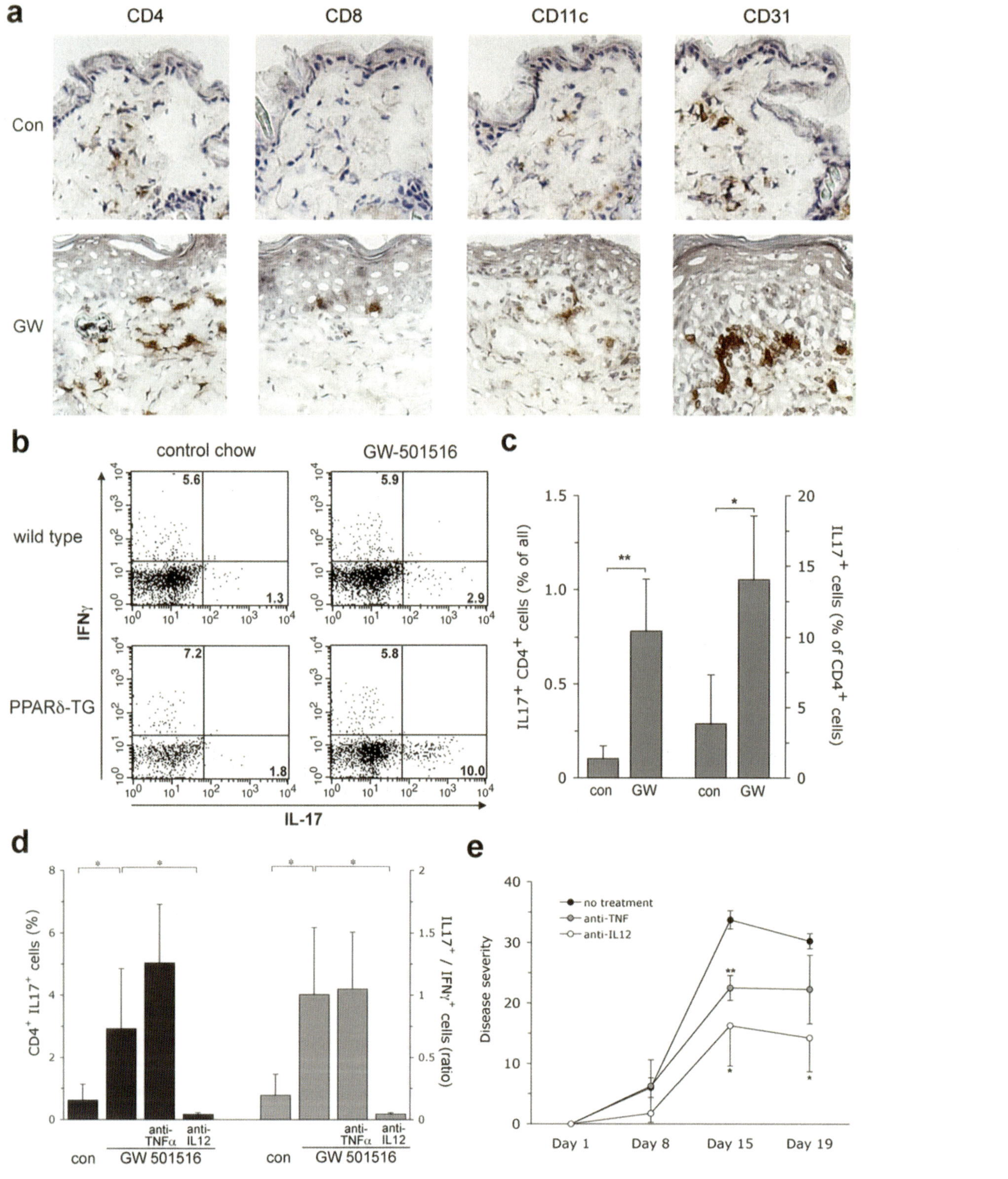

Figure 4. Immune activation in PPARβ/δ-mediated skin disease. (a) Immunohistochemistry for CD4, CD8, CD11c, and CD31 (Pecam 31) of skin from PPARβ/δ transgenic mice maintained in the absence (top) or presence of GW501516. Magnification 200×, (b) flow cytometry analysis showing intracellular FACS-staining for IFNγ and IL17 of skin cells (gated for CD4) from wild type and PPARβ/δ transgenic mice maintained in the presence or absence of GW501516, respectively. Numbers in quadrants indicate frequency of positive cells, (c) frequency of $CD4^+IL17^+$ of $IL17^+$ cells (expressed as percent of all $CD4^+$ gated cells) in PPARβ/δ transgenic and C57Bl/6 wild type mice maintained in the presence or absence of GW501516 (n = 4 per group), as determined by flow cytometry. * $p<0.01$; ** $p<0.001$, (d) frequency of $CD4^+IL17^+$ Th17 cells (left y-axis, black columns) and ratio of $IL17^+$ and $IFN\gamma^+$ cell frequencies (righ y-axis, grey columns) in the skin of PPARβ/δ mice maintained in the absence or presence of GW501516 with or without i.p. injection of anti-TNFα, or αIL12/23p40 (n = 4, see Methods), (e) disease severity, expressed as mean ± s.d., assessed by the degree of erythema, thickening, scaling, and hair loss (see Methods, representative photographs of mice on day 19 post induction are shown in figure S6) in PPARβ/δ transgenic mice GW501516 – containing chow with or without additional intraperitoneal injection of anti-TNFα or αIL12/23p40 (anti-IL12). * $p<0.01$, ** $p<0.001$ (treatment vs. control).

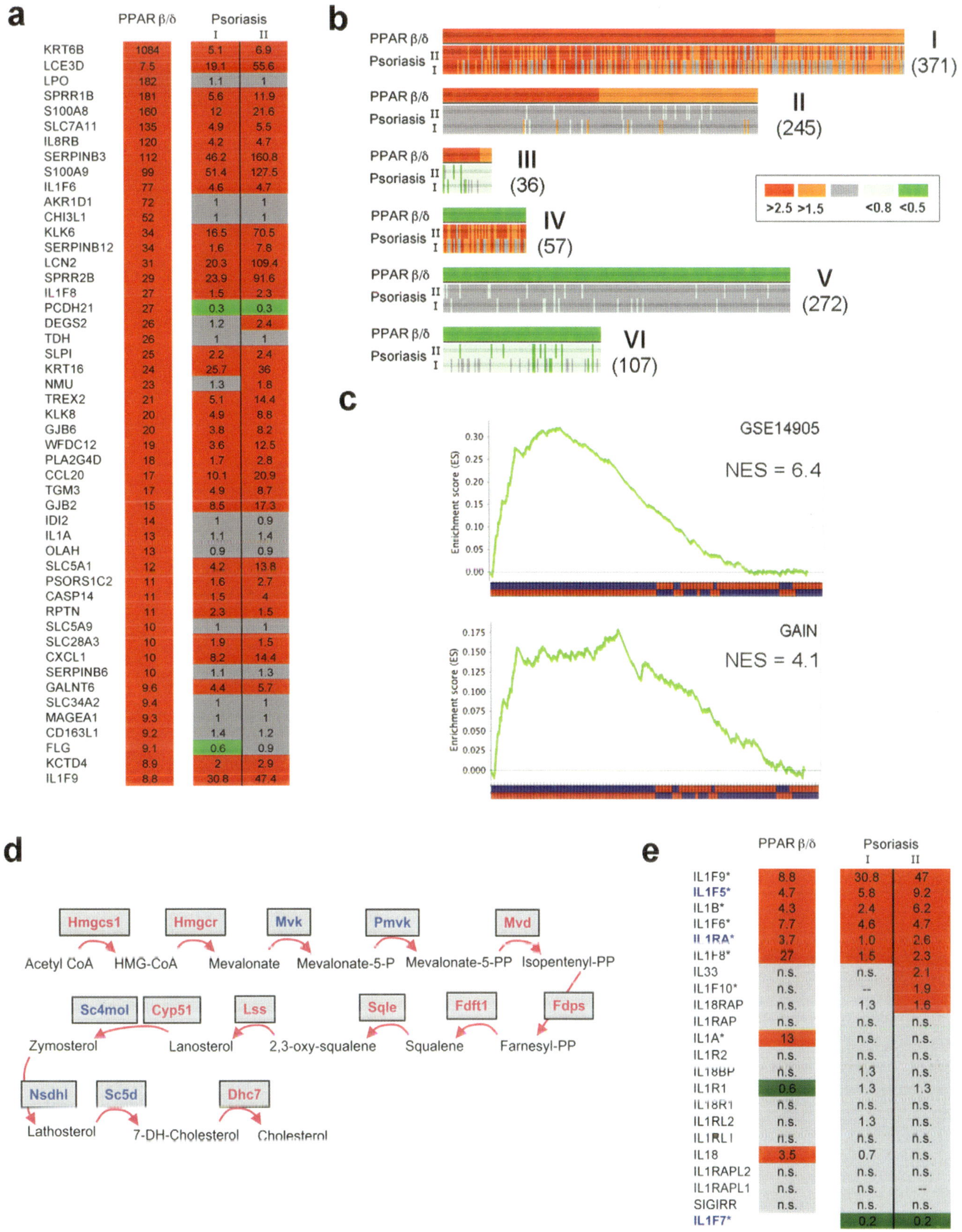

a

	PPAR β/δ	Psoriasis I	Psoriasis II
KRT6B	1084	5.1	6.9
LCE3D	7.5	19.1	55.6
LPO	182	1.1	1
SPRR1B	181	5.6	11.9
S100A8	160	12	21.6
SLC7A11	135	4.9	5.5
IL8RB	120	4.2	4.7
SERPINB3	112	46.2	160.8
S100A9	99	51.4	127.5
IL1F6	77	4.6	4.7
AKR1D1	72	1	1
CHI3L1	52	1	1
KLK6	34	16.5	70.5
SERPINB12	34	1.6	7.8
LCN2	31	20.3	109.4
SPRR2B	29	23.9	91.6
IL1F8	27	1.5	2.3
PCDH21	27	0.3	0.3
DEGS2	26	1.2	2.4
TDH	26	1	1
SLPI	25	2.2	2.4
KRT16	24	25.7	36
NMU	23	1.3	1.8
TREX2	21	5.1	14.4
KLK8	20	4.9	8.8
GJB6	20	3.8	8.2
WFDC12	19	3.6	12.5
PLA2G4D	18	1.7	2.8
CCL20	17	10.1	20.9
TGM3	17	4.9	8.7
GJB2	15	8.5	17.3
IDI2	14	1	0.9
IL1A	13	1.1	1.4
OLAH	13	0.9	0.9
SLC5A1	12	4.2	13.8
PSORS1C2	11	1.6	2.7
CASP14	11	1.5	4
RPTN	11	2.3	1.5
SLC5A9	10	1	1
SLC28A3	10	1.9	1.5
CXCL1	10	8.2	14.4
SERPINB6	10	1.1	1.3
GALNT6	9.6	4.4	5.7
SLC34A2	9.4	1	1
MAGEA1	9.3	1	1
CD163L1	9.2	1.4	1.2
FLG	9.1	0.6	0.9
KCTD4	8.9	2	2.9
IL1F9	8.8	30.8	47.4

e

	PPAR β/δ	Psoriasis I	Psoriasis II
IL1F9*	8.8	30.8	47
IL1F5*	4.7	5.8	9.2
IL1B*	4.3	2.4	6.2
IL1F6*	7.7	4.6	4.7
IL1RA*	3.7	1.0	2.6
IL1F8*	27	1.5	2.3
IL33	n.s.	n.s.	2.1
IL1F10*	n.s.	--	1.9
IL18RAP	n.s.	1.3	1.6
IL1RAP	n.s.	n.s.	n.s.
IL1A*	13	n.s.	n.s.
IL1R2	n.s.	n.s.	n.s.
IL18BP	n.s.	1.3	n.s.
IL1R1	0.6	1.3	1.3
IL18R1	n.s.	n.s.	n.s.
IL1RL2	n.s.	1.3	n.s.
IL1RL1	n.s.	n.s.	n.s.
IL18	3.5	0.7	n.s.
IL1RAPL2	n.s.	n.s.	n.s.
IL1RAPL1	n.s.	n.s.	--
SIGIRR	n.s.	n.s.	n.s.
IL1F7*		0.2	0.2

Figure 5. Congruent gene dysregulation in PPARβ/δ mice and psoriasis. (**a**) Fold-change between the lesional skin of PPARβ/δ mice after administration of GW501516 and control mice (n = 3 per group), and between lesional and non-lesional skin samples from psoriasis obtained through the GAIN (I) and the GSE14905 (II) datasets, respectively, as detailed in Methods. Red: FC >1.5, Green: FC <0.8. Shown are the top 50 upregulated genes. The complete dataset is given in table S1. (**b**) Heat map showing all genes dysregulated in GW501516-fed PPARβ/δ mice (n = 1077), clustered

by congruence with psoriasis. Color codes for –fold change are indicated. The genes in all clusters are detailed in table S2. (**c**) gene-set enrichment analysis (GSEA), performed using the top 500 genes upregulated in psoriasis lesions from the GSE14905 dataset (top), or the GAIN dataset (bottom), as genesets, respectively, and the complete mouse array collapsed to single genes as expression dataset. Analysis was run with 100 permutations and a classic statistic, NES = normalized enrichment score. The blue-red lines on the bottom represent heat-map of human genes found to be upregulated (blue on top) or downregulated in the mouse set. (**d**) Induction of cholesterol biosynthesis, conjugation, and channeling by PPARβ/δ. Red: upregulated in psoriasis and PPARβ/δ transgenic mice, blue: upregulated only in PPARβ/δ transgenic mice. Shaded boxes: repressed by Foxo1. (**e**) Induction of IL-1 signalling by PPARβ/δ. Datasets and color codes are as in (a). "n.s.": $p>0.01$; "--": fold change between 0.8–1.2., blue print: anti-inflammatory. * gene located within the IL1 cluster on chr. 2q between 113.2–113.7 Mb. (IL1F7 has only been identified in *homo sapiens* and *bos taurus*, the closest homologue in mice is IL1F5.).

confirms a large overlap in gene regulation between psoriasis and the skin disease in PPARβ/δ mice, strongly suggesting that the phenotype similarities described above are not a phenocopy but involve overlapping signalling pathways.

PPARβ/δ-dependent regulation of specific pathways

When extending analysis of gene expression to functional processes, we found that processes concordantly regulated in psoriasis and PPARβ/δ transgenic mice included lipid-metabolism, differentiation, and proliferation (table S4), which confirmed the expected, given the known activity profile of PPARβ/δ. Likewise, the complete set of genes involved in cholesterol biosynthesis was strongly co-upregulated (fig. 5d, table S6), as were a number of proliferation-associated kinases (table S8). Unexpectedly, however, both the human and the murine datasets exhibited a highly consistent upregulated IL1-signalling module, which, remarkably, not only includes pro-inflammatory transcripts but also the anti-inflammatory components IL1F5, and the IL1-receptor antagonist (fig. 5e, table S7). Importantly, wild type C57Bl/6 mice administered GW501516 did not exhibit these changes (table S1), but did show the expected upregulation of genes involved in lipid metabolism (table S5), thereby confirming that the observed induction of IL1-signalling was triggered by the transgene rather than endogenous murine PPARβ/δ. These results strongly suggest that a number of transcriptional programs known to be dysregulated in psoriasis are regulated by PPARβ/δ.

Critical role of STAT3 in PPARβ/δ dependent skin disease

STAT3 is phosphorylated in psoriasis [34], as well as in a wound-response type model of psoriasis induced by serum response factor-deficiency [35]. Accordingly, we analyzed STAT3 activation in PPARβ/δ mice. Tyr-705 phosphorylation of STAT3 was markedly increased in lesional skin of PPARβ/δ transgenic mice (figure 6a) and localized to the nuclei of suprabasal cells in the epidermis (figure 6b). Moreover, inhibition of STAT3 phosphorylation by the JAK2 inhibitor WP1066 led to a marked attenuation of skin disease, demonstrating the relevance of this pathway for the development of clinical disease, further demonstrating the overlap in pathogenesis between psoriasis and the current model (figure 6c).

STAT3 activation mediates suppression of interferon-target genes

As described above, the single group of genes upregulated in psoriasis but downregulated in PPARβ/δ mice were the interferon response genes (fig.5b, cluster IV). Strikingly, precisely this set of genes was previously shown to be repressed by STAT3 in vivo (fig. 6d, dark shaded columns). We therefore hypothesized that the notable repression of interferon-response genes in the skin of PPARβ/δ transgenic mice with skin disease was mediated by activation of STAT3. Indeed, repression of STAT3 activation by use of the JAK2 inhibitor significantly blocked the down-regulation of one of the most repressed transcripts, IFI27 (fig. 6e). This STAT3-dependent effect was specific to interferon-response genes, since the dysregulation of another inflammatory pathway, exemplified by IL1β, remained unaltered by STAT3 inhibition (fig. 6e). These data show the inhibition of IFN signalling in PPARβ/δ transgenic mice is mediated by STAT3 as part of what has previously been termed the "anti-inflammatory response" [36].

Discussion

We here show that PPARβ/δ is activated in the upper epidermis of human psoriatic skin and that recapitulation of this event in mice is sufficient to elicit major elements of psoriasis. PPARβ/δ transgenic mice exhibit not only down-stream immunological changes but also psoriasis – specific gene dysregulation, thereby defining subsets of genes regulated by PPARβ/δ in psoriasis. Although the current transgenic model exhibits important differences to psoriasis (see below) and cannot recapitulate all features of a polygenetic disease, it does thus indicate that activation of PPARβ/δ in the upper spinous layer of the epidermis initiates a number of inflammatory and immunological changes seen in psoriasis.

One major implication of the present results is that they suggest a molecular explanation for the clinical overlap between psoriasis and metabolic, as well as cardiovascular disease [37]. Thus, PPARβ/δ expression is increased in chronic inflammation and regulated by caloric intake [38,39]. Specifically, factors such as TNFα which are known to directly induce PPARβ/δ expression are increased in the chronic inflammation accompanying metabolic syndrome [40]. Therefore, obesity, chronic inflammation, and dyslipidemia may increase the penetrance of psoriasis by inducing PPARβ/δ expression. Conversely, it is tempting to speculate that weight reduction or correction of other PPARβ/δ - inducing factors leads to suppression of PPARβ/δ expression in the skin, thus dampening disease severity. This may well be a contributory factor in the clinical observation that the response to low-dose cyclosporin, an established psoriasis treatment, is improved in psoriasis patients undergoing weight loss [41].

The role of PPARβ/δ in inflammation has been extensively and controversially studied, several papers suggesting anti-inflammatory properties (e.g. [42]), while others find that it stimulates pro-inflammatory cytokine synthesis including IL-8 and IL1β in macrophages [43]. Here, we show that, in the skin, PPARβ/δ induces a specific IL-1 signalling "module" both in human psoriasis and in PPARβ/δ transgenic mice. This module includes pro-inflammatory mediators such as IL1β, which is known to stimulate Th17 differentiation [44], and IL1F8, which stimulates pro-inflammatory mediators in fibroblasts [45], but also anti-inflammatory cytokines such as IL-1F5, which actually inhibits inflammatory skin disease [46], as well as the IL1 receptor antagonist (IL1RA). The latter has recently been shown to be a direct target of PPARβ/δ [47] and to be upregulated in psoriasis [48], thereby corroborating our findings. Thus, the PPARβ/δ - mediated induction of IL1-family cytokines in psoriasis defies a

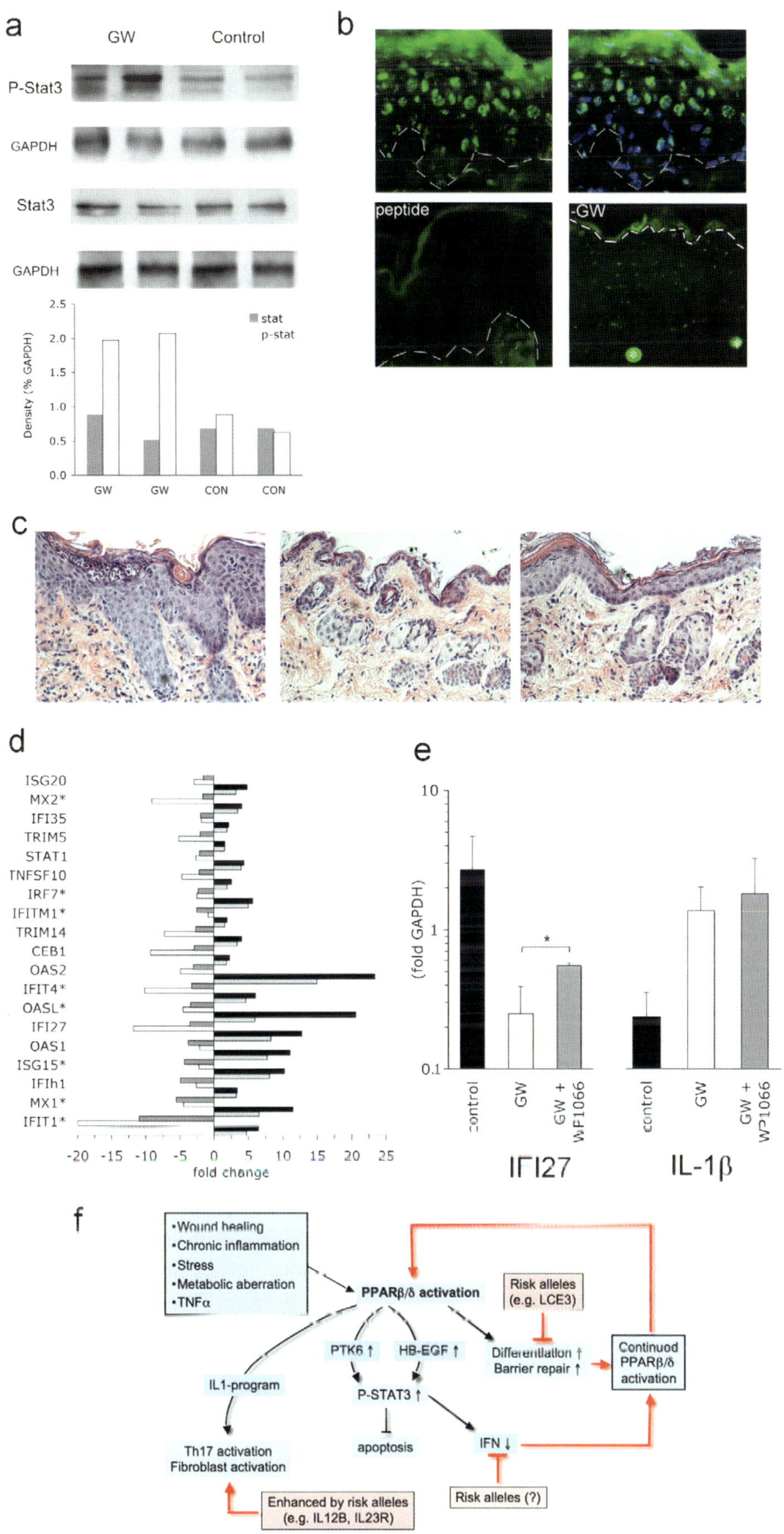
a
GW
Control
P-Stat3
GAPDH
Stat3
GAPDH
Density (% GAPDH)
stat
p-stat
GW
GW
CON
CON
b
peptide
-GW
c
d
ISG20
MX2*
IFI35
TRIM5
STAT1
TNFSF10
IRF7*
IFITM1*
TRIM14
CEB1
OAS2
IFIT4*
OASL*
IFI27
OAS1
ISG15*
IFIh1
MX1*
IFIT1*
fold change
e
(fold GAPDH)
control
GW
GW + WF1066
IFI27
IL-1β
f
•Wound healing
•Chronic inflammation
•Stress
•Metabolic aberration
•TNFα
PPARβ/δ activation
Risk alleles (e.g. LCE3)
PTK6 ↑
HB-EGF ↑
Differentiation ↑
Barrier repair ↑
Continued PPARβ/δ activation
IL1-program
P-STAT3 ↑
apoptosis
IFN ↓
Th17 activation
Fibroblast activation
Enhanced by risk alleles (e.g. IL12B, IL23R)
Risk alleles (?)

Figure 6. Activation of STAT3 by PPARβ/δ. (**a**) Western blot of whole skin samples from two GW501516-treated (GW) and two control PPARβ/δ transgenic mice, respectively, probed with anti phospho-STAT3 (top) and anti-STAT3 (bottom) along with anti-GAPDH loading controls (top-band of the STAT3 doublet represents STAT3α, bottom-band STAT3β, respectively), semi-quantitative densitometry performed using ImageJ is included on the bottom, (**b**) immunofluorescence with anti phospho-STAT3 of GW-treated skin (upper left), upper right: same with DAPI counterstain to verify nuclear localisation, bottom left: control stain performed in the presence of blocking peptide, lower right: PPARβ/δ transgenic mouse not treated with GW. White dashed lines mark the dermo-epidermal bounday; all samples at 400× magnification. * = hair shaft (**c**) H&E histology of skin from GW-treated (left panel), untreated (middle), GW-treated mice concurrently receiving intraperitoneal injections of the STAT3 inhibitor WP1066 (right) at 200× magnification, (**d**) fold change of genes previously shown to be repressed by activated STAT3 (dark grey columns, data taken from [56]) and their regulation in GW501516-fed vs. control PPARβ/δ transgenic mice (white), lesional vs. non-lesional skin from psoriasis patients in the GSE14905 (black), as well as the GAIN (light grey) datasets, respectively. * denotes genes that are not contained in cluster IV (table S2) since they did not meet the $p<0.01$ cut-off. (**e**) Taqman-based qPCR of IFI27 and IL1β from whole skin of untreated (black columns), GW-fed (white), and GW-fed + WP1066-injected PPARβ/δ mice (grey), respectively (n = 3 mice per group), * $p<0.05$; (**f**) schematic illustrating the PPARβ/δ /STAT3 /IL-1 pathway identified here, the role of PPARβ/δ in maintaining chronically active psoriasis, as well as disease-enhancing role of predisposing genomic risk alleles. The box on the upper left lists factors known to trigger both PPARβ/δ induction as well as clinical psoriasis flares.

simplified concept of purely "pro-" or "anti-" inflammatory. Clearly, these results would signal some caution regarding the proposed use of PPARβ/δ agonists to treat a variety of conditions [49].

We here identify activation of STAT3 as a novel pathway targeted by PPARβ/δ. PPARβ/δ activation evidently causes psoriasis-like disease not solely through STAT3 activation since (i) the phenotype is not completely reversed by inhibition of STAT3 and (ii) overexpression of STAT3 alone causes a less widespread psoriasis-like phenotype with a much longer latency [34]. Regarding the mechanism of STAT3 activation, STAT3 can be phosphorylated by a number of kinases. Of these, at least two appear to be involved. First, the two EGF-family ligands TGFα and HB-EGF, previously identified as a direct transcriptional target of PPARβ/δ [12], are highly upregulated in PPARβ/δ as well as in psoriasis, suggesting that EGF-receptor activation contributes to STAT3 phosphorylation. Second, PTK6 kinase, which also phosphorylates STAT3 [50], is the most highly upregulated kinase in psoriasis and PPARβ/δ mice (table S8). Thus, at least two kinase pathways converge on STAT3 phosphorylation both in psoriasis and PPARβ/δ mice.

An obvious difference between the skin disease induced by activation of PPARβ/δ and psoriasis in humans is the regulation of IFN signalling. While IFN response genes are strongly induced in psoriasis they are repressed in PPARβ/δ transgenic mice. On the other hand, subsequent downstream events, including CD4+ and CD8+ T-cell influx, endothelial activation, dendritic cell accumulation, as well as Th17 activation are all recapitulated preserved in this model. Therefore, the present data suggest that upregulation of interferon response genes is not, as commonly assumed, required for sustained disease. Furthermore, while the upregulation of IFN response genes could be taken for granted in the milieu of a wound-response, our data show that they should actually be repressed by the so-called anti-inflammatory response mediated by STAT3 [36,51]. Their continuous upregulation despite STAT3 activation suggests the existence of as yet to be identified factors actively inhibiting STAT3 repression of IFN target genes (schematically shown in fig. 6f).

Psoriasis is a genetically determined disease and genomic variants at the PPARβ/δ genomic locus have not so far been associated with psoriasis. Although this might be regarded as evidence against a role for PPARβ/δ in psoriasis, our data clearly show that overexpression of PPARβ/δ in psoriasis skin lesions is a common phenomenon occuring in the vast majority of psoriasis patients (fig. 1). Thus, upregulation of PPARβ/δ appears to occur downstream of individually variable genomic risk, offering a potential target for treatment relevant for most patients.

Apart from interferon response genes, the other major difference in gene expression between psoriasis and the phenotype in PPARβ/δ mice is terminal epidermal differentiation, which is blocked in psoriasis, but increased in the mouse model, which confirms the established pro-differentiation activity of PPARβ/δ [52] and the fact that it triggers differentiation in wound healing [28,53]. In psoriasis, on the other hand, late epidermal differentation is disturbed and the skin barrier disrupted. Based on the data presented here, one may speculate that the suppression of terminal differentiation and the block in skin barrier repair, aggravated by genomic risk alleles such as the recently described LCE3 variant [54], act as stimuli to maintain sustained upregulation of PPARβ/δ in the upper epidermal layers. The net effect would be the establishment of a vicious cycle, schematically shown in fig.6f, which is able to account for the chronic persistent course typical of psoriasis.

In conclusion, we here identify a central role for PPARβ/δ in the pathogenesis of psoriasis and identify IL1 and STAT3 signalling as novel pathways regulated by PPARβ/δ. Our data suggest novel approaches to psoriasis treatment. Finally, our results underscore that PPARβ/δ activation as a treatment strategy for metabolic diseases might harbour the risk of pro-inflammatory effects or autoimmune activation.

Methods

Ethics Statement

All work involving animals was approved by the Tayside Ethics Committee. Storage and use of all tissues included in the work presented here was approved by the Tayside Committee on Medical Research Ethics B (REC ref. Nr. 07/S1402/90).

PPARβ/δ immunohistochemistry

Paraffin-embedded samples were obtained from the Tayside Tissue bank. Prior to biopsy, patients gave written consent to storage and analysis of biopsy samples. Sections from paraffin embedded tissue (nominally 4 microns thick) were cut onto superfrost plus slides (VWR International Ltd) and dried for 1 hr at 60 °C before being de-paraffinised in Histoclear (National Diagnostics) and then rehydrated through a graded alcohol series. 10 mM Citric acid buffer, pH 6.0 was used as standard microwave-based antigen retrieval methods. Sections were microwaved in a pressure cooker for 15 min before being immunostained on a DAKO autostainer using Vectastain® ABC kits (Vector Labs) according to the manufacturer's protocol. Briefly, sections were blocked in either normal goat, rabbit or horse serum containing 10%(v/v) from stock avidin solution (Vector Labs) for 20 min followed by 1 hr incubation with anti-PPARβ/δ (R&D, PP-K9436) at 1:100 overnight at 4°C for human samples (incubation for 1 h at room temperature yielded comparable results.), and 1:1000 for murine samples. Sections were washed 3× for 15 min in TBS, pH 7.6, followed by anti-mouse-biotin, antibody for 30 min followed by Vectastain Elite ABC reagent for another 30 min. Liquid Diaminobenzidine (DAB) (DAKO) was applied for 5 min and sections were counterstained with Mayer's haematoxylin.

H&E histology

Paraffin-embedded samples were heated for 15 minutes. Samples were treated with 3 washes of Xylene, followed by a series of graded alcohol washes. Samples were washed with water followed with staining with Harris' Haematoxylin. Wash 2 with water. Samples incubated in 0.1% acid alcohol for 1 minute followed by a 3rd wash with water. Samples were then incubated in STWS for 1 minute followed by a 4th wash with water. Samples stained with Shandon Eosin for 30 seconds followed by a 5th wash. Samples were re-hydrated with a series of graded alcohol washes followed by 3 washes with Xylene. Sections were mounted with DPX.

Generation of PPARβ/δ transgenic mice

PPARβ/δ transgenic mice were generated by cloning full-length human PPARδ downstream of the human CYP1A1 promoter. Plasmids encoding human PPARδ were prepared as follows. The PPARδ coding sequence was amplified using primers PRMG15 (5′-CTAGTCTAGA**ATG**GAGCACCCACAGGAGGAAGC-3′) and PRMG3 (5′-CTAGTCTAGATTAGTACATGTCCTTG-TAGATCTCCTG-3′), respectively (*Xba*I-sites underlined, ATG start codon in bold). PCR products were cleaved with *Xba*I and cloned in plasmid pUHD10-3 (M. Gossen, unpublished, Genbank accession number U89931) creating pMGD7 (PPARδ). The integrity of the inserts was confirmed by sequencing and cleaved out using *Bam*HI and ligated into plasmid pAHIR1-β-gal (Campbell, 1996} cleaved with *Bgl*II, resulting in the plasmid pMGD72 (PPARδ). Proper insert orientation was confirmed by restriction endonuclease analysis and sequencing. Transgenic mice were generated by microinjection of the expression unit (*Not*I fragment) of the plasmid pMGD72 into pro-nuclei of C57BL/J6 x CBA F1 fertilized eggs. Mice were maintained under standard animal house conditions.

Disease induction

PPARβ/δ mediated skin disease was induced either by administration of powdered standard RMI-chow containing 0.003% GW501516 (w/w, custom – synthesized by AF-Pharmaceuticals, UK, to ≥98% purity), or topical application of 0.3% (w/w) GW501516 in 10% (w/w) DMSO in Hydromol ointment (Alliance, UK); for topical induction, control mice received 10% DMSO in Hydromol.

Flow cytometry and intracellular measurement of IL17

Skin samples were shaved, trimmed of associated fat, cut to appr. 10–15 mm^3 size using a scissor, incubated in 2 mg/ml collagenase IV (Roche, cat-nr. 11088085001), 1.1 U/ml dispase I (Roche, cat-nr. 04942086001) in HBSS for 30′ at 37°C. Subsequently, samples were incubated in RPMI incl. Pen/Strep and 10% FCS, 0.5 µg/ml PMA, 0.5 µg/ml ionomycin for 3 h. For the last hour, Brefeldin A was added at 2 µg/ml. Surface and intracellular staining for CD4-FITC (Pharmingen, clone RM4-4), CD8-PerCP/Cy5.5b (Pharmingen, 53–6.7), IFNγ-APC (Pharmingen, cat-nr. 554413), and IL17-PE (Pharmingen, cat-nr. 559502) and analysis on a FACS-Calibur was done according to standard procedures.

TNFα and IL-12 antibody treatment

70 µg of anti-TNFα (Millipore, cat-nr 05-168), anti-IL12/23p40 (BioLegend, Clone C17.8, cat-nr. 505304), or PBS, respectively, were injected on three times per week, beginning on day 1 of GW501516 administration. Mice were sacrificed on day 22 for tissue analysis. For disease severity, erythema, scaling, palpable hyperkeratosis, and hair loss were scored as absent (0), weak (1), moderate (2), or severe (3), respectively, and the sum calculated for index regions (chin, forepaws, abdomen) chosen in order to allow hand-held analysis of mice during on-going treatment.

Expression profiling was performed as detailed in the supporting information (Method S1).

Western blot STAT3, P-STAT3

Nuclear extracts were made using the NE-PER kit (Pierce). Protein concentration was determined by Bradford assay. 40 µg of protein loaded per well, subjected to SDS-PAGE gel and transferred to nitrocellulose membrane. Primary antibodies: 1:1000 dilution of Phospho-Stat3 (Tyr705) Antibody (New England BioLabs UK, 9131S) and 1:1000 dilution of anti-Stat3 (New England BioLabs UK, 9132) followed by HRP– conjugated anti-rabbit Ig, ECL Plus (GE Healthcare, Amersham), and detection using a CCD camera.

Immunofluorescence P-STAT3

5 µm thick sections of snap-frozen skin were fixed in methanol, followed by incubation with anti-Phospho-Stat3 (Tyr705) (D3A7) (New England Biolabs UK, 9145S) with or without blocking peptide (New England Biolabs UK, 1195) for 1 hour at RT. Secondary antibody was Alexa Fluro® 488 donkey anti-rabbit IgG (H+L) (Invitrogen). Coverslips were mounted using ProLong® Gold antifade reagent with DAPI (Invitrogen, Cat.no.: P-36931).

Treatment with WP1066

WP1066 (Calbiochem, order-nr 573097) was dissolved in DMSO/PEG 600 (20/80) according to [55] at 1.25 µg/µl. Mice were injected with WP1066 or vehicle at 75 µl intraperitoneally three times a week.

Supporting Information

Table S1 Synopsis of dysregulated genes in PPARβ/δ transgenic mice and psoriasis. Sheet "Changed in PPARd mice": all genes found dysregulated in PPARd mice, as detailed in the file Method S1. Sheet "PPARd mice vs psoriasis": all genes dysregulated in PPARβ/δ mice (orange shaded cells) that are also present on the two gene expression sets representing psoriasis (green shaded cells). FC = fold change lesional vs. non-lesional (psoriasis), or induced vs. non-induced (PPARβ/δ transgenic mice).

Found at: doi:10.1371/journal.pone.0009701.s001

Table S2 Clustering of genes dysregulated in PPARβ/δ transgenic mice. The table contains all 1077 genes listed in the synopsis between dysregulated genes in PPARβ/δ transgenic mice and psoriasis, color-coded as up- (red/orange) or down- regulated (light-green/dark green), as shown in Figure 5b.

Found at: doi:10.1371/journal.pone.0009701.s002

Table S3 Concordance of gene dysregulation between psoriasis and PPARβ/δ transgenic mice.

Found at: doi:10.1371/journal.pone.0009701.s003

Table S4 Genes concordantly regulated between PPARβ/δ transgenic mice and psoriasis, listed for the functional categories lipid-metabolism, differentiation, and cell-cycle.
Found at: doi:10.1371/journal.pone.0009701.s004

Table S5 Genes induced by the PPARβ/δ agonist GW501516 in the skin of C57Bl/6 wild type mice.
Found at: doi:10.1371/journal.pone.0009701.s005

Table S6 Expression of genes involved in cholesterol biosynthesis in PPARβ/δ transgenic mice and psoriasis.
Found at: doi:10.1371/journal.pone.0009701.s006

Table S7 Interleukin-1 related genes in PPARβ/δ transgenic mice and psoriasis.
Found at: doi:10.1371/journal.pone.0009701.s007

Table S8 Expression of kinase genes in PPARβ/δ transgenic mice and psoriasis.
Found at: doi:10.1371/journal.pone.0009701.s008

Table S9 PPAR isoforms and ligands.
Found at: doi:10.1371/journal.pone.0009701.s009

Method S1 Expression profiling.
Found at: doi:10.1371/journal.pone.0009701.s010

Figure S1 (a) Immunohistochemistry of PPARβ/δ in a panel of eight paraffin-embedded samples from psoriasis skin lesions, counterstained with hematoxilin. The inset in the right upper panel in addition demonstrates expression in dermal fibroblasts and endothelial cells. Magnification 200× in each case. (b) Immunohistochemistry of PPARβ/δ in PPARβ/δ- transgenic mice treated with GW501516 for seven days, counterstained with hematoxilin. Panels in lower row were taken fom slides stained with secondary antibody only. Magnification 200× for all panels.
Found at: doi:10.1371/journal.pone.0009701.s011

Figure S2 Macroscopic changes in PPARβ/δ transgenic mice upon ligand-mediated activation of PPARβ/δ by administration of the ligand GW501516 in the chow. Pictures shown were taken 14 (left) or 20 days (middle, right) after disease induction. Note the sharp demarcation of hyperkeratosis on the abdomen (middle). Panel on upper right represents illustrates the scalp, exhibiting heavy scaling, but no marked erythema.
Found at: doi:10.1371/journal.pone.0009701.s012

Figure S3 Confinement of PPARβ/δ transgene expression to suprabasal epidermal keratinocytes. Co-immunofluorescence with anti-PPARβ/δ visualized with Alexa288 and either CD11c, visualized with TexasRed, was performed as described in Methods. The white dashed line indicates the dermo-epidermal boundary. Magnification 400×.
Found at: doi:10.1371/journal.pone.0009701.s013

Figure S4 Expansion of Th17 cells upon activation of PPARβ/δ. PPARβ/δ transgenic mice were maintained in the presence (black columns) or absence (dark shaded) of GW501516, as were C57Bl6/j wild type (light shaded: GW; white: control) and Th17 cell frequencies determined by intracellular FACS, as described in Methods. Data show mean ± s.d. of Th17 cells (top), as well as the ratio between $IL17^+$ and $IFN\gamma^+$ cells (bottom) in the lymphocyte gate for n = 3 mice per group. * $p<0.05$.
Found at: doi:10.1371/journal.pone.0009701.s014

Figure S5 Inhibition of PPARβ/δ-mediated skin disease by depletion of Th17 cells. PPARβ/δ transgenic mice were maintained in the absence (control) or presence (all other groups) of GW501516 and additionally treated by injection of either anti-IL12/23p40, or anti-TNFα, as described in Methods. Pictures shown were taken nineteen days after disease induction. Mice were manually restrained to allow for comparable positioning during photography, thereby causing artificial tightening of abdominal skin.
Found at: doi:10.1371/journal.pone.0009701.s015

Figure S6 Reproducibility of gene dysregulation in psoriasis. Fold-change of gene expression between lesional and non-lesional skin in two independent datasets. The left panel shows all genes, the right panel all genes significantly upregulated ($p<0.001$) in both datasets. R2 = 0.93 for both panels. The dashed line indicates theoretically equal up-regulation in the two datasets. Both datasets were obtained using the same platform (using the Affymetrix HU133 Plus 2.0 array). The dataset from the GAIN cohort was obtained from the dbGaP website (www.ncbi.nlm.nih.gov/sites/entrez?db = gap). The CEL files are also available at the GEO website of NCBI (GEO dataset GSE13355). In the initial release, whole-skin expression profiles from paired lesional/non-lesional samples of 31 psoriasis patients were available which was used for the present analysis. The CEL files containing the dataset GSE14905 (n = 28 patients) were also downloaded from the GEO website. The data show the extend of reproducibility of gene dysregulation across patients and also indicate that -fold changes obtained with the GSE14905 dataset are consistently slightly higher than those observed in the GAIN data.
Found at: doi:10.1371/journal.pone.0009701.s016

Figure S7 Upregulation of psoriasis-associated genes in lesional skin of PPARβ/δ transgenic mice. The expression level for the representative genes shown, previously found to be upregulated in the skin of PPARβ/δ mice treated with GW501516 by microarray-based expression profiling (see main text), was quantified using TaqMan-based real-time PCR using Assays-on-Demand kits obtained from ABI according to the manufacturer's instruction (LCE3f: Mm02605425, Il1β: Mm01336189, Hb-EGF: Mm00439305, CRABPII: Mm00801693, ALOX12b: Mm00507782, ml: MM00436999, ATP12a: Mm00446786). The data shown represent mean ± s.d. of GAPDH-calibrated expression levels obtained from n = 3 mice for each group (GW-fed, red columns, vs. control, blue columns). For all genes, $p<0.001$ in a two-sided independent t-test.
Found at: doi:10.1371/journal.pone.0009701.s017

Figure S8 Expression of transgenically overexpressed PPARβ/δ in murine skin. Whole skin samples from C57Bl/6j wild type (WT) or PPARβ/δ transgenic mice fed control chow (Tg) or GW501516-containing chow (TG+GW) were taken, genomic DNA digested, and total RNA isolated, followed by cDNA synthesis. RT-PCR was performed for the indicated number of cycles using primers specific for the transgene. Two mice for each condition were used.
Found at: doi:10.1371/journal.pone.0009701.s018

Author Contributions

Conceived and designed the experiments: MR JF. Performed the experiments: MR LR JF. Analyzed the data: MR LR JF. Contributed reagents/materials/analysis tools: CNAP MCUG. Wrote the paper: JF.

References

1. Gelfand JM, Stern RS, Nijsten T, Feldman SR, Thomas J, et al. (2005) The prevalence of psoriasis in African Americans: results from a population-based study. J Am Acad Dermatol 52: 23–26.
2. Dubertret L, Mrowietz U, Ranki A, van de Kerkhof PC, Chimenti S, et al. (2006) European patient perspectives on the impact of psoriasis: the EUROPSO patient membership survey. Br J Dermatol 155: 729–736.
3. Wu Y, Mills D, Bala M (2008) Psoriasis: cardiovascular risk factors and other disease comorbidities. J Drugs Dermatol 7: 373–377.
4. Poikolainen K, Karvonen J, Pukkala E (1999) Excess mortality related to alcohol and smoking among hospital-treated patients with psoriasis. Arch Dermatol 135: 1490–1493.
5. Finlay AY, Coles EC (1995) The effect of severe psoriasis on the quality of life of 369 patients. Br J Dermatol 132: 236–244.
6. Schmitt JM, Ford DE (2006) Work limitations and productivity loss are associated with health-related quality of life but not with clinical severity in patients with psoriasis. Dermatology 213: 102–110.
7. Sommer DM, Jenisch S, Suchan M, Christophers E, Weichenthal M (2006) Increased prevalence of the metabolic syndrome in patients with moderate to severe psoriasis. Arch Dermatol Res 298: 321–328.
8. Naldi L, Chatenoud L, Linder D, Belloni Fortina A, Peserico A, et al. (2005) Cigarette smoking, body mass index, and stressful life events as risk factors for psoriasis: results from an Italian case-control study. J Invest Dermatol 125: 61–67.
9. Barish GD, Narkar VA, Evans RM (2006) PPAR delta: a dagger in the heart of the metabolic syndrome. J Clin Invest 116: 590–597.
10. Short B (2009) Time (and PPARbeta/delta) heals all wounds. J Cell Biol 184: 767.
11. Michalik L, Auwerx J, Berger JP, Chatterjee VK, Glass CK, et al. (2006) International Union of Pharmacology. LXI. Peroxisome proliferator-activated receptors. Pharmacol Rev 58: 726–741.
12. Romanowska M, al Yacoub N, Seidel H, Donandt S, Gerken H, et al. (2008) PPARdelta enhances keratinocyte proliferation in psoriasis and induces heparin binding EGF-like growth factor. J Invest Dermatol 128: 110–124.
13. Westergaard M, Henningsen J, Johansen C, Rasmussen S, Svendsen ML, et al. (2003) Expression and localization of peroxisome proliferator-activated receptors and nuclear factor kappaB in normal and lesional psoriatic skin. J Invest Dermatol 121: 1104–1117.
14. Tan NS, Michalik L, Noy N, Yasmin R, Pacot C, et al. (2001) Critical roles of PPAR beta/delta in keratinocyte response to inflammation. Genes Dev 15: 3263–3277.
15. Di-Poi N, Michalik L, Tan NS, Desvergne B, Wahli W (2003) The anti-apoptotic role of PPARbeta contributes to efficient skin wound healing. J Steroid Biochem Mol Biol 85: 257–265.
16. Icre G, Wahli W, Michalik L (2006) Functions of the Peroxisome Proliferator-Activated Receptor (PPAR) alpha and beta in Skin Homeostasis, Epithelial Repair, and Morphogenesis. J Invest Dermatol 126 Suppl: 30–35.
17. Piqueras L, Reynolds AR, Hodivala-Dilke KM, Alfranca A, Redondo JM, et al. (2006) Activation of PPAR{beta}/{delta} Induces Endothelial Cell Proliferation and Angiogenesis. Arterioscler Thromb Vasc Biol.
18. van der Vleuten CJ, de Jong EM, van de Kerkhof PC (1996) Epidermal differentiation characteristics of the psoriatic plaque during treatment with calcipotriol. Arch Dermatol Res 288: 366–372.
19. Lowes MA, Chamian F, Abello MV, Fuentes-Duculan J, Lin SL, et al. (2005) Increase in TNF-alpha and inducible nitric oxide synthase-expressing dendritic cells in psoriasis and reduction with efalizumab (anti-CD11a). Proc Natl Acad Sci U S A 102: 19057–19062.
20. Di Cesare A, Di Meglio P, Nestle FO (2009) The IL-23/Th17 axis in the immunopathogenesis of psoriasis. J Invest Dermatol 129: 1339–1350.
21. Sabat R, Philipp S, Hoflich C, Kreutzer S, Wallace E, et al. (2007) Immunopathogenesis of psoriasis. Exp Dermatol 16: 779–798.
22. Nair RP, Duffin KC, Helms C, Ding J, Stuart PE, et al. (2009) Genome-wide scan reveals association of psoriasis with IL-23 and NF-kappaB pathways. Nat Genet 41: 199–204.
23. Di-Poi N, Ng CY, Tan NS, Yang Z, Hemmings BA, et al. (2005) Epithelium-mesenchyme interactions control the activity of peroxisome proliferator-activated receptor beta/delta during hair follicle development. Mol Cell Biol 25: 1696–1712.
24. Campbell SJ, Carlotti F, Hall PA, Clark AJ, Wolf CR (1996) Regulation of the CYP1A1 promoter in transgenic mice: an exquisitely sensitive on-off system for cell specific gene regulation. J Cell Sci 109 (Pt 11): 2619–2625.
25. Robertson RW, Zhang L, Pasco DS, Fagan JB (1994) Aryl hydrocarbon-induced interactions at multiple DNA elements of diverse sequence–a multicomponent mechanism for activation of cytochrome P4501A1 (CYP1A1) gene transcription. Nucleic Acids Res 22: 1741–1749.
26. Rowe JM, Welsh C, Pena RN, Wolf CR, Brown K, et al. (2008) Illuminating role of CYP1A1 in skin function. J Invest Dermatol 128: 1866–1868.
27. Kaufman CK, Sinha S, Bolotin D, Fan J, Fuchs E (2002) Dissection of a complex enhancer element: maintenance of keratinocyte specificity but loss of differentiation specificity. Mol Cell Biol 22: 4293–4308.
28. Michalik L, Wahli W (2007) Peroxisome proliferator-activated receptors (PPARs) in skin health, repair and disease. Biochim Biophys Acta 1771: 991–998.
29. Rosenfield RL, Kentsis A, Deplewski D, Ciletti N (1999) Rat preputial sebocyte differentiation involves peroxisome proliferator-activated receptors. J Invest Dermatol 112: 226–232.
30. Trivedi NR, Cong Z, Nelson AM, Albert AJ, Rosamilia LL, et al. (2006) Peroxisome proliferator-activated receptors increase human sebum production. J Invest Dermatol 126: 2002–2009.
31. Machado FS, Johndrow JE, Esper L, Dias A, Bafica A, et al. (2006) Anti-inflammatory actions of lipoxin A4 and aspirin-triggered lipoxin are SOCS-2 dependent. Nat Med 12: 330–334.
32. Chiaro CR, Morales JL, Prabhu KS, Perdew GH (2008) Leukotriene A4 metabolites are endogenous ligands for the Ah receptor. Biochemistry 47: 8445–8455.
33. Schmuth M, Jiang YJ, Dubrac S, Elias PM, Feingold KR (2008) Thematic review series: skin lipids. Peroxisome proliferator-activated receptors and liver X receptors in epidermal biology. J Lipid Res 49: 499–509.
34. Sano S, Chan KS, Carbajal S, Clifford J, Peavey M, et al. (2005) Stat3 links activated keratinocytes and immunocytes required for development of psoriasis in a novel transgenic mouse model. Nat Med 11: 43–49.
35. Koegel H, von Tobel L, Schafer M, Alberti S, Kremmer E, et al. (2009) Loss of serum response factor in keratinocytes results in hyperproliferative skin disease in mice. J Clin Invest 119: 899–910.
36. Murray PJ (2006) STAT3-mediated anti-inflammatory signalling. Biochem Soc Trans 34: 1028–1031.
37. Azfar RS, Gelfand JM (2008) Psoriasis and metabolic disease: epidemiology and pathophysiology. Curr Opin Rheumatol 20: 416–422.
38. Sun L, Ke Y, Zhu CY, Tang N, Tian DK, et al. (2008) Inflammatory reaction versus endogenous peroxisome proliferator-activated receptors expression, re-exploring secondary organ complications of spontaneously hypertensive rats. Chin Med J (Engl) 121: 2305–2311.
39. Masternak MM, Al-Regaiey KA, Del Rosario Lim MM, Bonkowski MS, Panici JA, et al. (2005) Caloric restriction results in decreased expression of peroxisome proliferator-activated receptor superfamily in muscle of normal and long-lived growth hormone receptor/binding protein knockout mice. J Gerontol A Biol Sci Med Sci 60: 1238–1245.
40. Sutherland JP, McKinley B, Eckel RH (2004) The metabolic syndrome and inflammation. Metab Syndr Relat Disord 2: 82–104.
41. Gisondi P, Del Giglio M, Di Francesco V, Zamboni M, Girolomoni G (2008) Weight loss improves the response of obese patients with moderate-to-severe chronic plaque psoriasis to low-dose cyclosporine therapy: a randomized, controlled, investigator-blinded clinical trial. Am J Clin Nutr 88: 1242–1247.
42. Barish GD, Atkins AR, Downes M, Olson P, Chong LW, et al. (2008) PPARdelta regulates multiple proinflammatory pathways to suppress atherosclerosis. Proc Natl Acad Sci U S A 105: 4271–4276.
43. Hall JM, McDonnell DP (2007) The molecular mechanisms underlying the proinflammatory actions of thiazolidinediones in human macrophages. Mol Endocrinol 21: 1756–1768.
44. Kryczek I, Wei S, Vatan L, Escara-Wilke J, Szeliga W, et al. (2007) Cutting edge: opposite effects of IL-1 and IL-2 on the regulation of IL-17+ T cell pool IL-1 subverts IL-2-mediated suppression. J Immunol 179: 1423–1426.
45. Magne D, Palmer G, Barton JL, Mezin F, Talabot-Ayer D, et al. (2006) The new IL-1 family member IL-1F8 stimulates production of inflammatory mediators by synovial fibroblasts and articular chondrocytes. Arthritis Res Ther 8: R80.
46. Blumberg H, Dinh H, Trueblood ES, Pretorius J, Kugler D, et al. (2007) Opposing activities of two novel members of the IL-1 ligand family regulate skin inflammation. J Exp Med 204: 2603–2614.
47. Chong HC, Tan MJ, Philippe V, Tan SH, Tan CK, et al. (2009) Regulation of epithelial-mesenchymal IL-1 signaling by PPARbeta/delta is essential for skin homeostasis and wound healing. J Cell Biol 184: 817–831.
48. Debets R, Hegmans JP, Croughs P, Troost RJ, Prins JB, et al. (1997) The IL-1 system in psoriatic skin: IL-1 antagonist sphere of influence in lesional psoriatic epidermis. J Immunol 158: 2955–2963.
49. Kang K, Hatano B, Lee CH (2007) PPAR delta agonists and metabolic diseases. Curr Atheroscler Rep 9: 72–77.
50. Liu L, Gao Y, Qiu H, Miller WT, Poli V, et al. (2006) Identification of STAT3 as a specific substrate of breast tumor kinase. Oncogene 25: 4904–4912.
51. El Kasmi KC, Holst J, Coffre M, Mielke L, de Pauw A, et al. (2006) General nature of the STAT3-activated anti-inflammatory response. J Immunol 177: 7880–7888.
52. Schmuth M, Haqq CM, Cairns WJ, Holder JC, Dorsam S, et al. (2004) Peroxisome proliferator-activated receptor (PPAR)-beta/delta stimulates differentiation and lipid accumulation in keratinocytes. J Invest Dermatol 122: 971–983.
53. Michalik L, Desvergne B, Tan NS, Basu-Modak S, Escher P, et al. (2001) Impaired skin wound healing in peroxisome proliferator-activated receptor (PPAR)alpha and PPARbeta mutant mice. J Cell Biol 154: 799–814.
54. de Cid R, Riveira-Munoz E, Zeeuwen PL, Robarge J, Liao W, et al. (2009) Deletion of the late cornified envelope LCE3B and LCE3C genes as a susceptibility factor for psoriasis. Nat Genet 41: 211–215.

14

The Flavonoid Luteolin Inhibits Fcγ-Dependent Respiratory Burst in Granulocytes, but Not Skin Blistering in a New Model of Pemphigoid in Adult Mice

Eva Oswald[1,2,4], Alina Sesarman[2], Claus-Werner Franzke[2], Ute Wölfle[3], Leena Bruckner-Tuderman[2,5,6], Thilo Jakob[1], Stefan F. Martin[1], Cassian Sitaru[2,5]*

1 Allergy Research Group, Department of Dermatology, University Freiburg Medical Center, Freiburg, Germany, **2** Molecular Dermatology, Department of Dermatology, University Freiburg Medical Center, Freiburg, Germany, **3** Competence Centre Skintegral, Department of Dermatology, University Freiburg Medical Center, Freiburg, Germany, **4** Faculty of Biology, University of Freiburg, Freiburg, Germany, **5** BIOSS Centre for Biological Signalling Studies, Freiburg, Germany, **6** Freiburg Institute for Advanced Studies, Freiburg, Germany

Abstract

Bullous pemphigoid is an autoimmune blistering skin disease associated with autoantibodies against the dermal-epidermal junction. Passive transfer of antibodies against BP180/collagen (C) XVII, a major hemidesmosomal pemphigoid antigen, into neonatal mice results in dermal-epidermal separation upon applying gentle pressure to their skin, but not in spontaneous skin blistering. In addition, this neonatal mouse model precludes treatment and observation of diseased animals beyond 2–3 days. Therefore, in the present study we have developed a new disease model in mice reproducing the spontaneous blistering and the chronic course characteristic of the human condition. Adult mice were pre-immunized with rabbit IgG followed by injection of BP180/CXVII rabbit IgG. Mice pre-immunized against rabbit IgG and injected 6 times every second day with the BP180/CXVII-specific antibodies (n = 35) developed spontaneous sustained blistering of the skin, while mice pre-immunized and then treated with normal rabbit IgG (n = 5) did not. Blistering was associated with IgG and complement C3 deposits at the epidermal basement membrane and recruitment of inflammatory cells, and was partly dependent on Ly-6G-positive cells. We further used this new experimental model to investigate the therapeutic potential of luteolin, a plant flavonoid with potent anti-inflammatory and anti-oxidative properties and good safety profile, in experimental BP. Luteolin inhibited the Fcγ-dependent respiratory burst in immune complex-stimulated granulocytes and the autoantibody-induced dermal-epidermal separation in skin cryosections, but was not effective in suppressing the skin blistering *in vivo*. These studies establish a robust animal model that will be a useful tool for dissecting the mechanisms of blister formation and will facilitate the development of more effective therapeutic strategies for managing pemphigoid diseases.

Editor: Dominik Hartl, University of Tübingen, Germany

Funding: The authors acknowledge support by grants from the Deutsche Forschungsgemeinschaft SI-1281/4-1 (CS), MA-1567/9-1 (SM), SFB850-B6 (LB-T, C-WF), and BIOSS (LB-T,CS), from the Medical Faculty of the Freiburg University (CS) and by the Freiburg Institute for Advanced Studies (LB-T). The funders had no role in study design, data collection and analysis, decision to publish, or preparation of the manuscript.

Competing Interests: The authors have declared that no competing interests exist.

* E-mail: cassian.sitaru@uniklinik-freiburg.de

Introduction

Pemphigoids are autoimmune blistering disorders associated with autoimmunity against hemidesmosomal proteins [1]. Collagen XVII (CXVII) is a major autoantigen in different pemphigoid diseases, including bullous pemphigoid (BP), pemphigoid gestationis, linear IgA disease, mucous membrane pemphigoid and lichen planus pemphigoides [1]. BP is a prototypical organ-specific autoimmune diseases of the skin associated with subepidermal blisters and autoimmunity against the hemidesmosomal proteins CXVII and BP230 at the dermal-epidermal junction (DEJ) [1,2]. While the plakin protein BP230 is an intracellular hemidesmosomal component [3,4], CXVII also known as the bullous pemphigoid antigen of 180 kDa (BP180) is a transmembrane collagen with its N-terminus intracellularly located, its ectodomain spanning the lamina lucida, and its C-terminus reaching the lamina densa of the basement membrane [5,6]. The ectodomain of BP180/CXVII consists of 15 interrupted collagenous regions and contains major epitopes of pemphigoid autoantibodies and autoreactive T cells within its 16th non-collagenous (NC16A) region [7–9]. Further antigenic determinants in pemphigoid diseases were shown on both intra- and extracellular domains of BP180/CXVII [10,11].

The pathogenic significance of autoantibodies against BP180/CXVII is supported by several lines of evidence: (1) serum levels of circulating autoantibodies against BP180/CXVII correlate with disease activity in patients with BP [12–15]; (2) pemphigoid autoantibodies and rabbit antibodies generated against BP180/CXVII recruit leukocytes to the DEJ and induce dermal-epidermal separation of human skin [16,17]; (3) rabbit antibodies generated against BP180/CXVII induce subepidermal blistering when injected into mice and hamsters [18,19]; (4) the passive transfer of autoantibodies from BP patients into CXVII-humanized mice induces dermal-epidermal separation [20,21]; (5) the transfer of maternal antibodies against human BP180/CXVII induces spontaneous skin blistering in pups humanized for the autoantigen [22]; (6) the transfer of splenocytes from mice immunized against human BP180/CXVII into Rag2$^{-/-}$/CXVII-humanized mice results in a sustained production of blister-inducing autoantibodies, partially mimicking the features of the disease in humans [23]. While the pathogenic role of autoantibodies to BP230 was suggested by several observations in patients and experimental animals, the contribution of anti-BP230 reactivity to disease pathogenesis still needs further investigation [15,24–26].

Previous attempts to induce blistering by injecting BP patient IgG into wildtype mice have failed [27,28]. To circumvent this problem, elegant alternative models have been developed using the passive transfer of antibodies generated against the murine autoantigens or, more recently, by the use of patients' autoantibodies in transgenic mice expressing human BP180/CXVII [18–21]. These ingenious models reproduce most of the major disease features and offer unique opportunities to elucidate the pathomechanisms underlying autoantibody-induced tissue damage in pemphigoid diseases. However, major shortcomings of these models are: 1) the fact that neonatal mice injected with BP180/CXVII-specific antibodies do not develop spontaneous skin blistering and 2) by their experimental design, the models in neonatal mice have a short observation period and do not allow for adequately reproducing the course of the chronic pemphigoid disease for pathogenic and therapeutic studies.

Therefore, in the present study we set out to develop a pemphigoid disease model in adult mice reproducing the spontaneous blistering and the chronic course characteristic of human condition. In a model of progressive antibody-induced glomerulonephritis it has been shown that pre-immunization with rabbit IgG in complete Freund's adjuvant several days prior to injection of rabbit anti-mouse glomerular basement membrane (GBM) antiserum results in strong inflammation with deposition of IgG and complement C3 and glomerular lesions [29]. Using this information, we pre-immunized mice with rabbit IgG before passively transferring rabbit IgG generated against BP180/CXVII. Mice pre-immunized against rabbit IgG and repeatedly injected with the BP180/CXVII-specific IgG developed spontaneous sustained blistering of the skin. In addition, blistering was associated with complement activation and recruitment of inflammatory cells and partly dependent on Ly-6G-positive cells. In further *ex vivo* and animal experiments, we investigated the therapeutic potential of luteolin, a plant flavonoid with potent anti-inflammatory and anti-oxidative properties [30]. Luteolin inhibited the Fcγ-dependent respiratory burst in immune complex (IC)-stimulated granulocytes and the autoantibody-induced dermal-epidermal separation in skin cryosections, but was not effective in suppressing the skin blistering in the new animal model of BP.

Results

Generation and characterization of rabbit antibodies against murine BP180/CXVII

Rabbit antibodies were generated against different fragments of murine BP180/CXVII by immunizing the animals with a mixture of the respective recombinant proteins. These antibodies were shown to bind to the basement membrane zone of murine skin by indirect immunofluorescence (IF) microscopy (**Figure S1A and B**). By immunoblotting, we showed that the generated antibodies recognized a 180 kDa protein band in extracts of BP180/CXVII-expressing COS-7 cells (**Figure S1C**).

Complement-activating capacity of rabbit IgG specific for murine BP180/CXVII

The complement-activating capacity of BP180/CXVII-specific IgG was evaluated by an *in vitro* complement-binding test (**Figure 1**). BP180/CXVII-specific IgG (**Figure 1A**), in contrast to normal rabbit IgG (**Figure 1B**), fixed complement at the epidermal basement membrane.

Granulocyte-activating capacity of rabbit IgG specific for murine BP180/CXVII

To analyze the ability of ICs composed of rabbit IgG and murine BP180/CXVII to activate granulocytes, we performed luminol chemiluminescence assays with granulocytes from healthy donors (**Figure 2A**). Incubation of granulocytes with BP180/CXVII-specific IgG complexed with the antigen, but not with the antigen alone, resulted in the production of reactive oxygen species (ROS) (**Figure 2A**). To assess the capacity of BP180/CXVII-specific rabbit antibodies to induce granulocyte-dependent dermal-epidermal separation in human skin, IgG from pre-immune rabbits and animals immunized with murine BP180/CXVII was incubated with skin cryosections, and subsequently with leukocytes. After the addition of leukocytes, BP180/CXVII-specific IgG induced subepidermal splits in skin cryosections (**Figure 2B**), in contrast normal rabbit IgG failed to induce dermal-epidermal separation in cryosections (**Figure 2C**).

Pre-immunization of mice against rabbit IgG

To accelerate and increase the inflammatory reaction triggered by binding of IgG autoantibodies at the DEJ of murine skin, we pre-immunized mice with purified rabbit IgG mixed with complete Freund's adjuvant. Subsequently, mice were injected with BP180/CXVII-specific or control rabbit IgG. The immunization induced the production of high levels of mouse IgG against rabbit IgG as shown by ELISA (**Figure S2A**). None of the mice pre-immunized with rabbit IgG showed skin disease clinically and histologically nor deposition of mouse IgG or complement C3 at the DEJ. However, injection of mice with BP180/CXVII-specific IgG, but not with normal rabbit IgG, resulted in deposition of mouse IgG at the murine epidermal basement membrane as detailed below.

Adult mice injected with BP180/CXVII-specific IgG develop spontaneous skin blistering

Adult SJL (n = 2), BALB/c (n = 31), C57BL/6 (n = 3) and C57BL/10 (n = 2) mice pre-immunized with rabbit IgG were

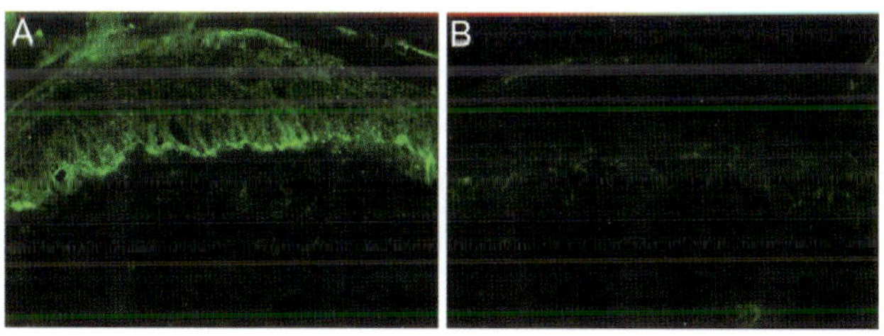

Figure 1. Complement-binding capacity of BP180/CXVII-specific rabbit antibodies. Frozen murine skin sections were incubated with rabbit antibodies and subsequently with fresh human serum as a source of complement. Bound C3 was visualized at the dermal-epidermal junction by fluorochrome-labeled antibody. (**A**) Deposits of C3 in sections incubated with BP180/CXVII-specific rabbit antibody. (**B**) No C3 deposition in sections incubated with normal rabbit IgG (magnification, ×400).

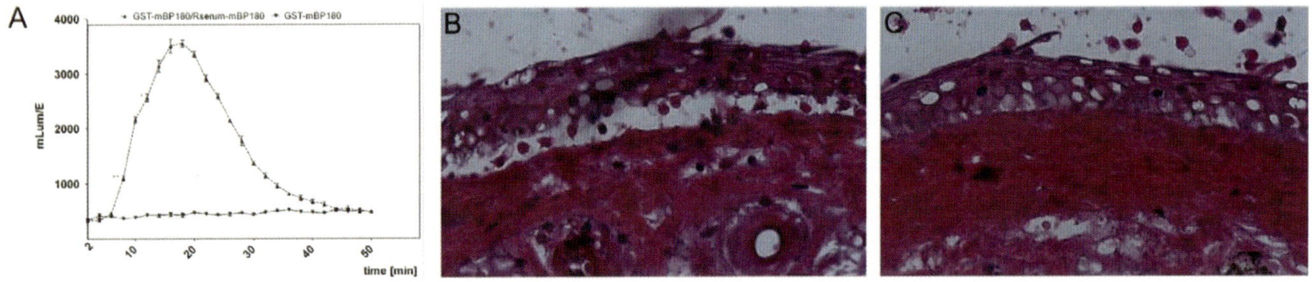

Figure 2. *Ex vivo* granulocyte-activation capacity of BP180/CXVII-specific rabbit IgG antibodies. (**A**) Leukocytes (3×10^7/ml) were stimulated with rabbit ICs consisting of 5 µg recombinant BP180/CXVII/well and 100 µl of 50-fold diluted BP180/CXVII-specific rabbit serum. ROS production was measured over a period of 60 min. Data are represented as mean ± SD; $p<0.001$. (**B, C**) Frozen skin sections were incubated with IgG and with 3×10^7 leukocytes/ml. Dermal-epidermal separation was observed in sections treated with (**B**) BP180/CXVII-specific IgG, but not with (**C**) normal rabbit IgG (magnification, ×400).

injected intraperitoneally (i.p.) or subcutaneously (s.c.) every second day with 15 mg of IgG purified from rabbit serum for 12 days. Mice (n = 35) injected i.p. (**Figure 3**) or s.c. (**Figure 4**) with IgG from rabbits immunized against murine BP180/CXVII developed skin lesions, including erythema, blisters and erosions. In contrast, mice injected with normal rabbit IgG (n = 5) did not show signs of skin disease (**Figure 3D–F and 4D**). Interestingly, the blistering phenotype induced by the i.p. injection was different when compared with the one triggered by the s.c. injection. While administration of BP180/CXVII-specific IgG by the i.p. route induced blisters at distant sites, including the ears, paws, eyes and snouts (**Figure 3A–C**), the s.c. injections of the BP180/CXVII-specific IgG resulted in lesions mainly restricted to skin areas in the proximity of the injection site (**Figure 4A–C**). Histologically dermal-epidermal separation of the skin with infiltration of inflammatory cells is found (**Figure 5A–C**). Infiltrates were dominated by neutrophils, with few eosinophils (**Figure 5A–B**).

The blistering phenotype in mice is associated with tissue-bound immunoreactants

Direct IF microscopy of perilesional skin revealed linear deposits of rabbit IgG (**Figure 6A**) and murine complement C3 (**Figure 6B**) at the epidermal basement membrane in adult mice that received IgG specific for BP180/CXVII. In addition, deposition of murine IgG was found at the basement membrane in mice injected with BP180/CXVII-specific IgG (**Figure 6C**), but not in animals treated with normal rabbit IgG (**Figure 6F**). In mice injected with normal rabbit IgG no deposition of IgG (**Figure 6D**) and complement C3 (**Figure 6E**) was detected by IF microscopy.

Repeated injection of antibodies induces stable extensive blistering skin disease in mice

In mice injected with rabbit IgG against murine BP180/CXVII, blistering of the skin started at 3–5 days after the first injection and developed during the observation period of 19 days to a full-blown skin blistering disease (**Figure 7**). The extent of the skin disease was scored and serum samples were obtained before the first injection of rabbit IgG (day 0) at day 3 as well as every second day thereafter. Circulating BP180/CXVII-specific rabbit IgG was detected in serum samples by ELISA (**Figure S2B**). During the observation time, disease activity was increasing until it reached a plateau around day 10. Subsequently, while new lesions continued to appear, some areas re-epithelized showing alopecia without scarring.

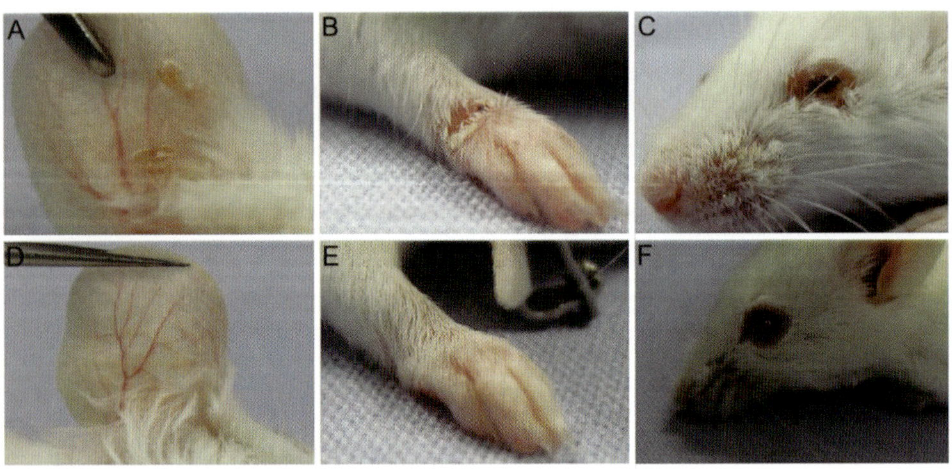

Figure 3. Intraperitoneal injection of BP180/CXVII-specific IgG induces blister formation in adult mice. Skin lesions, including blisters, erosions, and crusts developed on the (**A**) ear, (**B**) front leg and (**C**) periocular area in a BALB/c mouse pre-sensitized with rabbit IgG and subsequently receiving, over a period of 10 days, 6 i.p. injections of IgG, each containing 15 mg of IgG, from a rabbit immunized against murine BP180/CXVII. (**D, E, F**) A control mouse pre-sensitized with rabbit IgG and challenged with the same dose of normal rabbit IgG showed no skin alterations.

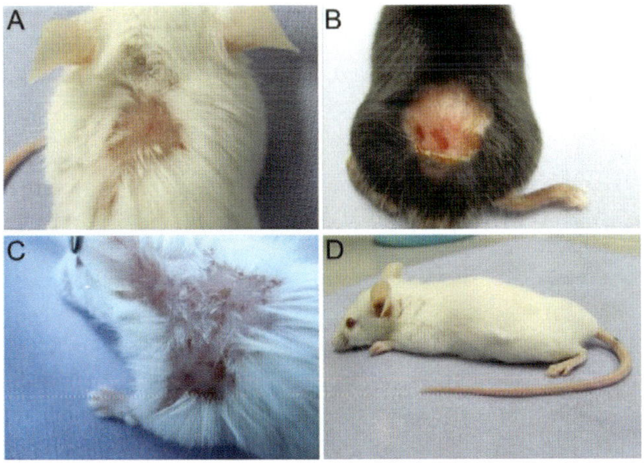

Figure 4. Subcutaneous injection of BP180/CXVII-specific IgG induces blister formation in adult mice. Skin lesions, including blisters, erosions crusts, and alopecia developed in (**A**) BALB/c, (**B**) C57BL6, and (**C**) SJL-1 mice pre-sensitized with rabbit IgG and subsequently receiving, over a period of 10 days, 6 s.c. injections of IgG, each containing 15 mg of IgG, from a rabbit immunized against murine BP180/CXVII. (**D**) A control mouse pre-sensitized with rabbit IgG and challenged with the same dose of normal rabbit IgG showed no skin alterations.

Neutrophil depletion partly inhibits blister formation *in vivo*

Since inflammatory infiltrates in our model were mostly composed of neutrophils, we supposed that these cells mediate tissue damage. Therefore, to deplete neutrophils we have used a Ly-6G-specific monoclonal antibody, which induced a severe reduction of neutrophils from around 30% prior to depletion to less than 6% of leukocytes in the peripheral blood. The depletion was maintained for 4 days with a subsequent increase of

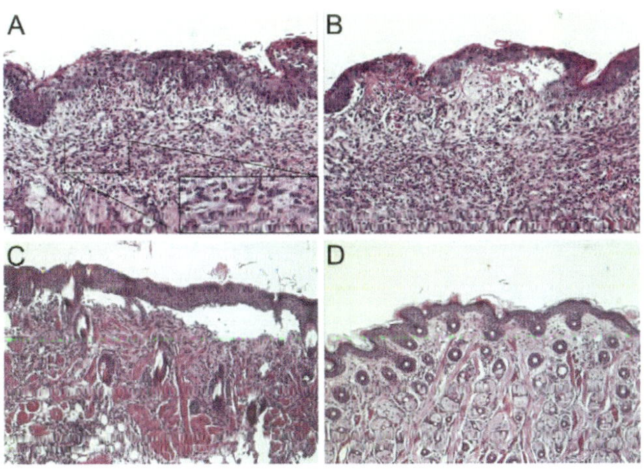

Figure 5. Dermal-epidermal separation in mice injected with BP180/CXVII-specific antibodies. Skin biopsies from mice pre-sensitized with rabbit IgG and subsequently injected with rabbit IgG were stained with hematoxylin and eosin. (**A**) Dense inflammatory infiltrates dominated by granulocytes in a BALB/c mouse receiving BP180/CXVII-specific IgG; (**B**) Subepidermal split and dense inflammatory infiltrates dominated by granulocytes; (**C**) Extensive dermal-epidermal separation; (**D**) Normal histological appearance in a control mouse receiving normal rabbit IgG (magnification, ×400).

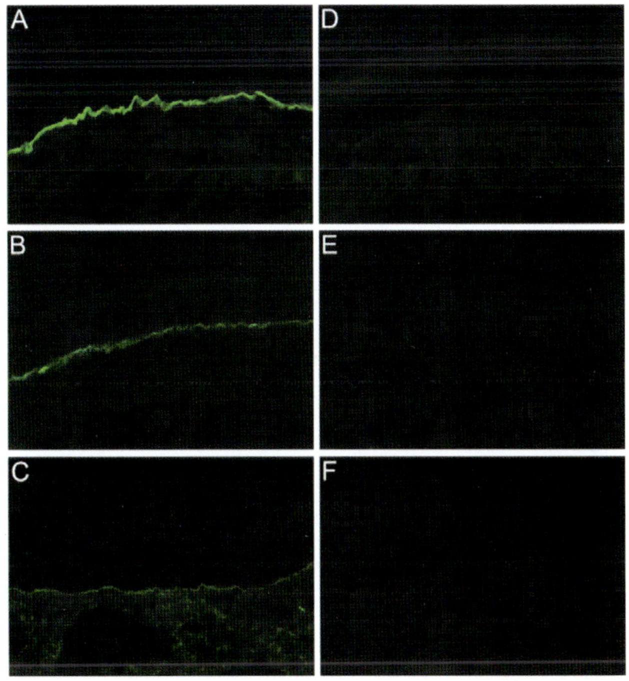

Figure 6. IgG and complement C3 deposition at the basement membrane in experimental bullous pemphigoid. IF microscopy, performed on frozen sections of a perilesional mouse skin biopsy reveals linear deposition of (**A**) rabbit IgG, (**B**) murine C3, and (**C**) murine IgG at the epidermal basement membrane in a diseased mouse. No deposits of (**D**) rabbit IgG, (**E**) murine C3, and (**F**) murine IgG of a control mouse showing no skin lesions (magnification, ×400).

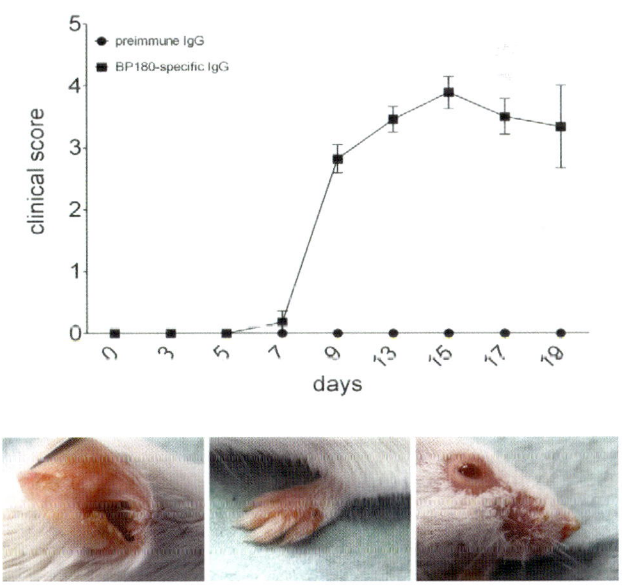

Figure 7. Repeated injections of antibodies against murine BP180/CXVII induce extensive skin blistering. The extent of disease was scored as described in Methods. Means of individual clinical scores of mice injected with BP180/CXVII-specific antibodies (n = 9) and mice injected with normal rabbit IgG (n = 5) are shown before the first injection as well as every subsequent second day for 19 days. The lower panel shows BALB/c mice at day 12 after the first i.p. injection.

neutrophils to normal frequency in the peripheral blood within 1 day. Mice pre-immunized with rabbit IgG and injected with rabbit IgG specific for BP180/CXVII developed skin blisters (**Figure 8A and B**). The transient depletion of neutrophils significantly reduced the skin blistering disease in the group of mice treated with the LyG6-specific compared with group treated with the mock antibody (n = 5/group; **Figure 8C**).

Luteolin inhibits IC-induced ROS production by leukocytes

Luteolin, a plant-derived flavonoid with potent anti-oxidative and anti-inflammatory properties, is a promising, small molecule for the treatment in several inflammatory diseases both by systemic and local application [30]. Therefore, we have addressed the effects of luteolin on the autoantibody-induced granulocyte activation and tissue damage in our model. Human leukocytes were stimulated with ICs consisting of BP180/CXVII-specific antibodies and antigen and treated with different concentrations of luteolin (50–200 µg/ml). Under these conditions, we have observed an inhibition of ROS production in a dose-dependent manner (**Figure 9A**). ROS production may play an important role in the secretion of gelatinase B (MMP-9) from activated neutrophils and is believed to be involved in tissue damage in BP. Therefore, we have asked whether luteolin also inhibits the release of MMP-9 from leukocytes stimulated with ICs. We show that the *in vitro* stimulation of human leukocytes for 3 h with ICs and different concentrations of luteolin does not inhibit the production and activation of MMP-9 in the supernatant of these cultures as detected and quantified by gelatine zymography (**Figure 9B**).

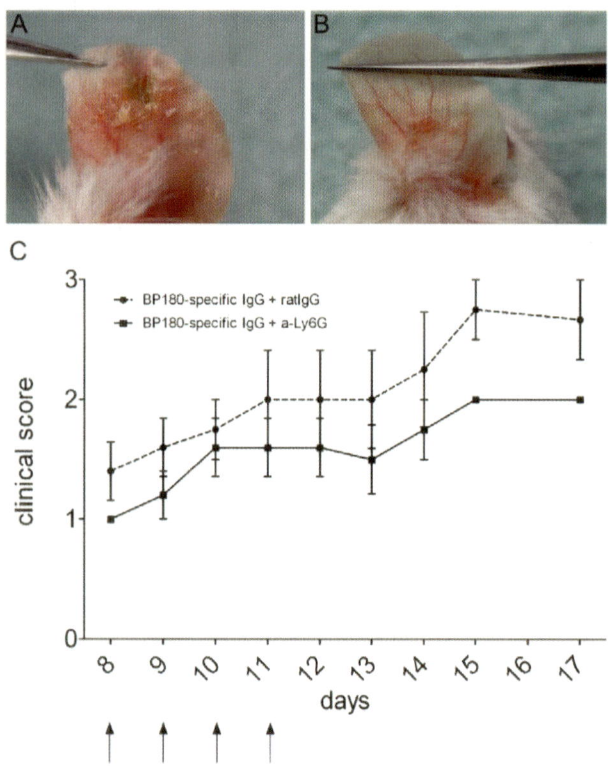

Figure 8. Neutrophil depletion partly inhibits skin blistering induced by BP180/CXVII-specific IgG in mice. Mice pre-immunized with rabbit IgG and injected i.p. with BP180/CXVII-specific rabbit IgG were treated with (**A**) a Ly-6G-specific monoclonal or (**B**) a mock antibody as described in Materials and Methods (arrows). (**C**) Disease activity during the depletion of Ly-6G-positive cells is significantly reduced in the group of mice treated with Ly-6G-specific antibody (n = 5) compared with the group treated with mock antibody (n = 5; $p<0.05$). Data are shown as mean ± SD.

Luteolin inhibits partly autoantibody-induced granulocyte-dependent dermal-epidermal separation *ex vivo*

We have investigated the effects of luteolin on tissue damage using an *ex vivo* cryosection model of autoantibody-induced granulocyte-dependent dermal-epidermal separation. Cryosections were treated either with sera from BP patients and BP180/CXVII-specific rabbit serum or with control sera from healthy donors and pre-immune rabbits followed by incubation with granulocytes from healthy donors. Addition of luteolin, but not vehicle alone, resulted in a significant reduction of the autoantibody-induced dermal-epidermal separation (**Figure 9C**).

Systemic and local application of luteolin does not significantly impact antibody-induced blistering *in vivo*

Based on the promising *ex vivo* results, we have extended the investigation of the luteolin effects on the autoimmune injury in our mouse model of BP. We pre-sensitized BALB/c mice with rabbit IgG and injected them every second day s.c. with BP180/CXVII-specific IgG or with pre-immune IgG. These mice were treated every day i.p. either with vehicle alone (n = 8) or with 1 mg of luteolin (n = 8). Luteolin administration did not significantly influence the antibody-induced skin blistering. Mice in both groups showed similar disease scores and antibodies to rabbit IgG throughout the experiment (**Figure 10C and Figure S3**). In a subsequent experiment, we have also evaluated the effects of a luteolin-rich topical preparation on the blistering induced in the ears of mice. For this purpose, we have injected s.c. 1.5 mg BP180/CXVII-specific (n = 14) or control IgG (n = 3) into the mouse ears and applied the luteolin-containing RF-40 (n = 10) preparation or vehicle alone (n = 7) every day for 4 days (**Figure 10A and B**). No significant changes were observed in mice topically treated with luteolin compared to those receiving vehicle alone.

Discussion

Pemphigoid diseases are associated with autoantibodies against BP180/CXVII and BP230. Data from experimental pemphigoid models suggest that BP180/CXVII-specific autoantibodies induce subepidermal skin blistering. Current pemphigoid disease models use neonatal mice injected with antibodies to BP180/CXVII. However, in these models, skin blistering does not occur spontaneously and is only induced when mechanical stress is applied to the skin. In addition, the experimental design using the neonatal mouse model of BP allows for observation periods of only up to 3 days. To address these shortcomings, in the present study we generated a pemphigoid disease model in adult mice pre-immunized against rabbit IgG, which developed a spontaneous extensive blistering skin disease upon injection of murine BP180/CXVII-specific rabbit antibodies and allowed for longer observation times.

The passive transfer of pemphigoid patients' autoantibodies into mice does not result in skin blistering. This is likely due to both a limited cross-reactivity of human autoantibodies with the murine autoantigens and to their lower capacity to activate mouse complement and leukocytes [28,31]. Therefore, alternative models using the passive transfer of murine BP180/CXVII-specific antibodies generated in rabbits into neonatal mice or neonatal

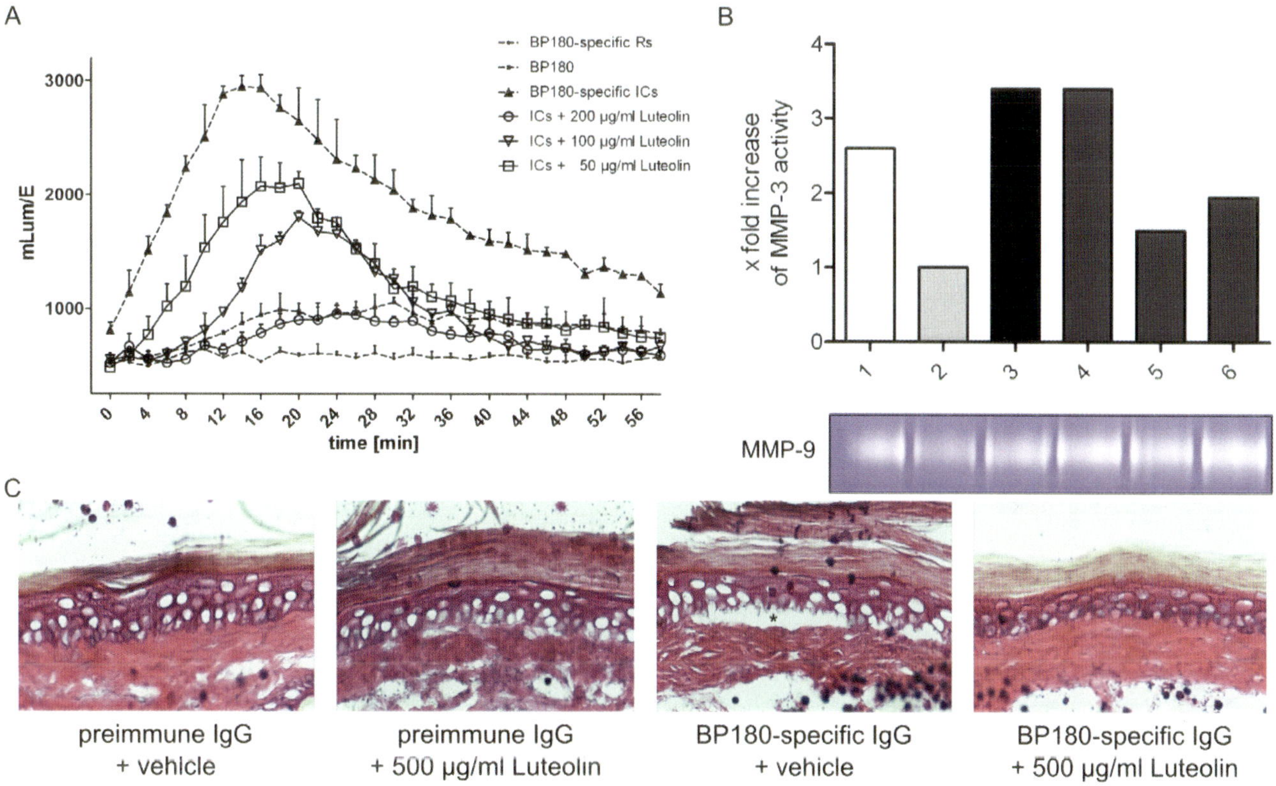

Figure 9. Luteolin inhibits ROS production, but not the release of MMP-9 from IC-stimulated leukocytes. (**A**) Leukocytes (3×10^7/ml) were pre-incubated with luteolin in different concentrations or vehicle alone and stimulated with rabbit ICs consisting of 5 µg recombinant BP180/CXVII/well and 100 µl of 50-fold diluted rabbit serum. ROS production was measured over a period of 60 min. Data are represented as mean ± SD; $p<0.05$. (**B**) 3×10^7/ml leukocytes were stimulated with rabbit ICs consisting of 5 µg recombinant BP180/CXVII/well and 100 µl of 50-fold diluted rabbit serum for 3 h at 37°C. MMP-9 activation was evaluated by zymography in 50-fold diluted supernatants of these cultures of cells stimulated with BP180/CXVII (lane 1), BP180/CXVII-specific rabbit IgG (lane 2), ICs (lane 3), ICs with 1000, 500 and 200 µg/ml Luteolin (lanes 4, 5, and 6 respectively). (**C**) Luteolin inhibits dermal-epidermal separation in cryosection assays *ex vivo*. Frozen murine skin sections were incubated with pre-immune rabbit serum or BP180/CXVII-specific rabbit serum. Significantly less dermal-epidermal separation was observed in sections treated with 500 µg/ml luteolin compared with those treated with vehicle alone (magnification, ×400).

human CXVII-transgenic mice injected with patient IgG have been devised [18,20,21]. In a separate study, we could show that purified rabbit IgG antibodies generated against murine BP180/CXVII transferred into adult mice results indeed in spontaneous blistering [32]. However, the disease onset was slower and the overall disease activity lower compared with other models for autoimmune subepidermal blistering disease [33] and typical patients with full-blown disease. To further improve the model, in the present study, we have applied an approach initially devised for the autoantibody-induced glomerulonephritis [29,34]. This progressive nephrotoxic serum nephritis in mice is a prototypic type II hypersensitivity response in the kidney induced by antibodies directed against the GBM. Pre-sensitization of mice with rabbit IgG prior to challenge with rabbit nephrotoxic serum results in IC formation leading to accelerated glomerular injury and renal dysfunction that resembles aspects of Goodpasture syndrome in humans [29]. In our pemphigoid model in adult mice, pre-sensitization with rabbit IgG resulted in accelerated onset and enhanced activity of the induced pemphigoid disease most likely due to IC formation of mouse anti-rabbit IgG and the tissue-bound rabbit anti-BP180/CXVII.

Our results show the induction of spontaneous skin blisters by the passive transfer of BP180/CXVII-specific IgG. For the induction of subepidermal skin blistering, we used purified rabbit IgG antibodies with high reactivity against the epidermal basement membrane. Similar to autoantibodies from BP patients [35] or to rabbit antibodies against collagen VII [33], our rabbit antibodies fixed complement *ex vivo* as assessed by an *in vitro* complement-binding assay, which measures complement activation by the classical pathway [36]. We also observed complement C3 deposits *in vivo* in our model reproducing the immunopathological finding of C3 deposits in BP patients.

The infiltration of leukocytes, dominated by granulocytes, into the upper dermis of the lesional skin is a further major pathological feature of human BP. We have seen constantly inflammatory infiltrates consisting predominantly of granulocytes in the skin of our mice. We could also show that *in situ*-bound and soluble ICs of rabbit IgG and BP180/CXVII activated granulocytes resulting in respiratory burst and dermal-epidermal separation *ex vivo*. However, while in approximately 50% of BP patients' eosinophils represent the major fraction of recruited cells, in our present model neutrophils were the main cell type observed. Thus similar to previous *in vivo* studies [18–21], eosinophil infiltration, an important histopathological feature of human BP, is not fully reproduced in our present model and should be addressed in further studies.

An interesting observation relates to the different clinical phenotypes induced in mice injected with BP180/CXVII-specific IgG depending on the administration route. The i.p. injection of antibodies resulted in generalized skin blistering with predilection

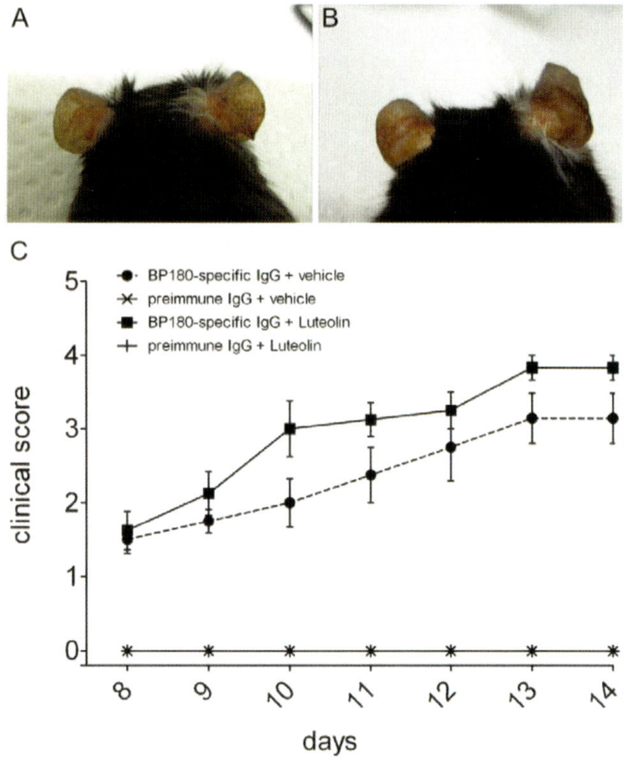

Figure 10. *In vivo* luteolin treatment does not significantly inhibit blistering in adult mice. BALB/c mice were pre-immunized with rabbit IgG and injected s.c. with BP180/CXVII-specific IgG. Control mice were pre-sensitized with rabbit IgG and challenged with the same dose of normal rabbit IgG showed no skin alterations. Topical treatment of mice with (**A**) luteolin at concentrations of 5.24 μM/ear did not result in different outcome compared with (**B**) animals treated topically with vehicle alone. (**C**) Treatment of mice with 1 mg luteolin i.p. daily (n = 8) did not significantly influence disease activity when compared to mice treated with vehicle alone (n = 8, p>0.5). Data are shown as mean ± SEM.

on the ears, legs, snout and periocular areas. The s.c. injection of the same IgG preparation triggered extensive skin disease mainly limited to the proximity of the injection area, although a few lesions at distant sites were also observed. The cause of this phenomenon is not known, but is not likely related to a lower systemic availability of pathogenic antibodies, since the levels of circulating BP180/CXVII-specific IgG in the two groups were similar. A further unresolved issue is why lesions develop at predilection sites when the pathogenic IgG is injected intraperitoneally. This site-specificity of the autoimmune attack, which resembles findings in the passive transfer model of epidermolysis bullosa acquisita [33], may be explained by the obvious exposure to increased mechanical trauma and/or by particularities of the vasculature at these sites that were shown to be relevant in antibody-dependent models of rheumatoid arthritis [37].

Results from a neonatal model of BP and our previous data from the *ex vivo* cryosection model of BP showed that granulocyte activation is a prerequisite for autoantibody-induced dermal-epidermal separation [16,38]. In our present study, depletion of neutrophils using a Ly-6G-specific antibody only partly inhibited skin blistering induced by BP180/CXVII-specific IgG. While a straightforward explanation for the relatively modest effect of neutrophil depletion on skin blistering in the adult model of BP is difficult to give at this time, a combination of factors is likely to have contributed to this outcome. First, the *ex vivo* cryosection model has an obvious limitation due to the fact that the skin sections are dead tissue containing damaged cells precluding more active, keratinocyte-dependent mechanisms to be reproduced in this model. Second, in the neonatal model granulocytes are needed for inducing the "epidermal wrinkling" sign by rubbing the mouse skin. It is however, not known how these cells impact the development of spontaneous blistering reproduced in the new animal model presented here. Importantly, as recently suggested, different mechanisms of autoantibody-induced blister formation may be in place in BP [39,40], which due to the longer observation time in the new BP model may have become apparent in our present study.

Luteolin (3′,4′,5,7-tetrahydroxyflavone), a plant flavonoid with potent anti-inflammatory and anti-oxidative properties and a good safety profile is being investigated as new therapy in inflammatory autoimmune disease and allergy [30]. Therefore, the aim of a further set of experiments was to investigate the therapeutic potential of luteolin in exprimental BP. Initial *ex vivo* experiments demonstrated that luteolin inhibited the FcγR-dependent production of ROS by leukocytes and partly the pemphigoid autoantibody-induced granulocyte-dependent dermal-epidermal separation of skin sections. However, mice treated with luteolin i.p. or by topical application did not show a lower pemphigoid disease activity upon challenge with blister-inducing rabbit IgG. Taken together these results suggest that luteolin is not acting on key pathogenic mechanisms in experimental BP *in vivo* and therefore do not qualify this compound for further exploring its therapeutic potential for the human pemphigoid disease.

In conclusion, this study demonstrates that the passive transfer of BP180/CXVII-specific IgG antibodies induces spontaneous blistering in adult mice and recapitulates the main clinical, histological, and immunopathological features of human pemphigoid disease. A further salient feature of this model is the fact that it allows longer observation times of the diseased mice. Using this model we could show that granulocytes significantly contribute to the autoantibody-triggered tissue damage. Promising *ex vivo* results using the anti-inflammatory flavonoid luteolin were not validated as effective systemic or topical therapy in the experimental pemphigoid model *in vivo*. These studies establish an animal model that will be a useful tool for dissecting the cellular and molecular mechanisms of blister formation in BP. In addition, this experimental system will facilitate the development of more effective therapeutic strategies for managing this chronic autoimmune disorder.

Materials and Methods

Mice

The animal's welfare is checked regularly, and the University Freiburg Medical Center animal facility complies with the national and international laws and regulations. The experiments were approved by the Animal Care and Use Committee (Regierungspräsidium Freiburg, Germany; no. G-10/14 and G-10/84) and performed by certified personnel. 6 to 8-week-old BALB/c, C57BL/6J, C57BL/10 and SJL female mice with a body weight of approximately 20 g were obtained from Charles River, Germany. All injections and bleedings were performed on mice narcotized by inhalation of isoflurane or intraperitoneal administration of a mixture of ketamine (100 μg/g) and xylazine (15 μg/g).

Generation of antibodies against murine BP180/CXVII

Polyclonal antibodies were produced by immunizing rabbits with 200 μg of a mixture containing purified glutathione S-transferase (GST)-mCXVII-EC1, GST-mCXVII-EC3, GST-mCXVII-EC7 and GST-mCXVII-IC2 in a 2:1:1:1 molar ratio in complete Freund's adjuvant. The recombinant fragments designated GST-mCXVII-EC1, GST-mCXVII-EC3, GST-mCXVII-EC7 and GST-mCXVII-IC2 contain murine collagen XVII sequences stretching from amino acid positions 498–580, 856–901, 1030–1134, and 186–475, respectively [31]. These GST-fusion proteins containing sequences of murine BP180/CXVII were cloned and purified as previously described [31,41]. Briefly, recombinant GST fusion and His-tagged proteins were expressed in *E. coli* TOP10 and XL1-Blue and purified by gluthatione agarose and metallochelate affinity chromatography, respectively as described [16,42]. The animals were boosted twice (at 15-day interval) with the same protein preparation in incomplete Freund's adjuvant. Immune sera were obtained at regular intervals and characterized by IF microscopy on cryosections of murine skin.

Affinity purification of rabbit IgG

IgG from rabbit serum or Amicon Ultra-15 filter-concentrated supernatants from hybridoma cells (clone NIMP-R14) was purified using Protein G Sepharose Fast Flow affinity column chromatography (Amersham Biosciences) as described [43]. Briefly, antibodies were eluted with 0.1 M glycine buffer (pH 2.5), neutralized with 1.5 M Tris-HCl (pH 10), and concentrated under extensive washing with PBS (pH 7.2) using Amicon Ultra-15 filters (Millipore). Purified IgG was filter-sterilized (pore size, 0.22 μm; Millipore) and the protein concentration was measured spectrophotometrically at 280 nm. Reactivity of IgG fractions was analyzed by IF microscopy on murine skin.

Passive transfer experiments and clinical scoring of disease activity

Adult mice were pre-immunized on day 0 with 200 μg of rabbit IgG and injected starting with day 3 every second day subcutaneously (s.c.) or intraperitoneally (i.p.) six times with 15 mg of rabbit IgG against murine BP180/CXVII with end-titer on adult mouse skin of 1:16,000–32,000. Control mice received 15 mg of pre-immune IgG purified from rabbits. For neutrophil depletion *in vivo* BALB/c mice were injected i.p. with 0.125 mg of the depleting rat anti-Ly-6G antibody or control rat IgG starting 3 days after injection of BP180/CXVII-specific rabbit IgG on days 5, 7, 8, 9, 10, and 11. Luteolin 98 MM was obtained from International Development and Manufacturing (MMD), dissolved in 1 M NaOH and diluted 1:10 in PBS to produce a stock solution of 10 mg/ml (pH 8.5). For the luteolin treatment *in vivo*, BALB/c mice were injected i.p. with 1 mg of luteolin dissolved in PBS (pH 8.5) or vehicle alone every day. In mice the LD50 values are of >180 mg/kg by i.p. injection [44]. For topical therapy, mice were injected twice s.c. in the ears with 1.5 mg IgG and the luteolin-rich *Reseda luteola l.* extract (RF 40) was topically used at luteolin concentrations of 5.24 μM/site [45]. All skin samples were examined by IF microscopy for IgG and complement C3 deposition and by light microscopy (H&E staining) for signs of dermal-epidermal separation and/or inflammatory infiltrates, as previously described [46,47]. Mice were weighed daily and examined for their general condition and for evidence of cutaneous lesions (i.e., erythema, blisters, erosions, and crusts). Intact blisters or erosions were counted and the extent of skin disease was scored as follows: 0, no lesions; 1, fewer than 20 lesions or less than 10% of the skin surface; 2, more than 20 lesions or 10–20% of the skin surface; 3, 20–40% of the skin surface; 4, 40–60% of the skin surface; and 5, more than 60% of the skin surface.

To evaluate the correlation of antibody titers with the extent of disease, sera were obtained from adult mice at different time points, including before starting the treatment and 2 days after the last injection. Sera were assayed for antibody titers by ELISA. Biopsies of lesional and perilesional skin and esophagus were obtained 2–3 days after the last injection and prepared for examination by histopathology and IF microscopy.

IF microscopy

Indirect and direct IF microscopy using rabbit or mouse sera was performed as described previously [33]. Briefly, indirect IF was carried out on frozen murine skin sections from untreated mice, which were incubated 1 h with 100-fold diluted rabbit serum. Direct IF microscopy was performed using frozen skin sections from treated mice. Bound immunoreactants were visualized using a 100-fold diluted AlexaFluor 488-conjugated antibodies specific for rabbit IgG, mouse C3 and mouse IgG (all Invitrogen). Complement-fixing activity of antibodies to the DEJ was determined as described [43]. Briefly, sections of normal mouse skin were incubated 1 h with 1-fold diluted rabbit sera against BP180/CXVII or control IgG, followed by washing with PBS (pH 7.2), twice for 10 min. Subsequently, sections were treated for 1 h with fresh human serum as a source of complement, diluted 1:5 with Gelatin Veronal Buffer (Sigma). *In situ* complement deposition was visualized using a 100-fold diluted AlexaFluor-488-conjugated antibody specific for human C3 (Invitrogen).

ROS measurement by luminol chemiluminescence

Human leukocytes were isolated from the peripheral blood of healthy donors. For the experiments conducted with human leukocytes, we obtained approval from the Ethics Committee of the Medical Faculty of the University of Freiburg, Germany (Institutional Board Project no. 407/08). We obtained written informed consent from the donors whose material was used in the study, in adherence to the Helsinki Principles. After 3% dextran sedimentation erythrocytes were lysed using a hypotonic solution of 0.2% NaCl. Leukocytes were washed in DMEM medium without supplements and resuspended at a final density of 3×10^7 cells/ml. Cell viability was tested with trypan blue; only preparations with a viability greater than 95% were used. Plate bound murine ICs were formed using the recombinant fragments of murine collagen XVII (GST-mCXVII-EC1, -EC3, -EC7 and -IC2) and rabbit sera from rabbits immunized against BP180/CXVII. Briefly, 96-well microtiter plates were coated with 5 μg of equimolar amounts of GST-mCXVII-fragments in 0.1 M bicarbonate buffer (pH 9.6). The wells were washed five times with PBS (pH 7.2) containing 0.05% Tween 20, after each step. After blocking for 1 h with PBS-Tween containing 1% bovine serum albumin (fraction V; Sigma-Aldrich, Germany), wells were incubated for 2 h with a 50-fold diluted rabbit sera against mouse BP180/CXVII. ROS production was measured using luminol chemiluminescence. Leukocytes were pre-incubated for 5 min at 37°C with 150 μM luminol (Sigma) and, subsequently, 100 μl of cell suspension was added to each well. To study the effects of luteolin, leukocytes were pre-incubated with luteolin to a final concentration of 50, 100, 200 μg/ml or with vehicle alone for 10 min. All procedures were performed in the dark. Unless otherwise specified the chemiluminescence intensity was recorded continuously for 1 h. Kinetic measurement of ROS production in leukocytes stimulated with PMA (500 nM; Sigma) was conducted as control.

MMP-9 activity measurement by gelatine zymography

Human leukocytes were isolated from the peripheral blood of healthy donors and treated as described for ROS production. For the analysis of the effects of luteolin on MMP-9 release and activation by IC-stimulated leukocytes, the cells were pre-incubated with luteolin to a final concentration of 1000, 500 and 200 µg/ml or with vehicle alone in DMEM for 3 h at 37°C. The supernatant was collected, diluted 1:50 in PBS and sample buffer without reducing agents was added. All samples were loaded and separated for 1–2 h on a 8% SDS-PAGE gel containing 1% gelatine under non-reducing conditions. Subsequently, the gel was stained with Coomassie Brillant Blue staining solution for 1 h, followed by destaining the gel for 2 h as described [48].

Flow Cytometry

Blood samples were lysed with ACK lysis buffer, Fc-blocked with anti-mouse CD16/CD32 and then stained for FACS analysis with anti-mouse Ly-6G-FITC and anti-mouse Gr-1-PE or isotype controls as described previously [49,50]. Neutrophils were defined as $Gr\text{-}1^+$ $Ly\text{-}6G^+$ cells. All antibodies were from BD Pharmingen. FACS analysis was performed with FACS Canto II (Becton Dickinson).

Cryosection assay

IgG from rabbits or patients was diluted 1:5 in PBS and the protein concentration was measured using absorbance at 280 nm. Six-micrometer cryosections of murine or human skin were washed in PBS to remove embedding medium and incubated with 100 µl of diluted antibody preparations for 2–3 h at 37°C. Sections were washed twice with PBS and chambers were prepared as previously described [41]. Human leukocytes were isolated from the peripheral blood of healthy donors. For the experiments conducted with human leukocytes, we obtained approval from the Ethics Committee of the Medical Faculty of the University of Freiburg, Germany (Institutional Board Project no. 407/08). We obtained written informed consent from the donors whose material was used in the study, in adherence to the Helsinki Principles. After 3% dextran sedimentation erythrocytes were lysed using a hypotonic solution of 0.2% NaCl. Leukocytes were washed in DMEM medium without supplements and resuspended at a final density of 3×10^7 cells/ml. Cell viability was tested with trypan blue; only preparations with a viability greater than 95% were used. In some experiments, leukocytes were pre-incubated with luteolin to a final concentration of 1000, 500 or 200 µg/ml or with vehicle alone for 10 min. Leukocyte suspensions were injected into the chambers and incubated for 3 h at 37°C. Chambers were then disassembled and sections washed in PBS, air dried, and stained with hematoxylin and eosin.

Histology

Biopsies of lesional and perilesional skin and esophagus were fixed in 3.7% buffered formalin. Sections from paraffin-embedded tissues were stained with H&E.

Immunoblot analysis

For immunoblotting, subconfluent COS-7 cells transformed with murine full length BP180/CXVII cDNA or NIMP-R14 hybridoma cells were lysed for 30 min on ice in a buffer containing 1% Triton X-100, 0.137 M NaCl, 20 mM Tris/HCl pH 8.0 (pH 8.0), 2 mM EDTA, and 1 mM Na_3VO_4, 10% glycerol and 1 mM PMSF [33]. The samples were separated by SDS-PAGE on 6% polyacrylamide gels, followed by transfer onto nitrocellulose membrane. 200-fold diluted polyclonal rabbit antibodies directed against murine BP180/CXVII as described above were used. After incubation with a chicken anti-rabbit IgG HRP-conjugated secondary antibody (Novus biologicals), signals were visualized by 3,3′-diaminobenzidine (Merck) [41].

ELISA

ELISA was used to measure circulating mouse IgG against rabbit IgG following established protocols with minor modification [51]. Briefly, 500 ng purified normal rabbit IgG were immobilized on 96-well microtiter plates using 0.1 M bicarbonate buffer (pH 9.6). After each step, the wells were washed four times with PBS (pH 7.2) containing 0.05% Tween 20, unless otherwise specified. After blocking for 1–2 h with PBS-Tween containing 1% bovine serum albumin (fraction V; Sigma-Aldrich), wells were incubated for 2 h with a 250-fold dilution of mouse sera. Bound antibodies were detected using a 3,000-fold dilution of an HRP-labeled goat anti-mouse IgG antibodies (BioRad) and orthophenylene diamine (Dako) as a chromophore (490 nm).

ELISA was used to measure circulating rabbit IgG against BP180/CXVII following established protocols with minor modification [51]. Briefly, 300 ng of the purified His-tagged murine BP180/CXVII (EC1 fragment) was immobilized on 96-well microtiter plates using 0.1 M bicarbonate buffer (pH 9.6). After each step, the wells were washed four times with PBS (pH 7.2) containing 0.05% Tween 20, unless otherwise specified. After blocking for 2 h with PBS-Tween containing 1% bovine serum albumin (Sigma-Aldrich), wells were incubated for 2 h with a 100-fold dilution of mouse sera. Bound antibodies were detected using a 3,000-fold dilution of a chicken anti-rabbit IgG HRP (NOVUS biologicals) and orthophenylene diamine (Dako) as a chromophore (492 nm).

Statistical analysis

All analyzes were performed using GraphPad Prism Version 5.03. Continuous variables were compared using the Man-Whitney U or Students' t test. $P<0.05$ was considered statistically significant.

Supporting Information

Figure S1 Reactivity and specificity of IgG antibodies from rabbits immunized with murine BP180/CXVII. Frozen skin sections were incubated with 100-fold diluted serum from a rabbit (**A**) immunized against BP180/CXVII or (**B**) pre-immune rabbit serum. (**C**) Extracts of the NIMP-R14 hybridoma cell line (*lanes 1 and 3*) and of BP180/CXVII-expressing COS-7 cells (*lanes 2 and 4*) were separated by 6% SDS-PAGE and immunoblottted with 200-fold diluted pre-immune rabbit serum (*lanes 1 and 2*) or serum from a rabbit immunized against BP180/CXVII (*lanes 3 and 4*).

Figure S2 (A) Serum levels of mouse IgG antibodies against rabbit IgG. Levels of murine IgG in serum samples of pre-immunized mice, which were subsequently injected with BP180/CXVII-specific (n = 5) or control (n = 3) rabbit IgG were measured by an ELISA using rabbit IgG as antigen as described in Materials and Methods. Data are shown as mean ± SD. (**B**) **Serum levels of rabbit IgG against BP180/CXVII in mice.** Levels of rabbit IgG autoantibodies in serum samples of mice injected with BP180/CXVII-specific (n = 9) or control (n = 5) rabbit IgG were measured by an ELISA using recombinant BP180/CXVII, as described in Materials and Methods. Data are shown as mean ± SD.

Figure S3 Luteolin therapy does not influence levels of the injected pathogenic BP180/CXVII-specific IgG and of rabbit IgG-specific mouse IgG antibodies. (A) Serum levels of mouse IgG antibodies against rabbit IgG. Levels of murine IgG in serum samples of pre-immunized mice, which were subsequently injected with BP180/CXVII-specific (n = 16) or control (n = 11) rabbit IgG and treated with luteolin (n = 14) or vehicle (n = 13) were measured by an ELISA using rabbit IgG as antigen as described in Materials and Methods. Data are shown as mean ± SD. (**B**) **Serum levels of rabbit IgG against BP180/CXVII in mice**. Levels of rabbit IgG autoantibodies in serum samples of mice injected with BP180/CXVII-specific (n = 16) or control (n = 11) rabbit IgG and subsequently treated with luteolin (n = 14) or vehicle (n = 13) were measured by an ELISA using recombinant BP180/CXVII, as described in Materials and Methods. Data are shown as mean ± SD.

Acknowledgments

We thank Jessika Batt, Freiburg, Germany, for excellent technical assistance.

Author Contributions

Conceived and designed the experiments: EO CS. Performed the experiments: AS C-WF EO. Analyzed the data: LB-T SM TJ UW AS EO. Contributed reagents/materials/analysis tools: C-WF LB-T UW AS SM. Wrote the paper: EO CS LB-T SM TJ. Read and approved the final manuscript: CS EO AS C-WF LB-T TJ SM UW.

References

1. Mihai S, Sitaru C (2007) Immunopathology and molecular diagnosis of autoimmune bullous diseases. J Cell Mol Med 11: 462–81.
2. Sitaru C (2009) Bullous pemphigoid: a prototypical antibody-mediated organ-specific autoimmune disease. J Invest Dermatol 129: 822–4.
3. Stanley JR, Hawley-Nelson P, Yuspa SH, Shevach EM, Katz SI (1981) Characterization of bullous pemphigoid antigen: a unique basement membrane protein of stratified squamous epithelia. Cell 24: 897–903.
4. Stanley JR, Tanaka T, Mueller S, Klaus-Kovtun V, Roop D (1988) Isolation of complementary DNA for bullous pemphigoid antigen by use of patients' autoantibodies. J Clin Invest 82: 1864–70.
5. Diaz LA, Ratrie H, Saunders WS, Futamura S, Squiquera HL, et al. (1990) Isolation of a human epidermal cDNA corresponding to the 180-kD autoantigen recognized by bullous pemphigoid and herpes gestationis sera. Immunolocalization of this protein to the hemidesmosome. J Clin Invest 86: 1088–94.
6. Giudice GJ, Emery DJ, Diaz LA (1992) Cloning and primary structural analysis of the bullous pemphigoid autoantigen BP180. J Invest Dermatol 99: 243–50.
7. Giudice GJ, Emery DJ, Zelickson BD, Anhalt GJ, Liu Z, et al. (1993) Bullous pemphigoid and herpes gestationis autoantibodies recognize a common non-collagenous site on the BP180 ectodomain. J Immunol 151: 5742–50.
8. Büdinger L, Borradori L, Yee C, Eming R, Ferencik S, et al. (1998) Identification and characterization of autoreactive T cell responses to bullous pemphigoid antigen 2 in patients and healthy controls. J Clin Invest 102: 2082–9.
9. Lin MS, Gharia MA, Swartz SJ, Diaz LA, Giudice GJ (1999) Identification and characterization of epitopes recognized by T lymphocytes and autoantibodies from patients with herpes gestationis. J Immunol 162: 4991–7.
10. Egan CA, Taylor TB, Meyer LJ, Petersen MJ, Zone JJ (1999) Bullous pemphigoid sera that contain antibodies to BPAg2 also contain antibodies to LABD97 that recognize epitopes distal to the NC16A domain. J Invest Dermatol 112: 148–52.
11. Perriard J, Jaunin F, Favre B, Büdinger L, Hertl M, et al. (1999) IgG autoantibodies from bullous pemphigoid (BP) patients bind antigenic sites on both the extracellular and the intracellular domains of the BP antigen 180. J Invest Dermatol 112: 141–7.
12. Haase C, Büdinger L, Borradori L, Yee C, Merk HF, et al. (1998) Detection of IgG autoantibodies in the sera of patients with bullous and gestational pemphigoid: ELISA studies utilizing a baculovirus-encoded form of bullous pemphigoid antigen 2. J Invest Dermatol 110: 282–6.
13. Schmidt E, Obe K, Bröcker EB, Zillikens D (2000) Serum levels of autoantibodies to BP180 correlate with disease activity in patients with bullous pemphigoid. Arch Dermatol 136: 174–8.
14. Iwata Y, Komura K, Kodera M, Usuda T, Yokoyama Y, et al. (2008) Correlation of IgE autoantibody to BP180 with a severe form of bullous pemphigoid. Arch Dermatol 144: 41–8.
15. Di Zenzo G, Thoma-Uszynski S, Fontao L, Calabresi V, Hofmann SC, et al. (2008) Multicenter prospective study of the humoral autoimmune response in bullous pemphigoid. Clin Immunol 128: 415–26.
16. Sitaru C, Schmidt E, Petermann S, Munteanu LS, Bröcker E, et al. (2002) Autoantibodies to bullous pemphigoid antigen 180 induce dermal-epidermal separation in cryosections of human skin. J Invest Dermatol 118: 664–71.
17. Herrero-Gonzalez JE, Brauns O, Egner R, Rönspeck W, Mascaro JM, et al. (2006) Immunoadsorption against two distinct epitopes on human type XVII collagen abolishes dermal-epidermal separation induced in vitro by autoantibodies from pemphigoid gestationis patients. Eur J Immunol 36: 1039–48.
18. Liu Z, Diaz LA, Troy JL, Taylor AF, Emery DJ, et al. (1993) A passive transfer model of the organ-specific autoimmune disease, bullous pemphigoid, using antibodies generated against the hemidesmosomal antigen, BP180. J Clin Invest 92: 2480–8.
19. Yamamoto K, Inoue N, Masuda R, Fujimori A, Saito T, et al. (2002) Cloning of hamster type XVII collagen cDNA, and pathogenesis of anti-type XVII collagen antibody and complement in hamster bullous pemphigoid. J Invest Dermatol 118: 485–92.
20. Nishie W, Sawamura D, Goto M, Ito K, Shibaki A, et al. (2007) Humanization of autoantigen. Nat Med 13: 378–83.
21. Liu Z, Sui W, Zhao M, Li Z, Li N, et al. (2009) Subepidermal blistering induced by human autoantibodies to BP180 requires innate immune players in a humanized bullous pemphigoid mouse model. J Autoimmun 31: 331–8.
22. Nishie W, Sawamura D, Natsuga K, Shinkuma S, Goto M, et al. (2009) A novel humanized neonatal autoimmune blistering skin disease model induced by maternally transferred antibodies. J Immunol 183: 4088–93.
23. Ujiie H, Shibaki A, Nishie W, Sawamura D, Wang G, et al. (2010) A novel active mouse model for bullous pemphigoid targeting humanized pathogenic antigen. J Immunol 184: 2166–74.
24. Hall RP3, Murray JC, McCord MM, Rico MJ, Streilein RD (1993) Rabbits immunized with a peptide encoded for by the 230-kD bullous pemphigoid antigen cDNA develop an enhanced inflammatory response to UVB irradiation: a potential animal model for bullous pemphigoid. J Invest Dermatol 101: 9–14.
25. Kiss M, Husz S, Jánossy T, Marczinovits I, Molnár J, et al. (2005) Experimental bullous pemphigoid generated in mice with an antigenic epitope of the human hemidesmosomal protein BP230. J Autoimmun 24: 1–10.
26. Feliciani C, Caldarola G, Kneisel A, Podstawa E, Pfütze M, et al. (2009) IgG autoantibody reactivity against bullous pemphigoid (BP) 180 and BP230 in elderly patients with pruritic dermatoses. Br J Dermatol 161: 306–12.
27. Naito K, Morioka S, Ikeda S, Ogawa H (1984) Experimental bullous pemphigoid in guinea pigs: the role of pemphigoid antibodies, complement, and migrating cells. J Invest Dermatol 82: 227–30.
28. Anhalt GJ, Diaz LA (1987) Animal models for bullous pemphigoid. Clin Dermatol 5: 117–25.
29. Neale TJ, Wilson CB (1982) Glomerular antigens in glomerulonephritis. Springer Semin Immunopathol 5: 221–49.
30. Seelinger G, Merfort I, Schempp CM (2008) Anti-oxidant, anti-inflammatory and anti-allergic activities of luteolin. Planta Med 74: 1667–1677.
31. Sesarman A, Oswald E, Chiriac MT, Csorba K, Vuta V, et al. (2012) Interaction of human IgG autoantibodies with murine innate immunity factors: implications for disease models using the passive transfer of IgG in mice. submitted.
32. Chiriac MT, Licarete E, Rados AM, Sas AG, Lupan I, et al. (2012) A novel model of adult bullous pemphigoid in wild-type mice. submitted.
33. Sitaru C, Mihai S, Otto C, Chiriac MT, Hausser I, et al. (2005) Induction of dermal-epidermal separation in mice by passive transfer of antibodies specific to type VII collagen. J Clin Invest 115: 870–8.
34. Nagai H, Takizawa T, Nishiyori T, Koda A (1982) Experimental glomerulonephritis in mice as a model for immunopharmacological studies. Jpn J Pharmacol 32: 1117–24.
35. Mihai S, Chiriac M, Herrero-Gonzales J, Goodall M, Jefferis R, et al. (2007) IgG4 autoantibodies induce dermal-epidermal separation. J Cell Mol Med 11: 1117–28.
36. Katz SI, Hertz KC, Yaoita H (1976) Herpes gestationis. Immunopathology and characterization of the HG factor. J Clin Invest 57: 1434–41.
37. Binstadt BA, Patel PR, Alencar H, Nigrovic PA, Lee DM, et al. (2006) Particularities of the vasculature can promote the organ specificity of autoimmune attack. Nat Immunol 7: 284–92.
38. Liu Z, Giudice GJ, Zhou X, Swartz SJ, Troy JL, Fairley JA, Till GO, Diaz LA (1997) A major role for neutrophils in experimental bullous pemphigoid. J Clin Invest 100: 1256–1263.
39. Iwata Y, Komura K, Kodera M, Usuda T, Yokoyama Y, Hara T, Muroi E, Ogawa F, Takenaka M, Sato S (2008) Correlation of ige autoantibody to bp180 with a severe form of bullous pemphigoid. Arch Dermatol 144: 41–48.
40. Sitaru C (2009) Bullous pemphigoid: a prototypical antibody-mediated organ-specific autoimmune disease. J Invest Dermatol 129: 822–824.
41. Csorba K, Sesarman A, Oswald E, Feldrihan V, Fritsch A, et al. (2010) Cross-reactivity of autoantibodies from patients with epidermolysis bullosa acquisita with murine collagen VII. Cell Mol Life Sci 67: 1343–51.

42. Sesarman A, Sitaru AG, Olaru F, Zillikens D, Sitaru C (2008) Neonatal Fc receptor deficiency protects from tissue injury in experimental epidermolysis bullosa acquisita. J Mol Med 86: 951–9.
43. Sesarman A, Mihai S, Chiriac MT, Olaru F, Sitaru AG, et al. (2008) Binding of avian IgY to type VII collagen does not activate complement and leucocytes and fails to induce subepidermal blistering in mice. Br J Dermatol 158: 463–71.
44. Chen C, Peng W, Tsai K, Hsu S (2007) Luteolin suppresses inflammation-associated gene expression by blocking NF-kappaB and AP-1 activation pathway in mouse alveolar macrophages. Life Sci 81: 1602–14.
45. Woelfle U, Simon-Haarhaus B, Merfort I, Schempp CM (2010) Reseda luteola l. extract displays antiproliferative and pro-apoptotic activities that are related to its major flavonoids. Phytother Res 24: 1033–1036.
46. Sitaru C, Kromminga A, Hashimoto T, Bröcker EB, Zillikens D (2002) Autoantibodies to type VII collagen mediate Fcgamma-dependent neutrophil activation and induce dermal-epidermal separation in cryosections of human skin. Am J Pathol 161: 301–11.
47. Shimanovich I, Mihai S, Oostingh GJ, Ilenchuk TT, Bröcker E, et al. (2004) Granulocyte-derived elastase and gelatinase B are required for dermal-epidermal separation induced by autoantibodies from patients with epidermolysis bullosa acquisita and bullous pemphigoid. J Pathol 204: 519–27.
48. Liu Z, Zhou X, Shapiro SD, Shipley JM, Twining SS, et al. (2000) The serpin alpha1-proteinase inhibitor is a critical substrate for gelatinase B/MMP-9 in vivo. Cell 102: 647–55.
49. Shimanovich I, Mihai S, Oostingh GJ, Ilenchuk TT, Bröcker E, et al. (2004) Granulocyte-derived elastase and gelatinase b are required for dermal-epidermal separation induced by autoantibodies from patients with epidermolysis bullosa acquisita and bullous pemphigoid. J Pathol 204: 519–527.
50. Sitaru AG, Sesarman A, Mihai S, Chiriac MT, Zillikens D, et al. (2010) T cells are required for the production of blister-inducing autoantibodies in experimental epidermolysis bullosa acquisita. J Immunol 184: 1596–1603.
51. Sitaru C, Chiriac MT, Mihai S, Büning J, Gebert A, et al. (2006) Induction of complement-fixing autoantibodies against type VII collagen results in subepidermal blistering in mice. J Immunol 177: 3461–8.

Filaggrin Gene Defects Are Independent Risk Factors for Atopic Asthma in a Polish Population: A Study in ECAP Cohort

Joanna Ponińska[1], Bolesław Samoliński[2], Aneta Tomaszewska[2], Filip Raciborski[2], Piotr Samel-Kowalik[2], Artur Walkiewicz[2], Agnieszka Lipiec[2], Barbara Piekarska[2], Jarosław Komorowski[2], Edyta Krzych-Fałta[2], Andrzej Namysłowski[2], Jacek Borowicz[2], Grażyna Kostrzewa[1], Sławomir Majewski[3], Rafał Płoski[1]*

1 Department of Medical Genetics, Medical University of Warsaw, Warsaw, Poland, **2** Department of Prevention of Environmental Hazards and Allergology, Medical University of Warsaw, Warsaw, Poland, **3** Department of Dermatology and Venereology, Medical University of Warsaw, Warsaw, Poland

Abstract

Background: *FLG* null variants of which 2282del4 and R501X are the most frequent in Caucasians are established risk factors for atopic dermatitis (AD) with an effect probably mediated through impairment of epidermal barrier. Among subjects with AD *FLG* defects are also consistently associated with asthma and allergic rhinitis (AR) but it is less clear to what extent these associations are also present independently from skin disease. The aim of the present study was to evaluate the role of 2282del4 and R501X in predisposing to these allergic phenotypes in a Polish population.

Methodology: 2282del4 and R501X were typed among 3,802 participants of the Epidemiology of Allergic Diseases in Poland (ECAP) survey, a cross-sectional population-based study using ECRHS II and ISAAC questionnaires, and ambulatory examination.

Principal Findings: The *FLG* null variants were associated with AD (OR = 2.01, CI: 1.20–3.36, P = 0.007), allergic rhinitis (in particular persistent form, OR = 1.69, CI:1.12–2.54, P = 0.011), and asthma (in particular atopic asthma, OR = 2.22, CI:1.24–3.96, P = 0.006). Association with atopic asthma (but not persistent allergic rhinitis) was also present in the absence of AD, (OR = 2.02, CI: 1.07–3.81, P = 0.027) as well as in the absence of AD <u>and</u> history of broadly defined inflammatory skin disease (OR = 2.30, CI: 1.07–4.93, P = 0.03). Association to atopic asthma would have not been found if diagnosis was made by questionnaire only (OR = 1.15, CI: 0.58–2.32, P = 0.8). We did not observe an association between *FLG* variants and allergic sensitizations (P = 0.8) or total IgE. (P = 0.6).

Conclusions/Significance: In a Polish population *FLG* 2282del4 and R501X carriage increases risk for development of AD and atopic asthma (also in the absence of AD or history thereof). This suggests that interventions aimed at restoring epidermal barrier may have a general role in asthma prophylaxis/treatment.

Editor: Jacques Zimmer, Centre de Recherche Public de la Santé (CRP-Santé), Luxembourg

Funding: The work was financed by grants from Polish Ministry of Science and Higher Education, Ministry of Health grant nr 6P052005C/06572, and Warsaw Medical University grant nr 1WY/NK1W/2009. The funders had no role in study design, data collection and analysis, decision to publish, or preparation of the manuscript.

Competing Interests: The authors have declared that no competing interests exist.

* E-mail: rploski@wp.pl

Introduction

Filaggrin gene (*FLG*) is strongly expressed in the granular cells of the epidermis leading to production of a large precursor protein profilaggrin. In the process of differentiation profilaggrin is proteolytically cleaved into functional filaggrin peptides which bind and collapse the keratin cytoskeleton and subsequently are degraded into hydrophilic amino acids forming the natural moisturizing factor. The N-terminal domain of profilaggrin is likely to have an additional function as it specifically localizes to the nucleus. All these processes are critical for creation of epidermal barrier with appropriate mechanical and biochemical properties [1].

FLG null variants are strong risk factor for AD [2,3]. In Caucasians two such variants are particularly common: 2282del4 and R501X with originally reported carrier rates in general population of ~2 and 6%, respectively [2]. Both variants result in a complete loss of processed filaggrin due to premature termination codons within the first *FLG* repeat. Whereas several new *FLG* variants have been reported they are substantially less prevalent and qualitatively different with some residual function [4].

Among subjects with AD *FLG* defects are associated with other allergic disease such as asthma and allergic rhinitis (AR) however, it is less clear to what extent these associations are present independently from skin disease [5]. Two meta-analyses concluded that there was no association between *FLG* null variants and asthma among subjects without AD although the ORs from pooled estimates suggested a trend in the direction of association

[5,6]. Regarding association with AR in the absence of AD two studies reported conflicting results: Weideinger et al. [7] found an effect whereas Marenholz et al. did not [8].

Our purpose was to examine in a Polish population association of the 2282del4 and R501X *FLG* loss-of-function variants with AD, asthma and allergic rhinitis.

Materials and Methods

Ethics Statement

The study was approved by Ethical Committee of Medical University of Warsaw. All ECAP subjects gave an informed written consent including specific consent to genetic testing. Written consent for anonymous use of DNA was also obtained from subjects undergoing paternity tests whose samples were used to verify population prevalence of R501X.

Subjects

The study was based on participants of Epidemiology of Allergic Diseases in Poland (ECAP, www.ECAP.pl) living in major metropolitan areas of Poland (Katowice, Wrocław, Lublin, Gdańsk, Warszawa, Poznań and Białystok). ECAP is a continuation of the European Community Respiratory Health Survey II (ECRHS II) and International Study of Asthma and Allergy in Childhood (ISAAC). ECAP includes randomly selected population aged 20–44 y.o. (ECRHS standard) as well as 6–7 y.o. and 13–14 y.o. (ISAAC standard). The recruitment was done by a randomization procedure based on the personal identity number (PESEL). Out of the 25262 subjects who were approached by pollsters, 9446 refused participation (response rate −62.6%). In the present analysis two of the questionnaire's answers were used (i) "Have you ever had asthma?", (ii) "Have you ever had eczema, atopic dermatitis or other inflammatory skin condition".

Those who completed questionnaire were invited for an ambulatory examination. Four thousand thirty eight subjects (25.5%) have taken up the offer. The examination included medical history, physical examination, spirometry, PNIF (Peak Nasal Inspiratory Flow) and skin prick tests with 15 allergens: hazel, alder, birch, grasses/grain, rye, Artemisia, plantain, Alternaria, Cladosporium, molds I (Alternaria tenuis, Botrytis cinerea, Cladosporium herbarum, Culvularia lunata, Fusarium moniliforme, Helminthosporium), molds II (Aspergillus fumigatus, Mucor mucedo, Penicillium notatum, Rhizopus nigricans, Serpula lacrymans, Pullularia pullulans), Dermatophagoides pteronyssinus, Dermatophagoides farinae, dog, cat, negative control, histamine.

Concentration of total IgE in serum was determined with reagents of the Phadia CAP System [9] (N = 3440) or the Allergopharma-ELISA-Test [10] (N = 712). The obtained data were presented in IU/ml (international units per mililitre).

The clinical diagnoses of asthma (atopic or non atopic), intermittent allergic rhinitis (i.e. with symptoms present <4 days a week or for <4 consecutive weeks), persistent allergic rhinitis, (i.e. with symptoms present >4 days a week and for >4 consecutive weeks) and atopic dermatitis were based on the International Global Initiative for Asthma (GINA) guidelines [11], ARIA criteria [12,13], and criteria of Hanifin and Rajka [14], for asthma, allergic rhinitis and atopic dermatitis, respectively. In addition a history of food allergy, drug allergy, insect bite allergy, urticaria, Quincke's oedema or other chronic diseases was obtained. During the examination blood samples were collected.

While analyzing associations between *FLG* variants and allergic disorders comparisons were performed against a group of healthy controls (N = 1865), defined as individuals without any allergic disorder or other chronic disease (including ichtyosis vulgaris) based on performed clinical workup and history. Family history of atopy or other disease(s) was not an exclusion criterion.

Due to faulty blood sample collection (wrong labeling, degradation) the final genetic analysis was carried in 94% of those who underwent medical exam, i.e. 3802 subjects: 951 children 6–7 y.o. (47.6% females), 1054 children 13–14 y.o. (49.2% females) and 1797 adults (60.7% females).

Genetic analysis

Genomic DNA was extracted from whole blood. Typing for 2282del4 was performed by sizing of fluorescently labeled PCR product on ABI 3130 sequencer, typing for R501X was done by PCR-RFLP with *NlaIII* restrictase (1639 samples) or TaqMan allelic discrimination assay (2323 samples). One hundred sixty samples were typed for R501X by both methods with complete concordance. All these methods were described previously [2,8,15]. During typing every positive sample was repeated by reanalysis of DNA from the original stock. Whole screening was blinded to diagnoses.

Statistical analysis

In the analysis heterozygous and homozygous genotypes were pooled. Statistical significance of differences in genotype frequency among analyzed groups was assessed with chi square test or Fisher's exact test as appropriate. The strength of association was estimated by calculating Odss Ratio (OR) with 95% confidence interval (CI). Given the reports on the role of the *FLG* null variants in predisposing to AD, asthma and AR no correction for multiple testing was applied. Deviation from Hardy-Weinberg equilibrium was assessed by a Chi-square test with one degree of freedom. Total IgE concentration was log transformed to achieve normal distribution and presented means are geometric means (i.e. back transformed). In the analysis of *FLG* status vs. total IgE the adjustment for test-method, sex and age was performed by univariate ANOVA.

In our study we could detect the following effects with the power of 0.8 at alpha = 0.05: asthma–OR = 2.0, allergic rhinitis–OR = 1.7, atopic dermatitis–OR = 2.3 and allergic sensitization–OR = 1.5.

Calculations were performed with *Statistica* package.

Results

The FLG R501X variant is rare in a Polish population

While analyzing the 3802 subjects from ECAP cohort we identified 3629 wild type, 140 heterozygous and three homozygous 2282del4 genotypes (carriage rate: 3.76%, CI: 3.20–4.41) as well as 30 heterozygous R501X genotypes (carriage rate: 0.8%, CI: 0.55–1.12). There were no compound heterozygotes. In order to verify relatively low frequency of R501X vs. 2282del4 variant in a Polish population we also tested 510 samples randomly selected from an anonymous bank containing DNA isolated for the purpose of paternity tests [16]. We found 19 samples positive for 2282del4 (carriage rate: 3.79%, CI: 2.44–8.85) and five positive for R501X (carriage rate: 1.0%, CI: 0.43–2.31). The distribution of *FLG* variants did not deviate from Hardy-Weinberg equilibrium in either cohort (P = 0.5 in both cases).

Associations between FLG variants and studied phenotypes

When analyzing distribution of combined *FLG* variants we found an association with AD (OR = 2.01, P = 0.007), asthma (OR = 1.70, P = 0.024) and AR (OR = 1.43, P = 0.046, Table 1). Analysis of individual variants showed statistically significant associations between 2282del4 and AD (OR = 1.92, P = 0.022), asthma (OR = 1.97, P = 0.005), and AR (OR = 1.47, P = 0.047, Table 1).

Further analysis indicated that the statistically significant associations between 2282del4 or combined genotype and asthma as well as AR were limited, respectively, to atopic asthma (AA) and persistent AR (pAR, Table 1).

We noted that when subjects were stratified according to the answer to the question: 'Have you ever had asthma' the frequency of *FLG* variants was statistically significantly increased only among those who were diagnosed with asthma by a physician during the present study but who were not aware of having the disease as judged by questionnaire data (OR = 1.81, P = 0.03 and OR = 3.53, P = 0.00005, for the comparison of combined genotype frequency vs. healthy controls, for all asthma and AA, respectively, Table 2). Had the study been based solely on questionnaire data, only a trend for association between combined *FLG* variants and asthma would have been found (OR = 1.15, P = 0.83, Table 2).

In ECAP cohort there was no association between *FLG* variants and allergic sensitizations or total IgE concentration. The prevalence of the combined genotype was 4.7% (78/1676) vs. 4.5% (95/2126) among those with a positive skin-prick test to at least one allergen and the remaining group, respectively (OR = 1.04, CI:0.77–1.42, P = 0.8). Mean concentration of total IgE was 9.08 (CI: 7.38–11.17) vs. 9.62 (CI: 9.20–10.06) for those with and without *FLG* defects, respectively (P = 0.6, analysis adjusted for test-method, sex and age category).

The association between FLG null variants and atopic asthma (AA) is also found among those without atopic dermatitis (AD) or history thereof

Although the OR for AA conferred by 2282del4 or the combined genotype was higher among those with than those without AD (OR = 4.37 vs. OR = 2.23, and OR = 3.61 vs. OR = 2.02, respectively) the associations were statistically significant in both subgroups (P<0.03, Table 3). Analysis of pAR showed similar trends although the statistical significance of these associations among those without AD was borderline (P = 0.049 and P = 0.053, for 2282del4 and combined *FLG* variants, respectively (Table 4).

The frequency of the combined genotype showed a trend for increase among subjects who were not diagnosed with AD but who reported history of an inflammatory skin condition in the questionnaire (OR = 1.38, CI: 0.96–2.0, P = 0.08, comparison vs. healthy controls). Thus, we were interested whether the observed associations between *FLG* variants and AA among those without AD could be caused by an association among those with a history of AD or other inflammatory skin disease. However, this was not apparent since there was an association between 2282del4 or combined genotype and AA also among subjects without AD according to both clinical diagnosis and self reported history of an inflammatory skin condition: 7.1% (7/99) vs. 3.1% (55/1790), OR = 2.40 (CI: 1.06–5.42), P = 0.03 and 8.1% (8/99) vs. 3.7% (66/1790), OR = 2.30 (CI: 1.07–4.93), P = 0.03, for 2282del4 and combined genotype, respectively.

Since the chances of AD resolution increase with age we also analyzed the association between AA and *FLG* variants among those without AD in the youngest age group (i.e. children 6–7 y.o.). Among those with AA the prevalence of 2282del4 and the combined genotype was 12.9% (4/31) which was higher than among controls (OR = 4.53, CI: 1.54–13.38, P = 0.018 and OR = 3.74, CI: 1.28–10.98, P = 0.032, for 2282del4 and the combined genotype, respectively).

Conversely, analysis of pAR did not show associations with *FLG* variants among those without AD according to both the questionnaire and clinical diagnosis: 3.8% (13/340) vs. 3.1% (55/1790), OR = 1.25 (CI: 0.68–2.32, P = 0.5), and 4.7% (16/340) vs. 3.7% (66/1790), OR = 1.29 (CI: 0.74–2.26, P = 0.4) for prevalence of 2282del4 and the combined genotype among pAR and healthy controls, respectively.

Discussion

While studying a population based cohort of subjects we observed that the *FLG* defects conferred an increased risk for development of AD, AR (in particular pAR) and asthma (in particular AA). Whereas both associations were particularly strong among subjects with AD, the association with AA remained after exclusion of subjects with current AD even when analysis was limited to the youngest age group, i.e. a group with the lowest chance of complete resolution of skin disease. Association between AA and *FLG* variants was also present among those without current AD or history of AD or other inflammatory skin disease.

The association between *FLG* defects and AA in the absence of AD contrasts with conclusions of two recent meta-analyses

Table 1. Prevalence of *FLG* variants according to clinical diagnosis.

		2282del4			R501X			2282del4 or R501X		
Diagnosis	**n**	**n (%)**	**OR (95%CI)**	**P**	**n (%)**	**OR (95%CI)**	**P**	**n (%)**	**OR (95%CI)**	**P**
Atopic Dermatitis	271	16 (5.9)	1.92 (1.09–3.39)	0.022	4 (1.5)	2.31 (0.74–7.22)	0.14	20 (7.4)	2.01(1.20–3.36)	0.007
Asthma										
All	414	25 (6.0)	1.97 (1.22–3.18)	0.005	1 (0.2)	0.37 (0.05–2.89)	0.3	26 (6.3)	1.70 (1.07–2.69)	0.021
Atopic	186	14 (7.5)	2.49 (1.36–4.56)	0.002	1 (0.5)	0.84 (0.11–6.46)	0.9	15 (8.1)	2.22 (1.24–3.96)	0.006
Non-atopic	228	11 (4.8)	1.55 (0.8–3.0)	0.19	0	NA	0.2	11 (4.8)	1.28 (0.67–2.46)	0.5
Allergic Rhinitis										
All[1]	1114	51 (4.6)	1.47 (1.01–2.15)	0.047	8 (0.7)	1.22 (0.49–3.04)	0.7	59 (5.3)	1.43 (1.01–2.04)	0.046
persistent	591	33 (5.6)	1.81 (1.17–2.8)	0.007	4 (0.7)	1.05 (0.34–3.28)	0.9	37 (6.3)	1.69 (1.12–2.54)	0.011
intermittent	497	17 (3.4)	1.08 (0.63–1.88)	0.7	4 (0.8)	1.37 (0.43–4.31)	0.59	21 (4.2)	1.31 (0.69–1.86)	0.63
Healthy controls	1865	59 (3.2)			12 (0.6)			71 (3.8)		

[1]In 24 subjects allergic rhinitis could not be classified as intermittent or persistent; NA not applicable; All comparisons vs. healthy controls.

Table 2. Prevalence of the *FLG* variants vs. concordance between diagnosis of asthma (all kinds or atopic asthma) by a physician (i.e. diagnosed during the present study) and individual awareness of having asthma (all kinds) according to questionnaire data.

Diagnosis:			2282del4	R501X	2282del4 or R501X	OR (CI) P *
Physician	**Questionnaire**	**N**	**n (%)**	**n (%)**	**n (%)**	
All asthma						
+	+	127	7 (5.5)	0	7 (5.5)	1.47 (0.68–3.22) 0.34
+	-	269	17 (6.3)	1 (0.4)	18 (6.7)	**1.81 (1.07–3.07) 0.03**
Atopic asthma						
+	+	61	2 (3.3)	0	2 (3.3)	0.86 (0.23–3.25) 0.9
+	-	116	12 (10.3)	1 (0.9)	13 (11.2)	**3.53 (1.86–6.72) 0.00005**
Asthma (all) by questionnaire irrespective of physician's diagnosis		206	9 (4.4)	0	9 (4.4)	1.15 (0.58–2.32) 0.83
Healthy controls		1865	59 (3.2)	12 (0.6)	71 (3.8)	

* Calculated for the comparison of the frequency of the combined genotype (2282del4 or R501X) vs. healthy controls. Cells with P values <0.05 are **boldfaced**; Questionnaire data were not available in 18 subjects with asthma including 9 with AA.

although it should be noted that both these studies reported trends in the direction of association (OR = 1.11 and OR = 1.30) [5,6].

On one hand, some cases of resolved AD might have been missed in our study due to lack of patients'/parents' recall. Recall errors regarding history of allergic diseases have been demonstrated [17] and are likely to exist also in our cohort. On the other hand, the discrepancy with pervious studies [5,6] might also be caused by population specific genetic, environmental and/or life style factors as well as methodological issues. In our cohort the association between *FLG* null variants and asthma (in particular AA) was found preferentially (exclusively?) among those who were not aware of having the disease. This suggests that AA associated with *FLG* defects in the absence of AD may have a subtle phenotype being particularly difficult to diagnose by family practitioners. Notwithstanding the precise reasons for the discussed discrepancies, our results indicate that in a Polish population *FLG* defects represent a risk factor for asthma, irrespective of apparent skin disease or history thereof which it is possible to elicit in a clinical setting.

Interestingly, association between *FLG* defects and asthma without eczema has also been found in a cohort of Danish children prospectively followed from birth [18]. Furthermore, similar longitudinal follow-up methodology which should maximize the diagnosis rate was also employed in a study of German cohort where a relatively distinct trend towards an association was found (OR = 2.47, P = 0.11) [8]. Further evidence implicating epidermal barrier function in asthma pathogenesis came recently from a large genome-wide study showing that a locus with a likely function in keratinocytes (*RORA*) was among ten loci most strongly associated with this disease [19]. These findings suggest that at least in some cohorts epidermal barrier defects may play a role in asthma pathogenesis among those without AD.

In contrast to studies in other populations [5,6] we did not observe an association between *FLG* null variants and allergic sensitization(s) as judged by analysis of skin prick test results or concentration of total IgE. This result is consistent with recent observations in a Danish cohort where the risk of sensitization among *FLG* defect carriers increased only after onset of asthma and/or eczema [18] and suggests that the effect of *FLG* null variants on AD or AA development is not likely to be primarily mediated through allergic sensitizatibn.

The association between *FLG* variants and AD confirms the findings in other populations [3,6]. However, the association found in our study had only moderate statistical significance and effect size. This is consistent with suggestions that *FLG* variants are associated with severe forms of AD which are more readily ascertained in hospital based studies [20–23].

Our results also add to data on differences in population specific prevalence of *FLG* variants. We showed that in a Polish population the prevalence of the R501X variant (~1%) was distinctly lower than the prevalence of ~6% reported for Irish and Scottish populations [2]. An intermediate R501X frequency in German population (~2.5% as estimated from pooled data of Stemmler et al. [24] and Weidinger et al. [20]) suggests a clinal variation in prevalence of this variant in Europe.

In conclusion, we show that in a Polish population *FLG* null variants 2282del4 and R501X are risk factors for AD, and independently from it, for AA. A methodological observation is that in a Polish population AA associated with *FLG* defects may

Table 3. Distribution of the *FLG* variants in subjects with atopic asthma (AA) stratified by diagnosis of atopic dermatitis.

		2282del4			R501X			Combined genotype		
Atopic dermatitis	**n**	**n (%)**	**OR (CI)**	**P**	**n (%)**	**OR (CI)**	**P**	**N (%)**	**OR (CI)**	**P**
-	162	11 (6.8)	2.23 (1.15–4.33)	0.015	1 (0.6)	0.96 (0.12–7.42)	0.97	12 (7.4)	2.02 (1.07–3.81)	0.027
+	24	3 (12.5)	4.37 (1.27–15.07)	0.011	0	NA	0.69	3 (12.5)	3.61 (1.05–12.38)	0.029

All comparisons vs. healthy controls (Table 1), NA: not available.

Table 4. Distribution of the *FLG* variants in subjects with persistent allergic rhinitis (pAR) stratified by diagnosis of atopic dermatitis.

		2282del4			R501X			Combined genotype		
Atopic dermatitis	**n**	**n (%)**	**OR (CI)**	**P**	**n (%)**	**OR (CI)**	**P**	**n (%)**	**OR (CI)**	**P**
-	523	26 (5.0)	1.6 (1.0–2.57)	0.049	4 (0.8)	1.19 (0.38–3.71)	0.76	30 (5.7)	1.54 (0.99–2.38)	0.053
+	68	7 (10.3)	3.51 (1.54–8.01)	0.001	0	NA	0.51	7 (10.3)	2.9 (1.28–6.57)	0.008

All comparisons vs. healthy controls (Table 1), NA: not available.

have a subtle phenotype being difficult to diagnose by a questionnaire.

Acknowledgments

We would like to thank Andrzej Emeryk (Lublin), Ewa Niżankowska-Mogilnicka (Kraków), Andrzej Fal (Wrocław), Wojciech Silny (Poznań), Anna Bodzenia-Łukaszyk (Białystok), Ewa Jassem (Gdańsk), Anna Bręborowicz (Poznań), Jurek Kruszewski, Marek Kulus (Warszawa), Piotr Kuna (Łódź), Barbara Rogala and Radosław Gawlik (Katowice) for help in carrying out the study.

Author Contributions

Conceived and designed the experiments: RP BS SM JP. Performed the experiments: JP GK. Analyzed the data: RP JP BS. Contributed reagents/materials/analysis tools: AT FR PS-K AW AL BP JK EK-F AN JB. Wrote the paper: RP BS JP SM.

References

1. O'Regan GM, Sandilands A, McLean WHI, Irvine AD (2008) Filaggrin in atopic dermatitis. Journal of Allergy and Clinical Immunology 122: 689–693.
2. Palmer CNA, Irvine AD, Terron Kwiatkowski A, Zhao Y, Liao H, et al. (2006) Common loss-of-function variants of the epidermal barrier protein filaggrin are a major predisposing factor for atopic dermatitis. Nat Genet 38: 441–446.
3. Baurecht Hr, Irvine AD, Novak N, Illig T, Buhler B, et al. (2007) Toward a major risk factor for atopic eczema: Meta-analysis of filaggrin polymorphism data. Journal of Allergy and Clinical Immunology 120: 1406–1412.
4. Sandilands A, Terron-Kwiatkowski A, Hull PR, O'Regan GM, Clayton TH, et al. (2007) Comprehensive analysis of the gene encoding filaggrin uncovers prevalent and rare mutations in ichthyosis vulgaris and atopic eczema. Nat Genet 39: 650–654.
5. van den Oord RAHM, Sheikh A (2009) Filaggrin gene defects and risk of developing allergic sensitisation and allergic disorders: systematic review and meta-analysis. BMJ 339: b2433.
6. Rodriguez E, Baurecht H, Herberich E, Wagenpfeil S, Brown SJ, et al. (2009) Meta-analysis of filaggrin polymorphisms in eczema and asthma: Robust risk factors in atopic disease. Journal of Allergy and Clinical Immunology 123: 1361–1370.
7. Weidinger S, O'Sullivan M, Illig T, Baurecht Hr, Depner M, et al. (2008) Filaggrin mutations, atopic eczema, hay fever, and asthma in children. Journal of Allergy and Clinical Immunology 121: 1203–1209.
8. Marenholz I, Nickel R, Ruschendorf F, Schulz F, Esparza-Gordillo J, et al. (2006) Filaggrin loss-of-function mutations predispose to phenotypes involved in the atopic march. Journal of Allergy and Clinical Immunology 118: 866–871.
9. Johansson GOS (1998) Clinical Workshop. IgE antibodies and the Pharmacia CAP System in allergy diagnosis. Lidkoping: Landstroms. 48 p.
10. Debelic M, Wahl R (1996) In vitro tests: immunoglobulins E and G. In: Fuchs E, Schulz KH, eds. Manuale allergologicum IV. Deisenhofen, Germany: Dustri-Verlag Dr Karl Feistle. pp 1–27.
11. Global Initiative for Asthma (2009) Global Strategy for Asthma. Management and Prevention NHLBI/WHO Workshop Report. http://www.ginasthma.com.
12. Bousquet J, van Cauwenberge P, Khaltaev N (2001) Allergic rhinitis and its impact on asthma. J Allergy Clin Immunol 108: S147–S334.
13. Bousquet J, Khaltaev N, Cruz AA, Denburg J, Fokkens WJ, et al. (2008) Allergic rhinitis and its impact on asthma (ARIA) 2008 update (in collaboration with the World Health Organization, GA(2)LEN and AllerGen). Allergy 63: 8–160.
14. Hanifin JM, Rajka G (1980) Diagnostic features of atopic dermatitis. Acta Derm Venereol (supl) 92: 44–47.
15. Smith FJ, Irvine AD, Terron-Kwiatkowski A, Sandilands A, Campbell LE, et al. (2006) Loss-of-function mutations in the gene encoding filaggrin cause ichthyosis vulgaris. Nat Genet 38: 337–342.
16. Mueller-Malesinska M, Nowak M, Ploski R, Waligora J, Korniszewski L (2001) Epidemiology of 35delG mutation in GJB2 gene in a Polish population. Journal of Audiological Medicine 10: 136–141.
17. Kulig M, Bergmann R, Edenharter G, Wahn U (2000) Does allergy in parents depend on allergy in their children? Recall bias in parental questioning of atopic diseases. Multicenter Allergy Study Group. J Allergy Clin Immunol 105: 274–278.
18. Bonnelykke K, Pipper CB, Tavendale R, Palmer CN, Bisgaard H (2010) Filaggrin gene variants and atopic diseases in early childhood assessed longitudinally from birth. Pediatr Allergy Immunol 21: 954–961.
19. Moffatt MF, Gut IG, Demenais F, Strachan DP, Bouzigon E, et al. (2010) A Large-Scale, Consortium-Based Genomewide Association Study of Asthma. New England Journal of Medicine 363: 1211–1221.
20. Weidinger S, Rodriguez E, Stahl C, Wagenpfeil S, Klopp N, et al. (2006) Filaggrin Mutations Strongly Predispose to Early-Onset and Extrinsic Atopic Dermatitis. J Invest Dermatol 127: 724–726.
21. Brown SJ, Sandilands A, Zhao Y, Liao H, Relton CL, et al. (2007) Prevalent and Low-Frequency Null Mutations in the Filaggrin Gene Are Associated with Early-Onset and Persistent Atopic Eczema. J Invest Dermatol 128: 1591–1594.
22. Barker JNWN, Palmer CNA, Zhao Y, Liao H, Hull PR, et al. (2006) Null Mutations in the Filaggrin Gene (FLG) Determine Major Susceptibility to Early-Onset Atopic Dermatitis that Persists into Adulthood. J Invest Dermatol 127: 564–567.
23. Henderson J, Northstone K, Lee SP, Liao H, Zhao Y, et al. (2008) The burden of disease associated with filaggrin mutations: A population-based, longitudinal birth cohort study. Journal of Allergy and Clinical Immunology 121: 872–877.
24. Stemmler S, Parwez Q, Petrasch-Parwez E, Epplen JT, Hoffjan S (2006) Two Common Loss-of-Function Mutations within the Filaggrin Gene Predispose for Early Onset of Atopic Dermatitis. J Invest Dermatol 127: 722–724.

Peristomal Skin Complications Are Common, Expensive, and Difficult to Manage: A Population Based Cost Modeling Study

Søren Meisner[1]*, Paul-Antoine Lehur[2], Brendan Moran[3], Lina Martins[4], Gregor Borut Ernst Jemec[5]

1 Stoma Care Clinic, Bispebjerg University Hospital, Copenhagen, Denmark, **2** Institute of Digestive Diseases, University Hospital of Nantes, Nantes, France, **3** Pelican Cancer Foundation, North Hampshire Hospital, Basingstoke, United Kingdom, **4** London Health Sciences Centre, London, Ontario, Canada, **5** Department of Dermatology, Health Sciences Faculty, Roskilde Hospital, University of Copenhagen, Copenhagen, Denmark

Abstract

Background: Peristomal skin complications (PSCs) are the most common post-operative complications following creation of a stoma. Living with a stoma is a challenge, not only for the patient and their carers, but also for society as a whole. Due to methodological problems of PSC assessment, the associated health-economic burden of medium to longterm complications has been poorly described.

Aim: The aim of the present study was to create a model to estimate treatment costs of PSCs using the standardized assessment Ostomy Skin Tool as a reference. The resultant model was applied to a real-life global data set of stoma patients (n = 3017) to determine the prevalence and financial burden of PSCs.

Methods: Eleven experienced stoma care nurses were interviewed to get a global understanding of a treatment algorithm that formed the basis of the cost analysis. The estimated costs were based on a seven week treatment period. PSC costs were estimated for five underlying diagnostic categories and three levels of severity. The estimated treatment costs of severe cases of PSCs were increased 2–5 fold for the different diagnostic categories of PSCs compared with mild cases. French unit costs were applied to the global data set.

Results: The estimated total average cost for a seven week treatment period (including appliances and accessories) was 263€ for those with PSCs (n = 1742) compared to 215€ for those without PSCs (n = 1172). A co-variance analysis showed that leakage level had a significant impact on PSC cost from 'rarely/never' to 'always/often' $p<0.00001$ and from 'rarely/never' to 'sometimes' $p = 0.0115$.

Conclusion: PSCs are common and troublesome and the consequences are substantial, both for the patient and from a health economic viewpoint. PSCs should be diagnosed and treated at an early stage to prevent long term, debilitating and expensive complications.

Editor: H. Peter Soyer, The University of Queensland, Australia

Funding: Coloplast A/S supported the work of this study by providing funding for external consultancy for unit cost collection, data analysis and preparation of the manuscript. The funders had no role in study design, data collection, analysis, decision to publish, or preparation of the manuscript.

Competing Interests: The authors have read the journal's policy and have the following conflicts: Meisner declares consultancy for Coloplast. Lehur, Jemec, Martins, and Moran previously received honaria from Coloplast. Jemec and Martins previously received a research grant from Coloplast. All authors have declared in individual letters, that can be mailed upon request, that the funding does not influence or alter their adherence to all PLoS ONE policies on sharing data and materials.

* E-mail: smei0001@bbh.regionh.dk

Introduction

Creation of a stoma is a commonly performed and crucial component of abdominal and general surgical practice. The consequences for the patient can however be both complex and life threatening [1]. Stoma complications occur with a high frequency in spite of careful pre-operative planning, continuously improving surgical technique and extensive surgical experience [2]. It has been suggested that the complication rate appears to have in fact remained the same for the last 50 years [3], despite major advances in other aspects of medical and surgical care over the same period. Stoma complications include necrosis, leakage, granuloma formation, retraction, stenosis, prolapsed and parastomal hernia, and peristomal skin diseases [4]. While considerable attention has been focused on the surgical complications in the published literature, the consequences of peristomal skin complications (PSCs) have attracted less notice. PSCs are a constant challenge for a great majority of individuals with a stoma. It is the most common post-operative complication following creation of a stoma. Various studies have reported a PSC rate ranging from 18–60% [5–8] and a recent study reported that peristomal skin problems account for about 40% of all visits to stoma care nurses [9], suggesting that these problems play a greater role in the life of people with stomas than generally acknowledged [10]. The risk is life long, but the incidence of complications is highest in the first five years after operation [11] where a considerable reduction in stoma diameter and height is generally the norm – hence requiring adjustment of the appliance to minimize the risk of leakage and PSCs.

There are several challenges in the assessment of PSCs, one being to define the exact prevalence. The wide variation in reporting the complications may be due to the less than systematic assessment of the peristomal skin by different groups of health care professionals who seldom communicate on aspects of PSCs. In 2008 Martins et al developed the Ostomy Skin Tool (OST) using a simple and standardized approach for assessing peristomal skin [12]. The intention was to improve patient monitoring and optimize communication between health care professionals. Currently, the OST is a widely used and accepted tool translated into several languages. In Japan, this instrument has been implemented as a national standard tool. Recently the tool was validated and shown to be reliable [13,14].

Another challenge is to objectively assess the impact of PSCs. One method of doing this could be to assess cost, either in terms of utilities such as time [15] or actual monetary cost. Therefore the aim of the present study was to create a model for cost assessment of PSCs using the OST as a reference. These costs are important to know for surgeons creating a stoma and for other stoma care professionals as the quality of stoma creation, function, and stoma care has a life-long direct impact on costs for the patients and health care systems at a level never previously defined in a similar approach. Finally the model was applied on a large real-life data set from people with ostomies to assess the prevalence and financial burden of PSCs.

Materials and Methods

Initially a literature search was performed to find published relevant costs, cost estimations or health economic models on PSCs, however no relevant data were identified. Hereafter it was decided to create a model for cost estimations of PSCs.

Model design for cost estimation of PSCs

The structure of the model (Figure 1) was based on contributions from three stoma expert panels using the validated OST as reference for determination of diagnosis categorization, severity and care of PSCs. A seven week treatment period was determined based on previous results from a recent study suggesting that clinically significant improvement of PSCs can be expected during a 6–8 week treatment period [7].

The Ostomy Skin Tool (OST)

The OST is a standardized assessment tool developed with the aim to help health care professionals in evaluating and monitoring the condition of peristomal skin reliably and accurately [12–14]. The OST generates an objective score based on clinical observation of three domains: discoloration (D), erosion/ulceration (E), and tissue overgrowth (T). The three domains are scored according to the extent of the involved peristomal area and the severity of change in the skin. The combined score, or DET score, is in the range from 0–15 where 0 represents normal skin and 15 the worst combination of severity and extent. The OST also contains a full description of clinical signs for five diagnostic categories of PSCs and a care guide for each of the categories..Contact dermatitis and allergic dermatitis are two subcategories of an overall 'chemical irritation' category and the last three diagnostic categories are: mechanical trauma, disease related, and infection related. A simplified use of the DET score has been suggested [14] introducing three levels of severity 'mild' (DET<4), 'moderate' (DET≥4<7), and 'severe' (DET≥7).

Consensus of appropriate PSC treatment (Step 1)

Best local practice varies from country-to-country and site-to-site. To develop an appropriate global understanding of a treatment algorithm to be used in a cost analysis, 11 highly skilled stoma care nurses from 9 countries were identified for interviews based on their daily practice with PSCs and their experience with the OST. The stoma care nurses were informed on the purpose of the study by e-mail and acceptance to participate were confirmed by e-mail. The nurses were interviewed face-to-face expressly for this study and informed consents were re-obtained verbally ahead of the interviews. The verbal consent was transcribed to interview notes. Before the interviews the stoma care nurses were introduced and trained in the simplified DET scale of 3 severity categories 'mild', 'moderate', and 'severe' which together with the OST care guide were used as a common framework in the interviews. The collection of interviews and analysis hereof were handled anonymously.

The stoma care nurses' recommendations for appropriate treatment for each case of 'irritant contact dermatitis', 'allergic dermatitis', 'mechanical trauma', 'disease related' or 'infection related' for all three levels of severity (mild, moderate and severe) were recorded (see example Table 1). Health care spending was captured for health care visits, changes in type or use of appliances, medication, and surgery. The same interview questions were given to a dermatologist with special expertise in stoma care and the compilation of all interviews formed a global understanding of average treatment for every diagnostic category and severity level of PSC (15 subcategories in total). Complete treatment algorithms are available in Table S1.

Assignment of cost for health care spending (step 2)

France was chosen as the country of reference because the cost of appliances is independent of the manufacturer. A unit cost was assigned for each treatment item to determine the cost induced by each subcategory of PSC. In France e.g., a typical treatment with topical corticosteroid costs 2.57€ and a stoma care nurse visit is estimated to cost 15€. The French unit costs for all products applied in this model can be found in Table S2.

The DialogueStudy

To determine the distribution of treatment costs for the different diagnostic categories of PSCs and level of severity, the model was applied on data from the DialogueStudy (DS). The DS is the largest study ever undertaken in stoma care practice with more than 3000 people with a stoma enrolled from 18 countries [16]. The results from the DS provided a wealth of data on PSCs combined with leakage, ostomy appliance performance and quality of life assessed with the validated Stoma-Quality of Life (QoL) questionnaire [17]. In the DS, the participants' PSCs were assessed using the OST. Baseline data of gender distribution, type of stoma (colo-, ileo- or urostomy), mean age and mean time since surgery and presence of PSCs are listed in Table 2 and Table 3. In the model patients with multiple causes of PSCs or cause recorded as 'other' were assigned an imputed cost equal to the weighted average cost for a patient with known causes of PSCs with the same level of severity.

Sensitivity analysis (Tornado diagram)

Treatment cost estimation of PSCs was based on typical treatment patterns and did not rely on observed health care

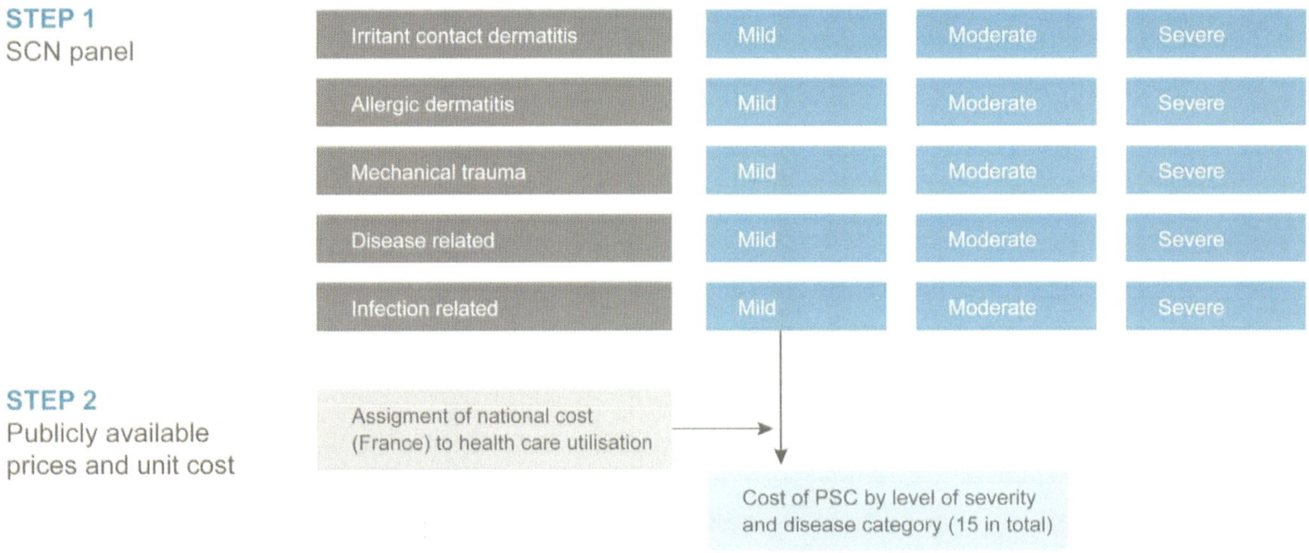

Figure 1. Model design for cost estimation of PSC.

utilization. In order to test how robust the PSC cost estimates were with respect to the unit cost established by this method, a sensitivity analysis was conducted. Each of the 15 categories listed in Table 4 were varied by ±20% and the PSC cost estimates were re-established for baseline population in the DS, freezing the cost for the 14 other categories. The resulting 2×15 estimates are depicted in a Tornado diagram Figure 2. The Tornado diagram illustrates which of the 15 estimated category cost has the largest impact on the overall PSC cost estimate.

Statistical methods

The baseline PSC treatment costs are analyzed using a linear normal based analysis of covariance (multivariate analysis). PSC treatment costs are furthermore analyzed using a logarithmic transformation. Transforming estimates back, relative differences are obtained instead of absolute differences.

The covariates considered were:

- Type of ostomy
- One or two piece appliance
- Convex or non-convex baseplate
- Frequency of clinic visit to SCN or doctor
- The baseline leakage level (on a 3-level scale)
- Time span since stoma creation
- Reason for the stoma creation
- Permanency of stoma
- Age and gender of the patient
- Country and center treating the patient

The same sets of covariates were used for total and PSC cost analysis.

Ethic statement

No ethic approval was obtained for the study as the study design is based on treatment algorithms, cost estimations and analysis of already published data from the Dialogue Study.

The stoma care nurses were informed on the purpose of the study by e-mail and acceptance to participate were confirmed by e-mail. The nurses were interviewed face-to-face expressly for this study and informed consents were re-obtained verbally ahead of the interviews. The verbal consent was transcribed to interview notes.

Results

The model created was used to estimate the treatment costs for managing an average case of PSC for all levels of severity and

Table 1. Example of recommended management of 'moderate' irritant contact dermatitis.*

Moderate irritant contact dermatitis	
Freq. (%)	**Health Care Intervention**
100	SCN consultation
51	2nd SCN consultation
15	3rd SCN consultation
6	Topical corticosteroid therapy

*Based on interviews of expert stoma care nurse (SCN).

Table 2. Patient characteristics DS.

		Participants (N)	%
Gender	Males	1474	49
	Females	1541	51
Type of stoma	Colostomy	2015	67
	Ileostomy	954	31
	Urostomy*	46	2
PSC	Yes	1742	60
	No	1175	40

*People with urostomies were not enrolled in all countries. DS = Dialogue Study. PSC = Peristomal Skin Complication.

Table 3. Patient characteristics DS.

	Mean ± SD
Mean age (years)	63.2±14.3
Time since surgery (years)	5.9±7.9

diagnostic categories of PSC for a 7 week treatment period. The results are listed in Table 4 and are presented in euros based on French unit costs in 2011.

The treatment cost of severe cases of PSC increased 2–5 fold for the different categories of PSCs compared with mild cases of PSCs. The change in cost from mild to moderate cases showed an additional cost ranging from 4–47€ with 'disease related' PSCs at the highest end.

The model was applied on the real-life baseline data from the DS. The treatment cost of a PSC was calculated for each patient where treatment of a patient with normal skin was assigned a treatment cost of zero. Based on the assumption that the numbers of appliance (baseplate and pouches) changes were the same for patients with and without PSCs, the total average cost for a 7 week treatment period (including appliances and accessories) was 263€ (n = 1742) for those with PSCs and 215€ (n = 1172) for those without PSC. Forty-three percent suffered from a 'mild' PSC, 42% had a 'moderate' PSC and 15% percent suffered from a severe PSC (Figure 3A). The treatment cost for the severe group was 6.1 fold higher compared with 'mild' cases and 4.5 fold higher compared with moderate cases (Figure 3B). The distribution of underlying causes of PSCs are shown in Figure 4A and the estimated treatment cost in Figure 4B. 'Allergic dermatitis', 'disease related' and 'infection related' had the highest estimated treatment cost (70.3€, 102.0€ and 60.4€ respectively).

In the DS, 58% of the participants had their stoma created as part of their treatment for cancer. The treatment cost of PSCs were in the same range [24–35.4€] independent of the underlying reason for stoma creation. DS participants with PSCs had an ileostomy or colostomy in 35% and 65% of the cases respectively. The average treatment cost for a patient with an ileostomy was 32.1€ and 24.0€ for a patient with a colostomy (Table 5).

Table 4. Cost of managing a case of PSC by cause and severity.*

Diagnostic category	Mild	Moderate	Severe
Irritant contact dermatitis	20.86	24.89	152.19
Allergic reaction	46.92	68.02	106.23
Mechanical trauma	18.63	23.30	113.93
Disease related	40.45	87.91	195.82
Infection	35.39	49.24	167.69

*Mild: DET score<4; Moderate: DET Score<7; Severe: DET score≥7.
DET = Discoloration, Erosion/Ulceration, Tissue-overgrowth. PSC = Peristomal Skin Complication. Cost estimations are based on French unit cost in 2011 (Euro).

Twenty-four percent of the participants in the DS experienced 'always/often leakage' and had the highest estimated cost (45.6€) compared with the group who 'sometimes' experienced leakage (20.3€) or 'rarely/never' (16.7€) (Figure 5A and B).

A co-variance analysis was performed to test for factors influencing the treatment cost of PSCs at baseline. Of the different variables tested leakage had a high statistically significant impact on the treatment cost of PSCs. From 'rarely/never' to 'always/often' there was a statistically significant impact on PSC treatment cost ($p<0.00001$) with a difference in an average cost of 29€ and from 'sometimes' to 'rarely/never', $p = 0.0115$ with an estimated difference in average cost of 11€. Furthermore, a borderline significant impact ($p = 0.0422$) was seen for 'year of age at baseline'.

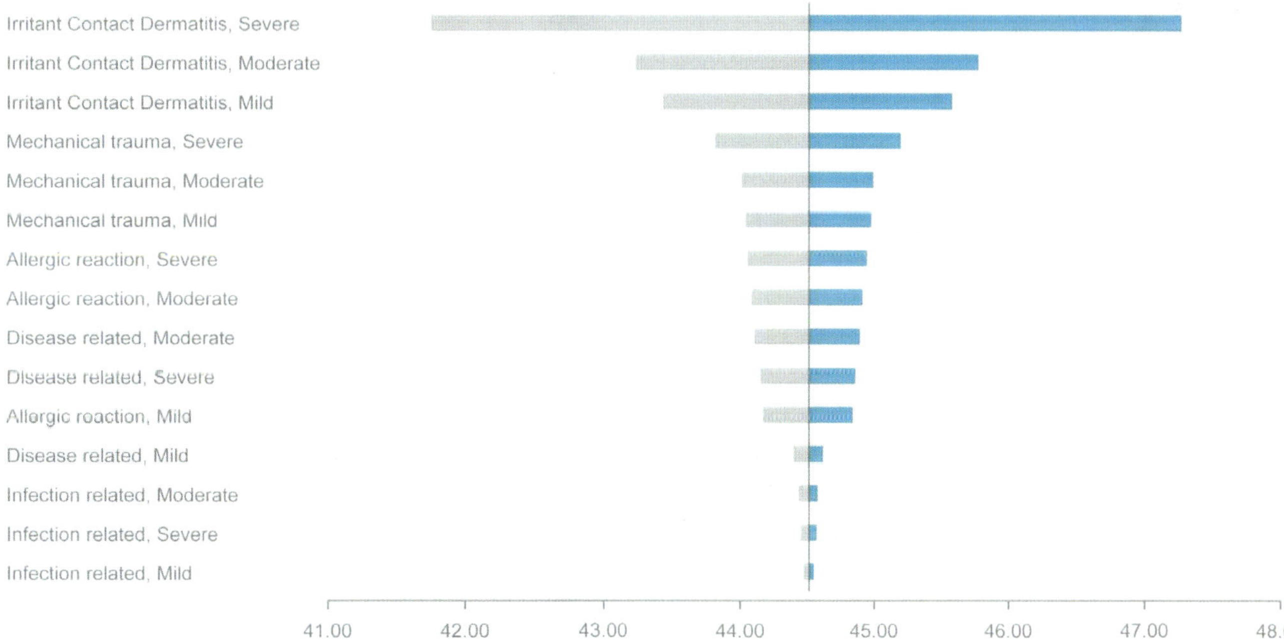

Figure 2. Sensitivity analysis of ±20% change in PSC cost presented in Tornado diagram.

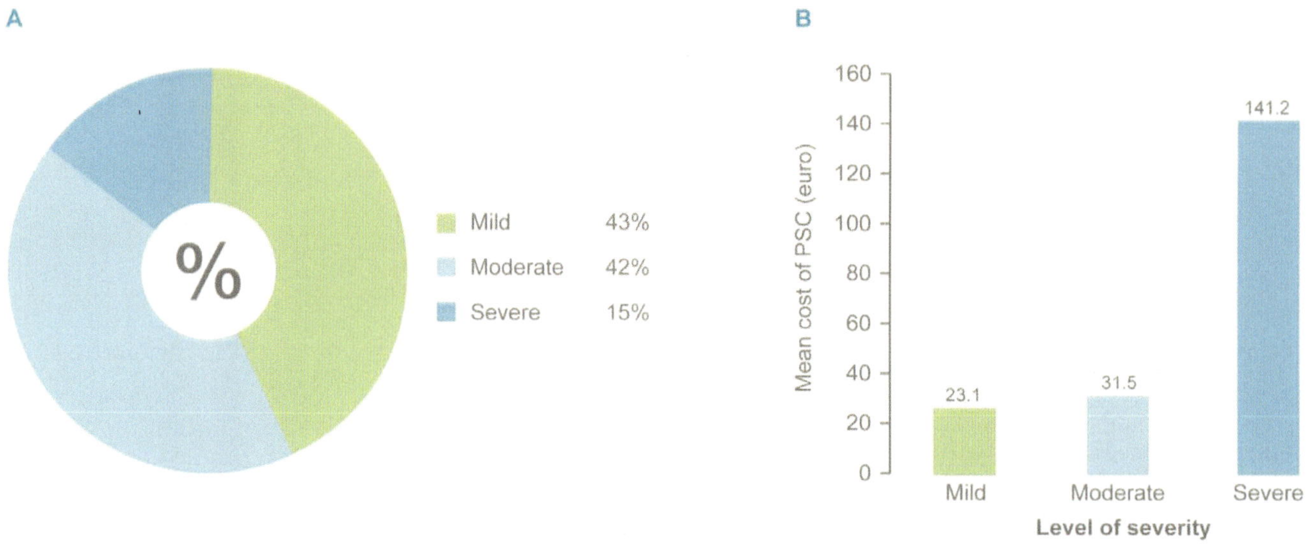

Figure 3. Cost of PSC according to level of severity (DS). PSC: Peristomal Skin Complication. DS: Dialogue Study.

A sensitivity analysis of ±20% change in treatment cost for the 15 categories of PSCs was performed to assess the robustness of the model and the estimated cost related to PSCs. The outcome of the analysis is presented as a Tornado diagram in Figure 2. The results show that changes in the cost of a severe irritant contact dermatitis has the largest impact on the cost of PSCs. However the PSC cost estimate is robust to changes in the 15 subcategories; for instance the PSC cost changed 0.3% for a 1% change in the cost of a severe irritant contact dermatitis (at the top of the Tornado diagram), and less with any of the other 14 subcategories.

Discussion

Surgical formation of a stoma is a significant clinical procedure in numerous ways, with stoma patients facing emotional, physical and social challenges. Stoma related complications occur frequently creating specific care problems and may have a major impact on the outcome in terms of patients' coping with their new life style. Living with a stoma is a challenge not only for the patient and their relatives and carers but also for society as a whole. In the long term it may be associated with increased absence from work due to illness, or to the need for early retirement, both significant health-economic burdens. The most common post-operative complication is PSCs [4]. The degree of peristomal skin irritation may range from that of a mild peristomal dermatitis to full-thickness skin necrosis and ulceration. A mild skin disorder if not taken seriously can rapidly progress into a more severe condition requiring medical action [6]. It is imperative that people with a stoma regularly check the peristomal skin and seek professional advice in a timely manner if deterioration in skin condition is observed.

In the current climate of limited available resources it is important to be aware of the most optimal use of resources. The aim of the present study was to create a model for cost estimation of PSCs. Interviews formed the basis for a model treatment algorithm for 'mild', 'moderate', and 'severe' cases of PSCs in five different underlying disease categories using the validated OST as a common reference tool. Not surprisingly there was a general

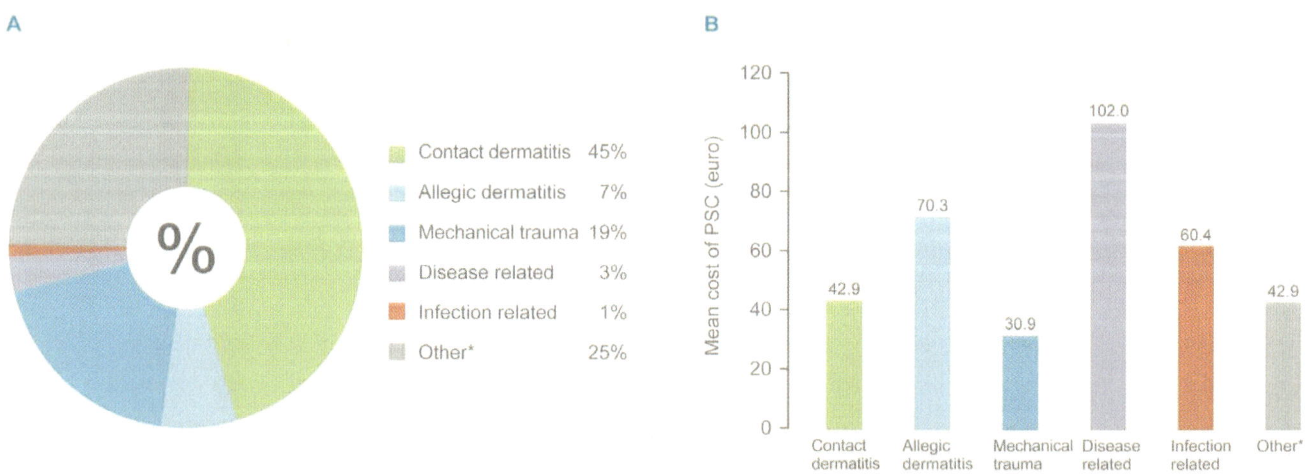

Figure 4. Cost of PSC according to diagnostic categories (DS). *Other: Was assigned an imputed cost equal to the weighted average cost for a patient with known cause of PSC with the same level of severity. PSC: Peristomal Skin Complication. DS: Dialogue Study.

Table 5. Cost of PSC (euro).

		N	%	Treatment cost mean (€)	Total treatment cost[1] mean (€)
Type of stoma	Colostomy	1125	65	24.0	244.2
	Ileostomy	617	35	32.1	241.6
Reason for stoma	Cancer	949	55	24.2	242.4
	Ulcerative colitis	211	12	26.9	236.2
	Crohns disease	170	10	34.1	246.3
	Diverticulitis	123	7	35.4	254.8
	Other	268	16	27.8	246.5

[1]Including appliances and accessories. PSC = Peristomal Skin Complication.

understanding that severe cases of PSCs needed a more comprehensive treatment and health care utilization than mild cases of PSCs. Usually patients with mild PSCs only have slight skin changes, involving a small area of the skin and requiring no active treatment. Based on French unit costs treatment of a 'mild' PSC was estimated to add extra cost in the range of 19–40€ per patient for a seven week period. The main primary cost is for consultation fees. For moderate PSC, definite skin changes are seen, e.g. ulcers in the peristomal region and usually a larger area is involved. Furthermore non-prescription treatment may be required. The model based estimated extra cost for a moderate PSCs was in the range of 23–88€ per patient over ostomies without PSCs. For severe PSCs immediate attention is often needed e.g. systemic steroids or anti-bacterial treatment [18]. A severe condition often involves the whole skin surface beneath the appliance system and complicates the adhesion of the baseplate to the skin. Therefore a severe PSC has a significantly higher estimated added cost in the range of 106–196€ per patient for a seven week treatment period.

To determine the distribution of treatment cost for the different diagnostic categories of PSCs and the level of severity, the created model was applied on the real-life baseline data from the DS study as it is a large and well described published study – the largest of its kind including 3017 participants with a colostomy, ileostomy or urostomy [16]. The results showed that the overall average cost for an estimated seven week treatment period (incl. appliances and accessories) was 263€ per patient (n = 1742) for those with PSCs and 215€ per patient for those without PSCs. This is an additional cost of almost 50€ for those with PSCs for a seven week treatment period. France has approximately 114,000 people with ostomies (according to survey conducted by the French association of stoma care nurses (A.F.E.T.)). Given the prevalence of PSCs of 60% in the Dialogue Study requiring PSC treatment, this represents 3.4 million euros of additional costs over seven weeks and 25.4 million euros yearly in France, assuming that all patients with a stoma have had adequate access to stoma care nursing. Fifteen percent of the participants from the DS suffered from severe PSCs. The treatment cost for this group was estimated to be 6.1 fold higher compared with 'mild' cases and 4.5 fold higher compared with 'moderate' cases. It is also the case for pre-existing skin diseases including atopic dermatitis and psoriasis that often become aggravated on the peristomal skin and exacerbate the severity of the complication and hereby the need for active treatment. The estimated treatment costs for the underlying diseases in the DS showed that 'Allergic dermatitis', 'disease related' and 'infection related' had the highest costs (70.3€, 102.0€ and 60.4€ respectively). People with stomas suffering from pre-existing skin

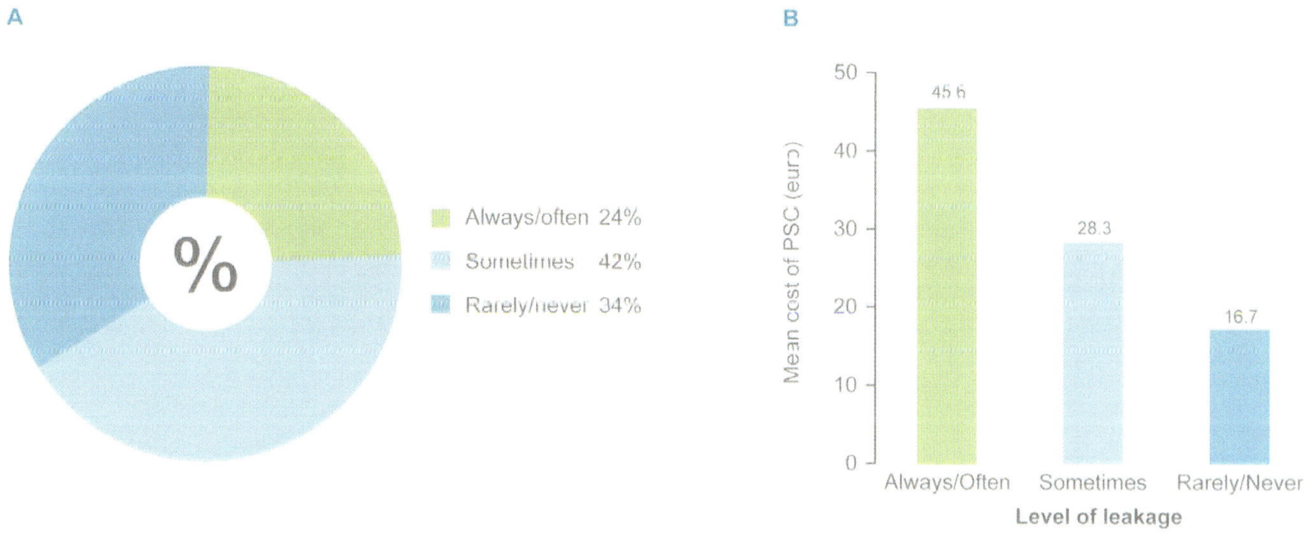

Figure 5. Cost of PSC according to leakage level (DS). PSC: Peristomal Skin Complication. DS: Dialogue Study.

diseases may benefit from more regular visits to a SCN to avoid more severe PSCs, subsequently reducing costs.

Unfortunately for many patients, PSCs may result in a vicious circle where the skin problem causes failure of the adhesive, which in turn gives rise to leakage and again can lead to more recalcitrant skin problems. Leakage is particularly problematic for patients with an ileostomy, because the condition of their skin is likely to deteriorate rapidly following leakage [18]. The absence of colonic function in patients with an ileostomy leads to more frequent stool, thus resulting in a greater risk of skin irritation compared with individuals with a colostomy [19]. Unsurprisingly, peristomal leakage, PSCs and overall QoL are interconnected [6,20] and the global results from the DS confirmed that leakage is a critical factor in the development of PSC [21]. Testing the influence of several co-variables on PSC costs, leakage turned out to have the highest impact in the present study. From a leakage perspective of 'rarely/never' to 'always/often' there was a statistical significant impact on PSC cost ($p<0.00001$) and from 'sometimes' to 'rarely/never', $p=0.0115$.

The management of leakage, the involvement and support of a SCN and the use of an appropriate appliance and accessories could potentially save money over the long term. In addition the frequency and severity of PSCs has a major impact on a patient's quality of life and overall daily living. A key aspect in optimal stomal function relates to stomal construction. Two recent papers have reported on the importance of high quality stoma construction, including adequate stoma length to minimize leakage under the adhesive and consequently the possibility of PSC [3,4].

The presented model gives an estimation of the cost associated with different forms of PSCs. A similar approach has not been published to date involving experts in the field from different professional perspectives. The sensitivity analysis of the model showed that the PSC cost estimate is robust to changes in all 15 diagnostic subcategories.

Limitations of the study

The model outlined, and the estimated costs, however has a number of limitations. All treatment estimates are based on a global understanding from expert experiences applied to average PSC cases and not on real-life observations. If local treatment differs significantly from the global understanding it should be considered to adjust the treatment algorithm accordingly. The estimated costs are for a seven week treatment nevertheless the analysis does not address the outcome of the PSC after this period. In France, only four out of the 12 accessories recorded in the DS are paid by the health care system and therefore only these are incorporated in the total cost estimations. As all costs are based on French unit cost a re-estimation should be considered if local unit cost deviates significantly from French costs.

Several of these limitations could be addressed by a future real-life study following stoma patients and their PSCs over a longer period e.g. six months to explore the precise effect of treatment, extent of recurrent PSC and the appropriate resources needed.

PSCs are a common post-operative complication. It affects the patient physically and psychologically, ultimately prolonging rehabilitation and adaptation to the stoma. Furthermore PSCs significantly increase the cost both for society but also for the individual living with a stoma. Ideally PSCs should be prevented and awareness of the data presented here is important to disclose to surgeons creating a stoma and to other stoma care professionals (e.g dermatologists) as the quality of stoma construction and management may have a life-long direct impact for the patient's well being and major financial implications for the health care system.

Conclusion

PSCs are common and both frequency and severity are under-recognized and under-reported. A key causative factor is undoubtedly peristomal leakage and individuals with an ileostomy are most at risk from a combination of the higher output and irritant nature of the effluent as compared with those people with a colostomy.

The consequences of PSCs are substantial, both from the patient and the health economy viewpoint. The extent of the problem warrants a major focus on methods to minimize the risk, detect PSCs at an early stage and institute optimal treatment to prevent the long-term, debilitating and expensive complications.

Supporting Information

Table S1 Health care interventions for the 5 diagnostic categories seen in a 6–8 week perspective. * 2× SCN, 50% 2× specialist consultations, infliximab, 25% week opiod.

Table S2 (A) French Unit Costs. [1] Nomenclature generale des actes professionnels infirmiers, Site de l'assurance maladie, www.ameli.fr. 2011. [2] Tarifs conventionnels médecins spécialistes. Site de l'assurance maladie, www.ameli.fr, 2011. [3] Arrêté du 1er mars 2011 fixant pour l'année 2011 les éléments tariffaires mentionnés aux I et IV de l'article L. 162-22-10 du code de la sécurité sociale. Secteur privé.(www.legifrance.gouv.fr) - Classification Commune des Actes Médicaux (C.C.A.M). www.ameli.fr. 2011. [4] Assistance Publique des Hôpitaux de Paris (APHP). Service Financiers, Paris 2008. [5] BCB drugs database. Groupe Cegedim, Boulogne-Billancourt.www.resip.fr, 2011. (B) French ostomy appliance and accessories cost. The cost varies with the type of product in accordance with the following: • reimbursement prices are regarded as independent of manufacturer. • individual components of the appliance are priced thus (arbitrary units): One piece convex appliances are not reimbursed in France. The relative difference between two piece flat and convex base plates has been added to the cost of a one piece appliance in the DialogueStudy dataset for one piece convex appliances. Refence: Liste des produits et prestations remboursables 2011 (www.ameli.fr).

Acknowledgments

The study would not have been possible without the dedicated help from the members of the Stoma Research Board (http://www.coloplast.com/ostomycare/stoma_research_board/resumes), Birgitte Dissing Andersen (Herlev Hospital, Herlev, Denmark), Janet Stoia Davis (Stoia Consultants, CA, USA), Kathy Tavernelli (Cleveland Clinic Home Care Services, Cleveland, OH, USA) and from the following interviewed stoma care nurses who provided expert input to the treatment algorithm:

Birgitte Dissing Andersen, (Herlev Hospital, Herlev, Denmark), Ineke Claessens (UMCU, Utrecht, The Netherlands), Kirsten Dahl, (Skånes universitetssjukhus, Malmö, Sweden), Adelina Fernández (Complejo Hospitalario Universitario de Vigo, Vigo, Spain), Karina Halff (The Netherlands Cancer Institute, Amsterdam, The Netherlands), Louise Forest-Lalande (CHU Sainte-Justine, Montreal, Quebec, Canada), Doris Kost (Medizinische Hochschule Hannover, Germany) Oirda Samai (Brignoles, France), Wendy Sansom (Box Hill Hospital, Melbourne, Australia) and Marie Waller (Cambridge University Hospitals NHS Foundation Trust, Cambridge, UK).

Lars K. Langkilde (Wickstrøm & Langkilde Aps, Denmark) contributed with health economic input to the model and performed the sensitivity analysis. Carsten Henrik Wachmann (Larix Aps, Denmark) did the statistical analyses. Xavier Colon (CemkaEval, France) did the unit cost collection. Martin Nottmeier (Coloplast A/S) performed the interviews.

Zenia M. Størling (Trial Form Support Aps, Denmark) contributed with medical writing of the manuscript.

Author Contributions

Analyzed the data: SM PAL BM LMM GBEJ. Wrote the paper: SM PAL BM LMM GBEJ. Provided expert input to the treatment algorithm: GBEJ LMM.

References

1. Robertson I, Leung E, Hughes D, Spiers M, Donnelly L, et al. (2005) Prospective analysis of stoma-related complications. Colorectal Dis 7: 279–285.
2. Shabbir J, Britton DC (2010) Stoma complications: a literature overview. Colorectal Dis 12: 958–964.
3. Wille-Jorgensen P, Meisner S (2010) Just another stoma - why have we not improved? Colorectal Dis 12: 957.
4. Persson E, Berndtsson I, Carlsson E, Hallen AM, Lindholm E (2010) Stoma-related complications and stoma size - a 2-year follow up. Colorectal Dis 12: 971–976.
5. Colwell JC, Goldberg M, Carmel J (2001) The state of the standard diversion. J Wound Ostomy Continence Nurs 28: 6–17.
6. Herlufsen P, Olsen AG, Carlsen B, Nybaek H, Karlsmark T, et al. (2006) Study of peristomal skin disorders in patients with permanent stomas. Br J Nurs 15: 854–862.
7. Martins L, Samai O, Fernández A, Urquhart M, Hansen AS (2011) Maintaining healthy skin around an ostomy: peristomal skin disorders and self-assessment. Gastrointestinal Nursing 9: 9–13.
8. Nybaek H, Jemec GB (2010) Skin problems in stoma patients. J Eur Acad Dermatol Venereol 24: 249–257.
9. Jemec GB, Nybaek H (2008) Peristomal skin problems account for more than one in three visits to ostomy nurses. Br J Dermatol 159: 1211–1212.
10. Davis JS, Svavarsdóttir MH, Pudlo M, Arena R, Lee Y, et al. (2011) Factors impairing quality of life for people with an ostomy. Gastrointestinal Nursing 9: 14–18.
11. Londono-Schimmer EE, Leong AP, Phillips RK (1994) Life table analysis of stomal complications following colostomy. Dis Colon Rectum 37: 916–920.
12. Martins L, Tavernelli K, Serrano JLC (2008) Introducing a peristomal skin assessment tool: The Ostomy Skin Tool. World Council of Enterostomal Therapists 28.
13. Jemec GB, Martins L, Claessens I, Ayello EA, Hansen AS, et al. (2011) Assessing peristomal skin changes in ostomy patients: validation of the Ostomy Skin Tool. Br J Dermatol 164: 330–335.
14. Martins L, Ayello EA, Claessens I, Steen HA, Hentze PL, et al. (2010) The ostomy skin tool: tracking peristomal skin changes. Br J Nurs 19: 960, 932–960, 934.
15. Holm EA, Jemec GB (2004) Time spent on treatment of atopic dermatitis: a new method of measuring pediatric morbidity? Pediatr Dermatol 21: 623–627.
16. Andersen BD, van Keizerswaard P, Castro MM, English E, Carter D (2011) Introduction to the DialogueStudy: methods and baseline demographic findings. Gastrointestinal Nursing 9: 4–8.
17. Prieto L, Thorsen H, Juul K (2005) Development and validation of a quality of life questionnaire for patients with colostomy or ileostomy. Health and quality of life outcome 3.
18. Nybaek H, Bang KD, Norgaard LT, Karlsmark T, Jemec GB (2009) Skin problems in ostomy patients: a case-control study of risk factors. Acta Derm Venereol 89: 64–67.
19. Hellman J, Lago CP (1990) Dermatologic complications in colostomy and ileostomy patients. Int J Dermatol 29: 129–133.
20. Pittman J, Rawl SM, Schmidt CM, Grant M, Ko CY, et al. (2008) Demographic and clinical factors related to ostomy complications and quality of life in veterans with an ostomy. J Wound Ostomy Continence Nurs 35: 493–503.
21. Porrett T, Nováková S, Schmotz K, Klimekova E, Aaes H (2011) Leakage and ostomy appliances: results from a large-scale, open-label study in clinical practice. Gastrointestinal Nursing 9: 19–23.

An A91V SNP in the *Perforin* Gene Is Frequently Found in NK/T-Cell Lymphomas

Rebeca Manso[1], Socorro María Rodríguez-Pinilla[1,2]*, Luis Lombardia[3], Gorka Ruiz de Garibay[2,4], Maria del Mar López[2,5], Luis Requena[6], Lydia Sánchez[7], Margarita Sánchez-Beato[2,8], Miguel Ángel Piris[2,9]

1 Pathology Department, Fundación Jiménez Díaz, Madrid, Spain, **2** Molecular Pathology Programme, Lymphoma Group, CNIO, Madrid, Spain, **3** Clinical Research Programme, Molecular Diagnostics Clinical Research Unit, CNIO, Madrid, Spain, **4** Clinical Immunology Department, Hospital Clínico de San Carlos, Madrid, Spain, **5** Biotechnology Programme, Monoclonal Antibodies Unit, CNIO, Madrid, Spain, **6** Dermatology Department, Fundación Jimenez Díaz, Madrid, Spain, **7** Biotechnology Programme, Immunohistochemistry Unit, CNIO, Madrid, Spain, **8** Oncology-Haematology Area, Instituto Investigación Sanitaria, Hospital Universitario Puerta de Hierro-Majadahonda, Madrid, Spain, **9** Pathology Department, Hospital Universitario Marqués de Valdecilla, Universidad de Cantabria, IFIMAV, Santander, Spain

Abstract

NK/T-cell lymphoma (NKTCL) is the most frequent EBV-related NK/T-cell disease. Its clinical manifestations overlap with those of familial haemophagocytic lymphohistiocytosis (FHLH). Since *PERFORIN* (*PRF1*) mutations are present in FHLH, we analysed its role in a series of 12 nasal and 12 extranasal-NKTCLs. 12.5% of the tumours and 25% of the nasal-origin cases had the well-known g.272C>T(p.Ala91Val) pathogenic SNP, which confers a poor prognosis. Two of these cases had a double-CD4/CD8-positive immunophenotype, although no correlation was found with perforin protein expression. p53 was overexpressed in 20% of the tumoral samples, 80% of which were of extranasal origin, while none showed *PRF1* SNVs. These results suggest that nasal and extranasal NKTCLs have different biological backgrounds, although this requires validation.

Editor: Ken Mills, Queen's University Belfast, United Kingdom

Funding: This study was supported by grants from the Ministerio de Ciencia e Innovación, Spain (RETICC, SAF2008-03871, FIS 08/0856) and the Spanish Association Against Cancer (AECC). MSB is supported by a Miguel Servet Contract (CP11/00018) from the Fondo de Investigaciones Sanitarias. RM is supported by the Conchita Rábago Foundation. The funders had no role in study design, data collection and analysis, decision to publish, or preparation of the manuscript.

Competing Interests: The authors have declared that no competing interests exist.

* E-mail: smrodriguez@fjd.es

Introduction

Extranodal NK/T-cell lymphomas (NKTCLs) are the main group of EBV-positive neoplasms that affect TNK cells, according to the recently revised WHO classification, which also includes aggressive NK cell leukaemia, chronic active EBV disease (CAEBV), severe mosquito bite allergy and hydroa vacciniforme. The precise role of EBV in the aetiology of the disease is poorly understood, although the incidence of NKTCL and the other EBV-associated lymphoproliferative disorders (LPDs) parallels the geographic distribution of EBV infection (in Asian and Central and South American populations) [1]. Most NKTCLs probably originate from mature NK cells, while a small proportion of cases, which express $\alpha\beta$ or $\gamma\delta$ TCR, appear to derive from cytotoxic T-lymphocytes (CTLs). They usually arise as tumours or destructive lesions in the nasal cavity, maxillary sinuses or palate. More rarely, they can appear in other extranodal sites, such as the skin, testis, lung or gastrointestinal tract. Despite their localised presentation in most patients, NKTCL is an aggressive lymphoma associated with a median survival for advanced-stage disease of only 6–12 months. NKTCL has a wide cytological spectrum and is characterised by angioinvasion and angiodestruction, leading to coagulative necrosis. Tumoral cells usually express cytoplasmic CD3, CD2 and, less frequently, CD56, and strongly express cytotoxic markers, including TIA-1, granzyme B and perforin [2,3,4].

Perforin is a 67-kDa pore-forming protein that, in mammals, is uniquely expressed in CTL [5,6]. The complete absence of *PRF1* function typically results in an aggressive, fatal immunoregulatory disorder of early childhood known as type 2 familial haemophagocytic lymphohistiocytosis (FHLH). The overall frequency of *PRF1* mutations in FHLH is between 15% and 50% and depends on the geographical and ethnic origin of the patients [7]. FHLH and EBV-associated haemophagocytic lymphohistiocytosis (EBV-HLH) have overlapping clinical manifestations, whereby CAEBV is often associated with EBV-HLH and some EBV-associated LPD patients eventually evolve into proper NKTCL cases [8,9]. Interestingly, a case of CAEBV with a mutated *PRF1* gene has been described [10], and a girl initially diagnosed with EBV-HLH carrying a *PRF1* gene mutation (S168N) finally developed an NKTCL [11].

The aim of the study reported in this paper was to establish whether *PRF1* mutations are present in NKTCLs. We analysed a series of 24 consecutive NKTCLs, 12 each of nasal and extranasal origin, and found two *PRF1* single-nucleotide variations (SNVs) in 16.6% of the cases. These SNVs were the well-known pathogenic SNP g.272C>T(p.Ala91Val) and the hitherto unreported c.289G>A(p.Ala97Thr). The p.Ala91Val SNV was present in 12.5% of all cases analysed, which is twice the percentage of cases expected for a Caucasian population (3% in heterozygosity according to http://www.ncbi.nlm.nih.gov/SNP/snp;rs = rs35947 132). These data are remarkable, since NKTCLs account for no more than 1% of all lymphomas in Europe. Furthermore, all positive cases were of nasal origin (33.3%), had a peculiar CD4/CD8-positive phenotype, exhibited no correlation with perforin expression, and conferred a poor prognosis on patients (median overall survival of 9.5 months compared with 25.54 and 10.6 months for nasal and extranasal-NKTCLs, respectively). Interestingly, in the present series, p53 was overexpressed in 20% of the tumoral samples, of which 80% were of extranasal origin, and none exhibited *PRF1* SNVs. These data suggest a specific background susceptibility to the development of this subgroup of tumours, at least in the Spanish population. However, a larger series of patients are needed to validate this finding.

Materials and Methods

Tissue samples

We analysed a series of 24 consecutive NKTCL cases submitted for diagnosis or a second opinion to the CNIO Pathology Laboratory between 2000 and 2010. Criteria for the diagnosis of NKTCLs were based on the WHO classification [12]. Complete clinical data were obtained from 21 patients. All patients who were alive at the end of the study or the direct relatives of deceased patients provided their written consent to participate. This specific project was supervised and approved by the Ethical Committee of the Hospital Carlos III, Madrid, and Hospital Universitario Marqués de Valdecilla, Santander.

Tissue microarray construction

Representative areas from formalin-fixed, paraffin-embedded lymphomas were carefully selected on H&E-stained sections and two 1-mm-diameter tissue cores were obtained from each specimen. The tissue cores were precisely arrayed into a new paraffin block using a tissue microarray (TMA) workstation (Beecher Instruments, Silver Spring, MD), following previously described methods [13].

Immunohistochemistry

TMA sections were immunohistochemically stained using the Endvision method with a heat-induced antigen-retrieval step. Sections were immersed in boiling 10 mM sodium citrate at pH 6.5 for 2 min in a pressure cooker. A panel of eight antibodies (CD3, CD4, CD8, CD56, p53, CD117, beta-catenin and perforin) were analysed (Table 1). Cases were considered positive whether the protein was present in more than 10% of the neoplastic cells. Perforin was analysed with respect to the presence or absence of the protein, the intensity of staining and the pattern of distribution of the granules. Three categories were created based on the intensity of staining: low, intermediate and high. Two groups were recognised, based on the distribution of the granules: a granular pattern limited to the Golgi region or one diffusely distributed throughout the cytoplasm. EBER-positive cells were considered to be neoplastic. Consecutive EBER-positive sections of each case were evaluated to quantify perforin staining. Reactive tonsil tissue was included as a control. The primary antibodies were omitted to provide negative controls.

EBV *in situ* hybridisation (EBER)

The presence of EBV RNA was established by non-isotopic *in situ* hybridisation with EBV-encoded RNA (EBER) 1 and 2 oligonucleotide probes (Dakocytomation) in paraffin-embedded tissue sections, as previously described [14].

PRF1 gene sequencing

Exons 2 and 3 of the *PRF1* gene have been amplified and sequenced with the primer sets shown in Table 2. Tissue sections from all cases contained between 50% and 80% tumoral cells. The 50-μl PCR reaction volume contained 0.2 mM of each dNTP, 1 unit Taq full DNA polymerase (Clontech Laboratories, Inc.), 0.2 μM of each of the forward and reverse primers and 100 ng of genomic DNA. After initial denaturation at 94°C for 2 min, 35 cycles of 15 s at 94°C, 30 s at 60°C and 30 s at 72°C were run in an MBS Satellite Thermal Cycler (Thermo Scientific). The expected size of the amplified PCR products (Table 2) was determined on an agarose gel with a 100-bp high-range ladder DNA size standard, and the amplified fragments were purified using the MSB Spin PCRapace (Invitek) system and sequenced by means of the dideoxy procedure with the BigDye Terminator v3.1 Cycle Sequencing kit (Life Technologies) and the same primers as for PCR, and analysed with a 3130XL ABI Genetic Analyzer and SeqScape v2.5 software (Life Technologies). PCR products from all cases were sequenced in duplicate from both strands and only cases with changes in both were considered as positive for each different SNV.

Results

Clinical features

There were 11 males and 13 females, with a median age at diagnosis of 56.6 years (range, 31–89 years). In 12 cases the lesion was initially nasal, two cases each had oropharingeal tumours or involvement of the gastrointestinal tract, six cases involved skin and subcutis, and one case each affected pleura and testis, respectively. We obtained complete clinical data from 21 cases, whose median follow-up was of 18.4 months (range, 1–121 months). None of the patients was referred with haemophagocytic syndrome or leukaemic involvement of the peripheral blood. One patient had previously had a renal transplant, one was HIV-positive and another was HCV-positive. At initial diagnosis the Ann Arbor Stage was low (I–II) in seven and two, and high (III–IV) in five and six nasal and extranasal lymphoma patients, respectively. The frequencies of IPI classes for nasal and extranasal cases at diagnosis were: low (four and two patients, respectively), low-intermediate (four and one), intermediate-high (zero and three) and high (two and two). The frequency across PIT classes at presentation was low (eight nasal and three extranasal cases), low-intermediate (one and four), intermediate-high (one and one) and high (zero and zero). First-line therapy was with CHOP or CHOP-like regimens (CHOP-14, CHOP-21, Mega-CHOP) in 18 patients, followed by local radiotherapy in four patients. Three patients received radiotherapy alone and another one underwent local excision and was administered steroids. Two patients received further autologous stem cell transplantation, and in five cases other second line chemotherapeutic regimens, such as SMILE, alemtuzumab, HPER-CVAD, ESHAP and IEV, were also applied. Seventeen patients died of the disease (nine of nasal and eight of extranasal origin) while four remained alive at last follow-up. The median overall survival for patients with nasal and extranasal NKTCLs was 25.54 (range, 2–121) and 10.6 (range, 1–80) months, respectively (Table 3).

Immunohistochemical and *in situ* hybridisation characteristics

EBER and CD3 were positive in all cases, 75% expressed CD56 and there were six CD8-positive, two double-CD8/CD4-positive and 14 double-CD8/CD4-negative cases. Perforin was expressed in 23 (95.8%) of the 24 cases, the intensity of staining being strong in 26.1%, moderate in 43.5% and low in 30.4% of them. Neither CD117 nor beta-catenin was positive in any of the cases, while p53

Table 1. Antibodies used in this series.

Antibody	Clone	Source	Dilution	Method (Automated)	Antigen Retrieval
CD3 FLEX	Polyclonal Rabbit	Dako	Ready to use	AUTOSTAINER (Dako Cytomation)	TRIS EDTA, 20 MIN
CD4 FLEX	4b12	Dako	Ready to use	AUTOSTAINER (Dako Cytomation)	TRIS EDTA, 20 MIN
CD8 FLEX	C8/144b	Dako	Ready to use	AUTOSTAINER (Dako Cytomation)	TRIS EDTA, 20 MIN
CD56 FLEX	1b6	Dako	Ready to use	AUTOSTAINER (Dako Cytomation)	TRIS EDTA, 20 MIN
PERFORINA	5d10	Novocastra	1:25	AUTOSTAINER (Dako Cytomation)	TRIS EDTA, 20 MIN
P53	Do7 (mouse)	Dako	Ready to use	AUTOSTAINER (Dako Cytomation)	TRIS EDTA, 20 MIN
BETA-CATENIN	Beta-catenin-1 (mouse)	Dako	Ready to use	AUTOSTAINER (Dako Cytomation)	TRIS EDTA, 20 MIN
CD117 (C-KIT)	Rabbit polyclonal	Dako	1/200	AUTOSTAINER (Dako Cytomation)	CITRATE, 20 MIN

was intensively positive in five of 22 (22.7%) cases (Table 3 and Figure 1).

Mutational studies

Three cases were heterozygous for the g.272C>T, p.Ala91Val SNV (12.5%). This is a well-known SNP and the most common base substitution identified in the *PRF1* gene [5]. Interestingly, the substitution of c.289G>A resulting in the amino acid residue change p.Ala97Thr in the *PRF1* gene was found in one other case (2.16%). This SNV was not found in any of the SNP databases (dbSNP137; Hapmap; 1000 genomes) or in the COSMIC database (Table 3). Unfortunately, we did not have normal DNA of the patient to rule out the possibility of it being present in the germline. Additionally, 25% of patients showed other SNPs; four patients had the c822C>T; pAla274Ala SNV (all heterozygous), while six showed the g.900C>T; p.His300His SNV (five heterozygous and one homozygous).

All cases with potential pathological *PRF1* SNVs were of nasal origin, representing 25% (3 of 12) of all nasal cases, or 33.3% when considering all the *PRF1* SNVs. Moreover, three of the four cases with *PRF1* SNV died of the disease, following an overall survival of 9.5 months (range, 2–21 months). These data are more in accordance with the outcome of extranasal than with nasal patients. Two of these cases were those that were double-positive for CD4 and CD8, and one appeared in the tumoral tissue of the renal posttransplant patient. Neither intensity of staining nor the pattern of granule distribution was related to the presence of *PRF1* SNVs.

Table 2. Primers used to amplify most of the exon 2 and 3 coding regions of the *PRF1* gene.

EXON 2	Primer Name	Sequence 5′-3′	Amplicon Length (bp)
	PRF_1_F	CATCCTTCTCCTGCTGCTG	221
	PRF_1_R	CCTCCTGTAGGGCATTTTCA	
	PRF_2_F	GCTCCTTCCCAGTGGACA	265
	PRF_2_R	ACATGCACATTGCTGGTG	
	PRF_3_F	ATCCGCAACGACTGGAAG	241
	PRF_3_R	CTTTCCAGGGCTCCTAGACC	
EXON 3	PRF_4_F	TCTCTCTCTTCTCGCAGTTTCC	231
	PRF_4_R	GTCCGTGAGCCCTTCCAG	
	PRF_5_F	CATATCGGCCCTCACTGC	248
	PRF_5_R	GCAGGTCGTTAATGGAGGTG	
	PRF_6_F	GCCTCCTTCCACCAAACCTA	248
	PRF_6_R	GCCCTGTCCGTCAGGTACT	

On the other hand, none of the p53-positive cases showed *PRF1* SNVs, and 80% were of extranasal origin. All cases were double-CD4/CD8-negative, and mainly had a cytoplasmic pattern of perforin expression. All these patients died after a median period of 4.2 months (Table 3).

Discussion

We report for the first time the presence of the g.272C>T, p.Ala91Val SNV of the *PRF1* gene in NKTCLs. We found it in 12.5% of our cases, which is more than twice the percentage of cases expected in a Caucasian population (3% in heterozygosity according to http://www.ncbi.nlm.nih.gov/SNP/snp;rs=rs35947132). These frequencies are remarkable, since NKTCLs account for no more than 1% of all lymphomas in Europe.

The pathogenic role of the g.272C>T variant has long been controversial [15,16], although it is accepted that this SNV leads to reduced cytotoxic activity of the perforin protein due to incorrect folding that decreases its cleavage to the active form and increases its degradation [5,7,17,18,19]. Such a reduction in the level of activity could predispose an individual to late or atypical FHLH, and the development of anaplastic large cell lymphomas, B- and T-cell lymphomas and acute childhood lymphoblastic leukaemia carrying the BCR-ABL fusion gene [7,20,21,22,23]. Except for the ALCL cases described by Cannella et al [21] none of the other T-cell lymphoma cases exhibiting A91V SNV have been correctly categorised according to the current WHO classification. Cannella et al [21] described this SNV in heterozygosity in eight of the 12 patients in which they found other *PRF1* gene mutations. Clementi et al reported a series of eight cases with equal numbers showing *PRF1* gene mutations in homozygosis and heterozygosity. A91V SNV was heterozygous in three of them, one of the cases being a T-cell non-Hodgkin lymphoma (NHL) [24]. Moreover, a *PRF1* gene mutation was described in two cases of subcutaneous panniculitis-like T-cell lymphoma [24,25]. One patient presented the 1168C>T (Arg390stop) in a single allele and the other had two mutations, the 272C>T (A91V) and the 1262G>T (Phe 421Cys), in heterozygosity. Both patients suffered from HLH, a widely described phenomenon in both subcutaneous panniculitis $\alpha\beta$ and $\gamma\delta$ T-cell lymphomas [26].

Except for the double-CD4/CD8 positivity of two cases, which is rare [25,27], all other immunophenotypes of the cases presented

Table 3. Most relevant immunohistochemical and clinical data of these series.

CASE	MUTATION	SEX	AD	LDD	P53	CD56	CD8	CD4	PI	PG	STATUS	OS (months)
1	NMF	M	77	Nasal tissue	N	HI	N	N	N	NP	A	121
2	NMF	M	50	Skin	N	HI	HI	N	Mo	GR	NK	NK
3	NMF	M	57	Nasal tissue	N	LI	N	N	L	GR	D	10
4	***g.272C>T; Ala91Val***	**M**	**71**	**Nasal tissue**	**N**	**N**	**HI**	**P**	**Mo**	**GR**	**D**	**2**
5	NMF	M	47	Skin	N	N	LI	N	L	GR	A	80
6	NMF	F	75	Nasal tissue	N	N	N	N	Mo	GR	D	45
7	NMF	M	46	Testis	N	LI	N	N	Mo	TC	D	1
8	NMF	M	53	Nasal tissue	NV	HI	NV	N	Mo	TC	NK	NK
9	*NMF*	*F*	*69*	*Pleura*	*P*	*HI*	*N*	*N*	*Mo*	*TC*	*D*	*2*
10	NMF	F	31	Pharynx	N	HI	N	N	H	GR	NK	NK
11	NMF	F	53	Nasal tissue	N	N	N	N	L	GR	D	10
12	*NMF*	*F*	*43*	*Nasal tissue*	*P*	*HI*	*N*	*N*	*H*	*TC*	*D*	*6*
13	*NMF*	*F*	*68*	*Skin*	*P*	*HI*	*N*	*N*	*Mo*	*TC*	*D*	*6*
14	NMF	M	78	Nasal tissue	N	HI	N	N	H	GR	A	32
15	NMF	F	34	Intestine	NV	N	N	NV	H	GR	D	3
16	*NMF*	*F*	*31*	*Stomach*	*P*	*HI*	*N*	*N*	*Mo*	*TC*	*D*	*4*
17	*NMF*	*F*	*89*	*Soft tissues*	*P*	*HI*	*N*	*N*	*Mo*	*GR*	*D*	*3*
18	NMF	F	62	Oral cavity	N	N	HI	N	L	GR	D	1
19	NMF	M	78	Skin	N	LI	HI	N	L	GR	D	5
20	***g.272C>T; Ala91Val***	**F**	**48**	**Nasal tissue**	**N**	**HI**	**HI**	**N**	**M**	**TC**	**A**	**21**
21	**c.289G>A; pAla97Thr**	**M**	**64**	**Nasal tissue**	**N**	**HI**	**N**	**N**	**M**	**GR**	**D**	**13**
22	NMF	F	27	Skin	N	HI	N	N	M	TC	D	1
23	***g.272C>T; Ala91Val***	**F**	**52**	**Nasal tissue**	**N**	**HI**	**LI**	**P**	**H**	**GR**	**D**	**2**
24	NMF	M	57	Nasal tissue	N	HI	HI	N	H	GR	D	19

NMF:No mutation found; M:Male; F:F; AD:Age at Diagnosis; LDD:Location of the disease at Diagnosis; N:Negative; P:Positive; NV: Not evaluable; HI: High-Intensity; LI:Low-Intensity; L:Low; Mo:Moderate; NP: Not present; NK: Not Known; PI:Perforin Intensity; PG: Perforin Granules; GR: Golgi Region; TC: Troughout the cytoplasm; A: Alive; D:Dead; OS: Overall Survival.

here were in accordance with previous reports [4,28,29]. Interestingly, these two double-CD4/CD8-positive cases carried the A91V SNV. In the present study, perforin was present in all but one (95.8%) case, although the pattern and intensity of expression varied from case to case. In the various series reported, perforin-positive cases account for 65–86% of NKTCLs [27,30,31,32], perforin losses being related to poor outcome [27]. In the present study, neither intensity of staining nor the pattern of granule distribution was associated with the presence of the A91V SNV.

The expression of other genes frequently found mutated in cancer and NKTCLs were also investigated in these series. Intense p53 staining was found in 22.7% of cases, while none of them expressed either CD117 or beta-catenin. Interestingly, none of the p53-positive cases showed *PRF1* SNVs, all were double-CD4/CD8-negative, and mainly had a cytoplasmic pattern of perforin expression.

The frequencies of mutations of *p53*, *KIT* and *CTNNB1* genes in NKTCLs varied between Asian countries and the rest of the world, suggesting that the development of these mutations is influenced by geographical, environmental and ethnic differences, as has been discussed by many authors [33,34,35,36,37,38]. Moreover, there is a well-known discrepancy in the positive rates between mutational and expression studies [33,34,35,36,37, 38,39]. The highest percentages of cases with mutated *KIT* and *CTNNB1* genes have been found in China (11.1%) and Japan (30.0%). Recently, Huang et al were unable to demonstrate nuclear beta-catenin expression, a result that accords with our findings [40]. The highest known rates for p53 mutation are those for Japan and Indonesia, where it was found in 62% and 63% of cases, respectively. The lowest mutation rates have been found in Korea (31% of cases) and Mexico (24%) [3]. Moreover, Quintanilla et al showed that the *p53* mutation is related to large cell morphology and advanced disease stage [35]. Quintanilla et al reported 60% and 86% of p53-positive cases in Mexican and Peruvian populations, respectively [35,41]. Pongpruttipan et al [29] found 68% of their cases from the Thai population to be positive, while Ye et al [42] found 33.3% of cases to be positive in the Chinese population. The latter two groups exhibited close correlation between p53 expression and both prognosis and advanced disease stage. This and all previously reported studies were done with the same Dako antibody for p53 and using the same cut-off value (>10% positive tumoral cells) to define positivity, with the exception of Ye et al, who used a value of 5%. However, the Quintanilla et al study included exclusively nasal NKTCLs while the others combined nasal and extranasal NKTCL cases in their analyses. In the present series, only one of the five positive cases was of nasal origin, representing 8.3% (one out of 12) of them, while 33.3% of those NKTCLs of extranasal origin (four out of 12) had p53 expression. These data suggest that

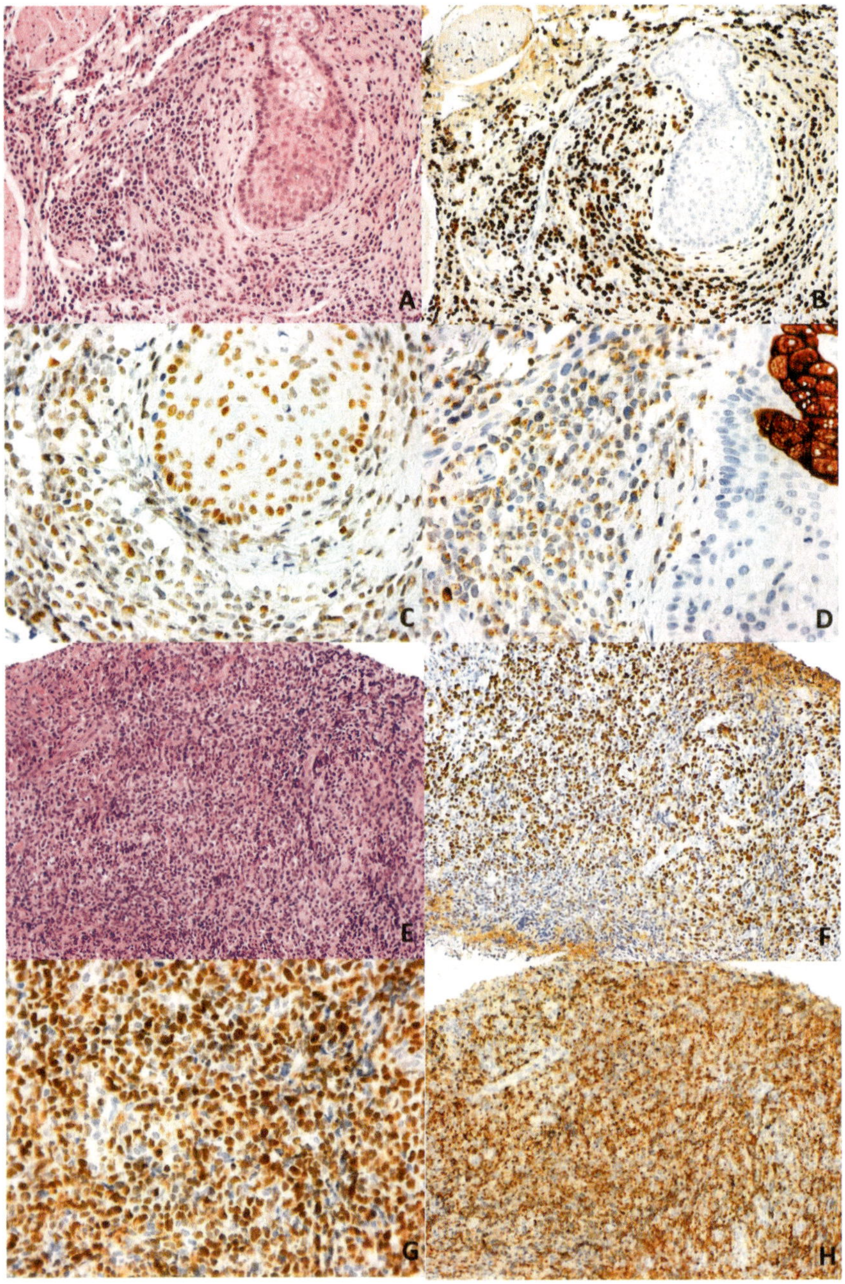

Figure 1. An A91V SNV-positive case (A-HE, staining, B-EBER-positive) showing negativity for p53 (C) and low-level of perforin expression (D). An A91V SNV-negative case (E-HE, staining, F-EBER-positive) showing intense expression of p53 (G) and perforin (H).

p53 expression in NKTCLs in the Spanish population is also different from that in other regions of the world. Nevertheless, in considering all the data from the present study, all of the positive cases were III/IV stage patients, while 52.9% and 29.4% of the negative cases were high- and low-stage patients, respectively.

We found the *PRF1* gene A91V SNV in 25% of nasal NKTCLs but in none of the extranasal ones, while 80% of p53-positive cases were extranasal in origin. Several papers have concluded that the clinical features and treatment response of extranasal and nasal NKTCLs are different [43,44,45,46,47,48], consistent with the results we present herein. Nevertheless, the underlying features responsible for these differences remain to be determined. On the other hand, some authors have suggested that nasal and extranasal NKTCLs behave alike at the same stage of the disease [46,47]. One publication addressing this subject has suggested that there are different genetic alterations in the two subgroups [49]. Nasal NKTCL patients with *PRF1* SNVs seem to behave more aggressively than those without it. The median overall survival of nasal NKTCL patients in our series was 25.5 months, while that of patients carrying *PRF1* SNVs was 9.5 months. On the other hand, p53-positive patients died after a median period of 3.7 months (4.2 months when nasal cases were included), while the value for the entire subgroup of extranasal NKTCLs was 10.6 months. Interestingly, only one of the three nasal NKTCLs carrying the *PRF1* SNVs for whom complete clinical data were available had stage IV disease, while the others were stage I and II.

In addition, the nasal case and three of the four cases positive for p53 for whom clinical data were complete were stage III and IV, respectively.

The pathogenic role of this *PRF1* SNV has been demonstrated and p53 expression is in most cases a surrogate marker for the *P53* gene mutation. The fact that none of the cases carrying *PRF1* SNVs showed p53 expression suggests the role of different pathways in the two diseases. Considering these findings together, leads us to conclude that nasal and extranasal NKTCLs may have different biological backgrounds. Our series was too short to warrant statistical analysis, so a larger series of patients is needed to confirm our findings.

In conclusion, we suggest that the g.272C>T *PRF1* gene SNV in combination with other gene alterations could increase the risk of developing nasal NKTCL, at least in a subgroup of the Spanish population. Moreover, the presence of p53 in 80% of extranasal NKTCLs not carrying the *PRF1* gene SNV suggests there is a different biological background in nasal and extranasal NKTCLs. However, a larger series of patients, stratified by origin and stage of disease and treated in a uniform way needs to be studied to validate our preliminary findings.

Acknowledgments

We thank IFIMAV and the staff of the CNIO Tumour Bank, especially Laura Cereceda and Maria Jesús Artiga.

Author Contributions

Conceived and designed the experiments: SMRP MSB MAP. Performed the experiments: RM GRG LL LS MML. Analyzed the data: RM SMRP LL MAP MSB. Contributed reagents/materials/analysis tools: LS LL LR. Wrote the paper: RM GRG SMRP MSB MAP.

References

1. Swerdlow SH CE, Harris NL, Jaffe ES (2008) WHO Classification of Tumours of Haematopoietic and Lymphoid Tissues. Mature T and NK-cell Neoplasm. Lyon: IARC Press.
2. Lee J, Kim WS, Park YH, Park SH, Park KW, et al. (2005) Nasal-type NK/T cell lymphoma: clinical features and treatment outcome. Br J Cancer 92: 1226–1230.
3. Aozasa K, Takakuwa T, Hongyo T, Yang WI (2008) Nasal NK/T-cell lymphoma: epidemiology and pathogenesis. Int J Hematol 87: 110–117.
4. Li S, Feng X, Li T, Zhang S, Zuo Z, et al. (2013) Extranodal NK/T-cell lymphoma, nasal type: a report of 73 cases at MD Anderson Cancer Center. Am J Surg Pathol 37: 14–23.
5. Brennan AJ, Chia J, Trapani JA, Voskoboinik I (2010) Perforin deficiency and susceptibility to cancer. Cell Death Differ 17: 607–615.
6. Pipkin ME, Rao A, Lichtenheld MG (2010) The transcriptional control of the perforin locus. Immunol Rev 235: 55–72.
7. Voskoboinik I, Trapani JA (2006) Addressing the mysteries of perforin function. Immunol Cell Biol 84: 66–71.
8. Isobe Y, Aritaka N, Setoguchi Y, Ito Y, Kimura H, et al. (2012) T/NK cell type chronic active Epstein-Barr virus disease in adults: an underlying condition for Epstein-Barr virus-associated T/NK-cell lymphoma. J Clin Pathol 65: 278–282.
9. Kimura H, Ito Y, Kawabe S, Gotoh K, Takahashi Y, et al. (2012) EBV-associated T/NK-cell lymphoproliferative diseases in nonimmunocompromised hosts: prospective analysis of 108 cases. Blood 119: 673–686.
10. Katano H, Ali MA, Patera AC, Catalfamo M, Jaffe ES, et al. (2004) Chronic active Epstein-Barr virus infection associated with mutations in perforin that impair its maturation. Blood 103: 1244–1252.
11. Lu G, Xie ZD, Zhao SY, Ye LJ, Wu RH, et al. (2009) Clinical analysis and follow-up study of chronic active Epstein-Barr virus infection in 53 pediatric cases. Chin Med J (Engl) 122: 262–266.
12. Chan KC Q-ML, Ferry JA, Peh SC (2008) Extranodal NK/T-cell lymphoma, nasal type. In: Swerdlow SH, Campo E, Harris NL, et al, eds. WHO Classification of Tumours of Haematopoietic and lymphoid Tissues. Lyon: IARC Press.
13. Garcia JF, Camacho FI, Morente M, Fraga M, Montalban C, et al. (2003) Hodgkin and Reed-Sternberg cells harbor alterations in the major tumor suppressor pathways and cell-cycle checkpoints: analyses using tissue microarrays. Blood 101: 681–689.
14. Kanavaros P, Lescs MC, Briere J, Divine M, Galateau F, et al. (1993) Nasal T-cell lymphoma: a clinicopathologic entity associated with peculiar phenotype and with Epstein-Barr virus. Blood 81: 2688–2695.
15. Molleran Lee S, Villanueva J, Sumegi J, Zhang K, Kogawa K, et al. (2004) Characterisation of diverse PRF1 mutations leading to decreased natural killer cell activity in North American families with haemophagocytic lymphohistiocytosis. J Med Genet 41: 137–144.
16. Zur Stadt U, Beutel K, Weber B, Kabisch H, Schneppenheim R, et al. (2004) A91V is a polymorphism in the perforin gene not causative of an FHLH phenotype. Blood 104: 1909; author reply 1910.
17. Voskoboinik I, Thia MC, Trapani JA (2005) A functional analysis of the putative polymorphisms A91V and N252S and 22 missense perforin mutations associated with familial hemophagocytic lymphohistiocytosis. Blood 105: 4700–4706.
18. Trambas C, Gallo F, Pende D, Marcenaro S, Moretta L, et al. (2005) A single amino acid change, A91V, leads to conformational changes that can impair processing to the active form of perforin. Blood 106: 932–937.
19. Risma KA, Frayer RW, Filipovich AH, Sumegi J (2006) Aberrant maturation of mutant perforin underlies the clinical diversity of hemophagocytic lymphohistiocytosis. J Clin Invest 116: 182–192.
20. Santoro A, Cannella S, Trizzino A, Lo Nigro L, Corsello G, et al. (2005) A single amino acid change A91V in perforin: a novel, frequent predisposing factor to childhood acute lymphoblastic leukemia? Haematologica 90: 697–698.
21. Cannella S, Santoro A, Bruno G, Pillon M, Mussolin L, et al. (2007) Germline mutations of the perforin gene are a frequent occurrence in childhood anaplastic large cell lymphoma. Cancer 109: 2566–2571.
22. Chia J, Yeo KP, Whisstock JC, Dunstone MA, Trapani JA, et al. (2009) Temperature sensitivity of human perforin mutants unmasks subtotal loss of cytotoxicity, delayed FHL, and a predisposition to cancer. Proc Natl Acad Sci U S A 106: 9809–9814.
23. Yang L, Liu H, Zhao J, Da W, Zheng J, et al. (2011) Mutations of perforin gene in Chinese patients with acute lymphoblastic leukemia. Leuk Res 35: 196–199.
24. Clementi R, Locatelli F, Dupre L, Garaventa A, Emmi L, et al. (2005) A proportion of patients with lymphoma may harbor mutations of the perforin gene. Blood 105: 4424–4428.
25. Chen RL, Hsu YH, Ueda I, Imashuku S, Takeuchi K, et al. (2007) Cytophagic histiocytic panniculitis with fatal haemophagocytic lymphohistiocytosis in a paediatric patient with perforin gene mutation. J Clin Pathol 60: 1168–1169.
26. Willemze R, Jansen PM, Cerroni L, Berti E, Santucci M, et al. (2008) Subcutaneous panniculitis-like T-cell lymphoma: definition, classification, and prognostic factors: an EORTC Cutaneous Lymphoma Group Study of 83 cases. Blood 111: 838–845.
27. Pongpruttipan T, Kummalue T, Bedavanija A, Khuhapinant A, Ohshima K, et al. (2011) Aberrant antigenic expression in extranodal NK/T-cell lymphoma: a multi-parameter study from Thailand. Diagn Pathol 6: 79.
28. Ng SB, Lai KW, Murugaya S, Lee KM, Loong SL, et al. (2004) Nasal-type extranodal natural killer/T-cell lymphomas: a clinicopathologic and genotypic study of 42 cases in Singapore. Mod Pathol 17: 1097–1107.
29. Pongpruttipan T, Sukpanichnant S, Assanasen T, Wannakrairot P, Boonsakan P, et al. (2012) Extranodal NK/T-cell lymphoma, nasal type, includes cases of natural killer cell and alphabeta, gammadelta, and alphabeta/gammadelta T-cell origin: a comprehensive clinicopathologic and phenotypic study. Am J Surg Pathol 36: 481–499.
30. Elenitoba-Johnson KS, Khorsand J, King TC (1998) Splenic marginal zone cell lymphoma associated with clonal B-cell populations showing different immunoglobulin heavy chain sequences. Mod Pathol 11: 905–913.
31. Gaal K, Sun NC, Hernandez AM, Arber DA (2000) Sinonasal NK/T-cell lymphomas in the United States. Am J Surg Pathol 24: 1511–1517.
32. Schwartz EJ, Molina-Kirsch H, Zhao S, Marinelli RJ, Warnke RA, et al. (2008) Immunohistochemical characterization of nasal-type extranodal NK/T-cell lymphoma using a tissue microarray: an analysis of 84 cases. Am J Clin Pathol 130: 343–351.
33. Li T, Hongyo T, Syaifudin M, Nomura T, Dong Z, et al. (2000) Mutations of the p53 gene in nasal NK/T-cell lymphoma. Lab Invest 80: 493–499.
34. Petit B, Leroy K, Kanavaros P, Boulland ML, Druet-Cabanac M, et al. (2001) Expression of p53 protein in T- and natural killer-cell lymphomas is associated with some clinicopathologic entities but rarely related to p53 mutations. Hum Pathol 32: 196–204.
35. Quintanilla-Martinez L, Kremer M, Keller G, Nathrath M, Gamboa-Dominguez A, et al. (2001) p53 Mutations in nasal natural killer/T-cell lymphoma from Mexico: association with large cell morphology and advanced disease. Am J Pathol 159: 2095–2105.
36. Hoshida Y, Hongyo T, Jia X, He Y, Hasui K, et al. (2003) Analysis of p53, K-ras, c-kit, and beta-catenin gene mutations in sinonasal NK/T cell lymphoma in northeast district of China. Cancer Sci 94: 297–301.
37. Hongyo T, Hoshida Y, Nakatsuka S, Syaifudin M, Kojya S, et al. (2005) p53, K-ras, c-kit and beta-catenin gene mutations in sinonasal NK/T-cell lymphoma in Korea and Japan. Oncol Rep 13: 265–271.
38. Kurniawan AN, Hongyo T, Hardjolukito ES, Ham MF, Takakuwa T, et al. (2006) Gene mutation analysis of sinonasal lymphomas in Indonesia. Oncol Rep 15: 1257–1263.

39. Takahara M, Kishibe K, Bandoh N, Nonaka S, Harabuchi Y (2004) P53, N- and K-Ras, and beta-catenin gene mutations and prognostic factors in nasal NK/T-cell lymphoma from Hokkaido, Japan. Hum Pathol 35: 86–95.
40. Huang Y, de Reynies A, de Leval L, Ghazi B, Martin-Garcia N, et al. (2010) Gene expression profiling identifies emerging oncogenic pathways operating in extranodal NK/T-cell lymphoma, nasal type. Blood 115: 1226–1237.
41. Quintanilla-Martinez L, Franklin JL, Guerrero I, Krenacs L, Naresh KN, et al. (1999) Histological and immunophenotypic profile of nasal NK/T cell lymphomas from Peru: high prevalence of p53 overexpression. Hum Pathol 30: 849–855.
42. Ye Z, Cao Q, Niu G, Liang Y, Liu Y, et al. (2013) p63 and p53 expression in extranodal NK/T cell lymphoma, nasal type. J Clin Pathol 66: 676–680.
43. Li YX, Fang H, Liu QF, Lu J, Qi SN, et al. (2008) Clinical features and treatment outcome of nasal-type NK/T-cell lymphoma of Waldeyer ring. Blood 112: 3057–3064.
44. Au WY, Weisenburger DD, Intragumtornchai T, Nakamura S, Kim WS, et al. (2009) Clinical differences between nasal and extranasal natural killer/T-cell lymphoma: a study of 136 cases from the International Peripheral T-Cell Lymphoma Project. Blood 113: 3931–3937.
45. Li YX, Liu QF, Fang H, Qi SN, Wang H, et al. (2009) Variable clinical presentations of nasal and Waldeyer ring natural killer/T-cell lymphoma. Clin Cancer Res 15: 2905–2912.
46. Suzuki R, Suzumiya J, Oshimi K (2009) Differences between nasal and extranasal NK/T-cell lymphoma. Blood 113: 6260–6261; author reply 6261–6262.
47. Li YX, Liu QF, Wang WH, Jin J, Song YW, et al. (2011) Failure patterns and clinical implications in early stage nasal natural killer/T-cell lymphoma treated with primary radiotherapy. Cancer 117: 5203–5211.
48. Jo JC, Yoon DH, Kim S, Lee BJ, Jang YJ, et al. (2012) Clinical features and prognostic model for extranasal NK/T-cell lymphoma. Eur J Haematol 89: 103–110.
49. Berti E, Recalcati S, Girgenti V, Fanoni D, Venegoni L, et al. (2010) Cutaneous extranodal NK/T-cell lymphoma: a clinicopathologic study of 5 patients with array-based comparative genomic hybridization. Blood 116: 165–170.

Hazard-Rate Analysis and Patterns of Recurrence in Early Stage Melanoma: Moving towards a Rationally Designed Surveillance Strategy

April K. S. Salama[1,2]☯, Nicole de Rosa[2,3]☯, Randall P. Scheri[2,3], Scott K. Pruitt[2,3], James E. Herndon II[2,4], Jennifer Marcello[4], Douglas S. Tyler[2,3], Amy P. Abernethy[1]*

1 Department of Medicine, Duke University Medical Center, Durham, North Carolina, United States of America, **2** Duke Cancer Institute, Duke University Medical Center, Durham, North Carolina, United States of America, **3** Department of Surgery, Duke University Medical Center, Durham, North Carolina, United States of America, **4** Department of Biostatistics and Bioinformatics, Duke University Medical Center, Durham, North Carolina, United States of America

Abstract

Background: While curable at early stages, few treatment options exist for advanced melanoma. Currently, no consensus exists regarding the optimal surveillance strategy for patients after resection. The objectives of this study were to identify patterns of metastatic recurrence, to determine the influence of metastatic site on survival, and to identify high-risk periods for recurrence.

Methods: A retrospective review of the Duke Melanoma Database from 1970 to 2004 was conducted that focused on patients who were initially diagnosed without metastatic disease. The time to first recurrence was computed from the date of diagnosis, and the associated hazard function was examined to determine the peak risk period of recurrence. Metastatic sites were coded by the American Joint Committee on Cancer (AJCC) system including local skin, distant skin and nodes (M1a), lung (M1b), and other distant (M1c).

Results: Of 11,615 patients initially diagnosed without metastatic disease, 4616 (40%) had at least one recurrence. Overall the risk of initial recurrence peaked at 12 months. The risk of initial recurrence at the local skin, distant skin, and nodes peaked at 8 months, and the risk at lung and other distant sites peaked at 24 months. Patients with a cutaneous or nodal recurrence had improved survival compared to other recurrence types.

Conclusions: The risk of developing recurrent melanoma peaked at one year, and the site of first recurrence had a significant impact on survival. Defining the timing and expected patterns of recurrence will be important in creating an optimized surveillance strategy for this patient population.

Editor: Andrzej T Slominski, University of Tennessee, United States of America

Funding: This study was funded through an Outcomes Research service agreement with Pfizer, Inc. The funders had no role in study design, data collection and analysis, decision to publish, or preparation of the manuscript.

Competing Interests: The authors have read the journal's policy and have the following conflicts. At the time of this study, Dr. Abernethy had a nominal consulting role with Pfizer, Inc., ($10,000); this has since discontinued. All other authors report no conflict of interest. This does not alter the authors' adherence to all the PLOS ONE policies on sharing data and materials.

* E-mail: amy.abernethy@duke.edu

☯ These authors contributed equally to this work.

Introduction

Melanoma is one of the few cancers whose incidence continues to rise, and in 2012, an estimated 76,250 new cases will be diagnosed in the United States [1]. Fortunately, the majority of these patients are diagnosed with localized disease and are considered cured. Despite this, approximately 20–30% of early stage melanoma patients develop a recurrence during their lifetime, with much higher rates seen in patients with regionally advanced disease [2]. The optimal timing and modality of surveillance after initial diagnosis and treatment is not known. Historically, routine imaging studies have not been shown to improve outcomes, and additional concerns have been raised regarding the risks of radiation exposure, the high false positivity rate and cost effectiveness [3,4,5,6]. Additionally, recent data suggests that frequent exams over an extended time period may be of limited benefit [7,8]. Currently, clinical practice varies widely and there is no consensus regarding the type, timing, or duration of radiologic or clinical evaluations. Timing of imaging surveillance is often guided by the data collection processes used in clinical trials, practical aspects of clinical care, experience in other cancers, and anecdote. Ideally, surveillance patterns would be matched to objective observations about metastatic patterns of spread in melanoma and risk for subsequent relapse. The lack of an improvement in outcomes with screening in historical series is likely influenced by the limited availability of systemic agents to alter the course of advanced disease, a landscape that has changed markedly over the past few years. The objective of this study was to determine high-risk periods of recurrence by metastatic site as a first step to designing practical surveillance care for patients with melanoma. For the over 800,000 people currently living in the United States with a previous diagnosis of melanoma, a rationally designed surveillance strategy could allow for improved disease outcomes, time savings, and a reduction in wasteful health resource utilization [9].

Methods

Population

All patients with melanoma at Duke University Medical Center were entered into a prospectively maintained computerized, single-institution registry database from 1970 to 2004. A retrospective review was conducted. All patients had histologically confirmed melanoma. Patient data including clinical characteristics, pathologic findings, date and status at last follow-up were entered prospectively into the database by trained data managers. Approval for this study was obtained from the Duke University Health System Institutional Review Board, and a waiver for written consent was granted. Because this study was a retrospective database review, it was felt to only represent a minimal risk of loss of confidentiality to any included patient. Precautions were taken to further minimize this risk, and all data were analyzed anonymously. Only the principal investigator and key personnel had access to the identified master file, which was stored in a secured location.

The Duke Melanoma Database is comprised of data from 14,029 patients. Exclusion criteria for this study included patients who presented with metastatic disease at diagnosis, who had a recorded recurrence within 30 days of initial diagnosis, or who were followed for less than 30 days; after these exclusions there were 11,615 patients included in the analysis.

Classification of recurrence

The first 3 sites of recurrence were summarized for each patient. Metastatic sites were categorized into 4 groups corresponding with American Joint Cancer Committee staging criteria: 1) local skin; 2) distant skin and lymph nodes including intransit nodes; 3) lung; and, 4) other distant sites which included adrenal glands, bone, central nervous system, eye, gastrointestinal, liver, other, and death due to metastases but not otherwise specified. If multiple recurrences occurred within 30 days of each other (in either direction) then recurrences were combined and counted as one event; the event was assigned the date of the earliest recurrence and the site was classified according to that site with the worst expected prognosis based on current staging criteria such that non-pulmonary visceral disease represented the poorest prognositc group, followed by patients with pulmonary metastases, distant skin and nodes, and local skin recurrence only.

Statistical methods

Patient characteristics and the pattern of metastatic spread from the first to third recurrence were summarized using basic descriptive statistics. Contingency tables were used to compare patient characteristics (sex, Clark's level, ulceration, Breslow thickness, primary site, and histology) and type of lymph node procedure between patients with and without recurrences. The mean age by recurrence status was computed. Kaplan-Meier survival estimates and plots were produced to summarize time from diagnosis to death by recurrence status (no recurrence vs. at least one recurrence). Among patients who had at least one recurrence, survival from time of first recurrence was summarized by site of first recurrence.

Table 1. Patient characteristics.

	No recurrences		At least one recurrence		Total	
Sex (%)						
Male	3592	(51.3)	2696	(58.4)	6288	(54.1)
Female	3407	(48.7)	1920	(41.6)	5327	(45.9)
Age at Diagnosis						
Mean (SD)	49 (15.1)		48 (14.9)		48.6 (15.0)	
Thickness of Invasion mm (%)						
≤1.00	2033	(29.0)	665	(14.4)	2698	(23.2)
1.01–2.0	2256	(32.2)	1237	(26.8)	3493	(30.1)
2.01–4.0	1076	(15.4)	1050	(22.7)	2126	(18.3)
>4.0	387	(5.5)	583	(12.6)	970	(8.4)
Missing/not recorded	1247	(17.8)	1081	(23.4)	2328	(20.0)
Clarks level of primary (%)						
Level I/In situ	281	(4.0)	58	(1.3)	339	(2.9)
Level II	691	(9.9)	205	(4.4)	896	(7.7)
Level III	2499	(35.7)	1322	(28.6)	3821	(32.9)
Level IV	2634	(37.6)	2015	(43.7)	4649	(40.0)
Level V	211	(3.0)	307	(6.7)	518	(4.5)
Unknown level	173	(2.5)	523	(11.3)	696	(6.0)
Does not apply	510	(7.3)	186	(4.0)	696	(6.0)
Ulceration (%)						
No	5496	(78.5)	2804	(60.7)	8300	(71.5)
Yes	712	(10.2)	1035	(22.4)	1747	(15.0)
Missing/not recorded	791	(11.3)	777	(16.8)	1568	(13.5)
Site of primary melanoma (%)						
Trunk	2586	(36.9)	1987	(43.0)	4573	(39.4)
Upper Extremity	1270	(18.1)	554	(12.0)	1824	(15.7)
Lower Extremity	1415	(20.2)	945	(20.5)	2360	(20.3)
Head/Neck	1176	(16.8)	885	(19.2)	2061	(17.7)
Eye	516	(7.4)	153	(3.3)	669	(5.8)
Other	36	(0.5)	91	(2.0)	127	(1.1)
Missing/not recorded	0	(0)	1	(0)	1	(0)

The period of highest risk for recurrence was evaluated by plotting the hazard function for time to 1st, 2nd and 3rd recurrence and noting the maximum hazard. The hazard function was estimated from the Kaplan-Meier survival function using the Epanechnikov Kernal smoothing method with a bandwidth of 8 and 101 grid points. Time to first recurrence was calculated from initial diagnosis and patients who did not have any recurrences were censored at their time of death or date last contact. Time to second recurrence was calculated for all patients who had at least one recurrence from date of first recurrence to date of 2nd recurrence or date of death/last contact if censored. Likewise, time to third recurrence was calculated among patients with at least 2 recurrences as time from 2nd recurrence to time to 3rd recurrence or date of death/last contact if censored. Since we defined a new recurrence to be at least 30 days from any previous recurrence, any patient who died or was otherwise lost to follow-up less than 1 month after their last recurrence was considered not to be at risk of recurrence and was excluded from calculation of the hazard function.

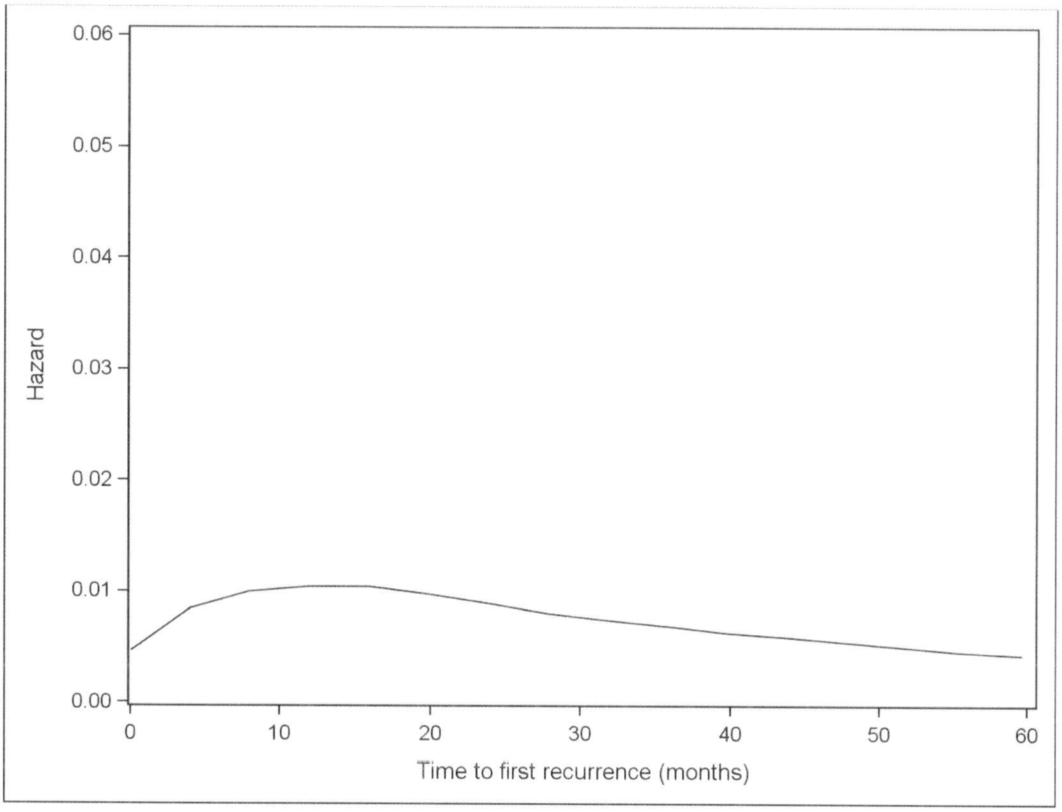

Figure 1. Hazard plot for first recurrence among all patients.

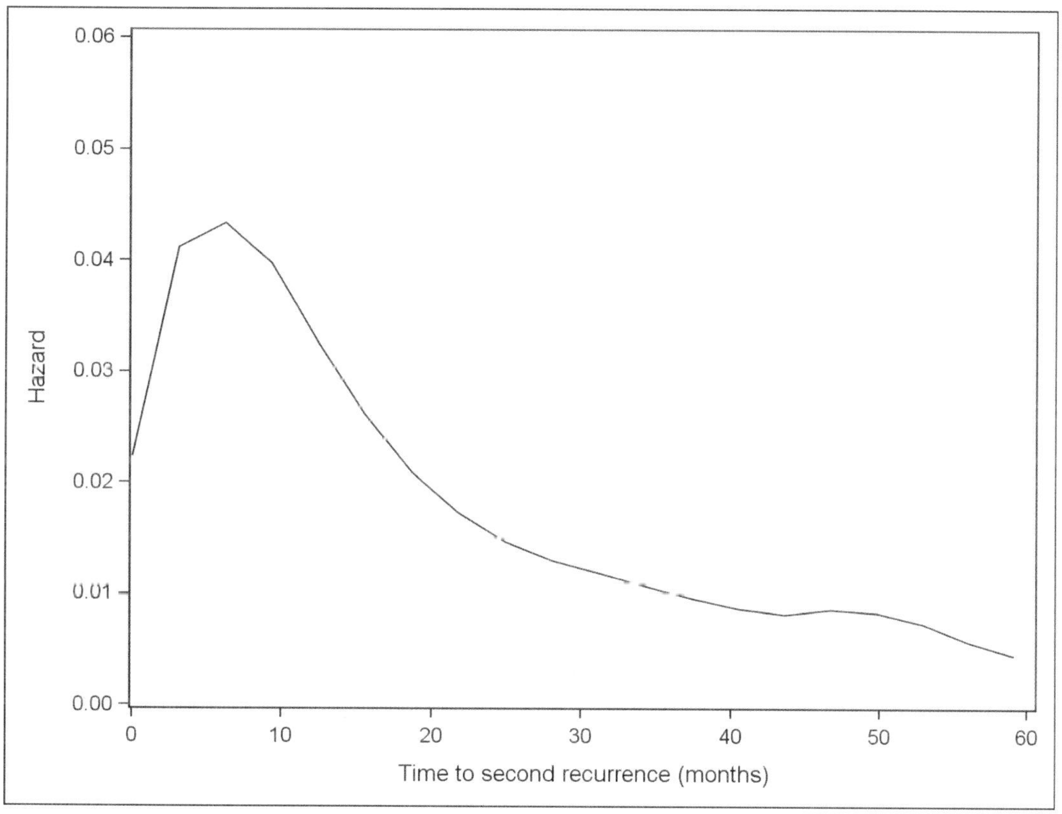

Figure 2. Hazard plot for 2nd recurrence among all patients with at least one recurrence.

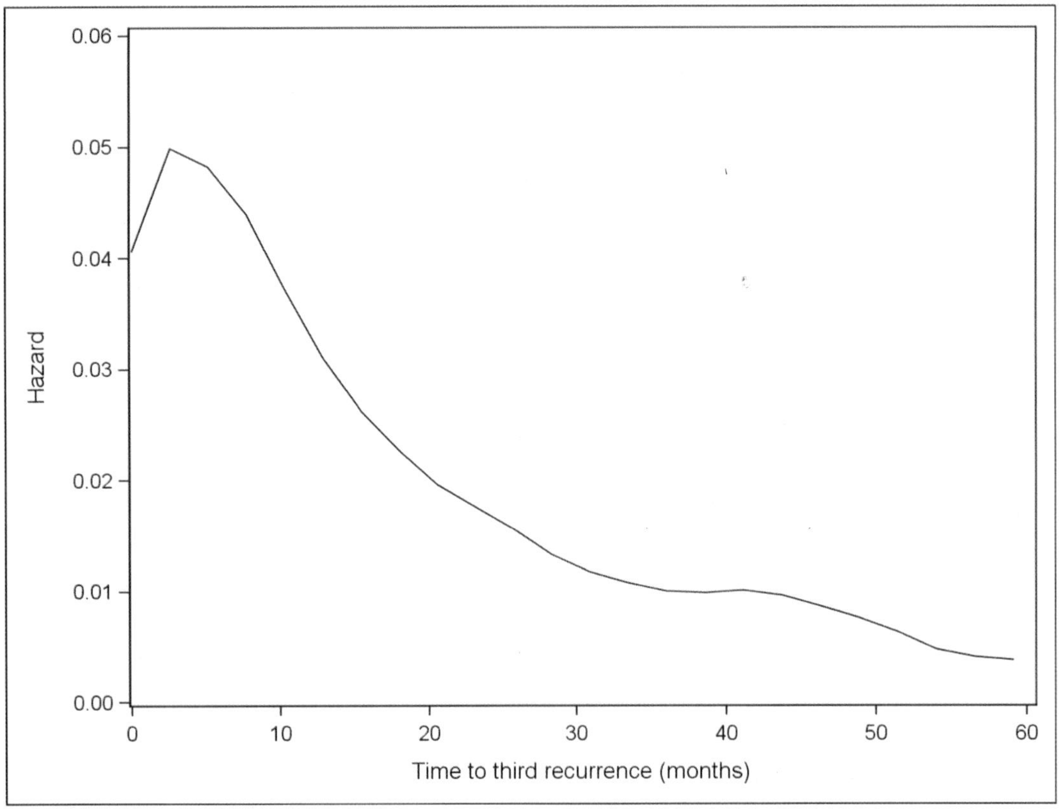

Figure 3. Hazard plot for 3rd recurrence among all patients with at least two recurrences.

The hazard of a first recurrence in local skin, distant skin/ nodes, lung, or other distant metastasis was estimated for each site separately and then plotted together for comparison. The definition for time to first recurrence remained the same when estimating each of the 4 hazard functions, however patients whose recurrence was not at the site being estimated were censored at the time of their first recurrence.

All data manipulation and analysis was performed with SAS v9.2 (Cary, NC).

Results

From 1970 to 2004, 14,029 patients with melanoma were treated at Duke Univerisity Medical Center. Patients who presented with metastatic disease at diagnosis, who had a recorded recurrence within 30 days of initial diagnosis, or who were followed for less than 30 days were excluded from this analysis. Of the 11,615 eligible patients, 4,616 (40%) had at least one recurrence during long-term follow-up. The clinicopathologic characteristics of these patients are shown in Table 1.

Hazard Risk of Recurrence

Overall, the risk of initial recurrence peaked at 12 months (Figure 1). The risk of initial recurrence at local skin, distant skin and nodes occurred early and peaked at 8 months while the risk of initial recurrence at lung and other distant sites occurred later and peaked at 24 months. After the initial recurrence, subsequent metastases appeared at progessively shorter intervals, with the time to development of second and third metastases peaking at 6.2 and 2.6 months, respectively (Figures 2 and 3). Although the risk of recurrence decreased over time, it did not reach zero.

Table 2. Summary of lymph node procedures performed.

	no recurrence		1+ recurrences (any site)		All	
	N	(%)	N	(%)	N	(%)
Had sentinel lymph node biopsy	255	(3.6)	79	(1.7)	334	(2.9)
Had full node dissection (no SLN)	1119	(16)	1917	(42)	3036	(26)
Had other lymph node procedure	152	(2.2)	1446	(31)	1598	(14)
No lymph node procedures recorded	5473	(78)	1174	(25)	6647	(57)

Table 3. Incidence of first recurrence by site.

	N	%
Local skin	742	16.1
Distant skin + nodes	2725	59.0
Nodes: 2487(91.3%)		
Distant Skin: 196(7.2%)		
Both: 42(1.5%)		
Lung	386	8.4
Other distant metastases	763	16.5
Total	4616	100.0

Patterns of Metastatic Disease

The most common site of initial recurrence was distant skin or nodes (59%). Of these patients, 91% experienced a nodal recurrence. One quarter of patients in this study had no lymph node assessment documented, while 42% of these patients underwent a completion lymph node dissection, 1.7% had a sentinel lymph node biopsy, and 31% had some type of other lymph node procedure, as listed in Table 2. The second most common site of metastasis was other distant metastases (16.5%), followed by local skin (16.1%), and lung (8.4%) (Table 3). In order to determine if the initial site of metastasis was predictive of future sites of recurrence, sites of second and third recurrences were analyzed. Patterns of spread varied widely across the melanoma population, and an appreciable pattern was not identified. Table 4 lists the incidence of second recurrence by site of first recurrence.

Survival

The median 5 and 10 year survival rates from the time of diagnosis were 92.5% (95% CI 91.7–93.2) and 84.3% (83.0–85.4) for patients without a recurrence, compared to 59.8% (58.3–61.2) and 38.9% (37.3–40.5) for patients whose disease had recurred. As expected, there was an association between survival and the initial site of recurrence. Among those who recurred, patients with an initial recurrence in the local skin had the best median survival from the time of recurrence (72 months), followed by distant skin and nodes (37 months), lung (12 months), and other distant metastasis (5 months; Figure 4).

Table 4. Incidence of second recurrence by site of first recurrence.

Site 1	**Site 2**	**N pts**
Local skin	None	200
	Local skin	176
	Distant skin + nodes	225
	Lung	65
	Other distant metastases	76
Distant skin + nodes	None	1089
	Local skin	163
	Distant skin + nodes	685
	Lung	225
	Other distant metastases	563
Lung	None	248
	Local skin	9
	Distant skin + nodes	23
	Lung	17
	Other distant metastases	89
Other distant metastases	None	659
	Local skin	2
	Distant skin + nodes	21
	Lung	17
	Other distant metastases	64

Discussion

Limited data is available regarding the optimal surveillance strategy for patients diagnosed with early stage melanoma. With over 11,000 patients, this study represents one of the largest cohorts reported to our knowledge. By using a hazard rate analysis, we sought to identify the highest risk period for recurrence in order to define a window where patients are most likely to benefit from surveillance.

In this study, we found that the risk of initial recurrence peaked at 12 months, which is consistent with current data showing that most metastases develop within the first few years after initial diagnosis [7,8]. The risk of recurrence at local skin, distant skin and nodes occurred early and peaked at 8 months, while distant metastasis to lung and other sites occurred later and peaked at 24 months. The risk of recurrence never returned to zero, as it is well documented that late recurrences can occur in a small percentage of patients, especially those with early stage disease [10,11,12,13,14,15,16]. The pattern of metastatic disease, in which most patients presented with a distant cutaneous or nodal recurrence, is similar to other reported series, and may be reflective of the fact that many patients were diagnosed prior to the routine use of sentinel lymph node biopsies [17,18]. Subsequent analyses in patients who have undergone a sentinel lymph node biopsy suggest that there is a lower proportion of regional nodal recurrences [19,20,21,22].

Furthermore, our data shows that once a metastatic lesion is identified, the remission period sequentially shortens with the risk of a second recurrence peakng at 6 months, and that of a third recurrence at 2.6 months. Survival, as expected, was also site dependent, with patients who initially developed metastases to the skin or lymph nodes having a longer median survival compared to patients who presented with metastases to visceral organs.

The driving force behind any surveillance strategy in oncology is that detecting a recurrence before a patient becomes symptomatic should have a favorable impact on survival. While case series have suggested that recurrences that are amenable to a surgical intervention (i.e., detected earlier) are associated with improved survival, this principle has not held true for most patients with melanoma [23]. The majority of recurrences are detected by patients themselves, and no imaging modality has provided a clear survival benefit [24,25]. An analysis by Turner et al showed that a less intensive monitoring schedule would likely only result in a small delay in the time to detect a recurrence, yet has the potential to save thousands of clinic visits over a 10 year course of follow up [7]. Despite the data, the desire to detect (and sometimes the fear of missing) these early recurrences has provided a rationale to adopt some type of surveillance strategy. With the landscape of systemic therapeutic options for advanced melanoma rapidly evolving, patients may stand to benefit from early treatment when they are asymptomatic, highlighting the importance of developing

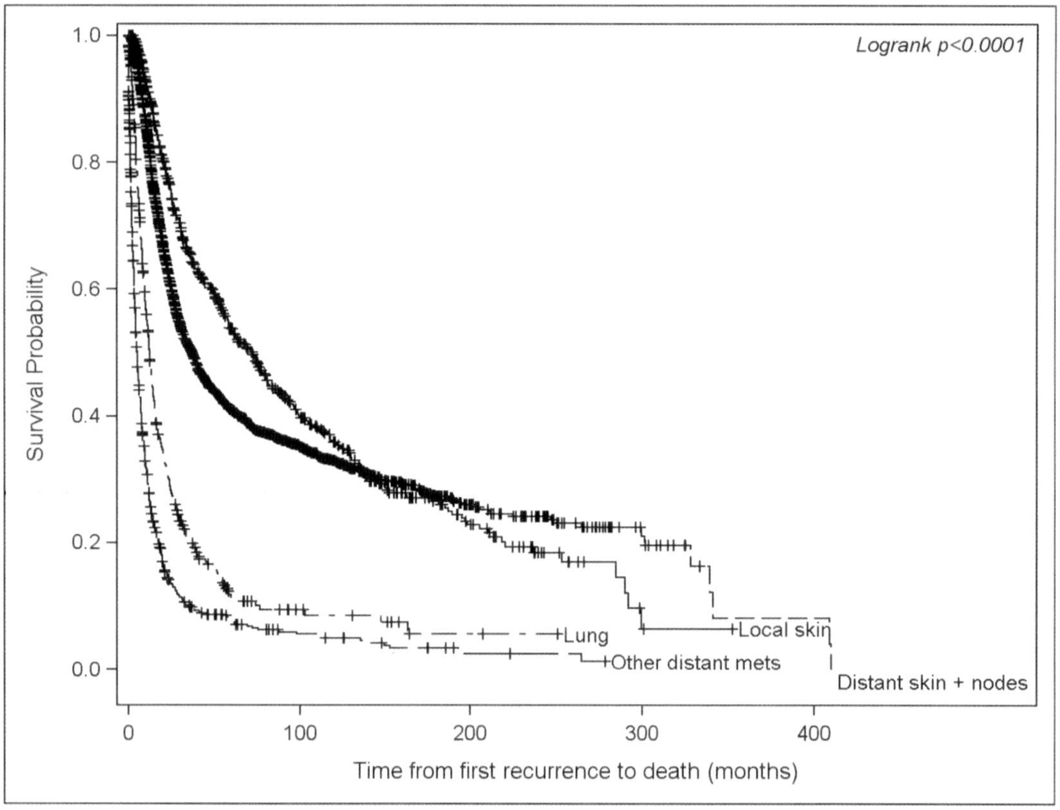

Figure 4. Kaplan-Meier survival from first recurrence by site.

a structured surveillance program that maximizes the potential advantages of early detection without placing an undue burden on patients or the healthcare system.

This study is limited by its retrospective design, and the lack of routine sentinel lymph node biopsies during the time period may influence timing and pattern of recurrence. Additionally, information regarding subsequent therapy and other patient related factors was not possible to identify in this retrospectively analyzed dataset. Nevertheless, this is a large cohort treated at a single institution and it serves to provide an initial framework for analyzing the pattern and timing of disease recurrence- a critical step to the development of any surveillance protocol.

In the absence of definitive data, opinions vary widely and currently no uniform standard exists regarding the appropriate follow up interval, use of imaging modalities, or optimal duration of follow up. The primary site of recurrence was not predictive of a pattern regarding the development of subsequent recurrences, suggesting that it may be difficult to tailor a surveillance strategy to an individual patient and that a standardized approach should be used for all patients once they recur. The initial site of metastasis directly correlated with prognosis in our population, consistent with the current AJCC staging system. Additionally, our study showed that recurrences tended to peak within the first 1–2 years after diagnosis, suggesting that intensive follow up beyond this period may be of lower yield.

Prospective surveillance protocols, designed to assess both the optimal follow-up interval and use of imaging modalities will be critical in order to move forward. Based on our data, structuring a program tailored to risk of recurrence based on the time since diagnosis is one approach for future work. A proposed strategy for surveillance might be to combine routine physical exam with more sensitive radiologic modalities, eg CT or PET/CT, for patients felt to be at high risk of recurrence based on current staging and prognostic information during the first year after diagnosis, as this was the highest risk period for in our overall population. Imaging and clinical exams could be performed at 3–6 month intervals depending on initial risk, and the follow up interval could subsequently be extended in the second and third years. With regards to specific subsets of patients, in this study, only a minority of patients underwent a sentinel lymph node biopsy. In the current era, sentinel lymph node assessment is considered at our institution for most patients with primaries >0.75 mm or thinner lesions with adverse features such as ulceration or an elevated mitotic rate. For patients who meet these criteria, but elect not to proceed with lymph node assessment, focused sonographic imaging and clinical exam of the lymph node basin may be a reasonable option, as a high proportion of nodal recurrences were seen in this study. The Multicenter Selective Lymphadenectomy Trial II (MSLT-2; NCT00297895), in which patients with a positive sentinel node are randomized to receive either serial ultrasound and clinical exams or completion lymph node dissection will hopefully address the utility of this strategy in patients with a positive sentinel lymph node. While the optimal follow up for patients who elect not to undergo any lymph node assessment remains undefined, the high rate of nodal relapse in this study suggests that this may be a reasonable option for this patient population as well. As the risk of recurrence peaked in the first two years in this study, intensive screening with radiologic studies and frequent physical exams beyond this point may be less useful, as relatively fewer recurrences would be detected. This study represents an initial step in creating a framework for future prospective evaluation of surveillance strategies by identifying high risk periods for recurrence. In the current era of resource management, a data driven method of surveillance for melanoma patients, as well as the determination of the most common sites of recurrence may allow for a defined surveillance strategy that is both cost effective and patient focused.

Author Contributions

Conceived and designed the experiments: DT AA. Analyzed the data: AS NR RS SP JH JM DT AA. Contributed reagents/materials/analysis tools: JH JM DT AA. Wrote the paper: AS NR AA.

References

1. Siegel R, Naishadham D, Jemal A (2012) Cancer statistics, 2012. CA Cancer J Clin 62: 10–29.
2. Balch CM, Gershenwald JE, Soong SJ, Thompson JF, Atkins MB, et al. (2009) Final version of 2009 AJCC melanoma staging and classification. J Clin Oncol 27: 6199–6206.
3. Morton RL, Craig JC, Thompson JF (2009) The role of surveillance chest X-rays in the follow-up of high-risk melanoma patients. Ann Surg Oncol 16: 571–577.
4. Xing Y, Bronstein Y, Ross MI, Askew RL, Lee JE, et al. (2011) Contemporary diagnostic imaging modalities for the staging and surveillance of melanoma patients: a meta-analysis. J Natl Cancer Inst 103: 129–142.
5. Brenner DJ, Hall EJ (2007) Computed tomography--an increasing source of radiation exposure. N Engl J Med 357: 2277–2284.
6. Weiss M, Loprinzi CL, Creagan ET, Dalton RJ, Novotny P, et al. (1995) Utility of follow-up tests for detecting recurrent disease in patients with malignant melanomas. JAMA 274: 1703–1705.
7. Turner RM, Bell KJ, Morton RL, Hayen A, Francken AB, et al. (2011) Optimizing the Frequency of Follow-Up Visits for Patients Treated for Localized Primary Cutaneous Melanoma. J Clin Oncol.
8. Romano E, Scordo M, Dusza SW, Coit DG, Chapman PB (2010) Site and timing of first relapse in stage III melanoma patients: implications for follow-up guidelines. J Clin Oncol 28: 3042–3047.
9. Howlader N, Noone AM, Krapcho M, Neyman N, Aminou R, et al. SEER Cancer Statistics Review, 1975–2008, National Cancer Institute. Bethesda, MD. Available: http://seer.cancer.gov/csr/1975_2008/.Based on November 2010 SEER data submission, posted to the SEER web site , 2011.
10. Crowley NJ, Seigler HF (1990) Late recurrence of malignant melanoma. Analysis of 168 patients. Ann Surg 212: 173–177.
11. Hansel G, Schonlebe J, Haroske G, Wollina U (2010) Late recurrence (10 years or more) of malignant melanoma in south-east Germany (Saxony). A single-centre analysis of 1881 patients with a follow-up of 10 years or more. J Eur Acad Dermatol Venereol 24: 833–836.
12. Shaw HM, Beattie CW, McCarthy WH, Milton GW (1985) Late relapse from cutaneous stage I malignant melanoma. Arch Surg 120: 1155–1159.
13. Callaway MP, Briggs JC (1989) The incidence of late recurrence (greater than 10 years); an analysis of 536 consecutive cases of cutaneous melanoma. Br J Plast Surg 42: 46–49.
14. Koh HK, Sober AJ, Fitzpatrick TB (1984) Late recurrence (beyond ten years) of cutaneous malignant melanoma. Report of two cases and a review of the literature. JAMA 251: 1859–1862.
15. McCarthy WH, Shaw HM, Thompson JF, Milton GW (1988) Time and frequency of recurrence of cutaneous stage I malignant melanoma with guidelines for follow-up study. Surg Gynecol Obstet 166: 497–502.
16. Reintgen DS, Cox C, Slingluff CL, Jr., Seigler HF (1992) Recurrent malignant melanoma: the identification of prognostic factors to predict survival. Ann Plast Surg 28: 45–49.
17. Tas F (2012) Metastatic Behavior in Melanoma: Timing, Pattern, Survival, and Influencing Factors. J Oncol 2012: 647684.
18. Tejera-Vaquerizo A, Barrera-Vigo MV, Fernandez-Canedo I, Blazquez-Sanchez N, Mendiola-Fernandez M, et al. (2007) [Longitudinal study of different metastatic patterns in the progression of cutaneous melanoma]. Actas Dermosifiliogr 98: 531–538.
19. Carlson GW, Page AJ, Cohen C, Parker D, Yaar R, et al. (2008) Regional recurrence after negative sentinel lymph node biopsy for melanoma. Ann Surg 248: 378–386.
20. Gershenwald JE, Colome MI, Lee JE, Mansfield PF, Tseng C, et al. (1998) Patterns of recurrence following a negative sentinel lymph node biopsy in 243 patients with stage I or II melanoma. J Clin Oncol 16: 2253–2260.
21. Dalal KM, Patel A, Brady MS, Jaques DP, Coit DG (2007) Patterns of first-recurrence and post-recurrence survival in patients with primary cutaneous melanoma after sentinel lymph node biopsy. Ann Surg Oncol 14: 1934–1942.
22. Zogakis TG, Essner R, Wang HJ, Foshag LJ, Morton DL (2007) Natural history of melanoma in 773 patients with tumor-negative sentinel lymph nodes. Ann Surg Oncol 14: 1604–1611.
23. Petersen RP, Hanish SI, Haney JC, Miller CC, 3rd, Burfeind WR, Jr., et al. (2007) Improved survival with pulmonary metastasectomy: an analysis of 1720 patients with pulmonary metastatic melanoma.[see comment]. Journal of Thoracic & Cardiovascular Surgery 133: 104–110.
24. Nieweg OE, Kroon BB (2006) The conundrum of follow-up: should it be abandoned? Surg Oncol Clin N Am 15: 319–330.
25. Francken AB, Shaw HM, Accortt NA, Soong SJ, Hoekstra HJ, et al. (2007) Detection of first relapse in cutaneous melanoma patients: implications for the formulation of evidence-based follow-up guidelines. Ann Surg Oncol 14: 1924–1933.

Clinic Attendances during the First 12 Months of Life for Aboriginal Children in Five Remote Communities of Northern Australia

Thérèse Kearns[1]*, Danielle Clucas[2], Christine Connors[3], Bart J. Currie[1,3], Jonathan R. Carapetis[4], Ross M. Andrews[1]

1 Child Health Division, Menzies School of Health Research, Charles Darwin University, Darwin, Northern Territory, Australia, **2** Department of Paediatrics, The University of Melbourne, Melbourne, Victoria, Australia, **3** Preventable Chronic Conditions, Northern Territory Department of Health and Families, Darwin, Northern Territory, Australia, **4** Telethon Institute for Child Health Research, Centre for Child Health Research, University of Western, Perth, Western Australia, Australia

Abstract

Background: The vast majority (>75%) of Aboriginal people in the Northern Territory (NT) live in remote or very remote locations. Children in these communities have high attendance rates at local Primary Health Care (PHC) centres but there is a paucity of studies documenting the reason and frequency of attendance. Such data can be used to help guide public health policy and practice.

Methods and Findings: Clinic presentations during the first year of life were reviewed for 320 children born from 1 January 2001–31 December 2006. Data collected included reason for infectious presentation, antibiotic prescription and referral to hospital. The median number of presentations per child in the first year of life was 21 (IQR 15–29) with multiple reasons for presentation. The most prominent infectious presentations per child during the first year of life were upper respiratory tract infections (median 6, IQR 3–10); diarrhoea (median 3, IQR 1–5); ear disease (median 3, IQR 1–5); lower respiratory tract infection (median 3, IQR 2–5); scabies (median 3, IQR 1–5); and skin sores (median 3, IQR 2–5).

Conclusions: Infectious diseases of childhood are strongly linked with poverty, poor living conditions and overcrowding. The data reported in our study were collected through manual review, however many remote communities now have established electronic health record systems, use the Key Performance Indicator System and are engaged in CQI (continuous quality improvement) processes. Building on these recent initiatives, there is an opportunity to incorporate routine monitoring of a range of infectious conditions (we suggest diarrhoea, LRTI, scabies and skin sores) using both the age at first presentation and the median number of presentations per child during the first year of life as potential indicators of progress in addressing health inequities in remote communities.

Editor: Martyn Kirk, The Australian National University, Australia

Funding: This work was supported by the Cooperative Research Council for Aboriginal Health (http://www.lowitja.org.au/), Rio Tinto Aboriginal Foundation (http://www.riotinto.com/), Ian Potter Foundation (http://www.ianpotter.org.au/), and the Australian Government Office of Aboriginal and Torres Strait Islander Health. The funders had no role in study design, data collection and analysis, decision to publish, or preparation of the manuscript.

Competing Interests: The authors have declared that no competing interests exist.

* E-mail: therese.kearns@menzies.edu.au

Introduction

Disparities in disease burden and life expectancy for Aboriginal and Torres Strait Islander people in Australia are well documented, even more so for those living in remote/very remote locations. [1] In the Northern Territory (NT), more than 75% of Aboriginal people live in remote or very remote locations. [1] Previously reported data from three remote communities highlighted very high clinic attendance rates and a previously unrecognized burden of skin infections commencing within the first few months of life. [2,3] We have now extended the study to include six birth cohorts (2001–2006) across five remote Aboriginal communities within the same region. We have focused our analyses using the presentations per child as the primary unit of measure and report clinic presentations for a range of infectious conditions.

Methods

We reviewed clinic presentations during the first year of life for children in five remote communities born from 1 January 2001 to 31 December 2006. The communities, located approximately 500–1000 km east of Darwin, were participating in the East Arnhem Regional Healthy Skin Project (EARHSP). [4] Children were recruited to the EARHSP by local researchers going house to house. Written informed consent was obtained from the parents/guardian to screen their child for clinical signs of scabies and skin sores and to conduct an audit of their clinic presentations.

Each community had a locally based Primary Health Care (PHC) centre, providing acute and chronic care as well as an after-hours emergency service. We estimated the total annual birth cohort for these five communities from 2001–2006 to be approximately 1500 (250 per year). For the purposes of this study,

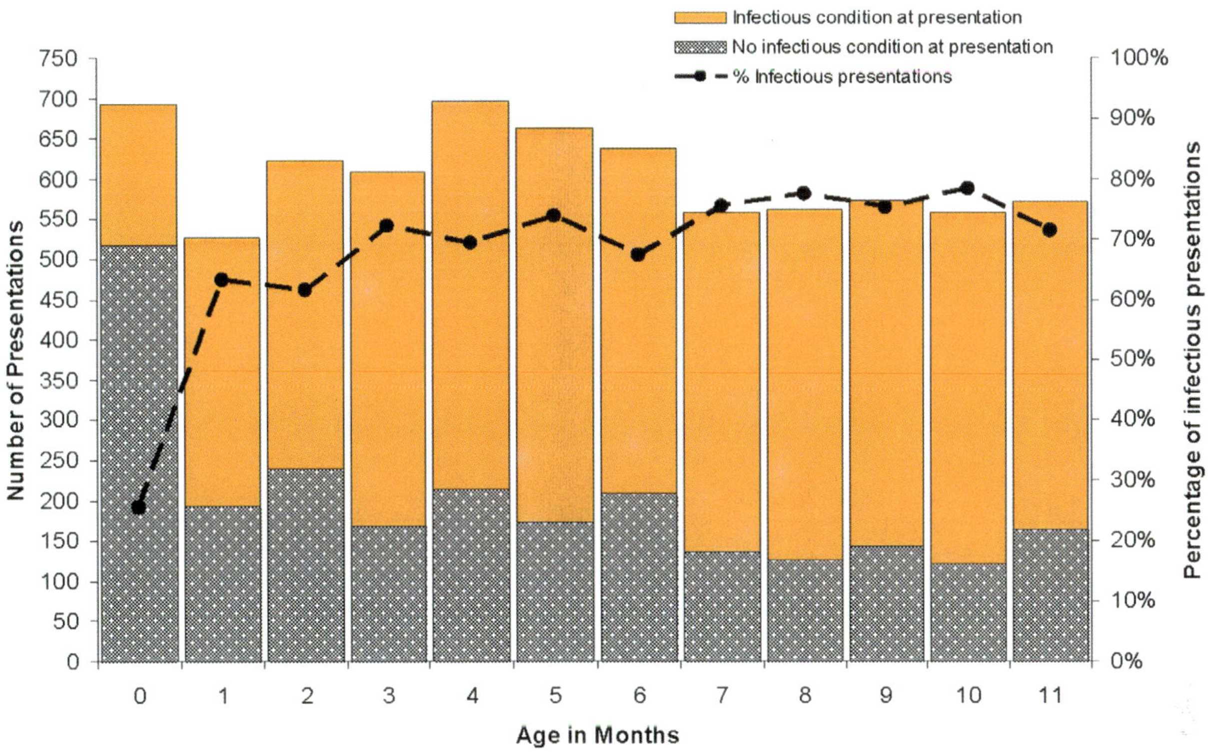

Figure 1. Presentations to health centre by age in months.

data for 320 children were included from a total of 450 from whom consent had been obtained. To be included in this study children had to have been seen at the PHC at least once in each age bracket of 0-<3months, 3-<6months, 6-<9 months and 9-<12 months. Multiple presentations on the same day were recorded as the one presentation. Presentations with missing or incomplete dates were excluded.

We utilized the same methods for review of presentations to PHC services as previously described. [2] We manually reviewed the clinic presentation records for each child and recorded: the date of each presentation, the child's height and weight, any infectious reason for presentation, antibiotic prescription and any referral to hospital. Each of the six communities had a designated clinic as the sole PHC service. One community also had a regional hospital nearby (within 20 km).

Ethics approval was obtained from The Human Research Ethics Committee of NT Department of Health and Families and Menzies School of Health Research (HREC ref 04/11).

Data were analysed in Stata version 12.1. [5] Data were examined per child and per presentation per child. Continuous skewed data were expressed as medians (interquartile range (IQR)) and dichotomous data as percentages. We assessed the contribution of scabies to the overall skin sore burden for presentations during the first year of life by calculating a risk ratio with 95% confidence interval (CI) of a diagnosis of skin sore infection at a presentation of scabies compared to no diagnosis of scabies at the same presentation. The method of generalized estimating equations was used with an exchangeable correlation structure in a log-binomial regression model to account for within-child correlation.

Results

The 320 children in the birth cohort (1 January 2001–10 May 2006) had a total of 7272 presentations to the PHC service during their first year of life; 53% were male. The median number of presentations per child in the first year of life was 21 (IQR 15, 29). The median number of presentations per child was 7 (IQR 5–10) for non-infectious causes in the first year of life, including routine health checks, and was 14 (IQR 9–20) for infectious conditions.

Other than the first month of life, almost two thirds of the presentations to the PHC service at each subsequent month of age included an infectious condition (Figure 1). There was a discernible but relatively moderate increase in presentations coded as being for non-infectious causes at 2, 4 and 6 months of age, coinciding with the childhood standard vaccination schedule.

As shown in Table 1, amongst our cohort the most prominent infectious presentations per child during the first year of life were: upper respiratory tract infection (median 6, IQR 3–10); diarrhoea (median 3, IQR 1–5); ear disease (median 3, IQR 1–5); lower respiratory tract infection (median 3, IQR 2–5); scabies (median 3, IQR 1–5); and skin sores (median 3, IQR 2–5). Overall, very few children managed to reach their first birthday without having at least one documented episode of an URTI (96%), scabies and/or skin sores (84%), ear disease (82%), diarrhoea (77%), or LRTI (75%). Recurrent presentations to the clinic for the same health condition were very common in a child's first year of life; 285 children (92.8%) represented for URTI, 229 (85.1%) for scabies or skin sores, 191 (73.2%) for ear disease, 174 (70.5%) for diarrhoea and 181 (75.7) for LRTI.

The median age of the first presentation was 1 month (IQR 0–3) for URTI (Figure 2A), 4 months (IQR 2–6) for LRTI (Figure 2B), 4 months (IQR 2–7) for scabies (Figure 2C), 5 months (IQR 2–7)

Table 1. Reasons recorded for presentation at the health centre during the first year of life for a cohort of 320 children born from 1 Jan 2001–31 Dec 2006 and living in one of five remote Aboriginal communities in East Arnhem land.

Reason for presentation	Number of Children Presenting (%)	Presentations per child median (IQR*)[†]	Children with more than one presentation n (%)[#]
Upper respiratory tract infections (URTI)	307 (95.9)	6 (3, 10)	285 (92.8)
Ear disease	261 (81.6)	3 (1, 5)	191 (73.2)
Scabies and/or skin sores	269 (84.1)	4 (2, 7)	229 (71.6)
Scabies	221 (69.0)	3 (1, 5)	156 (70.5)
Skin Sores	262 (81.9)	3 (2, 5)	200 (76.3)
Lower respiratory tract infections (LRTI)	239 (74.7)	3 (2, 5)	181 (75.7)
Diarrhoea	247 (77.2)	3 (1, 5)	174 (70.5)
Febrile Illness	158 (49.4)	2 (1, 4)	94 (59.5)
Throat Infection	88 (27.5)	1 (1, 2)	27 (30.7)
Tinea	53 (16.6)	1 (1, 2)	21 (39.6)
Acute post-streptococcal glomerulonephritis	0 (0.0)	–	–
Acute rheumatic fever	1 (0.0)	–	–
Non-infectious cause	319 (99.7)	7 (5, 10)	311 (97.5)
Total	**320 (100)**	**21 (15, 29)**	**320 (100)**

The proportion of children presenting for a specified reason is equivalent to the cumulative incidence of that condition/reason during the first year of life.
*IQR = Interquartile range.
[†]Median number of presentations per child, per condition in the first year of life.
[#]% of children with coded as having the same reason for presentation (recurrence) in the first year of life.

for skin sores (Figure 2D), 5 months (IQR 3–7) for ear disease (Figure 2E) and 5 months (IQR 4–8) for diarrhoea (Figure 2F).

Skin sores were 7.0 (95% CI 6.3, 8.0) times more likely to be concurrently diagnosed along with scabies than they were if there was not a scabies diagnosis.

Discussion

Worldwide, the health disparity between Indigenous and non-Indigenous people is well recognized as is the heavy infectious disease burden. [6] Within Australia, the leading cause of hospitalization for children under 2 years of age is infection with Aboriginal children having a significantly higher admission rate than non-Aboriginal children. [7] Infectious diseases of childhood are strongly linked with poverty, poor living conditions and overcrowding. [8,9].

Scabies is responsible for major morbidity worldwide as infestations facilitate skin sore infections by bacterial pathogens such as *Streptococcus pyogenes* and *Staphylococcus aureus*. [10] *Streptococcus pyogenes* can predispose children to secondary disease including rheumatic fever/heart disease which worldwide has the highest prevalence in Australian Aboriginal and Torres Strait Islander people. [11] In our study, the link between scabies and skin sore infections was illustrated by the finding that a child was 7.0 times more likely to have both scabies and skin sores than to have skin sores in the absence of scabies.

Within our cohort of 320 children, who were born from 2001–2006 and had spent the first year of their life in one of five remote Aboriginal communities in northern Australia, there were high rates of infectious disease presentations. We also observed frequent recurrences of the same infections among individual children. Upper respiratory tract infection was the most common with a median of 6 presentations per child in the first year of life. Diarrhoea, ear disease, lower respiratory tract infection, scabies and skin sores also predominated with a median of 3 presentations per child in the first year of life for each of these conditions. By one year of age 96% of the infants had attended the health service with at least one infectious episode.

Our findings support previously demonstrated high rates of clinic attendance in similar settings. [2,3] We acknowledge that our study cohort of 320 children, 21% of the estimated birth cohort, may not be representative of all children born in these communities and particularly those children who did not remain resident for the first year. In regards to internal validity, all members of our cohort were required to have attended the clinic on at least one occasion in each of four sequential 3-month periods. We adopted these eligibility criteria in order to define the population at risk during the first year of life and used this is a proxy indicator of presence within the community over that time. We required the child to have had at least one visit to the PHC across a range of age strata which coincided with the expected contact visits for standard immunisations and represented the minimum number of visits a well child would have if resident in the community during the first year of life. Given high immunisation rates of 85% for children aged <1 year, [1] we considered this would not unduly lead to bias towards sick children. Moreover, high clinic attendance rates had been documented by us in this region (median 23 presentations during the first year of life). [2,3] Of note, one third of presentations (a median of 7 per child) were for non-infectious causes, such as growth monitoring and immunisations, which again does not suggest a bias towards sick children.

The major strength of our study is in the utilization of existing datasets to monitor clinic presentations for infectious causes as a potentially useful indicator of progress towards improving health

e.

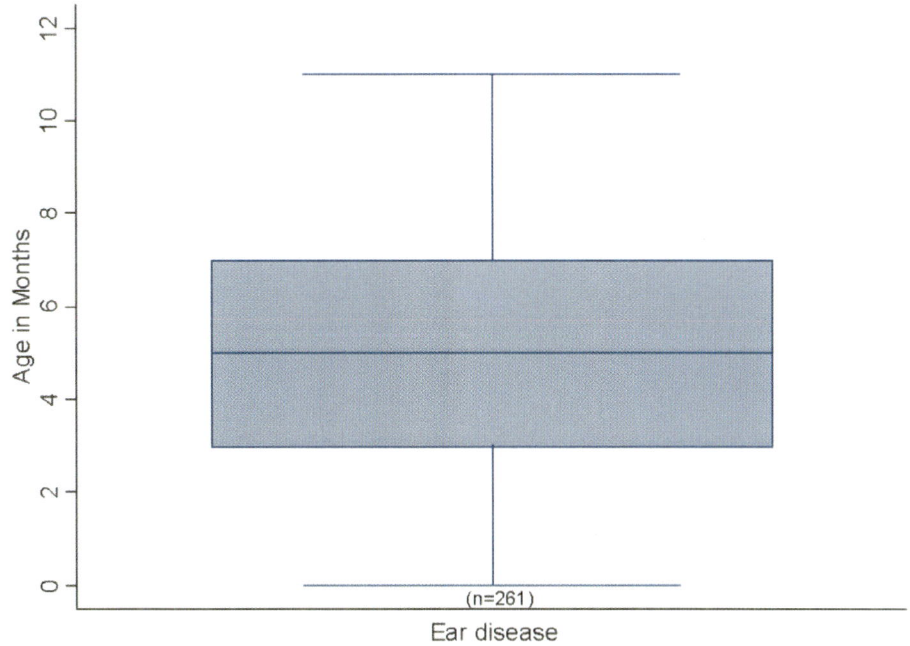

f.

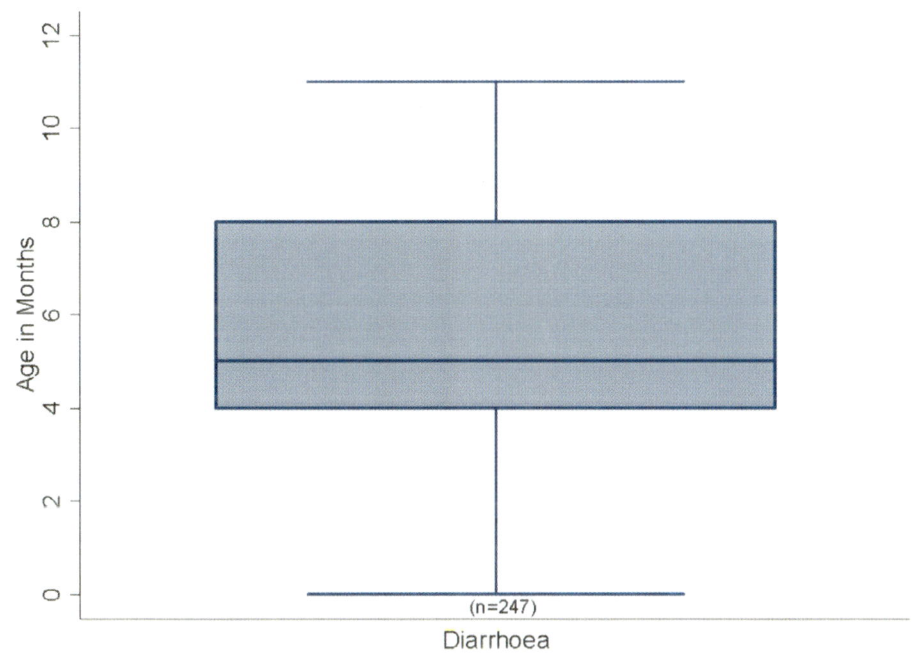

*Outliers in the box plots are defined as data lying more than 1.5 x IQR away from the box.

Figure 2. Median age at first clinic presentation for URTI, LRTI, scabies, skin sores, diarrhoea and ear disease in 5 remote communities in Northern Territory, Jan 01–Jan07.

outcomes during the first of year of life. Many remote communities now have established electronic health record systems, use the Key Performance Indicator System and are engaged in CQI (continuous quality improvement) processes. Building on these recent initiatives, there is an opportunity to incorporate routine monitoring of a range of infectious conditions (we suggest diarrhoea, LRTI, scabies and skin sores) using both the age at first presentation and the median number of presentations per child during the first year of life as potential indicators of progress in addressing health inequities in remote communities. For example, monitoring changes in the median number of diarrhoeal presentations to Primary Health Care centres for a range of birth cohorts before and after the introduction of routine rotavirus vaccination could fill a gap in the assessments of vaccine effectiveness in the field. Monitoring clinic presentations in the first year of life for diarrhoea, LRTI, scabies and skin sores would be consistent with the Australian and Northern Territory Governments commitments to closing the gap between Indigenous and non-Indigenous Australians. [12].

Acknowledgments

The authors gratefully acknowledge the five Primary Health Care Services that allowed us access to collect the information required from the health care records.

Author Contributions

Conceived and designed the experiments: DC CC BC JC RA. Performed the experiments: TK DC. Analyzed the data: TK RA. Contributed reagents/materials/analysis tools: TK DC CC BC JC RA. Wrote the paper: TK DC CC BC JC RA.

References

1. Australian Insititue of Health and Welfare (2011) Aboriginal and Torres Strait Islander Health Performance Framework 2010 report. Northern Territory.
2. Clucas D, Carville K, Connors C, Currie B, Carapetis J, et al. (2008) Disease burden and health-care clinic attendances for young children in remote Aboriginal communities of northern Australia. Bulletin of the World Health Organization 86: 241–320.
3. McMeniman E, Holden L, Kearns T, Clucas DB, Carapetis JR, et al. (2011) Skin disease in the first two years of life in Aboriginal children in East Arnhem Land. Australasian Journal of Dermatology 52: 270–273.
4. Andrews R, Kearns T, Connors C, Parker C, Carville K, et al. (2009) A Regional Initiative to Reduce Skin Infections amongst Aboriginal Children Living in Remote Communities of the Northern Territory, Australia. PLoS Negl Trop Dis 3: e554. doi:510.1371/journal.pntd.0000554.
5. StataCorpLP (2012) Stata/IC 12.1 for Windows. College Station, Texas: Stata Corporation.
6. Gracey M, King M (2009) Indigenous health part 1: determinants and disease patterns. The Lancet 374: 65–75.
7. Carville KS, Lehmann D, Hall G, Moore H, Richmond P, et al. (2007) Infection is the major component of the disease burden in aboriginal and non-aboriginal Australian children: a population-based study. Paediatr Infect Dis J 26: 210–216.
8. Amin TT, Ali A, Kaliyadan F (2011) Skin disorders among male primary school children in Al Hassa, Saudi Arabia: prevalence and socio-demographic correlates - a comparison of urban and rural populations. Rural And Remote Health 11: 1517–1517.
9. Munoz E, Powers JR, Nienhuys TG, Mathews JD (1992) Social and environmental factors in 10 aboriginal communities in the Northern Territory: relationship to hospital admissions of children. The Medical Journal Of Australia 156: 529–533.
10. Fischer K, Holt D, Currie B, Kemp D (2012) Chapter 5 - Scabies: Important Clinical Consequences Explained by New Molecular Studies. Advances in parasitology Volume 79: 339–373.
11. Carapetis J, Wolff D, Currie B (1996) Acute rheumatic fever and rheumatic heart disease in the top end of Australia's Northern Territory. Medical Journal of Australia 164: 146–149.
12. Australian Government (2012) Closing the Gap:Minister's Report.

ZNF750 Is Expressed in Differentiated Keratinocytes and Regulates Epidermal Late Differentiation Genes

Idan Cohen[1,2], Ramon Y. Birnbaum[3,4], Keren Leibson[1,2], Ran Taube[2], Sara Sivan[1,2], Ohad S. Birk[1,2,5]*

1 The Morris Kahn Laboratory of Human Genetics, National Institute for Biotechnology in the Negev, Ben Gurion University, Beer-Sheva, Israel, 2 Department of Molecular Genetics and Virology, Ben-Gurion University, Beer-Sheva, Israel, 3 Department of Bioengineering and Therapeutic Sciences, University of California San Francisco, San Francisco, California, United States of America, 4 Institute for Human Genetics, University of California San Francisco, San Francisco, California, United States of America, 5 Genetics Institute, Soroka Medical Center, Beer-Sheva, Israel

Abstract

Disrupted skin barrier due to altered keratinocyte differentiation is common in pathologic conditions such as atopic dermatitis, ichthyosis and psoriasis. However, the molecular cascades governing keratinocyte terminal differentiation are poorly understood. We have previously demonstrated that a dominant mutation in *ZNF750* leads to a clinical phenotype reminiscent of psoriasis and seborrheic dermatitis. Here we show that ZNF750 is a nuclear protein bearing a functional C-terminal nuclear localization signal. ZNF750 was specifically expressed in the epidermal suprabasal layers and its expression was augmented during differentiation, both in human skin and in-vitro, peaking in the granular layer. Silencing of *ZNF750* in Ca2+-induced HaCaT keratinocytes led to morphologically apparent arrest in the progression of late differentiation, as well as diminished apoptosis and sustained proliferation. ZNF750 knockdown cells presented with markedly reduced expression of epidermal late differentiation markers, including gene subsets of epidermal differentiation complex and skin barrier formation such as *FLG, LOR, SPINK5, ALOX12B* and *DSG1*, known to be mutated in various human skin diseases. Furthermore, overexpression of ZNF750 in undifferentiated cells induced terminal differentiation genes. Thus, ZNF750 is a regulator of keratinocyte terminal differentiation and with its downstream targets can serve in future elucidation of therapeutics for common diseases of skin barrier.

Editor: Johanna M. Brandner, University Hospital Hamburg-Eppendorf, Germany

Funding: This study was funded through a grant of the Israel Science Foundation (ISF) and through the generosity of the Morris Kahn Family Foundation. The funders had no role in study design, data collection and analysis, decision to publish, or preparation of the manuscript.

Competing Interests: The authors have declared that no competing interests exist.

* E-mail: obirk@bgu.ac.il

Introduction

Keratinocyte (KC) differentiation is an essential key process in formation and maintenance of the skin barrier. In fact, various common skin diseases such as psoriasis, atopic dermatitis (AD) and ichthyosis involve the disintegration of the epidermal skin barrier due to altered KC differentiation [1–3]. The major barrier resides within the exterior layers of the epidermis, which are constantly shed and replaced by inner layer cells that are committed to differentiate and move outwards in a columnar fashion. The epidermis maintains a single basal layer of proliferating cells that adhere to an underlying basement membrane, which retains the ability to self renew under both homeostatic and injury conditions [4]. Upon commitment to terminal differentiation, KCs undergo three distinct differentiation stages, forming the spinous, granular and stratum corneum layers. Each of these phases has specific characteristics in terms of transcription, morphology and function. In the first step of commitment to terminal differentiation, basal cells are withdrawn from the cell cycle, lose their ability to adhere to the basement membrane and migrate to the spinous layer. As cells enter the spinous layer, they switch off the expression of keratin 5 (*KRT5*) and *KRT14* that mark the stratified squamous epithelial cells which possess proliferative potential. Simultaneously, these cells initiate the expression of genes encoding KRT1 and KRT10, which reinforce cell–cell junctions and provide resistance against mechanical stresses at the body surface [5]. At a more advanced stage, granular layer cells begin to express *Filaggrin* (*FLG*) and acquire keratohyalin granules, which contain profilaggrin - the precursor of filaggrin. Filaggrin aggregates the keratin filaments into tight bundles, which collapse the cells into a flattened shape, forming the terminally differentiated cells that comprise the stratum corneum. Simultaneously, other structural genes, including *Involucrin* (IVL), *Loricrin* (LOR) and small proline-rich proteins (SPRRs), are expressed and subsequently crosslinked by transglutaminases to form the chemically resistant cornified envelope structure [6,7]. In addition, a complex series of lipids, such as ceramides, are synthesized and covalently attached to proteins of the cornified envelope, forming intercellular lamellae that help to produce a complete barrier of the skin. The resulting cornified layer is composed of terminally differentiated, dead, cornified, flattened KC cells that are known as corneocytes [1].

We have previously demonstrated that a dominant mutation in *zinc finger protein 750* (*ZNF750*) causes seborrhea-like dermatitis with psoriasiform elements [8]. The disease phenotype includes dramatically enhanced KC proliferation with parakeratosis, as well as dermal infiltrate of CD4 lymphocytes. The mutation causing this phenotype is within the *ZNF750* coding sequence, abrogating the zinc finger domain of the encoded protein [8]. There is some evidence that ZNF750 might play a role also in bone fide psoriasis since ZNF750 regulatory variants have been identified in classic forms of psoriasis [9]. ZNF750 encodes a novel C2H2 zinc finger protein that is highly expressed in human KCs, but not in dermal fibroblasts or CD4 leukocytes [8], suggesting that the human phenotype induced by *ZNF750* mutation stems from a primary defect in KCs. In the present work, studying both normal and ZNF750 silenced KCs, we determined that ZNF750 is a nuclear protein and characterized its expression pattern. Silencing of ZNF750 effected KCs terminal differentiation in terms of morphology, proliferation and gene expression.

Results

ZNF750 is Localized to the Nucleus as Determined by Its C-terminal Nuclear Localization Signals (NLS)

To determine the subcellular localization of ZNF750, we used western blot analysis of cytoplasmic and nuclear subcellular fractions as well as confocal microscopy with anti ZNF750 antibodies (Abs). Both assays demonstrated that ZNF750 is localized to the nucleus (Figure 1A, B). As ZNF750 is a relatively large protein of ~100 Kilo-Daltons (figures 1A, 2C), its entry through the nuclear envelope needs to be facilitated via a heterodimeric nuclear transport receptor comprising importin α and importin β, which enable nuclear import of functional NLS-bearing proteins [10]. Bioinformatic analysis of the 723 amino-acid sequence of ZNF750 using protein domain prediction programs NLS MAPPER and PSORT II, indicated the presence of three putative highly conserved NLSs: one bi-partite (BP) NLS at the C-terminal of the molecule and two mono-partite (MP) NLSs at both the N-terminal and C-terminal regions (Figure 1C). We investigated those putative NLS regulatory motifs of ZNF750 using GFP-tagged ZNF750 (GFP-ZNF750) full length or partial length (PL) constructs (Figure 1D). Similar to the endogenous ZNF750 protein, full length GFP-ZNF750 was localized to the nucleus (Figure 1E). Partial length ZNF750 lacking the N-terminal NLS showed similar localization to that of the full length ZNF750 (PL-A, Figure 1D, E). However, removal of the ZNF750 C-terminal NLSs fully abrogated its nuclear localization (PL-B, Figure 1D, E). As per bioinformatics analysis ZNF750 has no nuclear export signal motifs, ZNF750 localization is determined and controlled by its C-terminal bi-partite NLS.

ZNF750 Expression is Upregulated During Keratinocyte Differentiation

To determine the expression signature of *ZNF750* in KCs, we studied normal human epidermal KC (NHEK) cells and HaCaT cells [11] using Ca^{2+} induction to initiate a differentiation program which mimics the terminal differentiation that KCs undergo in vivo [12]. Through quantitative real-time PCR (QRT-PCR) and immunoblotting with Abs against both N-terminal and C-terminal regions of ZNF750, we showed that ZNF750 mRNA and protein levels increased during progression of KC differentiation in both NHEK and HaCaT cells, peaking at day 12 of Ca^{2+} induced differentiation (Figure 2A–C). Interestingly, this time line of *ZNF750* expression overlaps with that of *Filaggrin* (Figure 2A, B), a late differentiation marker of granular KCs [13]. As ZNF750 expression increased dramatically during KC differentiation (Figure 2A–C), we tested the effect of Phorbol 12-myristate 13-acetate (PMA) on *ZNF750* mRNA levels. PMA activates protein kinase C (PKC) proteins that function during terminal differentiation specifically in the transition from spinous to granular cells, inducing late differentiation markers including FLG [14]. Using QRT-PCR we measured the mRNA levels of *ZNF750* in proliferating KCs grown in low calcium media following 24 hours treatment with PMA. PMA treatment dramatically increased *ZNF750* mRNA levels in a dosage-dependent manner, similar to *FLG* expression, and had no effect on the early differentiation marker *KRT1* (Figure 2D). These in vitro findings are in line with ZNF750 studies of normal human skin sections, showing weak staining of nuclei in the suprabasal spinous layer as compared with strong staining in granular layer nuclei [15] and the sebaceous glands (Figure S1). The high expression of ZNF750 in differentiated KCs, which overlaps with that of the late differentiation marker *FLG*, suggests a role of ZNF750 in KC terminal differentiation.

ZNF750 Knockdown in Ca^{2+} Induced HaCaT Keratinocytes Leads to Sustained Cell Proliferation and Decreased Apoptosis

Assuming a possible role of ZNF750 in KC terminal differentiation, we generated stable HaCaT cell lines in which ZNF750 expression was silenced using small hairpin RNA (shRNA). Using five different shRNA sequences targeting *ZNF750* mRNA we identified three shRNAs (shRNAa, b, and c) that achieved efficient silencing as demonstrated by both QRT-PCR and western blot analysis (Figure 3A, B). A non-targeting scrambled shRNA was used as a control. To further examine the effect of ZNF750 knockdown, cells were Ca^{2+}-induced to differentiate until day twelve, when ZNF750 levels normally peak (Figure 2B, C). Compared with controls, Ca^{2+}-induced HaCaT cell cultures in which *ZNF750* expression was silenced showed morphological changes compatible with impaired late differentiation (Figure 3C). We next performed a cell proliferation assay using the cell proliferation marker Ki67 [16]. ZNF750 silenced cultures sustained proliferation activity at day twelve, which was ~10 fold higher ($p<0.0001$) than control cultures at that time point of late differentiation (Figure 3D,E). In addition, flow cytometry analysis of ZNF750 silenced cultures showed a ~4 fold ($p<0.0001$) decrease in apoptosis, as assessed by Annexin V assay (Figure 3F, G) and markedly reduced cell granularity (Figure 3H). Thus, ZNF750 knockdown affects the in-vitro terminal differentiation program, interfering with cell cycle withdrawal.

ZNF750 Regulates Molecular Pathways of Epidermal Terminal Differentiation

To identify ZNF750 downstream target genes, we performed whole genome expression microarray analysis of three HaCaT cultures in which ZNF750 was silenced (triplicates of ZNF750 shRNA-a) vs. three control cultures. Cultures were Ca^{2+} induced for twelve days prior to harvesting for microarray analysis, and ZNF750 silencing was validated (Figure 3A, B). ZNF750 silencing led to significant downregulation of 256 genes and upregulation of 381 genes (Table S1, corrected p-value<0.05, fold change≥2). Genes upregulated by ZNF750 silencing showed significant enrichment of Gene Ontology[17,18] terms related to cell cycle, cell cycle regulation, mitosis, proliferation, and cellular response to stress (corrected p-value<0.001; Figure S2). Genes downregulated by ZNF750 silencing included a subset of genes that were highly enriched in Gene Ontology terms related to KC terminal differentiation (corrected p-value<0.01; Figure 4A, Table S2). Microarray results were validated (QRT-PCR) using biological replicates (ZNF750 shRNA-a and b) for selected genes of this subset, namely *KRT1, INV, FLG, LOR, DSG1, DSC1, SPINK5,L-CE1C, LCE2B, LCE3D, SPRR1A* and *SPRR3* (Figure 4B). We further examined the effects of ZNF750 overexpression in HaCaT cells. Using pHR-CMV-ZNF750 lentiviral vector, we generated a stable cell line which overexpresses ZNF750. Undifferentiated cells that were transduced with an empty vector served as a control,

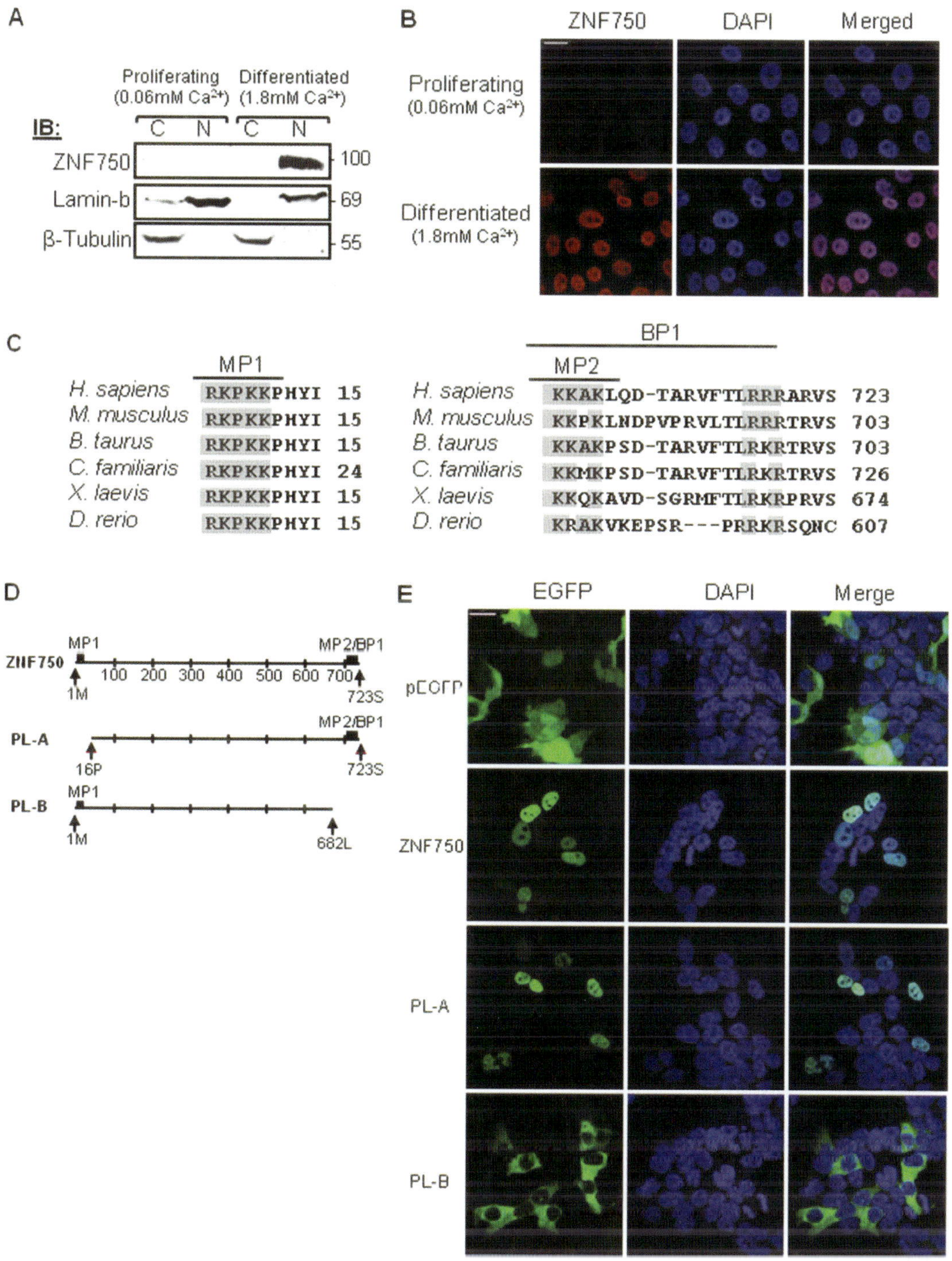

Figure 1. ZNF750 subcellular localization and functional NLS characterization. (A) Western blot analysis using cytoplasmic (C) and nuclear (N) fractions from HaCaT cells at proliferative/undifferentiated (0.06 mM Ca^{2+}) or differentiated (1.8 mM Ca^{2+}) state, analyzed by anti-ZNF750 Ab. (B) Confocal subcellular localization of ZNF750 in HaCaT cells. Cells at proliferative and differentiated states were fixed and immunostained by anti-ZNF750 Ab (red). DAPI (blue) was used to identify nuclei. Scale bar = 20 μm. (C) Sequence alignments representing the three putative NLSs of ZNF750 homologues in various organisms. Conserved amino acids of the predicted NLSs are shaded. (D) Schematic representation of EGFP-ZNF750 constructs. (E) Confocal subcellular localization of ZNF750 constructs in HEK293 cells. The expression of pEGFP-C2 (EGFP alone) is shown as a control. EGFP (green); DAPI (blue) was used to identify nuclei. Scale bar = 20 μm.

showing basal levels of late differentiation genes that were analyzed (Figure 4C). The undifferentiated state of the cells was confirmed by the early differentiation marker *KRT1*, and through analysis of *ZNF750* endogenous levels, using a primer set that targets the ZNF750 5′ untranslated region. Interestingly, overexpression of ZNF750 in undifferentiated KCs induced late differentiation genes that were downregulated by ZNF750 silencing, yet only ones belonging to the epidermal differentiation complex on chromosome 1q21 (Figure 4C). Thus, ZNF750 is both

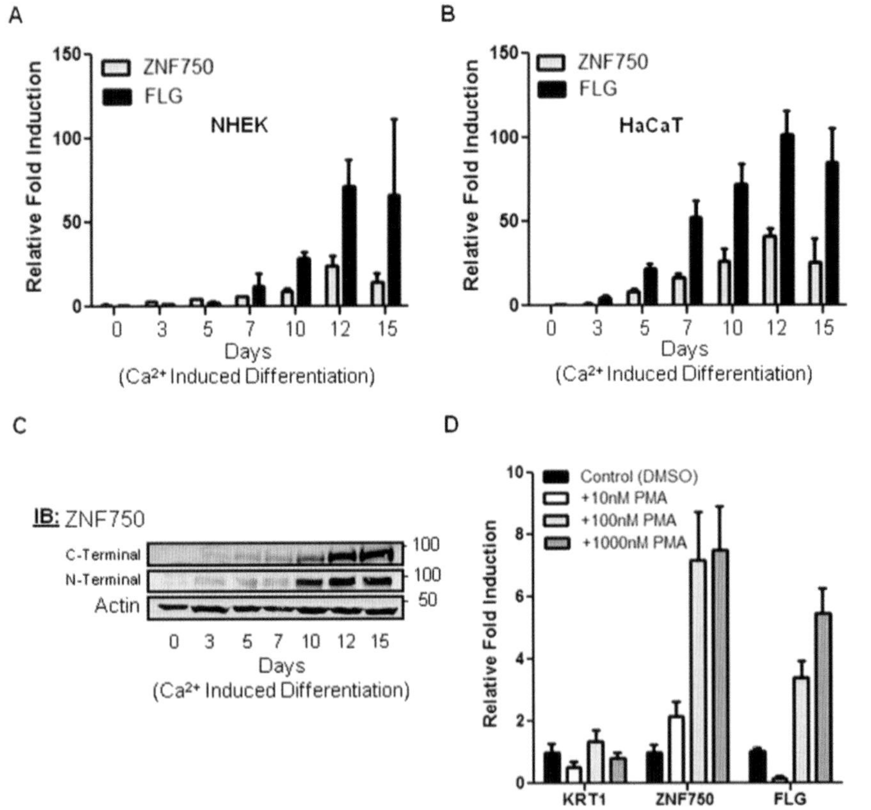

Figure 2. *ZNF750* mRNA and protein expression in Ca^{2+} induction and in human skin. (A) QRT-PCR of *ZNF750* mRNA expression during Ca^{2+} induction in NHEK cells. *Filaggrin* mRNA levels serve as internal control. Error bars represent mean values±SD, N = 3. (B) QRT-PCR of *ZNF750* mRNA expression during Ca^{2+} induction in HaCaT cells. Error bars represent mean values±SD, N = 3. (C) ZNF750 protein levels during Ca^{2+} induction in HaCaT cells, analyzed by anti-ZNF750 antibodies against both N-terminal and C-terminal regions. (D) QRT-PCR of *ZNF750, KRT1* and *FLG* mRNA expression in NHEK cells that were treated with PMA. Error bars represent mean values±SD, N = 2.

essential and sufficient for inducing those KC late differentiation genes.

Discussion

Our data, together with the recent publication by Sen et al. [15], demonstrate that ZNF750 is a nuclear effector that is strongly activated in and essential for terminal KC differentiation. We showed that ZNF750 expression in the cell nucleus is determined by its highly conserved functional NLS motif within its c-terminal region. Furthermore, ZNF750 acts in terminal KC differentiation: ZNF750 is expressed in suprabasal layers, and its expression is dramatically increased in the granular layer (Figure S1), [15]. These findings are in line with our demonstration that the expression of ZNF750 increased during Ca^{2+} induction of HaCaT KC and adult primary KC differentiation in vitro, reaching maximal levels just prior to terminal KC differentiation. These findings are in line with recent findings in primary neonatal KC [15], with different kinetics likely due to different experimental systems used. Moreover, we showed that PMA, a known inducer of late differentiation markers that promotes spinous to granular transition [14], markedly induced ZNF750 expression.

ZNF750 silencing experiments further substantiated the role of ZNF750 in terminal KC differentiation: ZNF750 knockdown in Ca^{2+}-induced HaCaT KCs led to arrest in the progression of late differentiation, as was evident morphologically (Figure 3C). In fact, in the silenced cells, morphological progression occurred only up to day 5–7 of in-vitro differentiation of HaCaT cells, the time point at which differentiation into spinous layer is described to be achieved at the molecular level [19–21], and the start point of further differentiation into granular cells. This arrest was also evident in the dramatically reduced granularity of day 12 ZNF750-silenced cells (Figure 3H). KCs in which ZNF750 was silenced demonstrated decreased apoptosis and continued proliferation into day 12 of Ca^{2+} induction. The arrested late differentiation, as evident per cell morphology at day 12, suggests that the relative enhanced proliferation of the ZNF750-silenced cells is likely due to abrogated progression into late differentiation. Our data are partly reminiscent of those seen in null mutants of Ikkα, a key regulator of KC and epidermal differentiation: Ikkα−/− mice present with a hyperproliferative and undifferentiated epidermis characterized by complete absence of a granular layer and stratum corneum [22]. Further studies are in place to unravel any molecular cascades that might link ZNF750 with Ikkα.

Molecular studies further supported the morphological findings. Using expression microarrays we demonstrated that ZNF750 knockdown depleted KC late differentiation markers such as FLG, LOR, SPINK5, SPRR3 and LCE genes, in line with similar findings recently reported by Sen et al. [15]. Many of those ZNF750 targets are mutated in various human skin diseases [2,23]. In fact, this explains in part the clinical phenotype of the ZNF750 human mutation we previously described [8], which combines elements of the phenotypes known to emerge from mutations in some of those downstream genes. Moreover, expression of ZNF750 in undifferentiated HaCaT cells was

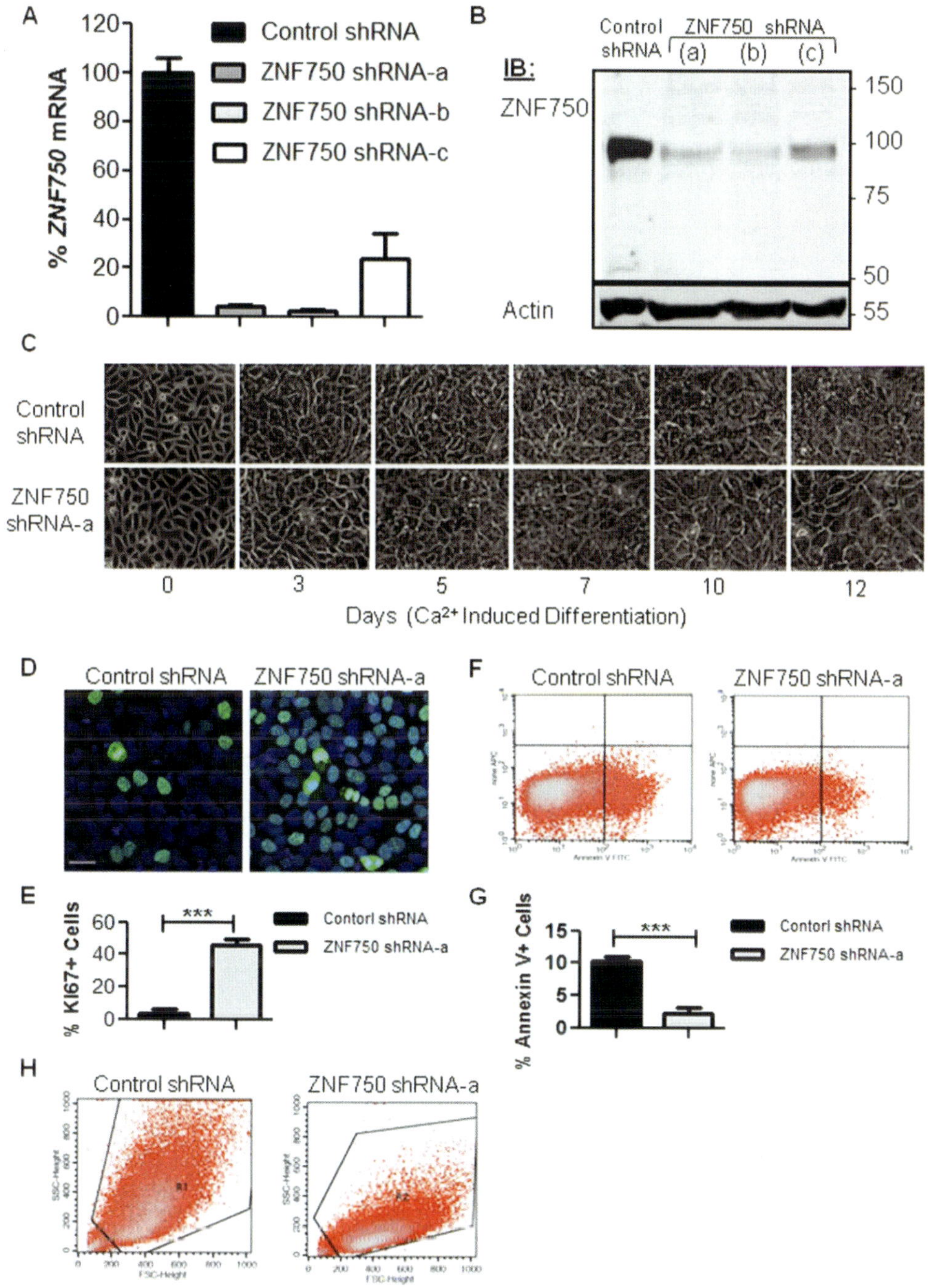

Figure 3. *ZNF750* silencing in HaCaT keratinocytes. HaCaT cells were transduced with scrambled shRNA (control) or with three different ZNF750 shRNAs (shRNA-a, b, and c). Cells were harvested and assayed at day 12 of Ca^{2+} induction. (A) QRT-PCR of *ZNF750* mRNA expression in the stable transduced cell lines. Error bars represent mean values±SD, N = 3. (B) western blot analysis showing ZNF750 protein levels in the stable transduced cell lines. A total of 50 µg of protein was loaded in each sample. Actin levels were measured to ensure equal amounts of loaded protein were loaded. (C) Morphological studies at different time points in HaCaT cell differentiation: control vs. *ZNF750* shRNA-a transduced cultures examined by phase contrast microscopy during Ca^{2+} induction. (D,E) *ZNF750* downregulation enhances cell proliferation. (D) Ki67 staining (green) followed by confocal microscopy. To-Pro 3 nuclear staining is shown in blue (E) quantification of Ki67 positive cells. More than 800 cells were counted for each slide. Error bars represent mean values±SD, N = 6 (***:P<0.0001). (F,G) Effects of *ZNF750* downregulation on apoptosis as assessed by Annexin V apoptosis assay. (F) Annexin V apoptosis assay using flow cytometry analysis. (G) quantification of Annexin V positive cells. More than 50,000 cells were counted in each sample Error bars represent mean values±SD, N = 4, (***:P<0.0001). (H) Effects on cell size (X axis) and granularity (Y axis) measured by flow cytometry.

sufficient to induce late differentiation genes, in line with similar recent findings by Sen et al. in primary keratinocytes [15]. It is interesting to note that those ZNF750-induced genes were all part of the epidermal differentiation complex (EDC), while other genes depleted by ZNF750 silencing were not induced by ZNF750 overexpression. Thus, the data provide additional evidence for a

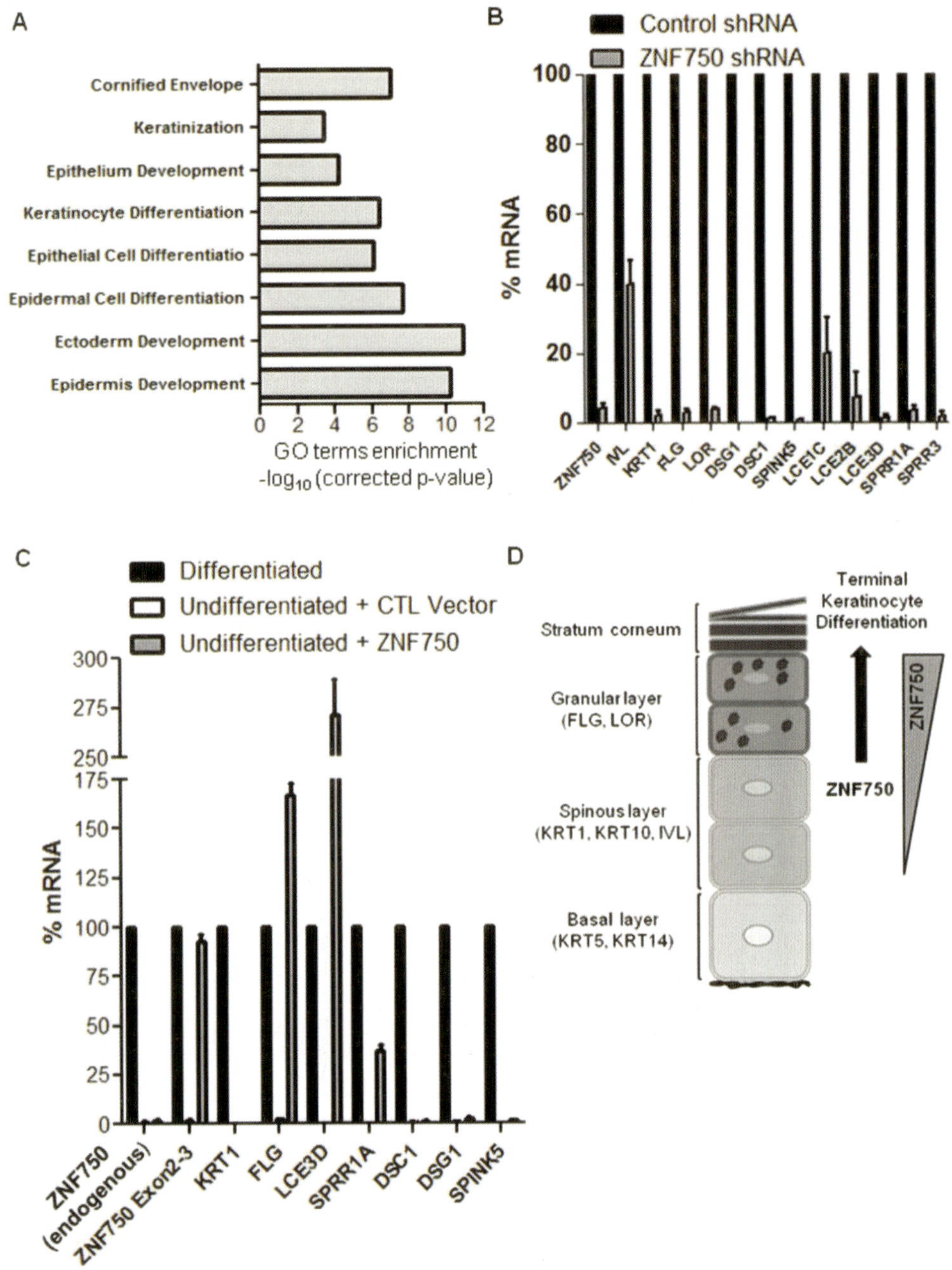

Figure 4. ZNF750 regulates keratinocyte terminal differentiation. (A) Gene Ontology terms for the 256 genes that were downregulated in *ZNF750* silenced cultures vs. control (P-value<0.05, FC≥2), with Bonferroni-corrected p-value<0.001. (B) QRT-PCR mRNA expression of a selected group of terminal differentiation genes in control vs. *ZNF750* silenced cultures, that showed downregulation fold change≥2. Error bars represent mean values±SD, N = 2. (C) mRNA expression (QRT-PCR) of a selected group of terminal differentiation genes in differentiated cells vs. undifferentiated HaCaT cells that overexpress *ZNF750* or an empty control vector (CTL). Cells in undifferentiated state were maintained at sub-confluence in low calcium media. Expression levels are shown relative to those of Ca^{2+}-induced differentiated HaCaT cultures at day twelve (100%). Two sets of primers targeting ZNF750 were used: "ZNF750 endogenous" PCR amplifies the ZNF750 5′ UTR, representing the ZNF750 endogenous expression only, and serves as an internal control demonstrating the cells' undifferentiated state. The ZNF750 Exon2-3 primer set PCR amplifies ZNF750 coding sequence common to the endogenous and exogenous ZNF750 molecules. Note that in the CTL control group mRNA levels of all tested markers were practically null. Error bars represent mean values±SD, N = 2. (D) Schematic representation: ZNF750 expression is gradually augmented throughout keratinocyte differentiation, inducing expression of late differentiation markers.

strong regulation of EDC by ZNF750. Taken together, our data suggest that ZNF750 is a regulator required for KC terminal differentiation, playing a pivotal role in this process (Figure 4D). A recent study by Sen et al. suggested that ZNF750 regulation of terminal keratinocyte differentiation is mediated by KLF4. However, overexpression of KLF4 in ZNF750 silenced keratinocytes only partially rescued expression of ZNF750-dependent terminal differentiation genes [15]. This is in line with our expression microarrays results showing that KLF4 was only slightly affected by ZNF750 silencing (failed to pass our significance terms filtering), suggesting that additional effectors that ZNF750 targets (highlighted by both studies) might mediate downstream pathways controlling terminal KC differentiation. It should be noted that the discrepancy in ZNF750-related KLF4 expression in our data as compared to the study of Sen et al. might be due to the different experimental systems used (HaCaT vs. primary KC). Further studies are warranted to determine the direct targets which mediate ZNF750 regulation of KC terminal differentiation process. Our study together with the recent findings of Sen et al. [15] highlight the essential role of ZNF750 in terminal KC differentiation, providing insights to the molecular pathways governing this process. ZNF750 and its downstream targets can serve in future elucidation of therapeutics for common diseases of impaired terminal KC differentiation and dysfunctional skin barrier.

Materials and Methods

Ethics Statement

We certify that the research in the manuscript "ZNF750 is expressed in differentiated keratinocytes and regulates epidermal late differentiation genes" describing immunohistochemistry studies of ZNF750 in normal human skin has been approved by the Soroka Medical Center institutional review board (IRB). No consent forms were needed as the samples were old archival samples analyzed anonymously, and most of each sample was kept for further use. The investigation approved is in accordance with the principles expressed in the Declaration of Helsinki. The Soroka Medical Center IRB waived the need for written informed consent for the use of the archival normal skin section.

Expression Constructs

ZNF750 cDNA reference sequence was derived from GenBank (NM_024702.2). pEGFP-ZNF750 expression vector was constructed by polymerase chain reaction (PCR) amplification of ZNF750 cDNA from HaCaT cell line, utilizing the oligonucleotide primers 5′- GAATTCGTTATGAGTCTCCTCAAAGAGCGGA -3′ (forward) and 5′- GGATCCTTAGGACACCCGGGCCCTCCT -3′ (reverse), and cloning into pGEM-T (Promega, WI, USA). This was sub-cloned into the mammalian expression vector pEGFP-C2 (Clontech, CA, USA) to yield ZNF750-EGFP. In addition, two partial length (PL) constructs (PL-A and B) were generated by the use of the following primers: PL-A 5′-GAATTCCCCAGGCCTCCAGGAAAGC-3′ (forward) and 5′-GGATCCTTAGGACACCCGGGCCCTCCT-3′ (reverse). PL-B 5′-GAATTCGTTATGAGTCTCCT-3′ (forward) and 5′-GGATCCGAGGTCACACTGGGCCTCTTGGCT-3′ (reverse). PL-A (amino acids 16–723) construct abrogates ZNF750 N-terminal NLS and PL-B (amino acids 1–682) abrogates ZNF750 C-terminal NLSs.

To generate ZNF750-FLAG expression vector, ZNF750 was PCR amplified using primers: 5′-GGATCCGCCACCATGAGTCTCCTCAAAGAGCG-3′ (forward) and 5′- TCTAGATTACTTGTCATCGTCATCCTTGTAATCGGACACCCGGGCCCTCCT -3′ (reverse), and was sub-cloned into pHR-CMV lentiviral vector [24], to generate pHR-CMV-ZNF750 that expresses C-terminal FLAG tagged ZNF750 under the control of CMV promoter and a puromycin resistance gene via IRES sequence. All constructs were sequenced to confirm their correct sequence and orientation.

Cell Cultures

Primary NHEK cells were purchased from Lonza (Walkersville, MD). Cells were grown in keratinocyte growth medium (KGM) containing 0.1 mM $CaCl_2$ supplemented with growth factor bullet kit (Lonza, Walkersville, MD). Medium was changed every 2–3 days. Cells were used at passage 3. For differentiation, cells were cultured in KC growth media containing 1.4 mM $CaCl_2$.

HaCaT cells [11], a spontaneously immortalized human KC line, were maintained in high-glucose DMEM medium containing 0.06 or 1.8 mM $CaCl_2$ supplemented with 10% fetal calf serum, 1% L -glutamine, and 1% penicillin/streptomycin (Biological Industries, Beit-Haemek, Israel).

HEK293 cells were grown on a high-glucose DMEM medium containing 1.8 mM $CaCl_2$ supplemented with 10% fetal calf serum, 1% L -glutamine, and 1% penicillin/streptomycin (Biological Industries).

Lentiviral Gene Transfer

VSV-G pseudotyped single round HIV particles were produced by co-transfection of the lentiviral vector, HIV gag/pol, pRev, pTat and VSV-G, into HEK293T cells by calcium phosphate. Supernatant was harvested 48 hrs post transfection, and filtered through 0.45 μ filter. Lentiviral particles were concentrated by ultracentrifugation for 2.5 hrs at 25,000 rpm and the pellet was re-suspended in cold DMEM. HaCaT cells were transduced with viral stock that expressed the ZNF750-FLAG or a control empty vector, supplemented with 8 mg/ml polybrene, for 4 hrs. Cells were then subjected to selection with 1 μg/ml puromycin for 1 week.

Immunohistochemistry

Formaldehyde-fixed 5-μm paraffin-embedded sections of normal human skin were obtained with Approval of the Institutional Review Board of Soroka Medical Center. Sections were deparaffinized in xylene, rehydrated in decreasing concentrations of ethanol, treated with 3% H_2O_2 in methanol for 15 minutes at room temperature, warmed in a microwave oven in citrate buffer for 15 minutes at 90°C, and stained with rabbit polyclonal anti-ZNF750 Abs (Sigma-Aldrich, St Louis, MO) for 1 hour at room temperature. After extensive washings in phosphate-buffered saline (PBS), the antibodies were revealed using the VECTRASTAIN ABC kit (Vector Laboratories, CA, USA). To identify nuclei, slides were counterstained with hematoxylin.

shRNA Lentiviral Transduction

We transduced HaCaT cells with *ZNF750* shRNA lentiviral particles (Table S3) or a scrambled shRNA as a control (Sigma-Aldrich) according to the manufacturer's recommendations. Briefly, 24 hours before transduction, cells were grown in six-well plates up to 5×10^4 cells per well. Viral stock (1–10 μl) and 2 μl of 8 mg/ml polybrene were added to the cells and incubated for 18–20 hours at 37°C in a 5% CO_2 humidified incubator. The amount of the viral stock was determined according to the desired multiplicity of infection (MOI = 5) and total transducing units (TU) per milliliter, per guidelines supplied by Sigma. At 24 hours after transduction, the cells were washed twice in 1× HBSS and maintained in DMEM containing 0.06 mM $CaCl_2$. Selection was performed in the presence of puromycin (2 μg/ml) for 1 week.

Quantitative Reverse Transcription PCR

Total RNA was isolated using TRI REAGENT (Molecular Research Center, Inc.) and subjected to DNase I (New England Bio-Labs) digestion to remove genomic DNA. RNA concentrations were determined by spectrophotometer at OD_{260}. First-strand cDNA was reverse transcribed from 500 ng of RNA by the Reverse-iT kit (ABgene, Epson, UK) using oligo-dT primers. cDNA PCR amplification was carried out using the SYBR Green JumpStart Taq ReadyMix (Sigma-Aldrich) on a Rotor-Gene RG-

3000 real-time PCR detection system (Corbett Research) with gene-specific intron-crossing oligonucleotide pairs listed in Table S4. To ensure the specificity of the reaction conditions, at the end of the individual runs, the melting temperature (Tm) of the amplified products was measured to confirm its homogeneity. Cycling conditions were as follows: 95°C for 10 minutes, 95°C for 20 seconds, 60°C for 15 seconds, and 72°C for 20 seconds for a total of 40 cycles. Each sample was analyzed in triplicate. Results were normalized to *GAPDH* mRNA levels. After the quantification procedure, the products were separated on 2% agarose gel electrophoresis to confirm that the reaction had amplified DNA fragments of expected size.

Expression Microarray Hybridization and Data Analysis

Microarray analysis was performed on biological triplicate samples. Labeled cRNA was hybridized to Affymetrix GeneChip HuGene-1_0-st-v1 arrays. Data have been deposited in GEO database compliance with MIAME guidelines. For gene expression analysis, arrays were RAM normalized [25] and differential expression was defined using the following filters: Statistical hypothesis testing for identification of differentially expressed genes was done using 2-Way ANOVA in Partek. P-values were adjusted for multiple testing by step-up FDR [26]. Fold change values are represented on linear scale, where positive and negative values indicate up- and down-regulation, respectively. Differentially expressed genes were defined as those having absolute expression signal >5 (log2 scale) in at least one of the arrays. Results were considered significant for FDR adjusted p-value<0.05 in any of the effects or interaction, and an average fold change ≥2. Gene Ontology term enrichment was performed using DAVID [17,18], and p-values represent a Bonferroni corrected p-value.

Subcellular Fractionation and Western Blot Analyses

Cells were washed with 1× PBS two times before addition of the cytoplasmic lysis buffer (10 mM Hepes at pH 8.0, 1.5 mM $MgCl_2$, 10 mM KCl, 0.5 mM DTT, 300 mM sucrose, 0.1% NP-40, 10 mM NaF, 10 mM Na 3 VO_4, 1× protease inhibitors, 0.5 mM PMSF). Cells were lysed for 10 min on ice and then quick-spun for 15 sec to collect cytosolic lysate. Pellets were washed two times with cytoplasmic lysis buffer and then lysed with nuclear lysis buffer (50 mM Hepes at pH 7.9, 250 mM KCl, 0.1 mM EDTA, 0.1 mM EGTA, 0.1% NP-40, 0.1% glycerol, 10 mM NaF, 10 mM Na_3VO_4 , 1 mM DTT, 1× protease inhibitors, 0.5 mM PMSF) for 30 min on ice. The lysates were spun for 20 min at 14,000 rpm at 4°C to collect nuclear lysates.

Cell lysates (50 µg) were used for immunoblotting, electrophrated on 8% SDS-PAGE and transferred to nitrocellulose membranes. Membranes were incubated in primary antibodies for 1 hr each. The primary Abs included Lamin-B1, β-Tubulin (Santa Cruz Biotechnology, Santa Cruz, CA) and ZNF750 (Sigma-Aldrich). After incubation with secondary horseradish peroxidase conjugated anti-goat or anti-rabbit antibodies (Santa Cruz Biotechnology), proteins were detected using the EZ-ECL chemiluminescence detection kit (Biological Industries). To compare the amount of protein in different samples, the blots were re-probed using anti β-actin Ab (Santa Cruz Biotechnology) and secondary horseradish peroxidase-conjugated anti-goat Ab (Santa Cruz).

Confocal Microscopy

HaCaT cells were cultured on glass coverslips to 60–80% confluence in media containing 0.06 mM or 1.8 mM CaCl2. Cells were washed with 1× PBS, fixed in 4% paraformaldehyde, permeabilized using Triton X-100 (0.5% v/v), incubated with primary rabbit anti-ZNF750 (Sigma-Aldrich) and secondary goat anti-rabbit AlexaFluor 546 (Invitrogen Corporation, CA,USA) antibodies, and then mounted with Vectashield (Vector Laboratories). HEK293 cells were cultured on a glass coverlips to 50–60% confluence, and transiently transfected with 1 µg DNA of an expression construct using lipofectamin2000 (Invitrogen). At 24 hours post transfection, cells were washed twice with 1× PBS, fixed in 4% paraformaldehyde, and permeabilized using Triton X-100 (0.5% v/v) and mounted with Vectashield (Vector Laboratories). The subcellular localizations were visualized using an Olympus confocal microscope with an ×40 and ×60 objective. Confocal images were recorded under identical conditions. Excitation was performed with a 488 nm (for EGFP), 504 nm (for DAPI) and a 543 nm (for AlexaFluor 546) laser and filtered accordingly.

Ki67 Proliferation Assay

HaCaT cells with stable expression of ZNF750 shRNA or a control shRNA were cultured on glass coverslips to 80–90% confluence in media containing 0.06 mM $CaCl_2$. Cells were induced to differentiate in media containing 1.8 mM $CaCl_2$. At day twelve of calcium induced differentiation, cells were washed twice with 1×PBS and fixed in 4% paraformaldehyde. Prior to staining, primary antibody diluting buffer (Biomeda Corp., Foster City, CA), containing Triton X-100 (0.5% v/v), was used to block nonspecific binding. Cells were incubated with rabbit anti Ki67 primary antibody (Cell Marque, Rocklin, CA) for 1 hour, followed by secondary goat anti rabbit AlexaFluor 488 (Invitrogen). To-Pro 3 (Molecular Probes, Invitrogen, USA) was used for nuclear staining. Cells were examined under an Olympus Fluoview FV1000 confocal laser scanning microscope using ×20 or ×60 objectives. Confocal images were recorded under identical conditions. Excitation was performed with a 488 nm (for AlexaFluor 488), and a 504 nm (for DAPI) laser and filtered accordingly. Ki67 positive cells were counted as a percent of total cells using Cell Profiler software. More than 800 cells were counted in each slide. N = 6 Differences in proliferation activity were considered significant at P-values<0.0001 calculated using a standard student's t-test.

Annexin V Assay

Annexin V assay was performed using MEBCYTO Apoptosis Kit (MBL CO., LTD. Nagoya, Japan) according to the manufacturer's protocol. Briefly, cells were incubated with Annexin V at room temperature for 15 minutes in the dark and then subjected to flow cytometry analysis. More than 50,000 cells were counted each time, N = 4. Differences in apoptotic activity were considered significant at P-values<0.0001, calculated using standard student's t-test.

Accession Numbers

Microarray data have been deposited into the GEO database with accession number GSE38039.

Supporting Information

Table S1 Genes that are upregulated or downregulated 2-fold or more in *ZNF750* silenced HaCaT cultures at day twelve of Ca^{2+} induction.

Table S2 Gene Ontology terms of selected ZNF750 target genes that were downregulated by ZNF750 silencing.

Table S3 shRNA sequences used for *ZNF750* silencing.

Table S4 Oligonucleotide sequences used in quantitative real-time PCR.

Figure S1 ZNF750 immunohistochemistry staining in normal human skin.

Figure S2 Genes whose expression was upregulated by ZNF750 silencing in HaCaT cells: Gene Ontology (GO) terms enrichment.

Author Contributions

Conceived and designed the experiments: IC RYB SS OSB. Performed the experiments: IC KL RT. Analyzed the data: IC RYB SS OSB. Contributed reagents/materials/analysis tools: RT OSB. Wrote the paper: IC OSB.

References

1. Candi E, Schmidt R, Melino G (2005) The cornified envelope: a model of cell death in the skin. Nat Rev Mol Cell Biol 6:328–340.
2. Segre AJ (2006) Epidermal barrier formation and recovery in skin disorders. J Clin Invest 116:1150–8.
3. Hoffjan S, Stemmler S (2007) On the role of the epidermal differentiation complex in ichthyosis vulgaris, atopic dermatitis and psoriasis. Br J Dermatol 157:441–447.
4. Fuchs E (2008) Skin stem cells: rising to the surface. J Cell Biol 180:273–284.
5. Fuchs E, Green H (1980) Changes in keratin gene expression during terminal differentiation of the keratinocyte. Cell 19:1033–1042.
6. Steven AC, Steinert PM (1994) Protein composition of cornified cell envelopes of epidermal keratinocytes. J Cell Sci 107:693–700.
7. Kalinin A, Marekov LN, Steinert PM (2001) Assembly of the epidermal cornified cell envelope. J Cell Sci 114:3069–3070.
8. Birnbaum RY, Zvulunov A, Hallel-Halevy D, Cagnano E, Finer G, et al. (2006) Seborrhea-like dermatitis with psoriasiform elements caused by a mutation in ZNF750, encoding a putative C2H2 zinc finger protein. Nat Genet 38:749–751.
9. Birnbaum RY, Hayashi G, Cohen I, Poon A, Chen H, et al. (2011) Association analysis identifies ZNF750 regulatory variants in psoriasis. BMC Med Genet 12:167.
10. Hodel MR, Corbett AH, Hodel AE (2001) Dissection of a nuclear localization signal. J Biol Chem 276:1317–1325.
11. Boukamp P, Petrussevska RT, Breitkreutz D, Hornung J, Markham A, et al. (1988) Normal keratinization in a spontaneously immortalized aneuploid human keratinocyte cell line. J Cell Biol 106:761–771.
12. Yuspa S, Kilkenny A, Steinert P, Roop DR (1989). Expression of murine epidermal differentiation markers is tightly regulated by restricted extracellular calcium concentrations in vitro. J Cell Biol 109:1207–1217.
13. Fuchs E, Byrne C (1994) The epidermis: rising to the surface. Curr Opin Genet Dev 4:725–736.
14. Dlugosz AA, Yuspa SH (1993) Coordinate changes in gene expression which mark the spinous to granular cell transition in epidermis are regulated by protein kinase C. J Cell Biol 120:217–225.
15. Sen GL, Boxer LD, Webster DE, Bussat RT, Qu K, et al. (2012) ZNF750 Is a p63 Target Gene that Induces KLF4 to Drive Terminal Epidermal Differentiation. Dev Cell 22(3):669–677.
16. Scholzen T, Gerdes J (2000) The Ki-67 protein: from the known and the unknown. J Cell Physiol 182:311–22.
17. Huang DW, Sherman BT, Lempicki RA (2009) Systematic and integrative analysis of large gene lists using DAVID Bioinformatics Resources. Nature Protoc 4(1):44–57.
18. Huang DW, Sherman BT, Lempicki RA (2009) Bioinformatics enrichment tools: paths toward the comprehensive functional analysis of large gene lists. Nucleic Acids Res 37(1):1–13.
19. Du L, Neis MM, Ladd PA, Lanza DL, Yost GS, et al. (2006) Effects of the differentiated keratinocyte phenotype on expression levels of CYP1–4 family genes in human skin cells. Toxicol Appl Pharmacol 213:135–144.
20. Deyrieux AF, Wilson VG (2007) In vitro culture conditions to study keratinocyte differentiation using the HaCaT cell line. Cytotechnology 54:77–83.
21. Micallef L, Belaubre F, Pinon A, Jayat-Vignoles C, Delage C, et al. (2008) Effects of extracellular calcium on the growth-differentiation switch in immortalized keratinocyte HaCaT cells compared with normal human keratinocytes. Exp Dermatol 18:143–151.
22. Descargues P, Sil AK, Karin M (2008) IKKa, a critical regulator of epidermal differentiation and a suppressor of skin cancer. EMBO J 27:2639–2647
23. Simpson CL, Patel DM, Green KJ (2011) Deconstructing the skin: cytoarchitectural determinants of epidermal morphogenesis. Nat Rev Mol Cell Biol 12(9):565–580.
24. Naldini LU, Blomer P, Gallay D, Ory R, Mulligan FH, et al. (1996) In vivo gene delivery and stable transduction of nondividing cells by a lentiviral vector. Science 272:263–267.
25. Irrizary RA, Hobbs B, Collin F, Beazer-Barclay YD, Antonellis KJ, et al. (2003) Exploration, normalization, and summaries of high density oligonucleotide array probe level data. Biostatistics 4:249–264.
26. Benjamini Y, Hochberg Y (1995) Controlling the False Discovery Rate: A Practical and Powerful Approach to Multiple Testing. J Roy Statist Soc Ser B 57:289–300.

21

Mathematical Modeling of Calcium Waves Induced by Mechanical Stimulation in Keratinocytes

Yasuaki Kobayashi[1,2], Yumi Sanno[3], Akihiko Sakai[3], Yusuke Sawabu[1], Moe Tsutsumi[4], Makiko Goto[4], Hiroyuki Kitahata[5], Satoshi Nakata[6], Junichi Kumamoto[2,4], Mitsuhiro Denda[2,4], Masaharu Nagayama[1,2]*

1 Research Institute for Electronic Science, Hokkaido University, Sapporo, Japan, **2** CREST, Japan Science and Technology Agency, Tokyo, Japan, **3** Graduate School of Science and Technology, Kanazawa University, Kanazawa, Japan, **4** Shiseido Research Center, Shiseido Co., Ltd., Yokohama, Japan, **5** Department of Physics, Graduate School of Science, Chiba University, Chiba, Japan, **6** Graduate School of Science, Hiroshima University, Higashi-Hiroshima, Japan

Abstract

Recent studies have shown that the behavior of calcium in the epidermis is closely related to the conditions of the skin, especially the differentiation of the epidermal keratinocytes and the permeability barrier function, and therefore a correct understanding of the calcium dynamics is important in explaining epidermal homeostasis. Here we report on experimental observations of in vitro calcium waves in keratinocytes induced by mechanical stimulation, and present a mathematical model that can describe the experimentally observed wave behavior that includes finite-range wave propagation and a ring-shaped pattern. A mechanism of the ring formation hypothesized by our model may be related to similar calcium propagation patterns observed during the wound healing process in the epidermis. We discuss a possible extension of our model that may serve as a tool for investigating the mechanisms of various skin diseases.

Editor: Attila Csikász-Nagy, Fondazione Edmund Mach, Research and Innovation Centre, Italy

Funding: This work was supported in part by a Grant-in-Aid for Scientific Research (B)(21340023) from The Ministry of Education, Culture, Sports, Science and Technology (MEXT), Japan. The funders had no role in study design, data collection and analysis, decision to publish, or preparation of the manuscript.

Competing Interests: The authors have declared that no competing interests exist.

* E-mail: nagayama@es.hokudai.ac.jp

Introduction

The barrier function of the skin is maintained by adjusting its state while sensing changes in chemical and physical stimuli received from internal and external environments [1]. In other words, keratinocytes are sensitive to such stimuli and are able to recover the damaged epidermal barrier. Recent studies have revealed that the calcium dynamics in the epidermal keratinocytes is strongly associated with cutaneous homeostasis: modulations in epidermal calcium concentration coordinately regulate events late in the epidermal differentiation that together form the barrier [2]. For example, Menon et al. [3] have demonstrated that alteration of the calcium gradient in the epidermis affects the exocytosis of the epidermal lamellar bodies. It is also known that the concentration of calcium is highest in the uppermost region of the epidermis (the epidermal granular layer) in healthy normal skin, and that the calcium gradient disappears immediately after barrier disruption [4,5]. Moreover, abnormal calcium gradients in the epidermis have been observed in a variety of skin diseases [6], and the mutation of the calcium pump or gap junctions is known to induce genetic skin diseases [7–9]. In addition, it has been reported that information regarding the stimuli, damage status, and the skin pathology are reflected in the features of calcium wave propagation and distribution in cultured keratinocytes [10,11]. Therefore, understanding the mechanisms of the dynamical behavior of the calcium distribution in the epidermal keratinocytes should provide us with clues regarding the possible treatment of various skin diseases.

Although individual phenomena regarding the spatio-temporal dynamics of calcium ions have been investigated, the relationships between these phenomena, and how they are related to the epidermal structure and the barrier function have not yet been clarified. Conventional research on dermatology usually adopts the methodology of biochemistry or molecular biology, and these approaches enable us to discuss the detailed relationship between the chemicals and the molecular functions. On the other hand, formulating a mathematical model for describing the global behavior of calcium waves enables us to discuss the functions of calcium-wave related phenomena within the cells, and should even show several guidelines for directing future dermatological research. Such a model would be incorporated into the mathematical model of the epidermis, where the interaction of the structure and the calcium dynamics could be simulated. Therefore, a mathematical approach may help us to understand not only individual functions but also the whole system as a hierarchical structure.

Calcium waves have been mathematically understood as traveling waves on excitable media [12–14]. A traveling wave on excitable media, once triggered by a sufficiently strong stimulus, propagates infinitely by exciting neighboring regions continuously. This excitable media picture, however, is insufficient to reproduce the features of calcium waves in keratinocytes; calcium waves in keratinocytes do not propagate infinitely but stop within a finite area. We have already obtained important results on the in vitro observation of calcium waves induced by mechanical stimulation on cultured keratinocytes [15]. The experimental results reproduced under a different condition (see Materials and Methods) is shown in Fig. 1. The concentration of calcium ions in the stimulated cell increases, followed by an increase in calcium concentration in the neighboring cells. However, the calcium wave propagates only in a restricted region, up to about five cell diameters away from the stimulated cell. Recently, Warren et al. has proposed a mathematical model of ATP-mediated calcium waves in mammalian airway epithelium with many internal variables and succeeded in reproducing finite range propagation of calcium waves [16]. Also, Edwards and Gibson introduced a similar model to explain calcium waves in astrocytes [17]. In contrast to their study, we need a simpler model for calcium waves in keratinocytes, in order to investigate the dynamical behavior of the in vivo three-dimensional structure of the epidermis, especially the barrier function of it.

In this paper, using known biochemical and dermatological results, we introduce a mathematical model that can account for the behavior of calcium waves in keratinocytes, especially a ring-shaped pattern recently observed by Tsutsumi et al. [18]. In order to compare our numerical simulations with experimental data, previous experiments are reproduced and the calcium levels are measured under several conditions. We discuss the relation of the ring pattern to skin diseases, and a possible extension to a mathematical model of the epidermal structure.

The Mathematical Model

Several mathematical models, such as the "one-pool" and "two-pool" models, have been proposed for describing intracellular calcium waves. In the former model, it is assumed that calcium ions and IP_3 both affect a single type of calcium ion pool [19–22]. In the latter model, it is assumed that there are two types of calcium ion pools in each cell, where one pool has receptors for calcium ions and the other has receptors for IP_3 [13,23]. The one-pool model has been often used in recent studies, due to its ability to reproduce several experimental results. We adopt the "one-pool model" proposed by Atri et al. [23] as the basis of our model, to which the following assumptions are added: (i) ATP diffuses in a culture solution. (ii) ATP can be detected by ATP-receptors on cell membranes, and IP_3 is synthesized inside each cell [24,25]. (iii) IP_3 and calcium ions inside cells can travel through gap junctions and excite neighboring cells. (iv) Gap junctions close when the Ca^{2+} gradient between cells becomes large.

Based on these assumptions, we propose a mathematical model consisting of ordinary and partial differential equations for the following variables; $A(\boldsymbol{x},t)$ (the ATP concentration in a culture solution), $P_i(t)$ (the IP_3 concentration in the ith cell), $c_i(t)$ (the calcium ion concentration in the ith cell), $w_{ij}(t)$ (the activity of the gap-junctions between cells i and j), and $h_i(t)$ (the inactivation factor of the ith cell, which is defined in the "one-pool model").

We consider a two dimensional space, where N cells with radius r are randomly distributed. The center of the ith cell is located at $\boldsymbol{x}_i$ and any two cells are connected through gap-junctions when their distance is less than R_{gj}. To calculate the ATP dynamics, we utilize the bi-domain method: we treat the space as cell-free when calculating the concentration field $A(\boldsymbol{x},t)$, and when calculating intracellular dynamics of the cell i, the value of the surrounding ATP concentration is represented by $A(\boldsymbol{x}_i,t)$. The mathematical model including all these features is as follows:

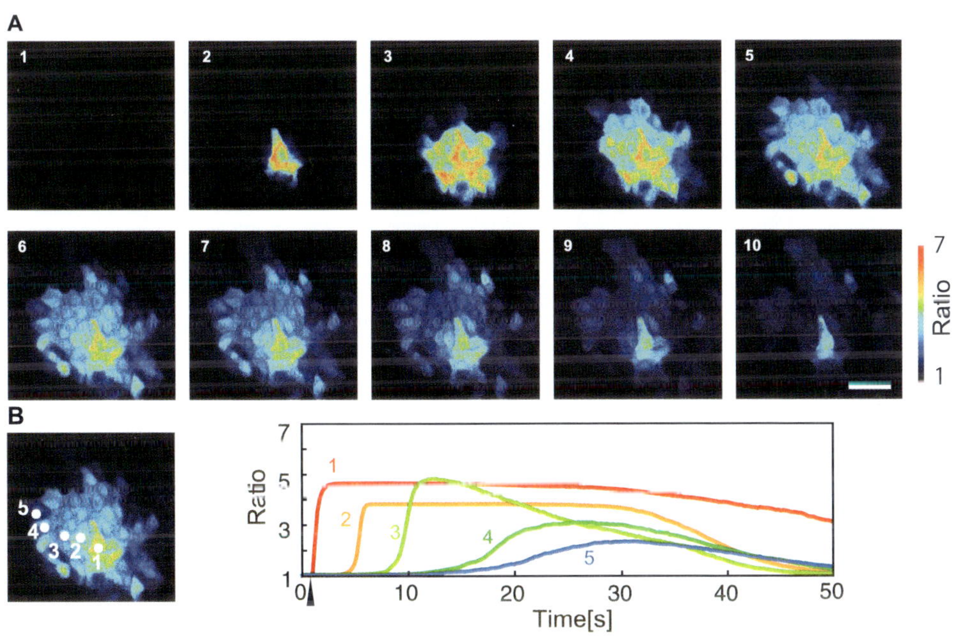

Figure 1. Experimental results on the calcium wave propagation induced by a mechanical stimulation to one cell. (A) Snapshots with an interval of 4.86 s. The scale bar is 100 μm. The ratiometric images (F/F_0) are shown in false color, where blue, green, yellow, and red indicate the increase in intracellular calcium concentration, in this order (see the scale bar on the right). (B) Time change in the calcium concentration is shown in each cell depicted in the left figure. The time when mechanical stimulus was applied is indicated by an upper arrowhead.

$$
\begin{cases}
\dfrac{\partial A}{\partial t} &= d_A \Delta A - K_{aa}A + \displaystyle\sum_{j=1}^{N} G\left(\boldsymbol{x}, \boldsymbol{x}_j, \frac{dc_j}{dt}\right),\\
\dfrac{dc_i}{dt} &= \displaystyle\sum_{j \neq i}^{N} w_{ij} d_c(\boldsymbol{x}_i, \boldsymbol{x}_j)(c_j - c_i) + F_c(P_i, c_i, h_i),\\
\dfrac{dP_i}{dt} &= \displaystyle\sum_{j \neq i}^{N} w_{ij} d_P(\boldsymbol{x}_i, \boldsymbol{x}_j)(P_j - P_i) + F_P(A) - K_{pp}P_i,\\
\dfrac{dh_i}{dt} &= \dfrac{1}{\tau_{h0}} F_h(c_i, h_i),\\
\dfrac{dw_{ij}}{dt} &= \dfrac{1}{\tau_{w0}} F_w(w_{ij}, c_i, c_j),
\end{cases} \tag{1}
$$

where

$$F_c(P,c,h) = K_F\left(\mu_0 + \frac{\mu_1 P}{K_\mu + P}\right)\left(\alpha_0 + \frac{(1-\alpha_0)c}{K_1 + c}\right)h - \frac{\gamma c}{K_\gamma + c} + \beta_0 c_{\text{out}},$$

$$F_P(A) = \frac{K_{pa}A}{H_0 + A}, \quad F_h(c,h) = \frac{K_2^2}{K_2^2 + c^2} - h,$$

$$F_w(w_{ij}, c_i, c_j) = -w_{ij} + \frac{1}{2}\left\{1 + \tanh\left(\frac{w_{d0} - |c_i - c_j|}{\epsilon_{w0}}\right)\right\},$$

$$G\left(\boldsymbol{x}, \boldsymbol{x}_j, \frac{dc_j}{dt}\right) = \chi_\delta(\boldsymbol{x}, \boldsymbol{x}_j, r) K_{ac} R\left(\frac{dc_j}{dt}\right),$$

$$d_P(\boldsymbol{x}_i, \boldsymbol{x}_j) = \chi_0(\boldsymbol{x}_i, \boldsymbol{x}_j; R_{\text{gj}}) d_P, \quad d_c(\boldsymbol{x}_i, \boldsymbol{x}_j) = \chi_0(\boldsymbol{x}_i, \boldsymbol{x}_j; R_{\text{gj}}) d_c,$$

$$\chi_\delta(\boldsymbol{x}, \boldsymbol{y}; r) = \frac{1}{2}\left(1 + \tanh\left(\frac{r - \|\boldsymbol{x} - \boldsymbol{y}\|}{\delta}\right)\right),$$

$$\chi_0(\boldsymbol{x}, \boldsymbol{y}; r) = \begin{cases} 1 & \|\boldsymbol{x} - \boldsymbol{y}\| \leq r, \\ 0 & \|\boldsymbol{x} - \boldsymbol{y}\| > r, \end{cases}$$

$$R(x) = \begin{cases} x & x \geq 0, \\ 0 & x < 0. \end{cases}$$

The relationships among the concentrations of calcium ions, IP_3, ATP, etc., are illustrated in Fig. 2.

The effect of the mechanical stimulation is described as an increase in the concentration of calcium ion, in the stimulated cell. Since it is known that the stimulated cell releases ATP to the culture solution [15,24], and that ATP release is observed even without the calcium excitation [10], the extracellular ATP concentration, near the stimulated cell is also increased independently of the calcium excitation. The mechanical stimulus is represented by the stimulus function $S(t)$. We assume that the effect of stimulation appears in the model equations as the time derivative of $S(t)$, not $S(t)$ itself, reflecting the fact that ATP release does not continue under continuous stimuli. By the same token, the function G, the ATP release due to the calcium excitation, depends not on the calcium concentration itself but on the time derivative of it. Also, following a recent experimental result [18], we further assume that when a cell is broken by a strong stimulus, a stimulant $B(\boldsymbol{x},t)$ is released that induces the influx of extracellular Ca^{2+} through calcium channels on the plasma membrane. These features are introduced to our mathematical model to reproduce the experimental findings of the mechanical stimulation:

$$
\begin{cases}
\dfrac{\partial A}{\partial t} &= d_A \Delta A - K_{aa}A + \displaystyle\sum_{j=1}^{N} G\left(\boldsymbol{x}, \boldsymbol{x}_j, \frac{dc_j}{dt}\right) + \sum_{j \in \Lambda} I_A\left(\boldsymbol{x}, \boldsymbol{x}_j, \frac{dS}{dt}\right),\\
\dfrac{dc_i}{dt} &= \displaystyle\sum_{j \neq i}^{N} w_{ij} d_c(\boldsymbol{x}_i, \boldsymbol{x}_j)(c_j - c_i) + F_c(P_i, c_i, h_i) + I_c^{(i)}\left(B, \frac{dS}{dt}\right),\\
\dfrac{dP_i}{dt} &= \displaystyle\sum_{j \neq i}^{N} w_{ij} d_P(\boldsymbol{x}_i, \boldsymbol{x}_j)(P_j - P_i) + F_P(A) - K_{pp}P_i,\\
\dfrac{dh_i}{dt} &= \dfrac{1}{\tau_{h0}} F_h(c_i, h_i),\\
\dfrac{dw_{ij}}{dt} &= \dfrac{1}{\tau_{w0}} F_w(w_{ij}, c_i, c_j),\\
\dfrac{\partial B}{\partial t} &= d_B \Delta B - K_{bb}B + \displaystyle\sum_{j \in \Lambda'} F_B(\boldsymbol{x}, \boldsymbol{x}_j),
\end{cases} \tag{2}
$$

where

$$I_A(\boldsymbol{x}, \boldsymbol{x}_k) = \chi_\delta(\boldsymbol{x}, \boldsymbol{x}_k, r) R\left(\frac{dS}{dt}\right),$$

$$I_c^{(i)} = \begin{cases} S_a R\left(\dfrac{dS}{dt}\right) + c_{\text{out}} \dfrac{K_{bc}B^2}{H_b^2 + B^2} & i \in \Lambda, \\ c_{\text{out}} \dfrac{K_{bc}B^2}{H_b^2 + B^2} & i \notin \Lambda, \end{cases}$$

$$S(t) = \frac{S_c}{4}\left\{1 + \tanh\left(\frac{t - t_0}{\delta_t}\right)\right\}\left(1 + \tanh\left(\frac{t_1 - t}{\delta_t}\right)\right)$$

$$F_B(\boldsymbol{x}, \boldsymbol{x}_j) = \begin{cases} \chi_\delta(\boldsymbol{x}, \boldsymbol{x}_j, r) B_0 \left(1 - \exp\left(-\dfrac{t - t_d^{(j)}}{t_b}\right)\right) & t > t_d^{(j)}, \\ 0 & t \leq t_d^{(j)}. \end{cases}$$

Here Λ and Λ' denote the set of mechanically stimulated and broken cells, respectively, and $t_d^{(j)}$ indicates the time that cell j is broken. All the other parameters not mentioned above are explained in Table 1.

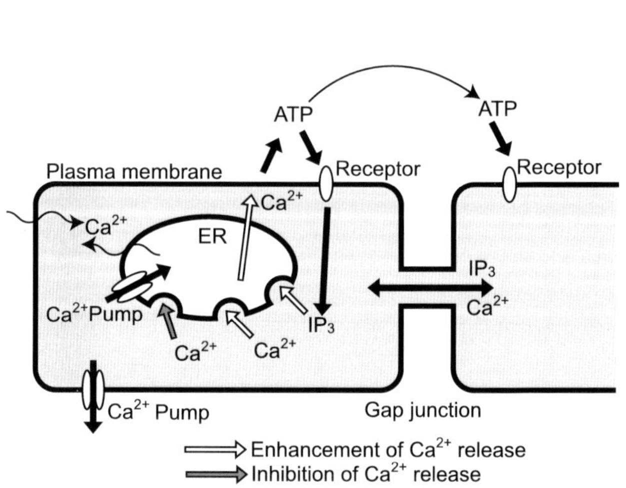

Figure 2. Schematic illustration of the relationship among concentrations of Ca^{2+}, IP_3, and ATP. White and gray arrows denote the enhancement and inhibition of Ca^{2+} release, respectively.

Table 1. List of parameters.

parameter	meaning
K_{aa}	degradation rate of ATP
K_{pp}	degradation rate of IP_3
$\tau_h 0$	typical timescale of the inactivation factor
$\tau_w 0$	typical timescale of the gap-junction activity
d_A	diffusion coefficient of ATP
d_P	diffusion rate of IP_3 through gap-junctions
d_c	diffusion rate of Ca^{2+} through gap-junctions
K_F	maximum Ca^{2+} flux through IP_3 receptors
μ_0	probability of the spontaneous activation at the IP_3 binding domain
μ_1	maximum probability of the activation at the IP_3 binding domain due to IP_3
K_μ	typical value of IP_3 at which the activation by IP_3 becomes effective
α_0	probability of the spontaneous activation at the first Ca^{2+} binding domain
K_1	typical value of IP_3 at which the activation by Ca^{2+} becomes effective
γ	maximum Ca^{2+} flux due to Ca^{2+} pumping out of the cytosol
K_γ	typical value of Ca^{2+} at which Ca^{2+} pumping becomes effective
β_0	coefficient of Ca^{2+} leaking into the cytosol from the extracellular Ca^{2+}
K_{pa}	maximum rate of the IP_3 production due to ATP
H_0	typical value of the ATP at which the IP_3 production becomes effective
K_2	typical value of Ca^{2+} at which activation of the second Ca^{2+} binding domain becomes effective
w_0	threshold of Ca^{2+} concentration difference for gap-junction closing
$_w 0$	sensitivity for gap-junction closing
K_{ac}	coefficient of ATP production due to Ca^{2+} increase
d_B	diffusion coefficient of the stimulant
K_{bb}	degradation rate of the stimulant
S_a	coefficient of the flux due to mechanical stimulation
K_{bc}	coefficient of the maximum flux due to the stimulant
H_b	typical value of the stimulant at which the stimulant-induced Ca^{2+} flux becomes effective
S	maximum strength of mechanical stimulation
δ_t	width of the transition layer between the on and off state of the stimulation
B_0	saturated value of the stimulant release rate
t_b	typical timescale of the stimulant release

When a stimulus is too strong and the Ca^{2+} level reaches a certain threshold c_{th}, we consider that the cell is broken, and set $\mu_1 = K_{pa} = 0$ for that cell, so that the Ca^{2+} and IP_3 levels relax to stationary states. At this point the stimulant B is released. We also assume that the stimulant B affects the Ca^{2+} level only when the extracellular calcium c_{out} exists [18].

We now turn to the normalization of our model equations. Let us introduce the following dimensionless variables:

$$u_i = \frac{c_i}{K_1}, \quad p_i = \frac{P_i}{K_\mu}, \quad a = \frac{A}{H_0}, \quad b = \frac{B}{H_B}, \quad \boldsymbol{y} = \frac{1}{r}\boldsymbol{x}, \quad \tau = \frac{t}{t^*}, \tag{3}$$

where $t^* = K_1/(K_F \alpha_0 \mu_0)$. Then the model equations are rewritten accordingly:

$$\begin{cases} \dfrac{\partial a}{\partial \tau} &= d_a \Delta a - k_{aa} a + \displaystyle\sum_{j=1}^{N} g\left(\boldsymbol{y}, \boldsymbol{y}_j, \frac{du_j}{d\tau}\right) + \sum_{j \in \Lambda} i_a\left(\boldsymbol{y}, \boldsymbol{y}_j, \frac{ds}{d\tau}\right), \\ \dfrac{du_i}{d\tau} &= \displaystyle\sum_{j \neq i}^{N} w_{ij} d_u(\boldsymbol{y}_i, \boldsymbol{y}_j)(u_j - u_i) + f_u(p_i, u_i, h_i) + i_u^{(i)}\left(b, \frac{ds}{d\tau}\right), \\ \dfrac{dp_i}{d\tau} &= \displaystyle\sum_{j \neq i}^{N} w_{ij} d_p(\boldsymbol{y}_i, \boldsymbol{y}_j)(p_j - p_i) + f_p(a) - k_{pp} p_i, \\ \dfrac{dh_i}{d\tau} &= \frac{1}{\tau_h} f_h(u_i, h_i), \\ \dfrac{dw_{ij}}{d\tau} &= \frac{1}{\tau_w} f_w(w_{ij}, u_i, u_j), \\ \dfrac{\partial b}{\partial \tau} &= d_b \Delta b - k_{bb} b + \displaystyle\sum_{j \in \Lambda'} f_b(\boldsymbol{y}, \boldsymbol{y}_j), \end{cases} \tag{4}$$

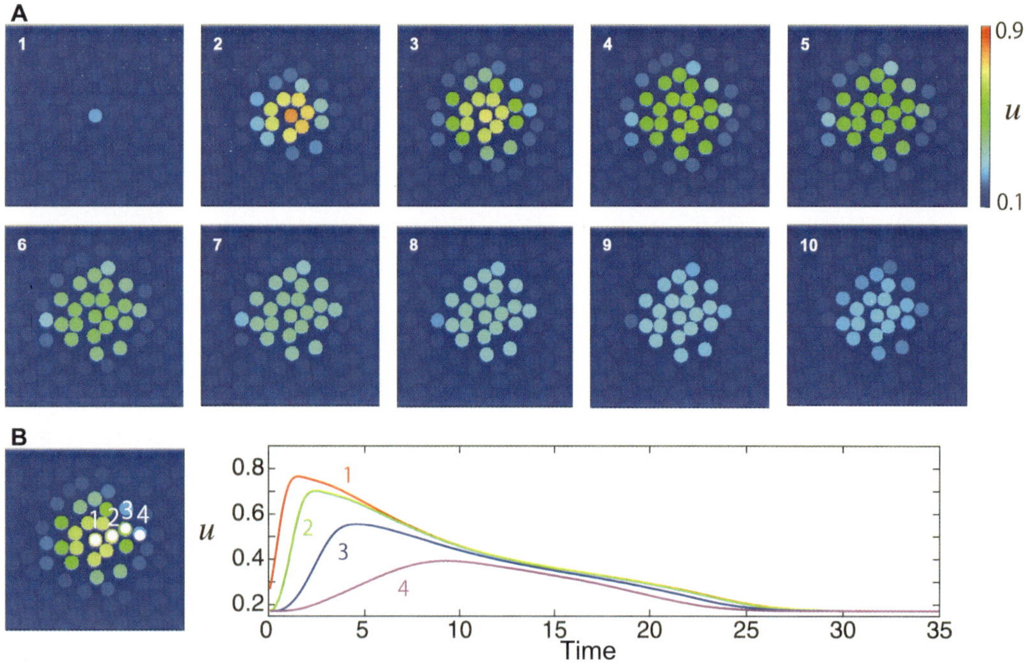

Figure 3. Numerical results of the mechanical stimulation. Stimulation is given to the cell located at the center at $t=0$. (A) Snapshots every 2 time units are shown. (B) Changes in the calcium concentration of the cells are specified in the left figure.

where

$$f_u(p,u,h)=\left(1+\frac{\mu p}{1+p}\right)\left(1+\frac{\alpha u}{1+u}\right)h-\frac{\gamma_1 u}{k_1+u}+\beta u_{\text{out}},$$

$$f_p(a)=\frac{k_{pa}a}{1+a},$$

$$f_h(u,h)=\frac{k_2^2}{k_2^2+u^2}-h,$$

$$f_w(w_{ij},u_i,u_j)=-w_{ij}+\frac{1}{2}\left\{1+\tanh\left(\frac{w_d-|u_i-u_j|}{\epsilon_w}\right)\right\},$$

$$f_b(\boldsymbol{y}_k)=\begin{cases}\chi_\delta(\boldsymbol{y},\boldsymbol{y}_k,1)b_0(1-\exp(-\frac{\tau-\tau_d}{\tau_b})) & \tau>\tau_d,\\ 0 & \tau\leq\tau_d,\end{cases}$$

$$g\left(\frac{du}{d\tau},\boldsymbol{y}_i\right)=\chi_\delta(\boldsymbol{y},\boldsymbol{y}_i,1)k_{ac}R\left(\frac{du_i}{d\tau}\right),$$

$$i_a\left(\frac{ds}{d\tau},\boldsymbol{y}_i\right)=\chi_\delta(\boldsymbol{y},\boldsymbol{y}_i,1)R\left(\frac{ds}{d\tau}\right),$$

$$i_u^{(i)}\left(b,\frac{ds}{d\tau}\right)=\begin{cases}s_aR\left(\frac{ds}{d\tau}\right)+u_{\text{out}}\frac{k_{bc}b^2}{1+b^2} & i\in\Lambda,\\ u_{\text{out}}\frac{k_{bc}b^2}{1+b^2} & i\notin\Lambda,\end{cases}$$

$$d_p(\boldsymbol{y}_i,\boldsymbol{y}_j)=\chi_0(\boldsymbol{y}_i,\boldsymbol{y}_j;r_{\text{gj}})d_p,$$

$$d_u(\boldsymbol{y}_i,\boldsymbol{y}_j)=\chi_0(\boldsymbol{y}_i,\boldsymbol{y}_j;r_{\text{gj}})d_u,$$

$$s(\tau)=\frac{\sigma_\epsilon}{4}\left\{1+\tanh\left(\frac{\tau-\tau_0}{\delta_\tau}\right)\right\}\left\{1+\tanh\left(\frac{\tau_1-\tau}{\delta_\tau}\right)\right\},$$

and the parameters are rescaled as $d_a=\frac{t^*d_A}{r^2}$, $d_p=\frac{t^*d_P}{r^2}$, $d_u=\frac{t^*d_c}{r^2}$, $d_b=\frac{t^*d_B}{r^2}$, $\mu=\frac{\mu_1}{\mu_0}$, $\alpha=\frac{1-\alpha_0}{\alpha_0}$, $\gamma_1=\frac{t^*\gamma}{K_1}$, $k_1=\frac{K_\gamma}{K_1}$, $u_{\text{out}}=\frac{c_{\text{out}}}{K_1}$, $\beta=t^*\beta_0$, $k_2=\frac{K_2}{K_1}$, $k_{aa}=t^*K_{aa}$, $k_{bb}=t^*K_{bb}$, $k_{ac}=\frac{K_1K_{ac}}{H_0}$, $k_{bc}=t^*K_{bc}$, $\sigma_\epsilon=\frac{S_\epsilon}{H_0}$, $w_d=\frac{w_d0}{K_1}$, $\epsilon_w=\frac{\epsilon_w0}{K_1}$, $s_a=\frac{H_0S_a}{K_1}$, $k_{pa}=\frac{t^*K_{pa}}{K_\mu}$, $k_{pp}=t^*K_{pp}$, $r_{\text{gj}}=\frac{R_{\text{gj}}}{r}$, $\tau_h=\frac{\tau_{h_0}}{t^*}$, $\tau_w=\frac{\tau_{w_0}}{t^*}$, $\tau_b=\frac{t_b}{t^*}$, $\tau_0=\frac{t_0}{t^*}$, $\tau_1=\frac{t_1}{t^*}$, and $\delta_\tau=\frac{\delta_t}{t^*}$.

It is noted that the effect of the diffusion of calcium ions is small, since the calcium ions can react with many kinds of proteins in the cells before diffusing through a gap junction. Hence we assume $d_p \gg d_u$.

We set the system size $L_x=L_y=25$. The equations for $a(\boldsymbol{y},t)$ and $b(\boldsymbol{y},t)$ are solved using the ADI method with a grid size of 0.125 under Neumann boundary conditions. The remaining equations are solved using an explicit Euler scheme with a time step of 0.001.

The initial conditions are assigned in such a way that all variables are in a steady state: $a(\boldsymbol{y},0)=0$, $u_i=u^*$, $P_i=0$, $h_i=k_2^2/(k_2^2+u^{*2})$, $wij=1$, and $b(\boldsymbol{y},0)=0$, where u^* is the solution to $f_u(p,u^*,k_2^2/(k_2^2+u^{*2}))=0$. The threshold $u_{\text{th}}=c_{\text{th}}/K_1$ is set to 1.0.

Unless otherwise noted, the remaining parameters are set with the following values: $d_a=1.38$, $d_p=0.138$, $d_u=0.0138$,

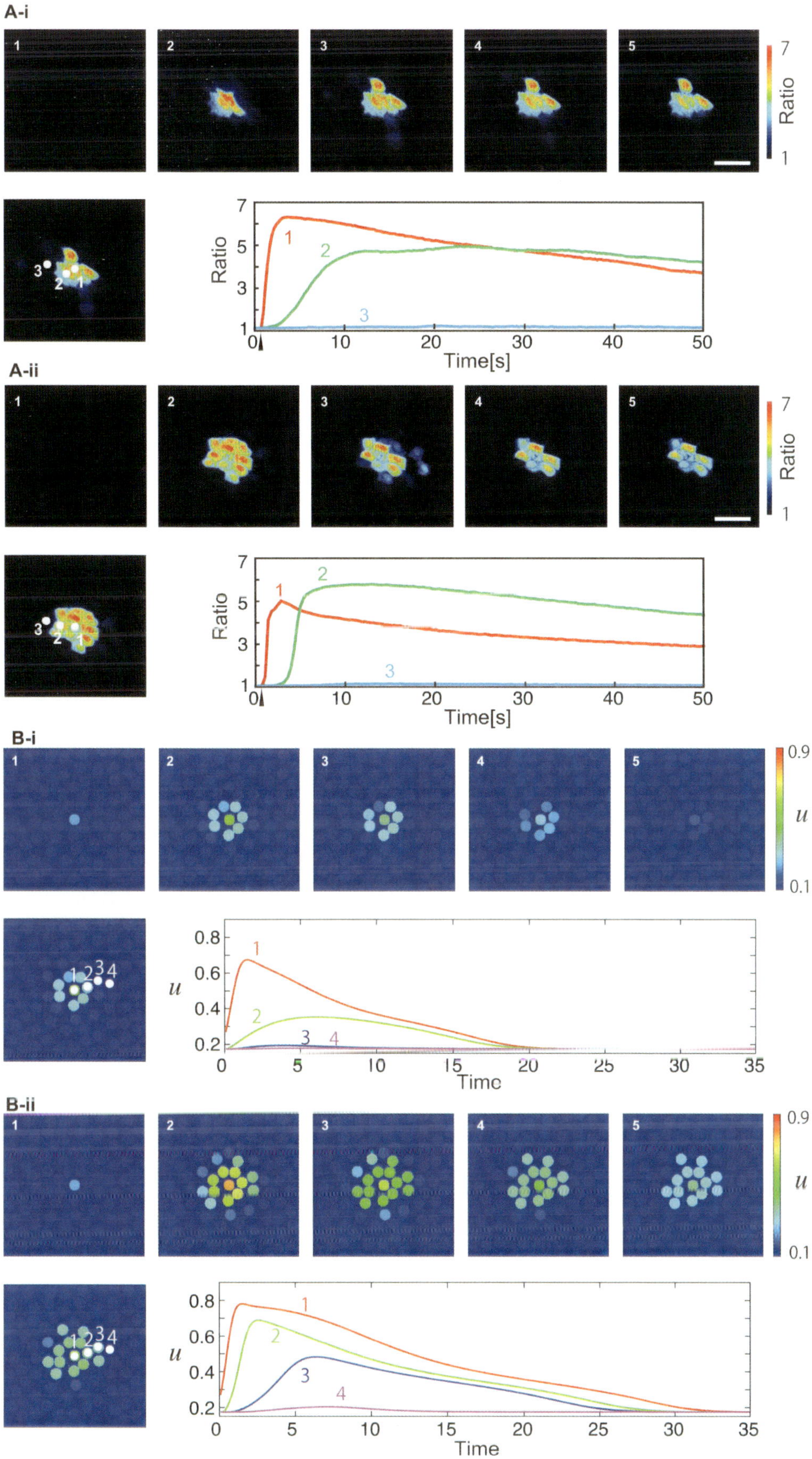
A-i
1
2
3
4
5
7
Ratio
1
7
5
3
1
Ratio
0
10
20
30
40
50
Time[s]
1
2
3
A-ii
1
2
3
4
5
7
Ratio
1
7
5
3
1
Ratio
0
10
20
30
40
50
Time[s]
1
2
3
B-i
1
2
3
4
5
0.9
u
0.1
0.8
0.6
0.4
0.2
u
0
5
10
15
20
25
30
35
Time
1
2
3
4
B-ii
1
2
3
4
5
0.9
u
0.1
0.8
0.6
0.4
0.2
u
0
5
10
15
20
25
30
35
Time
1
2
3
4

Figure 4. Experimental and numerical results with the addition of ATP-degrading enzyme and gap-junction-blocking reagent. (A-i) Experimental results with the addition of ATP-degrading enzyme (apyrase). In the upper figures, snapshots are shown with an interval of 10.7 s. The scale bars are 100 μm. The ratiometric images (F/F_0) are shown in false color, where blue, green, yellow, and red indicate increasing intracellular calcium concentration, in this order (see the scale bar on the right). In the figure below, change in the calcium concentration throughout time is shown for each cell depicted in the left figure. The time when the mechanical stimulus was applied is indicated by an upper arrowhead. (A-ii) Experimental results with the addition of gap-junction-blocking reagent (octanol). (B) The numerical results corresponding to the addition of (B-i) ATP degrading enzyme and (B-ii) gap-junction-blocking reagent. The parameters are the same as those used for Fig. 1 except for (B-i) $k_{aa}=13.8$, and (B-ii) $d_p=d_u=0.0$. Snapshots every 5 time units are shown. Below, change in u_i is shown throughout time in each cell depicted in the left figure.

$d_b=0.138$, $\mu=0.176$, $\alpha=8.09$, $\gamma_1=3.94$, $k_1=0.142$, $u_{\text{out}}=0.142$, $\beta=0.0276$, $k_2=1.0$, $k_{aa}=1.38$, $k_{bb}=2.07$, $k_{ac}=0.014$, $k_{bc}=0.788$, $\sigma_\epsilon=1.0$, $w_d=0.142$, $\epsilon_w=0.142$, $s_a=4.0$, $k_{pa}=165$, $k_{pp}=0.414$, $r_{gj}=3.75$, $\tau_h=0.144$, $\tau_w=0.724$, $\tau_b=7.24$, $\tau_0=0$, $\tau_1=0.724$, and $\delta_\tau=0.00724$. For these parameters we obtain $u^*=0.174$.

Results and Discussion

In the following numerical simulations, we apply a mechanical stimulation to a single cell which is located at the center of the domain. We first perform a simulation with a modest stimulation strength, $\sigma_\epsilon=1.0$, which implies that the stimulated cell is not broken and therefore that the stimulant B is not released. The results of the numerical simulation are shown in Fig. 3 A, which reproduces the experimentally observed finite-range wave propagation: the calcium wave only reaches a distance of several cells from the stimulated one.

Note that the finite-range wave propagation does not stem from a discrete nature of the cells, as is often found in discrete excitable media [26]: we have numerically checked that even when we take the continuous limit for all discrete variables, we still found finite range propagations.

The Effect of ATP-breaker and gap-junction blocker

To confirm the validity of our model, we compare the experimental and numerical results under the condition of an additional ATP-degrading enzyme and a gap-junction-blocking reagent. The experimental results, which are a reproduction of the previous work [15] under a different condition, are shown in Fig. 4, A-i and A-ii. We note that the area where the calcium wave propagates is smaller in comparison with the results shown in Fig. 1. In the numerical simulation, the addition of the ATP-degrading enzyme corresponds to an increased $k_a a$, and the gap-junction-blocking reagent corresponds to smaller d_p and d_u. The results of numerical simulation for such conditions are shown in Fig. 4, B-i and B-ii. The experimental results correspond well to the numerical ones.

Dependency on the strength of the mechanical stimulation

We have also compared an experimental and numerical results where the strength of the mechanical stimulation is varied. The experimental results, which are a reproduction of [27] under a different condition, are shown in Fig. 5 A, where we observe that the calcium wave propagates further when the stimulation is stronger. In the corresponding numerical simulation, we use a stronger stimulus $\sigma_\epsilon=5.0$, which is still weak so that the stimulant B is not released. The numerical results are shown in Fig. 5 B, which reproduces the expansion of the propagation range observed in the experiment.

Ring pattern

It has recently been reported that a strong mechanical stimulus, enough to break the cell, causes a ring-like Ca^{2+} localized pattern around the broken cell [18]. This experimental observation can also be reproduced by our model, by using an even stronger stimulus $\sigma_\epsilon=10.0$. The numerical results are shown in Fig. 6. We also reproduced the experiment [18] under a different experimental condition and measured the calcium levels for comparison with the simulation data (also shown in Fig. 6). In this case the Ca^{2+} level of the stimulated cell immediately crosses the threshold u_{th} and the cell is broken, leading to the release of the stimulant B. The gap junctions connecting the broken cell to the neighbors immediately close due to the dynamics of w_{ij}, so that the influx of Ca^{2+} from the broken cell is blocked. Also, since the gap junctions connecting the excited cells to the neighbors are closed for the same reason, the effect of excitation reaches only one cell diameter away, resulting in a ring pattern.

We have confirmed that the ring pattern is not formed when we set the extracellular calcium to zero, $u_{\text{out}}=0$. This means the stimulant B cannot affect the intracellular calcium dynamics. This is in accord with the experiment [18], where ring patterns were not observed when the mechanical stimulation was performed in the calcium-free medium.

General characteristics of calcium wave propagation in keratinocytes

From these results, it is confirmed that our mathematical model qualitatively reproduces the features of calcium wave propagation in cultured keratinocytes. Our model suggests that the essence of calcium wave propagation is ATP diffusion and transportation of IP_3 through gap junctions. The calcium waves created in our model propagate only within a limited area, in marked contrast to excitable waves in nerve cells, which is often represented by the Hodgkin-Huxley model [28] and the FitzHugh-Nagumo model [29,30]. In our model, the excited region expands not infinitely but finitely, and the excited region comes back to the steady state. Thus, the excited region looks like a disk, as is observed in the experiments.

We speculate that the finite range wave propagation, and especially the ring pattern formation might be used in vivo to define abnormal and damaged sites: when the damaged skin is repaired, information on the location of the damaged site must be detected, and the localized calcium excitation would serve as such a signal. We also hypothesize that the ring pattern-generating mechanism is responsible for the calcium localization beneath the stratum corneum in the epidermis: In the process of cornification, keratinocytes, undergoing denucleation, would release stimulants as we assumed, which would cause the experimentally observed localized calcium excitations just below the cornified layer, which then induces the differentiation into cornified cells. Hence we think that our calcium dynamics model can be incorporated into an

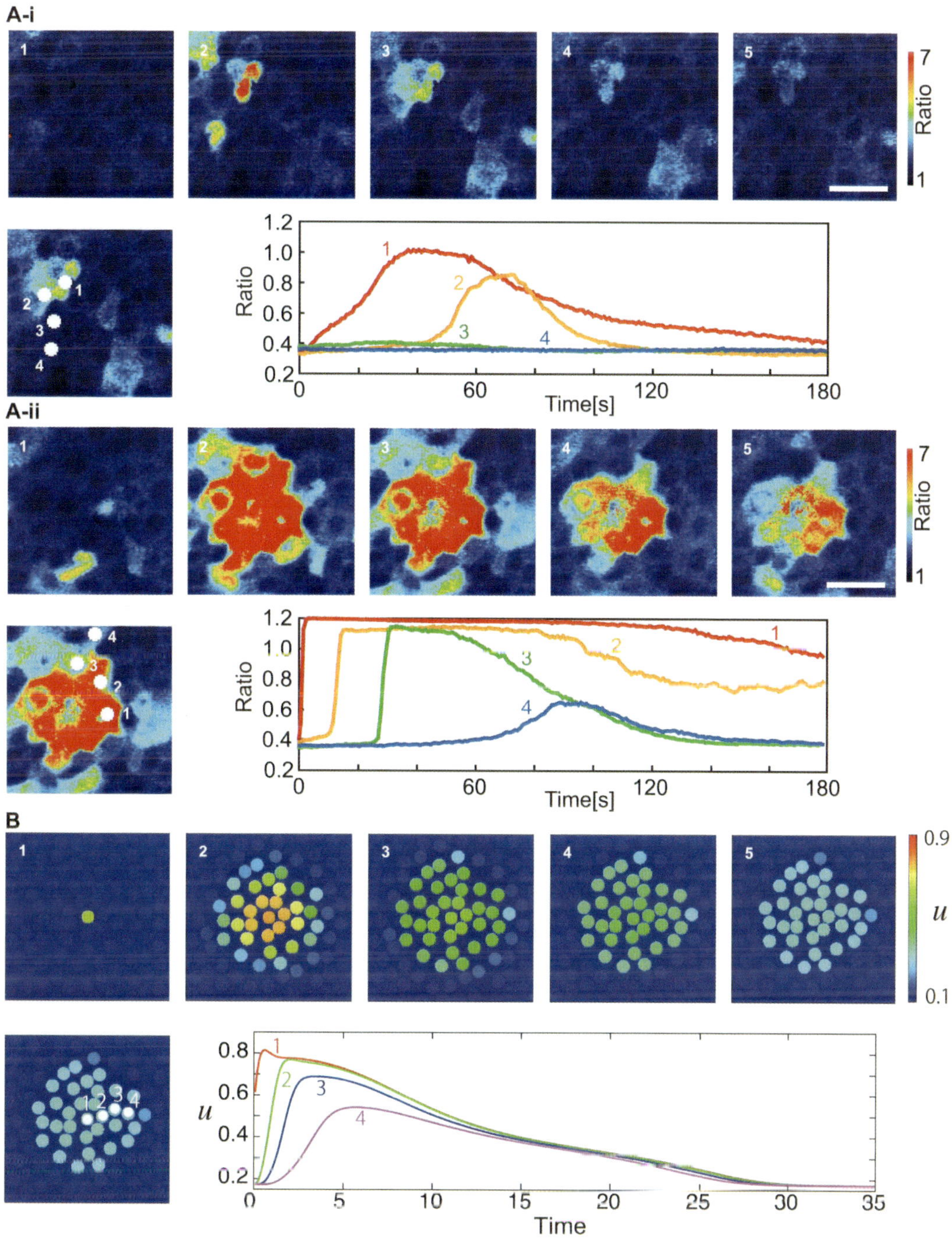

Figure 5. Comparison between (A) experimental and (B) numerical results when the strength of the stimulus is varied. (A) In the experiments, the pressure imparted on the cell was (A-i) 50 hPa and (A-ii) 100 hPa. In the upper figures in (A), snapshots are shown with the time intervals 40.0 s. The scale bars are 50 μm. The ratiometric images (F_{340}/F_{380}) are shown in false color, where blue, green, yellow, and red indicate increasing intracellular calcium concentration, in this order (see the scale bar on the right). Below, change in the calcium concentration is shown throughout time in each cell depicted in the left figure. The origin was set to be the time that the mechanical stimulus was applied. (B) Numerical results with the same settings as that of Fig. 3, except that the stimulus is five times stronger, $\sigma_c = 5.0$.

epidermal cell model to simulate epidermal homeostasis. Such a model can be used, for example, to study the importance of calcium dynamics for the structural stability of the epidermis.

Abnormal distribution of calcium in the epidermis is observed in atopic dermatitis, psoriasis [6], and the aged skin [31]. These skin problems can be characterized by the abnormal barrier function [1]. Since calcium distribution is strongly associated with the permeability barrier homeostasis [2], the extended model could also be used as a simulator of these skin diseases.

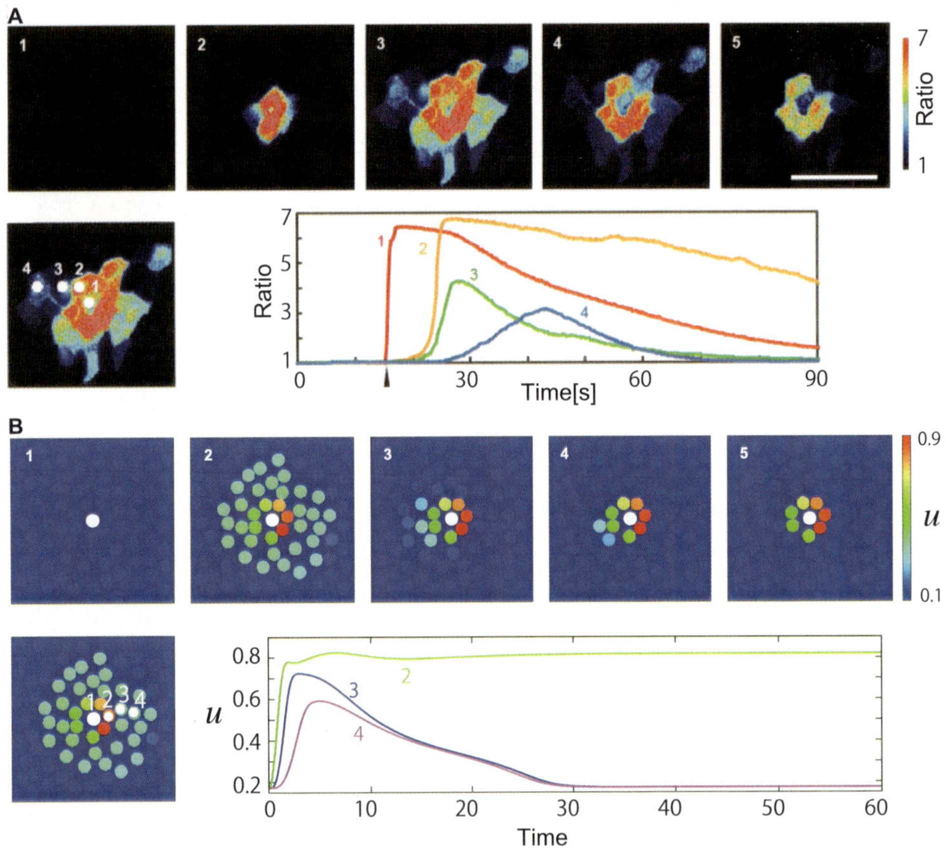

Figure 6. Ring patterns when a cell is broken by a strong mechanical stimulation. In experiment (A), a localized high-calcium-concentration region was observed around the broken cell. Snapshots are shown every 19.0 s. The scale bar is 100 μm. The ratiometric images (F/F_0) are shown in false color, where blue, green, yellow, and red indicate the increase in intracellular calcium concentration, in this order (see the scale bar on the right). Changes in the calcium concentrations are shown throughout time in the bottom right for the cells numbered in the left panel. The time that the mechanical stimulus was applied is indicated by an upper arrowhead. (B) Numerical results with the same settings as that of Fig. 3, except that the stimulus is ten times stronger, $\sigma_c = 10.0$. Snapshots every 15 time units are shown. The calcium level of cell 1, which immediately crosses u_{th} after stimulation, is not shown.

Materials and Methods

Cells and cell culture

Normal human epithelial keratinocytes were purchased from Kurabo (Osaka, Japan) and cultured in EPILIFE-KG2 (Kurabo). Keratinocytes were seeded onto collagen-coated glass coverslips (Matsunami, Osaka, Japan) and used within 5 days. Keratinocytes were grown to approximately 100%-120% confluency in the presence of 0.06 mM Ca^{2+}, and this was switched to 1.8 mM Ca^{2+} 24 h before experiments.

Measurement of intracellular calcium ions

Changes in intracellular calcium concentration in individual cells were measured with Fluo-4 AM (Molecular Probes Inc., OR, USA) for Figs. 1, 4 A and 6 A, and Fura-2 AM (Molecular Probes Inc., OR, USA) for Fig. 5 A. Cells were loaded with 5 μM Fluo-4 AM at 37°C for 40 min. After loading, cultures were rinsed in BSS containing (in mM): NaCl 150, KCl 5, $CaCl_2$ 1.8, $MgCl_2$ 1.2, HEPES 25, and D-glucose 10 (pH 7.4), and incubated for a further 10 min at room temperature to allow de-esterification of the loaded dye. The coverslip was mounted on an inverted epifluorescence microscope (Eclipse Ti, Nikon, Tokyo, Japan). The image data were obtained with a high-sensitivity CCD camera (ORCA-R2, Hamamatsu Photonics, Hamamatsu, Japan) under the control of analyzing system (AQUACOSMOS/RATIO, Hamamatsu Photonics). The fluorescence signals of Fluo-4 AM (for Figs. 1, 4 A and 6 A) were indicated by ratiometric images (F/F_0), where F_0 represents the initial level of fluorescence and F is the fluorescence recorded at different time points during the experiment. On the other hand, the fluorescence signals of Fura-2 AM (for Fig. 5 A) were represented as the ratio of fluorescence intensities at 340 and 380 nm (emission wavelength was 510 nm), i.e., F_{340}/F_{380}, where F_{340} and F_{380} are the fluorescence intensities at 340 and 380 nm, respectively.

Mechanical stimulation

A glass micropipette was made by pulling a glass capillary (Sutter Instrument, CA, USA) with a puller and mounted on a micromanipulator (Narishige, Tokyo, Japan). The micropipette was placed over a single cell and mechanical stimulation was applied to the cell by lowering the micropipette onto the surface of the cell, and then (i) rapidly returning it to its original position (Fig. 1), or (ii) keeping it in that position for an interval of time (Fig. 6). In case (i), if the stimulated cell shows any damage like dye leakage or abnormal morphology, or increase in fluorescence in the second stimulation, the experiment was eliminated. The same experiments were performed under the condition where an ATP degrading enzyme (apyrase) or gap-junction-blocking reagent (octanol) was added to the culture solution (Fig. 4 A). Apyrase and octanol were purchased from Sigma-Aldrich (St. Louis, MO, USA).

Hydraulic pressure stimulation was performed using a FemtoJet microinjector (Eppendorf, Hamburg, Germany) in BSS. A glass microtube was pulled from glass capillary and was filled with BSS or calcium-free BSS. It was connected with the microinjector and its tip was placed just over the cell. Pressure and injection time were controlled by the microinjector. First, the fluorescence intensity of the unstimulated cell was measured, and then the cell was stimulated with hydraulic pressure for 1 second. The fluorescence intensity was measured for more than 5 minutes (Fig. 5 A).

Conclusions

We have proposed a mathematical model for calcium wave propagation in keratinocytes considering the concentration of ATP as an extension of the "one-pool model" suggested previously. Using our model, we have reproduced experimental results of the calcium wave propagation in keratinocytes with the addition of an ATP-degrading enzyme or a gap-junction-blocking reagent, and achieved numerical results corresponding to the experimental observations where the strength of the mechanical stimulation is varied. By assuming the release of a stimulant from a broken cell, an experimentally observed ring pattern has also been reproduced. Through making our model, we suggest that the finite wave propagation is important for calcium waves in keratinocytes, i.e., calcium waves in keratinocytes do not propagate like traveling pulses, as in nerve cells, but propagate finitely while remaining in the shape of a disk. Although microscopic mechanism of the calcium propagation in the epidermis is still unknown, our model is expected to be used for studying of the role of calcium dynamics for the structural stability of the epidermis by incorporating it into epidermal cell models, which will be of great use for the cure of various skin diseases.

Acknowledgments

The authors acknowledge Dr. Yumihiko Ikura (Hokkaido University, Japan) for valuable comments.

Author Contributions

Conceived and designed the experiments: YK MT MG MD HK SN MN. Performed the experiments: YK Y. Sanno AS Y. Sawabu MT MG JK. Analyzed the data: YK MT HK. Contributed reagents/materials/analysis tools: MT MG MD. Wrote the paper: YK MT HK MD MN.

References

1. Elias PM, Feingold KR (2006) Stratum corneum barrier function: definitions and broad concepts. In: Elias PM, Feingold KR, editors. Skin Barrier. New York: Taylor & Francis.pp. 1–4.
2. Elias PM, Ahn SK, Denda M, Brown BE, Crumrine D, et al. (2002) Modulations in epidermal calcium regulate the expression of differentiation-specific markers. J Invest Dermatol 119:1128–1136.
3. Menon GK, Elias PM, Feingold KR (1994) Integrity of the permeability barrier is crucial for maintenance of the epidermal calcium gradient. Br J Dermatol 130:139–147.
4. Mauro T, Bench G, Sidderas-Haddad E, Feingold KR, Elias PM, et al. (1998) Acute barrier perturbation abolishes the Ca^{2+} and K^+ gradients in murine epidermis: quantitative measurement using PIXE. J Invest Dermatol 111:1198–1201.
5. Denda M, Hosoi J, Ashida Y (2000) Visual imaging of ion distribution in human epidermis. Biochem. Biophys. Res Commun 272:134–137.
6. Forslind B, Werner-Linde Y, Lindberg M, Pallon J (1999) Elemental analysis mirrors epidermal differentiation. Acta Derm Venereol (Stockh) 79:12–17.
7. Sakuntabhai A, Ruiz-Perez V, Carter S, Jacobsen N, Burge S, et al. (1999) Mutations in ATP_2A_2, encoding a Ca^{2+} pump, cause Darier disease. Nat Genet 21:271–277.
8. Hu Z, Bonifas JM, Beech J, Bench G, Shigihara T, et al. (2000) Mutations in ATP_2C_1, encoding a calcium pump, cause Hailey-Hailey disease. Nat Genet 24:61–65.
9. Meşe G, Richard G, White TW (2007) Gap junctions: basic structure and function. J Invest Dermatol 127:2516–2524.
10. Denda M, Denda S (2007) Air exposed keratinocytes exhibited intracellular oscillation. Skin Res Technol 13:195–201.
11. Tsutsumi M, Kitahata H, Nakata S, Sanno Y, Nagayama M, et al. (2010) Mathematical analysis of intercellular calcium propagation induced by adenosine triphosphate. Skin Res Technol 16:146–150.
12. Keener J, Sneyd J (1998) Mathematical Physiology. New York: Springer-Verlag.
13. Sneyd J, Wetton BTR, Charles AC, Sanderson MJ (1995) Intercellular calcium waves mediated by diffusion of inositol triphosphate: a two-dimensional model. Am J Physiol Cell Physiol 268:C1537–C1545.
14. Li P, Holden AV (2009) Intracellular Ca^{2+} nonlinear wave behaviours in a three dimensional ventricular cell model. Physica D 238:992–999.
15. Tsutsumi M, Inoue K, Denda S, Ikeyama K, Goto M, et al. (2009) Mechanical-stimulation-evoked calcium waves in proliferating and differentiated human keratinocytes. Cell Tissue Res 338:99–106.
16. Warren NJ, Tawhai MH, Crampin EJ (2009) Mathematical modelling of calcium wave propagation in mammalian airway epithelium: evidence for regenerative ATP release. Exp Physiol 95:232–249.
17. Edwards JR, Gibson WG (2010) A model for Ca^{2+} waves in networks of glial cells incorporating both intercellular and extracellular communication pathways. J Theor Biol 263:45–58.
18. Tsutsumi M, Goto M, Denda M (2013) Dynamics of intracellular calcium in cultured human keratinocytes after localized cell damage. Exp Dermatol 22:367–369.
19. Dupont G, Berridge MJ, Goldbeter A (1991) Signal-induced Ca^{2+} oscillations: properties of a model based on Ca^{2+}-induced Ca^{2+} release. Cell Calcium 12:73–85.
20. Girard S, Lückhoff A, Lechleiter J, Sneyd J, Clapham D (1992) Two-dimensional model of calcium waves reproduces the patterns observed in *Xenopus* oocytes. Biophys J 61:509–517.
21. Goldbeter A, Dupont G, Berridge MJ (1990) Minimal model for signal-induced Ca^{2+} oscillations and for their frequency encoding through protein phosphorylation. Proc Natl Acad Sci U S A 87:1461–1465.
22. Sneyd J, Girard S, Clapham D (1993) Calcium wave propagation by calcium-induced calcium release: an unusual excitable system. Bull Math Biol 55:315–344.
23. Atri A, Amundson J, Clapham D, Sneyd J (1993) A single-pool model for intracellular calcium oscillations and waves in the *Xenopus* laevis oocyte. Biophys J 65:1727–1739.
24. Koizumi S, Fujishita K, Inoue K, Shigemoto-Mogami Y, Tsuda M, et al. (2004) Ca2+ waves in keratinocytes are transmitted to sensory neurons: the involvement of extracellular ATP and $P2Y_2$ receptor activation. Biochem J 380:329–338.
25. Burnstock G, Williams M (2000) P2 purinergic receptors: modulation of cell function and therapeutic potential. J Pharmacol Exp Therap 295:862–869.
26. Keener JP (1987) Propagation and its failure in coupled systems of discrete excitable Cells. SIAM J Appl Math 47:556–572.
27. Goto M, Ikeyama K, Tsutsumi M, Denda S, Denda M (2010) Calcium ion propagation in cultured keratinocytes and other cells in skin in response to hydraulic pressure stimulation, J Cell Physiol 224:229–233.
28. Hodgkin AL, Huxley AF (1952) A quantitative description of membrane current and its application to conduction and excitation in nerve. J Physiol 117:500–544.
29. FitzHugh R (1961) Impulses and physiological states in theoretical models of nerve membrane. Biophys J 1:445–466.
30. Nagumo J, Arimoto S, Yoshizawa S (1962) An active pulse transmission line simulating nerve axon. Proc IRE 50:2061–2070.
31. Denda M, Tomitaka M, Akamatsu H, Matsunaga K (2003) Altered distribution of calcium in facial epidermis of aged adults. J Invest Dermatol 21:1557–1558.

Polymorphisms in the *CYP2E1* and *GSTM1* Genes as Possible Protection Factors for Leprosy Patients

Pablo Pinto[1], Claudio Guedes Salgado[2], Ney Santos[1], Dayse O. Alencar[1], Sidney Santos[1], Mara H. Hutz[3], Ândrea Ribeiro-dos-Santos[1]*

1 Laboratório de Genética Humana e Médica, Instituto de Ciências Biológicas, Universidade Federal do Pará, Belém, Pará, Brasil, **2** Laboratório de Dermatoimunologia, Instituto de Ciências Biológicas, Universidade Federal do Pará, Belém, Pará, Brasil, **3** Instituto de Biociências, Departamento de Genética, Universidade Federal do Rio Grande do Sul, Rio Grande do Sol, Brasil

Abstract

Background: The *CYP2E1* and *GSTM1* genes encode metabolic enzymes that have key functions in drug modification and elimination.

Methodology/Principal Findings: We investigated the possible effects of *CYP2E1* and *GSTM1* polymorphisms in 71 leprosy patients and in 110 individuals from the general population. The *GSTM1*0* null allele and INDEL *CYP2E1*1D* mutant genotypes were analyzed by conventional PCR, while *CYP2E1* SNPs (1053C>T, 1293G>C and 7632T>A) were determined by RT-PCR. In leprosy patients, the *GSTM1*0* and *CYP2E1*5* alleles and the combined alleles *GSTM1*0/CYP2E1*6* and *GSTM1*0/CYP2E1*5* were significantly related to a baciloscopic index (BI) (BI<3), while the *CYP2E1*6* allele was related to a better clinical evolution in the leprosy spectrum.

Conclusions/Significance: Therefore, *GSTM1*0*, *CYP2E1*5* and *CYP2E1*6* may be possible protection factors for leprosy patients.

Editor: Tanya Parish, Queen Mary University of London, United Kingdom

Funding: This study was supported by FINEP (Financiadora de Estudos e Projetos), CNPq/Casadinho (Conselho Nacional de Desenvolvimento Científico e Tecnológico), CAPES (Coordenação de Aperfeiçoamento Pessoal de Nível Superior) and PROPES/UFPA (Universidade Federal do Pará), FADESP (Fundação de Amparo a Pesquisa). The funders had no role in study design, data collection and analysis, decision to publish, or preparation of the manuscript.

Competing Interests: The authors have declared that no competing interests exist.

* E-mail: akely@ufpa.br

Introduction

Leprosy is an insidious infectious disease caused by the obligate intracellular bacteria *Mycobacterium leprae* that affects the skin and peripheral nerves, causing a chronic granulomatous infection [1].

Multidrug therapy (MDT), the treatment recommended by the World Health Organization (WHO), has healed millions of patients since it was implemented in 1980s. MDT consists of the use of dapsone and rifampicin for 6 months in paucibacilary (PB) patients, or both along with a third drug, clofazimine, for 12 months in multibacilary (MB) cases [2].

Patients are classified as PB or MB using a simple system introduced by the WHO in 1982. Patients with 5 skin lesions or less are classified as PB, and those with more than 5 lesions are classified as MB [3,4]. Although this simple classification scheme is adequate for remote sites where the population has little or no access to health care, it is not detailed enough for more in-depth research surveys.

Another way to classify leprosy patients is based on a skin smear test, for which a positive result is classified as MB, and a negative result as PB. A trained laboratory technician can readily identify AFB (acid fast bacillus), making this test a very reliable method. However, cases initially classified as PB (AFB negative) can evolve to MB in the natural course of the disease [5]. This phenomenon is especially true for those patients classified as indeterminate (MHI) using the Madrid classification system.

The use of the Ridley-Jopling clinical, histological and immunological criteria further improves case definitions, with TT (tuberculoid-tuberculoid) patients exhibiting a strong cellular immune response (CIR) and a negative skin smear test, while LL (lepromatous-lepromatous) patients have a weak or absent CIR and a highly positive skin smear [6]. In the middle of the spectrum are a large number of borderline patients, varying from weak to strong CIR and from negative to positive skin smears.

Interestingly, neither the CIR status nor the skin smear test is predictive of leprosy reactions or of the progression of each case through the physical disabilities caused by the disease. To date, little is known about which factors are crucial to the development of these disabilities. All types of patients, TT, borderline or LL, can progress with highly incapacitating disabilities and chronic neuropathies with no single marker or criteria to predict patient outcome [2,3].

Dapsone (4,4′-diaminodiphenyl sulfone, DDS) is one of the primary drugs used in anti-leprosy therapeutics. It is a bacteriostatic agent that competes with para-aminobenzoic acid (PABA), diminishing or blocking the production of bacterial folic acid [5,7]. Clofazimine is a riminophenazine dye that has bactericidal and anti-inflammatory effects. It inhibits bacterial proliferation by binding to bacterial DNA and blocking its replication [8,9]. Rifampicin, or rifampin (RIF) has a well-proven bactericidal effect on *M. leprae*. It is a semisynthetic drug, originally derived from *Streptomyces mediterranei*, and it is widely used for treating leprosy and tuberculosis. RIF prevents protein production by inhibition of RNA polymerase in bacterial cells [10–16].

CYP-450 members of the heme protein superfamily are notable for their large spectrum of action and the distribution of their biological structures. These proteins participate in critical processes including the biosynthesis of steroidal hormones and the detoxification by conjugation with cellular components, such as glutathione [17].

CYP2E1 is found in various tissues including brain, lungs and kidneys, but it is most concentrated in the liver, where the majority of biotransformation occurs. Four main SNPs in the *CYP2E1* gene have been investigated in different populations, including tuberculosis (TB) patients [18–20], who often show 1053C>T and 1293G>C mutations, which together form the compound allele *CYP2E1*1A*, CG; *CYP2E1*5*, TC. Another SNP, 7632T>A, is located in the sixth intron of the *CYP2E1* gene and has two alleles, wild-type *CYP2E1*1A* (T) and mutant *CYP2E1*6* (A). Additionally, a 96-bp INDEL polymorphism with two alleles, wild-type *CYP2E1*1C* (DEL) and mutant *CYP2E1*1D* (INS), has also been described [18,19].

There are different glutathione S-transferase (GST) isoforms, including *GSTM1*, which is located on chromosome 1. More than 51 SNPs have been described within *GSTM1*, among which are two functional alleles, *GSTM1*A* and *GSTM1*B*, that have the same detoxification efficacy; one null (deletion) allele, *GSTM1*0*; and one duplication [21,22].

Two GSTM1 polymorphisms, *GSTM1*1*, which has normal activity, and *GSTM1*0*, which has no enzymatic activity because it is a complete gene deletion, have been well studied in different populations [23–25]. The presence of the null allele seems to be related to substrate conjugation and excretion; therefore, its presence can be an indicator for more rational drug dosages for various groups of patients [26].

We investigated a sample of MDT-treated leprosy patients ascertained at the Dr. Marcello Candia Reference Unit in the Sanitary Dermatology of the State of Pará (UREMC) with the aim of identifying associations among ***CYP2E1*** polymorphisms [including 1053 C>T, 1293G>C (*CYP2E1*1A*, *CYP2E1*5*); 7632T>A (*CYP2E1*1A*, *CYP2E1*6*); 96-bp INDEL *CYP2E1*1C* (DEL) and *CYP2E1*1D* (INS)] and ***GSTM1*** polymorphisms (*GSTM1*1* and *GSTM1*0*) and possible protection factors for leprosy patients.

Methods

Sample

We investigated 71 leprosy patients who attended the Dr. Marcello Candia Reference Unit in the Sanitary Dermatology of the State of Pará (UREMC) in Marituba, Pará, Brazil, from January 2008 to December 2009. In UREMC there are about 40,000 yearly consultations on different medicine specialties as, among others, leprology, dermatology, ophthalmology and orthopedics, besides nursery, physical therapy and other health professionals sessions. Since 2002, UREMC registered between 308 and 472 leprosy patients (mean: 408 cases/year). During years 2008 and 2009, 765 leprosy cases were registered, from those, 71 (9,28%) were randomly selected for this study.

All patients were evaluated neurologically by Semmes-Weinstein monofilament examination (SWME) for sensory testing, and by voluntary motor testing (VMT) for function assessment of muscular force, as previously described [27]. They were classified according to the Ridley-Jopling system and were distributed in two groups depending on the progression of the disease: the positive (+) group consisted of PB patients skin smear negative Tuberculoid (TT) patients and MB skin smear negative Borderline-Tuberculoid (BT) patients, with or without leprosy reactions, with no sequel (defined by sensorial loss or motor deficit on hands or feet on Nerve Function Impairment (NFI) assessment), and the negative (−) group consisted of PB patients with or without leprosy reactions, but with sequel, together with all MB skin smear positive Borderline-Borderline (BB), Borderline-Lepromatous (BL) and Lepromatous-Lepromatous (LL) patients, regardless reactions or sequel. Additionally, in order to make other comparisons, patients were classified according to the baciloscopic index (BI), a group with a low (<3) BI (LBI), and a group with high (≥3) BI (HBI) [28]. A sample of 110 healthy individuals from the same geographic area were included in the study as controls. All patients were informed about the study before signing informed consent forms. The project was approved by the Pará Federal University ethics committee (N° 197/07).

DNA Extraction

DNA extraction was performed as previously described [29]. The DNA concentration was determined by spectrophotometry (Themo Scientific NanoDrop 1000, NanoDrop Technologies, Wilmington, US).

CYP2E1 Genotyping

Three *CYP2E1* polymorphisms, 1053C>T, 1293G>C and 7632T>A, were investigated using a TaqMan genotyping assay and analyzed by Real Time PCR 7500 (Life Technologies, CA, USA). The INDEL was investigated using conventional PCR methods, followed by visualization on an agarose gel. Specific PCR programs were established according to the annealing temperatures of the primers, and the amplifications were performed on a thermocycler Veriti 96 Well Thermal Cycler (Life Technologies, CA, USA). The alleles of the four *CYP2E1* polymorphisms investigated were defined using the official nomenclature, as described in http://www.cypalleles.ki.se/cyp2e1.htm.

GSTM1 Genotyping

For amplification, a set of primers for GSTM1F/GSTM1R was investigated using conventional PCR methods (thermocyclerVeriti 96 Well Thermal Cycler - Life Technologies, CA, US), followed by visualization on an agarose gel.

Ancestry Informative Markers (AIM)

Individual interethnic admixture was estimated using a panel of 48 ancestry informative markers (AIMs), as previously described [30].

Statistical Analyses

Estimations of linkage disequilibrium (D and D') and haplotypes and allelic frequencies were estimated with the M. Locus v. 2.0 software [31]. All other statistical analyses were performed using SPSS v. 12.0 (SPSS, Chicago, IL, USA), and results were considered statistically significant at $p<0.05$.

Results

Demographic and clinical characteristics of the patients are shown in Table 1. Age, gender, sequel and clinical forms were all statistically significant when LBI and HBI were compared. Sequel

Table 1. Demographic and clinical characteristic of the sample according with Baciloscopic Index.

Variables	Baciloscopic Index[c] (N = 71)		*p value* (IC-95%)
	LBI n(%) = 32	HBI n(%) = 39	
Age[a]	35.2± 2.97	62.5± 3.42	<0.001
Gender[b] (M/F)	15(46.8%)/17(53.2%)	32(82%)/7(12%)	0.003
Sequel[b] (YES/NO)	12(37.5%)/20(62.5%)	30(76.9%)/9(23.1%)	0.001
Clinical Forms (PB/MB)[b]	10(31.2%)/22(68.8%)	0/39(100%)	0.002

[a]*t*-Test of Student;
[b]Fisher's Exact Test;
[c]Baciloscopic Index (LBI = Baciloscopic Index Low; HBI = Baciloscopic Index High).

occurred in 76.9% of the HBI patients whereas in the LBI group only 37.5% of the patients presented sequel.

There were 19 patients classified in the positive (+) group, of which nine were designated PB (two with reaction) and 10 were MB (four with reaction and all without sequel), while 52 patients comprised the negative (−) group, two of which were PB (all with reaction and sequel), and 50 were MB (35 with reaction and 40 with sequel) (Table 2). Concerning genotypic and allelic distribution of SNPs, a high (42.3%), statistically significant, frequency of the heterozygous genotype for the *CYP2E1*6* allele was found among leprosy patients (Table 2). In the positive group, 63.2% (12 patients) exhibited this genotype, while in the negative group, a lower percentage (34.6%, 18 patients) was observed. The frequency of the wild-type *CYP2E1*1A* and mutant *CYP2E1*6* alleles in this population was 0.789 and 0.211, respectively, which was statistically significant when the positive and negative groups were compared (Table 2).

Leprosy patients were also divided into two groups according to the baciloscopic index (BI): a group with a low (<3) BI (LBI) and a group with high (≥3) BI (HBI). In addition to the analysis of the genotypic distribution of both *CYP2E1* and *GSTM1* markers in the LBI and HBI groups (Table 3), the combined effect of the two mutant alleles for the *CYP2E1* and *GSTM1* genes (*CYP2E1*6/GSTM1*0* and *CYP2E1*5/GSTM1*0*) was also analyzed. The mutant *CYP2E1*5* allele was present in 37.5% of the patients in the LBI group, while the wild-type *CYP2E1*1A* allele was observed in 92.3% of the patients in the HBI group. *GSTM1* gene analysis demonstrated that the mutant *GSTM1*0* allele was present in 56.2% of the LBI group patients and in 38.5% of the HBI group patients, while the wild-type *GSTM1*1* allele was present in 61.5% of the HBI group patients (Table 3). The analysis of the combined

Table 2. Genotypic and allelic distribution of SNPs on *CYP2E1* and *GSTM1* genes among patients grouped according to clinical evolution.

Genotype	Patients with Leprosy (%) (n = 71)	Group (+) (%) (n = 19)	Group (−) (%) (n = 52)	P*[1]	OR(95% IC)*[2]
CYP2E1 (96 INDEL)					
*1C/*1C	64 (90.1%)	16 (84.2%)	48 (92.3%)		1 (reference)
*1C/*1D	7 (8.9%)	3 (15.8%)	4 (7.7%)	0.375	0.444(0.09–2.202)
*CYP2E1*1C*	0.951	0.921	0.962		
*CYP2E1*1D*	0.049	0.079	0.038		
CYP2E1 (7632)					
*1A/*1A	41 (57.7%)	7 (36.8%)	34 (65.4%)		1 (reference)
*1A/*6	30 (42.3%)	12 (63.2%)	18 (34.6%)	**0.03**	0.309(0.103–0.922)
*CYP2E1*1A*	0.789	0.684	0.827		
*CYP2E1*6*	0.211	0.316	0.173		
CYP2E1 (1053/1293)					
*1A/*1A	56 (78.9%)	13 (68.5%)	43 (82.6%)		1 (reference)
*1A/*5	15 (21.1%)	6 (31.5%)	9 (17.4%)	0.206	0.453(0.135–1.513)
CYP2E1 1A*	0.894	0.842	0.914		
*CYP2E1*5*	0.106	0.158	0.086		
GSTM1					
*GSTM1*1*	38 (53.5%)	12 (63.2%)	26 (50%)		1 (reference)
*GSTM1*0*	33 (46.5%)	7 (36.8%)	26 (50%)	0.423	1.714 (0.583–5.043)

*[1]p-value;
*[2]OR-odds ratio, CI-confidence interval.

effect revealed that the *CYP2E1*6/GSTM1*0* genotypic combination was detected in 31.2% of the patients in the LBI group, while the *CYP2E1*5/GSTM1*0* genotypic combination was present in 28.1% of the patients in the LBI group; all were statistically significant when the different combinations were analyzed in the LBI or HBI groups.

Next, we performed a logistic regression analysis in which the two groups, LBI and HBI, were dependent variables and with covariables that could interfere with the results of PB and MB clinical forms. Although the results were not statistically significant for different variables, such as gender and sequel, they were significant when related to *CYP2E1*1A/*5* ($p = 0.0266$) and *GSTM1*0* ($p = 0.0500$) genotypes. These results suggest a strong association between both mutations and LBI (Table 4).

To evaluate the presence of population substructure, we compared the clinical progression of leprosy patients (positive and negative groups, as well as high and low baciloscopic index groups) with genomic ancestry, and the results showed no, significant. However, different frequencies were found for the investigated markers when leprosy patients were compared with a sample of healthy individuals from the same region (Table 5). The data showed that *CYP2E1*5* allele is more frequent among the healthy individuals than among patients (0.196 and 0.106, respectively; $X^2 = 6.85$; $p = 0.032$), while *CYP2E1*6* allele is more common among patients than in the control sample (0.211 e 0.090, respectively; $X^2 = 11.6$; $p = 0.003$).

Discussion

Loss of sensation is the hallmark of leprosy diagnosis. It is well known that both, MB and PB patients may evolve to nerve function impairment on the natural course of the disease [32]. It is usual - and comprehensible as an objective tool – to use BI to analyze the correlation between a specific gene or a genotypic combination and the evolution of leprosy. However, this cannot be the only parameter to evaluate in order to understand the disease behavior individually. HBI may indicate *M. leprae* ability to grow

Table 4. Logistic regression analysis of the association between genetic markers and LBI/HBI response in leprosy patients.

Variable	β	S.E.	Wald	df	*P*	O.R (95%CI)
Age	0.0363	0.0209	3.0109	1	**0.0012**	1.0562 (0.9953–1.0804)
Gender	0.8705	0.7327	1.4113	1	0.2348	2.3881 (0.5680–1.0407)
Sequel	0.8742	0.8405	1.0818	1	0.2983	2.3969 (0.4616–12.4468)
Clinical Form (PB/MB)	1.8598	1.1901	2.4421	1	0.1181	6.4226 (0.6233–66.1807)
*CYP2E1 *1A/*5*	−1.6341	0.8457	3.7339	1	**0.0266**	0.1198 (0.0184–0.7816)
*CYP2E1 *1A/*6*	1.0889	0.9079	1.4382	1	0.2304	2.9709 (0.5012–17.6087)
*GSTM1*0*	−1.3004	0.7025	3.4262	1	**0.05**	0.2724 (0.0687–1.0796)
African	−2.2083	1.8217	3.3266	1	0.4925	0.1099 (0.0002–60.2213)
European	0.9890	2.6275	0.1417	1	0.7066	2.6885 (0.0156–10.6548)
Amerindian	0.4674	2.5465	6.5769	1	0.8544	1.5958 (0.0108–11.0136)

β, Coefficient Stimation; **S.E.**, Standard Error; **df**, Degrees of Freedom; ***p***, p-value; **OR**, Odds Ratio; **CI**, Confident Interval.

Table 3. Combined and isolated genotypic distribution of *CYP2E1* gene (SNPs 1053T>C, 1293C>G and 7632T>A), and deletion (*GSTM1*1/GSTM1*0*) on gene *GSTM1* of patients classified accordingly to baciloscopic index BI (LBI and HBI).

Genotype	Leprosy patients (n = 71)	LBI (n = 32)	HBI (n = 39)	p*[1]	OR (95% IC)*[2]
***CYP2E1* (7632)**					
1A/*1A	41 (57.74%)	16 (50%)	25 (64.1%)		1 (reference)
1A/*6	30 (42.26%)	16 (50%)	14 (35.9%)	0.334	0.560 (0.216–1.452)
CYP2E1*1A	0.789	0.750	0.821		
CYP2E1*5	0.211	0.250	0.179		
***CYP2E1* (1053/1293)**					
1A/*1A	56 (78.87%)	20 (62.5%)	36 (92.3%)		1 (reference)
1A/*5	15 (21.13%)	12 (37.5%)	3 (7.7%)	**0.003**	0.139 (0.035–0.551)
CYP2E1*1A	0.894	0.813	0.962		
CYP2E1*5	0.106	0.187	0.038		
GSTM1					
GSTM1*1	38 (53.52%)	14 (43.8%)	24 (61.5%)		1 (reference)
GSTM1*0	33 (46.48%)	18 (56.2%)	15 (38.5%)	**0.0276**	0.486 (0.188–1.258)
***CYP2E1/GSTM1**[3]*					
CYP2E1*1A/GSTM1*1	58 (81.7%)	22 (68.8%)	36 (92.3%)		1 (reference)
CYP2E1*6/GSTM1*0	13 (18.3%)	10 (31.2%)	3 (7.7%)	**0.012**	0.183(0.045–0.740)
CYP2E1*1A/GSTM1*1	62 (87.3%)	23 (71.9%)	39 (100%)		1 (reference)
CYP2E1*5/GSTM1*0	9 (12.7%)	9 (28.1%)	–	**<0.005**	0.371 (0.27–0.513)

*[1]p-value;
*[2]OR-odds ratio, CI-confidence interval;
*[3]Combined effect of mutant alleles of distinct genes.

Table 5. Allele and genotype distributions of CYP2E1 and GSTM1 genes within two samples from leprosy patients and healthy individuals.

Genotype	Patients with Leprosy (%) (n = 71)	Healthy Population (%) (n = 110)	χ^2	p
CYP2E1 (96 INDEL)				
*1C/*1C	64 (90.1%)	96 (87.3%)		
*1C/*1D	7 (8.9%)	12 (10.9%)		
*1D/*1D	–	2 (1.8%)		
*CYP2E1*1C*	0.951	0.927	1.376	0.743
*CYP2E1*1D*	0.049	0.073		
CYP2E1 (7632)				
*1A/*1A	41 (57.7%)	90 (81.8%)		
*1A/*6	30 (42.3%)	20 (17.2%)		
*6/*6	–	–		
*CYP2E1*1A*	0.789	0.909	11.673	**0.003**
*CYP2E1*6*	0.211	0.091		
CYP2E1 (1053/1293)				
*1A/*1A	56 (78.9%)	70 (63.6%)		
*1A/*5	15 (21.1%)	37 (33.6%)		
*5/*5	–	3 (2.8%)		
*CYP2E1*1A*	0.894	0.805	6.855	**0.032**
*CYP2E1*5*	0.106	0.195		
GSTM1				
*GSTM1*1*	38 (53.5%)	53 (48.2%)		
*GSTM1*0*	33 (46.5%)	57 (51.8%)	1.136	0.722

inside the host in order to keep transmission chain and strain survival, or may indicate the inability of the host in constrain bacterial growth.

Notwithstanding, the capacity of the human host immune system in dealing with leprosy infection with no sequel is rarely addressed. In the present study two groups of patients were examined, and a striking difference when BI or disease evolution were evaluated were observed in relation to the genes investigated herein. While $CYP2E1^{7632}$*1A/*1A* was associated to a worse disease progression, and the presence of the mutant $CYP2E1^{7632}$*1A/*6* was associated with a good evolution, however, none of them were related to LBI or HBI. These findings suggest that different genes may be related to disease progression or bacterial growth inhibition mechanisms. Furthermore, $CYP2E1^{1053/1293}$*1A/*1A* was associated with HBI, while there no significant association was observed for clinical evolution analyses., $CYP2E1^{1053/1293}$*1A/*5* was significantly associated with LBI and a better disease progression.

The availability of modern antibiotics can help us to better understand the disease, and it is reasonable to think that pharmacogenomics related genes may also be related to disease outcome in human hosts. One of these key drugs is rifampicin.

Rifampicin can be bacteriostatic at lower concentrations or bactericidal at higher concentrations. When used alone, mycobacterium can readily develop resistance to RIF, and therefore, treatment should not rely solely on this drug [15]. Its biotransformation occurs through a process of hepatic deacetylation, giving rise to the active metabolite desacetylrifampicin [26]. RIF has a high capacity for inducing CYP450 isoforms, which contributes to a 40% reduction in half-life during the first half month of treatment and the acceleration of RIF deacetylation. Therefore, this drug is capable of intensifying its own biotransformation, diminishing its plasmatic half-life when administered in multiple doses [33]. Studies of the *CYP2E1* gene indicate that *CYP2E1*6* and *CYP2E1*5* alleles are associated with a higher level of transcription and microsomal enzyme activity; therefore, they are implicated in enzymatic biotransformation activity augmentation [34–36], consequently decreasing the half-life of RIF.

Our results show that among the patients grouped according to clinical progression, the heterozygous genotype *CYP2E1*1A/*6* was present in 63.2% of the individuals in the (+) group. The OR analysis of the *CYP2E1*6* allele demonstrated that this polymorphism provides protection to those individuals in the (+) group (Table 2).

We hypothesize that the *CYP2E1*6* allele could increased the rate of rifampicin metabolism. Augments the biotransformation by CYP450 enzymes and raising the levels of the active metabolite desacetylrifampicin, which has a higher bactericidal activity. Therefore, individuals with this mutation could more efficiently combat *M. leprae.*

A significant difference was found between healthy individuals and patients for the *CYP2E1*6* allele, which is more common among leprosy patients ($X^2 = 11.6$; $p = 0.003$). Since this association was unknown, more studies are necessary to confirm these results (Table 5).

Among leprosy patients, *CYP2E1*5* allele was more frequent in the LBI group. This allele was also more frequent in healthy subjects when compared to leprosy individuals. These results taken together suggest that *CYP2E1*5* is a protection factor that might be involved with bacterial growth inhibition (Table 5).

For the *GSTM1* gene, the null genotype *GSTM1*0* was present in 56.2% of the LBI group. The compound distribution of the two mutant alleles *CYP2E1*5/GSTM1*0* was present in 28.1% of LBI the patients, while *CYP2E1*6/GSTM1*0* was present in 31.2%. The estimated OR suggest that mutant alleles confer protection for LBI individuals.

Taken together, our results suggest that the *CYP2E1*5*, *CYP2E1*6* and *GSTM1*0* alleles may be considered as susceptibility markers for leprosy, and their distribution should be further investigated, as their presence seems to confer protection from *M. leprae*.

Acknowledgments

Special thanks the donors of samples (leprosy patients from northern Brazil), who enable this study to be carried out, CAPES (Coordenação de Aperfeiçoamento Pessoal de Nível Superior) and UFPA (Universidade Federal do Pará).

Author Contributions

Conceived and designed the experiments: CS SS MH ARS. Performed the experiments: PP CS DOA ARS. Analyzed the data: PP NS SS. Contributed reagents/materials/analysis tools: CS SS ARS. Wrote the paper: PP CS ARS.

References

1. Alcais A, Mira M, Casanova JI, Schurr E, Abel I (2005) Genetic dissection of immunity in leprosy. Current Opinion in Immunology 17: 44–48.
2. Moreira MBR, Pena GO, Pereira GFM, Madalena M (2002). Ministério da Saúde, Secretaria de Políticas de Saúde, Guia para o controle da hanseníase. ISBN 85-334-0346-1.
3. Stretch R (1999) Presentation and treatment of Hansen's disease. Nurs Times 95(29): 46–7.
4. Moreira AS, Ribeiro dos Santos RC, Bastos RR, Silva JV, Santos PM (2006) Conjunctival bacilloscopy in leprosy diagnosis and follow-up. Arq Bras Oftalmol 69(6): 865–9.
5. Goulart IMB, Arbex GL, Carneiro MH, Rodrigues MS, Gadia R (2002) Adverse effects of multidrug therapy in leprosy patients: a five-year survey at a Health. Rev Soc Bras Med Trop 35(5): 453–60.
6. Ridley DS, Jopling WH (1966) Classification of leprosy according to immunity: a five-group system. Inernational Journal of Leprosy Other Mycobact. Disease 34: 255–273.
7. Kaur MR, Lewis HM (2006) Hidradenitis suppurativa treated with dapsone: a case series of five patients. J Dermatol Treat 17: 211–213.
8. Morrison NE, Morley GM (1976) The mode of action of clofazimine: DNA binding studies. Int. J. Lepr 44: 133–135.
9. Yano T, Bratinova SK, Teh JS, Winkler J, Sullivan K, Isaacs A, et al. (2011) Reduction of Clofazimine by Mycobacterial Type 2 NADH:Quinone Oxidoreductase. Jour. Bio. Chem. 286: 10276–10287.
10. Jopling WH (1983) Side effects of antileprosy drugs in common use. Leprosy Review 54: 261–270.
11. Jopling WH (1985) References to "side-effects of antileprosy drugs in common use". Leprosy Review 56: 61–70.
12. Pfaltzgraff RE, Bryceson A (1985) Clinical Leprosy. In: Hastings RC. Leprosy. New York p.134–136.
13. Opromolla DVA (1997) Terapêutica da hanseníase. Medicina Ribeirão Preto 30: 345–350.
14. Souza CS (1997) Hanseníase: formas clínicas e diagnóstico diferencial. Medicina Ribeirão Preto 30: 325–334.
15. Rivers EC. Mancera RL (2008) New Anti-Tuberculosis Drugs with Novel Mechanisms of Action. Curr Med Chem; 15(19): 1956–67.
16. Rivera RC, López CR, Herranz AB, Cevallos MA (2010) Analysis of the Mechanism of Action of the Antisense RNA That Controls the Replication of the repABC Plasmid p42d. Journal of Bacteriology 192: 3268–3278.
17. -Hasler JA, Estabrook R, Murray M, Pikuleva I, Waterman M, Capdevila J, et al. (1999) Human cytochromes P450. Molecular Aspects of Medicine 20: 1–137.
18. Yamada S, Tang M, Richardson K, Halaschek-Wiener J, Chan M, et al. (2009) Genetic variations of NAT2 and CYP2E1 and isoniazid hepatotoxicity in a diverse population. Pharmacogenomics 10(9): 1433–45.
19. Kayaaltı Z, Söylemezoglu T (2010) Distribution of ADH1B, ALDH2, CYP2E1*6, and CYP2E1*7B genotypes in Turkish population. Alcohol 1: 9–12.
20. Uematsu F, Ikawa S, Kikuchi H, Sagami I, Kanamaru R, et al. (1994) Restriction fragment length polymorphism of the human CYP2E1 (cytochrome P450IIE1) gene and susceptibility to lung cancer: possible relevance to low smoking exposure. Pharmacogenetics 4(2): 58–63.
21. Widersten M, Pearson WR, Engstrom A, Mannervik B (1991) Heterologous expression of the allelic variant Mu-class glutathione transferases m and y. Biochemical Journal 276: 519–524.
22. Moyer AM, Salavaggione OE, Hebbring SJ (2007) Glutathione S-Transferase T1 and M1: Gene Sequence Variation and Functional Genomics. Clin Cancer Res 13: 7207–7216.
23. Li L, Yang L, Zhang Y, Xu Z, Qin T, et al. (2011) Detoxification and DNA repair genes polymorphisms and susceptibility of primary myelodysplastic syndromes in Chinese population. Leuk Res 35(6): 762–5.
24. Cho HR, Uhm YK, Kim HJ, Ban JY, Chung JH, et al. (2011) Glutathione S-transferase M1 (GSTM1) polymorphism is associated with atopic dermatitis susceptibility in a Korean population. Int J Immunogenet 38(2): 145–50.
25. Konwar R, Manchanda PK, Chaudhary P, Nayak VL, Singh V, et al. (2010) Glutathione S-transferase (GST) gene variants and risk of benign prostatic hyperplasia: a report in a North Indian population. Asian Pac J Cancer Prev 11(4): 1067–72.
26. Hardman JG, Limbird LE (2004) Goodman & Gilman as bases farmacológicas da terapêutica. Raven Press: Rio de Janeiro. 80 p.
27. Etienne D, Pieter F, Cairns S (2000) Report of theInternational Leprosy Association Technical Forum: Prevention of disabilities and rehabilitation. Lepr Rev73: S35–S43.
28. Vaishali BN, Usha BN, Swati M, Rao P (2011) Evaluation of significance of skin smears in leprosy for diagnosis follow-up, assessment of treatment outcome and relapse. Asiatic Jour. of Biotech. Resources 2(5): 547–552.
29. Sambrook J, Fritsch F, Maniatis T (1989) Molecular Cloning: A Laboratory Manual. Cold Spr Harb Laboratory, NY. 2nd edition.
30. Santos NPC, Ribeiro-Rodrigues EM, Ribeiro-dos-Santos AKC (2010) Assessing individual interethnic admixture and population substructure using a 48 insertion-deletion ancestry informative markers panel. Hum Mutat. 31(2): 184–90.
31. Long J (1999) Multiple Locus Haplotype Analysis, version 2.0. Software and documentation distributed by the author. Section on Population Genetics and Linkage, Laboratory of Neurogenetics, NIAAA, National Institutes of Health, Bethesda.
32. Crawford CL (2010) Historical aspects of leprosy. Clin Infect Dis 51: 476–7.
33. Douglas JG, Macleod MJ (1999) Pharmacokinetic factors in the modern drug treatment of tuberculosis. Clin Pharmacokinet 37: 127–46.
34. Tsutsumi M, Takada A, Wang JS (1994) Genetic polymorphisms of cytochrome P4502E1 related to the development of alcoholic liver disease. Gastroenterology 107: 1430–1435.
35. Yang BM, O'Reilly DA, Demaine AG, Kingsnorth AN (2001) Study of polymorphisms in the CYP2E1 gene in patients with alcoholic pancreatitis. Alcohol 23: 91–97.
36. Wang SM, Zhu AP, Li D, Wang Z, Zhang P, et al. (2009) Frequencies of genotypes and alleles of the functional SNPs in CYP2C19 and CYP2E1 in mainland Chinese Kazakh, Uygur and Han populations. J. Hum. Genet 54: 372–375.

23

Novel Sulfated Polysaccharides Disrupt Cathelicidins, Inhibit RAGE and Reduce Cutaneous Inflammation in a Mouse Model of Rosacea

Jianxing Zhang[1,2], Xiaoyu Xu[1,2], Narayanam V. Rao[3], Brian Argyle[1], Lindsi McCoard[1], William J. Rusho[4], Thomas P. Kennedy[3]*, Glenn D. Prestwich[1,2], Gerald Krueger[5]

1 Center for Therapeutic Biomaterials, University of Utah, Salt Lake City, Utah, United States of America, **2** Department of Medicinal Chemistry, University of Utah, Salt Lake City, Utah, United States of America, **3** Department of Internal Medicine, University of Utah, Salt Lake City, Utah, United States of America, **4** Department of Pharmaceutics and Pharmaceutical Chemistry, University of Utah, Salt Lake City, Utah, United States of America, **5** Department of Dermatology, University of Utah, Salt Lake City, Utah, United States of America

Abstract

Background: Rosacea is a common disfiguring skin disease of primarily Caucasians characterized by central erythema of the face, with telangiectatic blood vessels, papules and pustules, and can produce skin thickening, especially on the nose of men, creating rhinophyma. Rosacea can also produce dry, itchy eyes with irritation of the lids, keratitis and corneal scarring. The cause of rosacea has been proposed as over-production of the cationic cathelicidin peptide LL-37.

Methodology/Principal Findings: We tested a new class of non-anticoagulant sulfated anionic polysaccharides, semi-synthetic glycosaminoglycan ethers (SAGEs) on key elements of the pathogenic pathway leading to rosacea. SAGEs were anti-inflammatory at ng/ml, including inhibition of polymorphonuclear leukocyte (PMN) proteases, P-selectin, and interaction of the receptor for advanced glycation end-products (RAGE) with four representative ligands. SAGEs bound LL-37 and inhibited interleukin-8 production induced by LL-37 in cultured human keratinocytes. When mixed with LL-37 before injection, SAGEs prevented the erythema and PMN infiltration produced by direct intradermal injection of LL-37 into mouse skin. Topical application of a 1% (w/w) SAGE emollient to overlying injected skin also reduced erythema and PMN infiltration from intradermal LL-37.

Conclusions: Anionic polysaccharides, exemplified by SAGEs, offer potential as novel mechanism-based therapies for rosacea and by extension other LL-37-mediated and RAGE-ligand driven skin diseases.

Editor: H. Peter Soyer, The University of Queensland, Australia

Funding: This work was supported by a Centers of Excellence grant from the State of Utah to GlycoMira LLC, by the Center for Therapeutic Biomaterials, also a Utah Center of Excellence, and by NIH grant R43 AR057281 to Drs. Zhang, Prestwich and Kennedy. The funders had no role in study design, data collection and analysis, decision to publish, or preparation of the manuscript.

Competing Interests: Drs. Zhang, Rao, Krueger, Prestwich and Kennedy hold equity in GlycoMira, LLC, which licensed the SAGE technology from the University of Utah. Drs. Xu and Zhang, Ms. McCoard, and Mr. Argyle were employed in part by GlycoMira. This does not alter the authors' adherence to all the PLoS ONE policies on sharing data and materials.

* E-mail: tkennedy@mail.mcg.edu

Introduction

Rosacea is a common skin disease afflicting primarily Caucasian women of Celtic descent [1]. Rosacea is characterized by central erythema of the face, with telangiectatic blood vessels, papules and pustules, and can produce skin thickening, especially on the nose of men, creating rhinophyma. Rosacea can also produce dry, itchy eyes with irritation of the lids, keratitis and corneal scarring. The disease disfigures in a prominent manner, and its treatment is empiric and imperfect [2]. The pathogenesis of rosacea has been attributed in part to cutaneous over-production of a cationic anti-microbial cathelicidin peptide produced by the processing serine proteinase stratum corneum tryptic enzyme (SCTE) [3,4]. Cathelicidins are highly cationic 18 kDa propeptides cleaved to an active 37-amino acid C-terminal anti-microbial peptide, LL-37 [5]. LL-37 induces interleukin-8 (IL-8) secretion by human keratinocytes, and injection of LL-37 into mouse skin recapitulates rosacea-like redness and PMN infiltration [3].

We have evaluated a family of sulfated and metabolically stabilized anionic polysaccharide derivatives known as semi-synthetic glycosaminoglycan ethers (SAGEs). We hypothesized that a topically-applied SAGE could be used as a novel therapy for rosacea by binding and inhibiting the inflammatory activity of excess cationic cathelicidins. We show that one SAGE, GM-1111, exhibits substantial anti-inflammatory activities at nanomolar concentrations, including inhibition of cationic PMN proteases, inhibition of the leukocyte adhesion receptor P-selectin, and inhibition of the interaction of the receptor for advanced glycation end-products (RAGE) with its disparate ligands. GM-1111 avidly bound LL-37 and inhibited IL-8 secretion in cultured human keratinocytes in response to LL-37 stimulation. When mixed with LL-37, SAGEs prevented the extensive erythema and PMN infiltration produced by direct intradermal injection of LL-37 into mouse skin [3]. More importantly, topical application of a 1% SAGE-containing emollient to overlying injected skin also substantially reduced the redness and cutaneous PMN infiltration induced by intradermal LL-37. Herein, data demonstrate anionic polysaccharides, exemplified by SAGEs, as the first mechanism-based therapy that targets the proposed molecular etiology of rosacea.

Results

SAGEs are non-animal derived

Twenty-five novel derivatives of hyaluronic acid (HA) were obtained from GlycoMira, LLC (Salt Lake City, UT). HA is an immunoneutral skin polysaccharide consisting of long polymers (up to 10 MDa) of the disaccharide N-acetylglucosamine (GlcNAc) and glucuronic acid (GlcA) linked GlcNacβ1-3GlcAβ1-4 in repeating units along the chain. Fermentation-derived HA was chemically alkylated to provide lipophilicity to both improve dermal penetration and reduce hydrolysis by hyaluronidases [6]. Subsequently, the HA ethers were sulfated to adjust polyanionic charge and anti-inflammatory properties. The HA used as a starting material varied from 50 kDa to 950 kDa. A representative SAGE structure is illustrated in Figure 1. For further study, we chose the SAGE GM-1111, which was produced from 53 kDa HA and had a final molecular weight of 5.5 kDa.

SAGEs bind P-selectin, Mac-1 and RAGE, and potently inhibit P-selectin, cationic PMN proteases and interaction of RAGE with its disparate ligands

The SAGE GM-1111 showed anti-inflammatory activities similar to those of heparin or its low anticoagulant analogs [6] in a number of *in vitro* assays.

First, SAGEs avidly bound to the adhesion molecule P-selectin, the Mac-1 integrin (CD11b/CD18) and the multi-ligand immunoglobulin superfamily receptor RAGE. Figure 2 shows that GM-1111 exhibited saturable binding to P-selectin with a K_D of 0.0036 nM (Figure 2A), to Mac-1 with a K_D of 0.175 nM (Figure 2B) and to RAGE with a K_D of 1.69 nM (Figure 2C).

Second, SAGEs were potent inhibitors of the leukocyte adhesion molecule P-selectin [7]. Competitor-mediated displacement of U937 human monocytes, which loosely adhere to P-selectin through P-selectin glycoprotein ligand-1 (PSGL-1), was studied using fluorescent-labeled U937 cells. Table 1 and Figure 3A show that the SAGE GM-1111 inhibited U937 binding

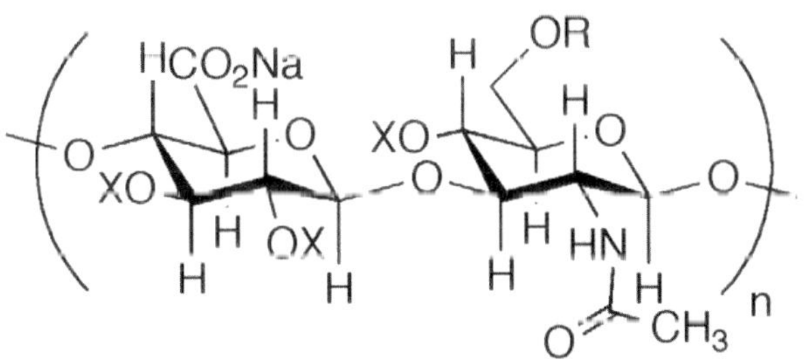

Figure 1. Structure of semi-synthetic glycosaminoglycan ethers (SAGEs). SAGEs can vary in molecular size, and in extent of alkylation and sulfation. GM-1111 is a low-molecular weight SAGE with an average molecular weight of 5.5 kDa.

to P-selectin with a 50% inhibitory concentration (IC_{50}) of 24.9 nM, approximately three times higher than the IC_{50} for heparin (7.9 nM).

Third, as sulfated polyanions, SAGEs were potent inhibitors of cationic PMN proteases such as human leukocyte elastase [8]. GM-1111 inhibited the PMN protease human leukocyte elastase (HLE) with an IC_{50} of 44.7 nM (Table 1 and Figure 3B), approximately three times higher than the IC_{50} of 14.9 nM for heparin. Thus, the polyanionic nature of the SAGEs would be expected to reduce protease activity in part *via* electrostatic interactions. However, this simplistic explanation cannot account for the totality of observed SAGE pharmacology *in vitro* [6].

Fourth, SAGEs were found to be potent inhibitors of RAGE binding with its ligands. The advanced glycation end-product (AGE) carboxymethyl lysine-modified (CML) protein is prominently formed in the dermis as the consequence of sun exposure, and avidly ligates and activates RAGE inflammatory signaling [9]. RAGE binds to immobilized CML-bovine serum albumin (BSA) in a dose dependent manner with an equilibrium constant (K_D) of 0.43 nM [10]. GM-1111 potently inhibited interaction of CML-BSA with RAGE (Table 1 and Figure 3C) with an with an IC_{50} of 413 nM. Once PMNs have migrated into inflamed dermis, PMN secretion of S100 calgranulins provides an active RAGE ligand to perpetuate inflammatory signaling even in the absence of AGE products [11]. RAGE engages immobilized S100b in a dose-dependent manner with a K_D of 0.45 nM [10]. GM-1111 inhibited ligation of RAGE by S100b calgranulin with an IC_{50} of 275 nM, compared with IC_{50} of 92 nM for heparin (Table 1 and Figure 3D) Likewise, RAGE binds immobilized human high mobility box group protein-1 (HMGB-1) in a saturable fashion with a K_D of 0.64 nM [10]. HMGB-1 is secreted by monocytes and macrophages as an inflammation producing cytokine and is also released by necrotic cells into areas of injury [12]. GM-1111 inhibited ligation of RAGE by HMGB-1 with an IC_{50} of 80 nM, compared with an IC_{50} of 2.9 nM for heparin (Table 1 and Figure 3E). Finally, using the Mac-1 (CD11b/CD18) as a counter-ligand, leukocytes ligate RAGE on vascular endothelium as an adhesion molecule essential for exiting the circulation into areas of inflammation [13]. GM-1111 inhibited binding of U937 monocytes to RAGE with an IC_{50} of 7.6 nM, essentially equipotent with the IC_{50} of 7.9 nM for heparin (Table 1 and Figure 3F). Taken together, these results suggest that SAGEs may provide considerable anti-inflammatory activity in diseases mediated by RAGE-ligand interactions, including the skin, where RAGE likely plays a role in lymphocyte-mediated diseases such as atopic dermatitis and psoriasis, as well as photo-ageing.

SAGEs are safe when administered topically

When applied to cultured human dermal fibroblasts (nHDF) and keratinocytes (nHEK), GM-1111 did not inhibit proliferation or cause cell toxicity up to 1 mg/ml (data not shown). Furthermore, none of the SAGEs tested, including GM-1111, elicited any skin reaction in Draize tests up to 10 mg/ml [14] (data not shown). SAGEs are also effectively non-anticoagulant in nature; for example, GM-1111 has approximately 0.2–0.5% of the anticoagulant activity of heparin. Specifically GM-1111 shows values of 0.3 IU/mg anti-Xa activity and 0.8 IU/mg anti-IIa activity, compared to 150–160 IU/mg each for unfractionated heparin. Unlike heparin, many highly charged polyanionic polymers are potent activators of Factor XII (Hagemann factor), secondarily producing kinins [15]. GM-1111 failed to show any activation of Factor XII [16], even at concentrations 10 to 100-fold higher than needed to achieve pharmacologic inhibition of

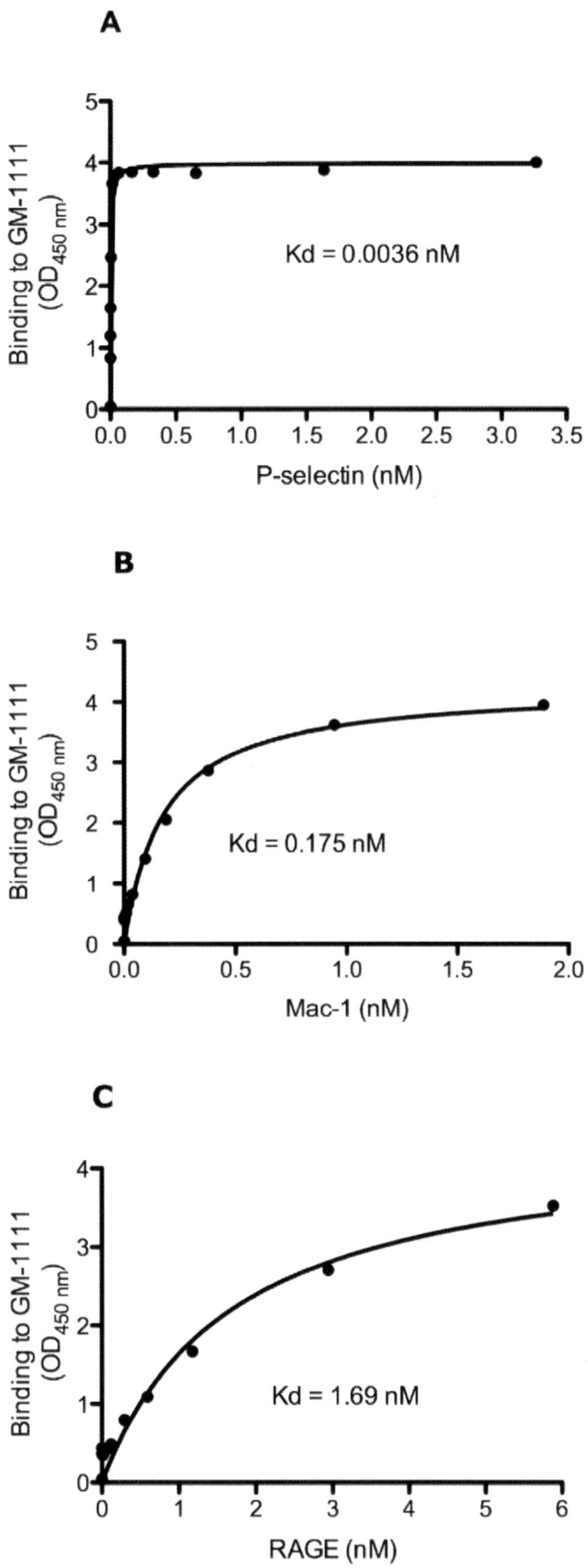

Figure 2. SAGEs bind to vascular adhesion proteins. GM-1111 was studied to determine binding affinity for P-selectin (**A**), Mac-1 (**B**), and RAGE (**C**). Binding affinity (K_D) values were 0.0036 nM for GM-1111 binding to P-selectin, 0.175 nM for GM-1111 binding to Mac-1 and 1.69 nM for GM-1111 binding to RAGE.

inflammation (data not shown). From these data, we concluded that the GM-1111 was safe as a lead candidate for topical use.

SAGEs bind to LL-37 and inhibit the biologic activity of LL-37 *in vitro*

The SAGE GM-1111 bound to the polycationic LL-37 peptide in a saturable fashion with a K_D of 0.225 nM (Figure 4A). This suggests that at least some of the biologic activity of the polyanionic SAGEs could be due to saturable, charge-neutralization of the cationic cathelicidins. However, electrostatic interactions alone cannot account for the overall SAGE pharmacology. For example, similar to previous reports [3], LL-37 induced IL-8 secretion by cultured human keratinocytes (Figure 4B). Addition of GM-1111 to the medium in addition to LL-37 significantly reduced IL-8 production by cultured keratinocytes (Figure 4B).

SAGEs inhibit cutaneous inflammation from intradermal LL-37

Intradermal injection of LL-37 into Balb/c mice at four 12-h intervals for 48 h produced cutaneous erythema with central necrosis (Figure 5A), prominent intradermal PMN infiltration (Figure 5C and Figure 6B), marked edema of the dermis (Figure 5C) and increased tissue myeloperoxidase (MPO) activity (Figure 5E). This reproduced the previously described murine model of rosacea [3]. The area of erythema (Figures 5B and F) and redness score (3.8±0.5 after LL-37 alone vs 1.2±0.5 after LL-37+ SAGE, $P<0.05$) were both significantly reduced by co-injection of GM-1111 with LL-37. Simultaneous injection of GM-1111 with LL-37 also significantly decreased PMN infiltration, as assessed by histology (Figure 5D) or tissue MPO activity (Figure 5E). Thus, at a minimum, charge neutralization of LL-37 by SAGE co-injection results in a significant reduction of LL-37-induced inflammation.

To determine if topical SAGEs were effective topical anti-inflammatory agents in this rosacea model, we formulated GM-1111 into a standard triglyceride-based transdermal emollient that contained 20% (w/w) water and 1% (w/w) of active drug. LL-37 was injected intradermally every 12 h for 48 h. In treated animals (n = 6 per group), the injected skin was gently rubbed with

Table 1. Anti-Inflammatory Activities of SAGE, GM-1111, *In Vitro*[1].

Anti-Inflammatory Assay	IC_{50} values (nM)	
	SAGE*	Heparin*
[1]U937 monocyte binding to P-selectin	24.9	7.9
[2]Human Leukocyte Elastase activity	44.7	14.9
[3]CML-BSA binding to RAGE	412.7	27.8
[3]S100b binding to RAGE	274.5	92.1
[3]HMGB-1 binding to RAGE	79.6	2.9
[1]U937 monocyte binding to RAGE	7.6	7.9

*The average molecular mass of SAGE is 5.5 kDa and heparin is 14 kDa. Details of [1]cell surface binding assays, [2] inhibition of human leukocyte elastase (HLE) and [3]solid phase binding assays are found in Methods. Detailed graphical plots of the results from cell surface binding assays, inhibition of HLE and solid phase binding assays are shown in Figure 3.

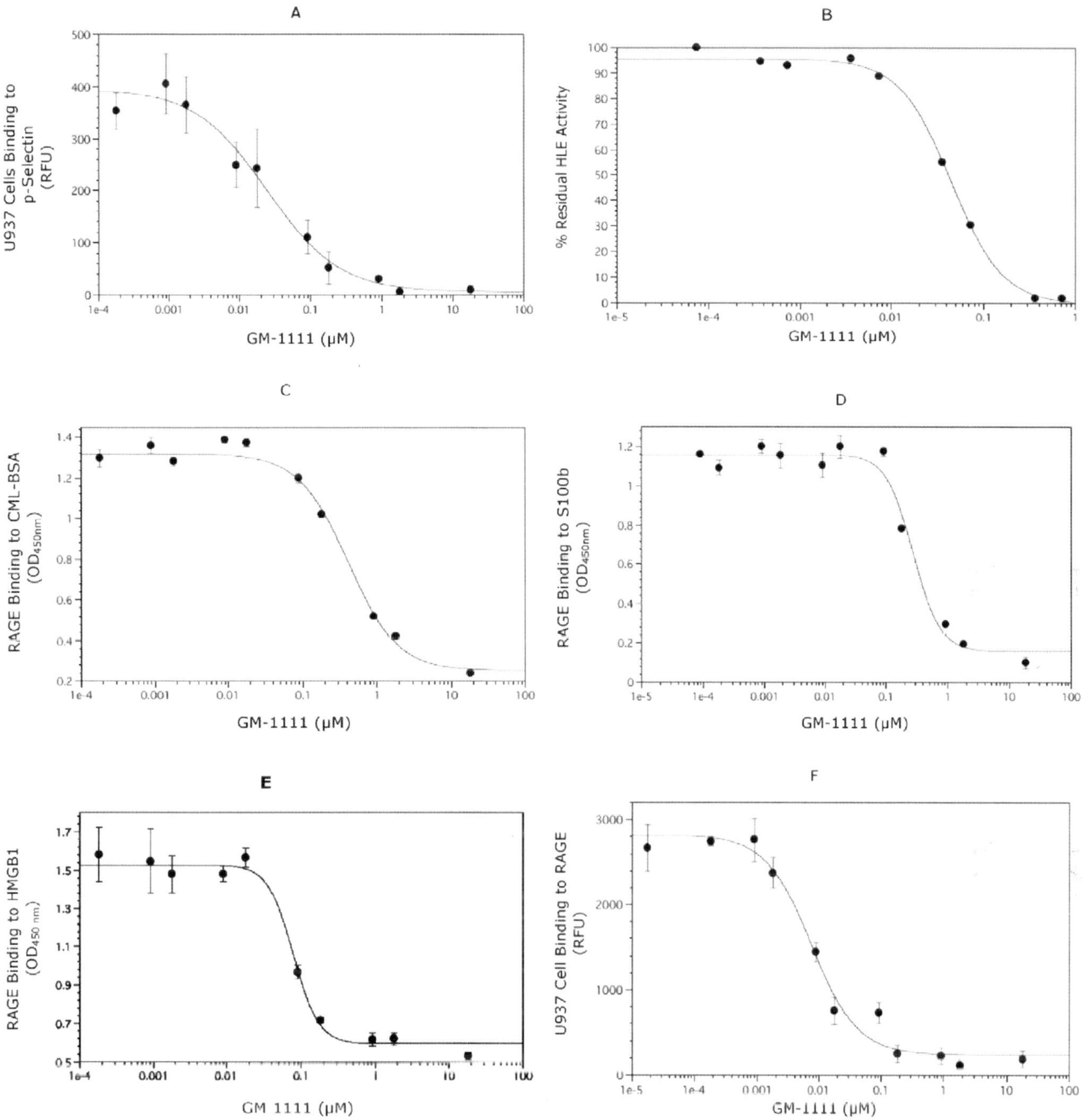

Figure 3. SAGEs inhibit P-selectin, HLE, interaction of RAGE with its many ligands. Data points in each figure represent the average value ± standard deviation of quadruplicate wells for each concentration of SAGE. **A.** SAGEs inhibit P-selectin. Inhibition of P-selectin glycoprotein ligand-1 (PSGL-1) binding to P-selectin by SAGEs was studied using calcein-labeled U937 cells incubated in microwells coated with P-selectin. After 1 h, plates were washed, bound cells were lysed with Triton-X100 buffer and bound cells were quantified using an excitation of 494 nm and emission of 517 nm. GM-1111 inhibits PSGL-1 attachment to P-selectin with an IC_{50} of 25 nM. **B.** SAGEs inhibit HLE. HLE (100 nM) was incubated with GM-1111 at 1 100 nm concentrations in 0.5 M HEPES buffer for 15 min. Following incubation, the elastase substrate, Suc-Ala-Ala-Val-*p*NA was added to the reaction mixture to the final concentration of 0.3 mM. Absorbance due to *p*-NA hydrolysis was monitored for 15 min at absorbance of 405 nm. GM 1111 inhibits HLE with an IC_{50} of 45 nM. **C–E.** SAGEs inhibit interaction of the AGE product CML-BSA, the calgranulin S100b and the alarmin HMGB-1 with RAGE. Microwell plates coated with CML-BSA (**C**), S100b calgranulin (**D**) or HMGB-1 (**E**) were incubated with RAGE-Fc chimera with or without GM-1111 for 2 h. Plates were washed, incubated with anti-RAGE antibody, incubated for 1 h, washed again four times and incubated with horse-radish peroxidase conjugated secondary for 1 h. A colorimetric reaction was produced by addition of tetramethyl benzidine chromogen (TMB) and quantified by absorbance at 450 nm. GM-1111 inhibits interaction of RAGE with CM-BSA, S100b and HMGB-1 with IC_{50} values of 413, 275 and 80 nM, respectively. **F.** SAGEs inhibit function of RAGE as an adhesion ligand. Inhibition of Mac-1-dependent ligation of RAGE by U937 cells was studied as in **A**, but using microwells coated with RAGE. GM-1111 inhibits Mac-1 attachment to RAGE with an IC_{50} of 7.6 nM.

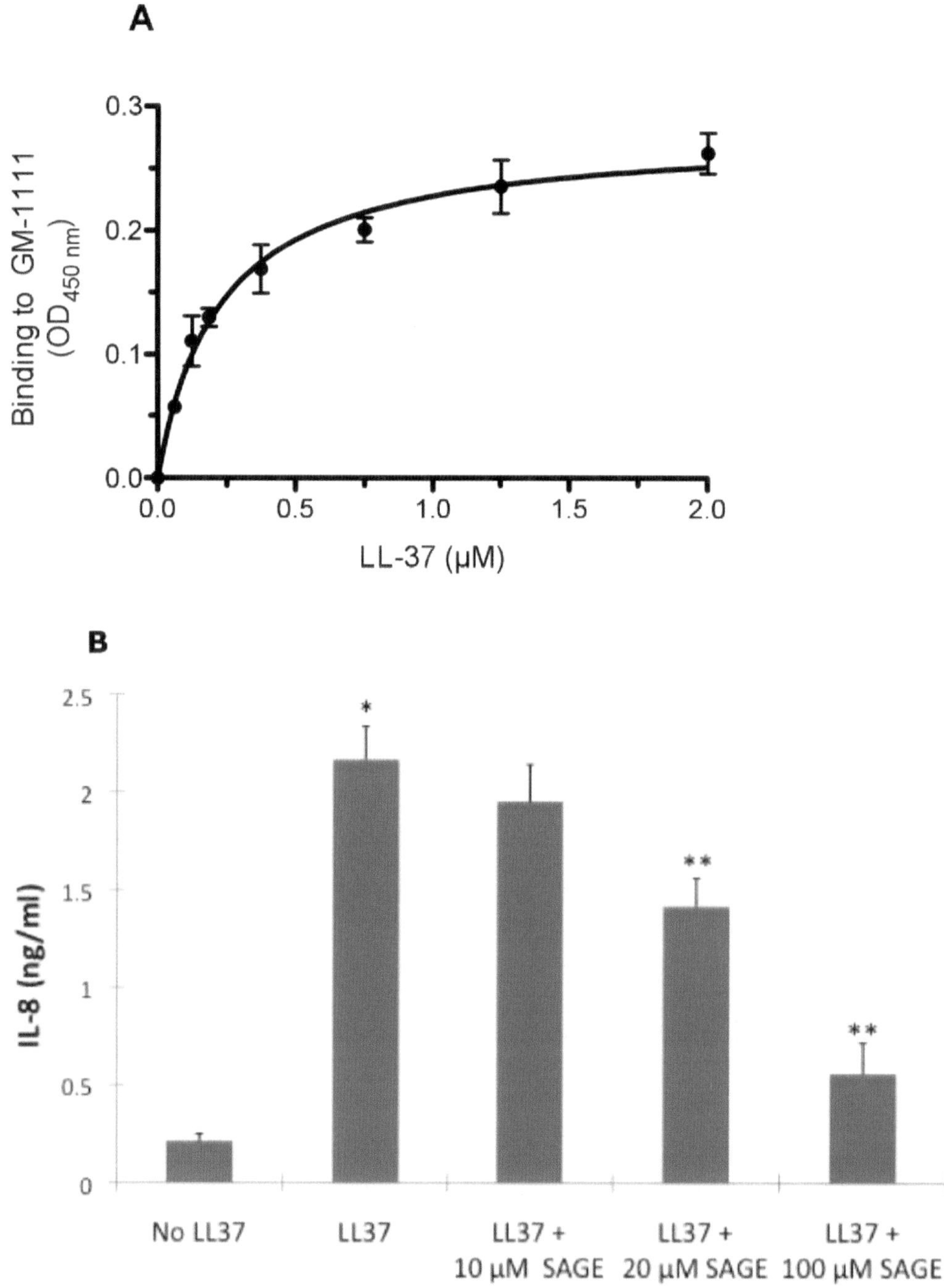

Figure 4. SAGE binds LL-37 and inhibits LL-37-induced interleukin-8 (IL-8) expression *in vitro*. A. SAGE binds LL-37. Microwell plates coated with GM-111 were incubated with LL-37 at 37°C for 2 h. Plates were washed, incubated with anti-LL-37 antibody, incubated for 1 h, washed again four times and incubated with peroxidase-conjugated secondary antibody for 1 h. A colorimetric reaction was produced by addition of TMB and quantified by absorbance at 450 nm. LL-37 binds to GM-1111 with a K_D of 0.225 nM. **B.** SAGE inhibits IL-8 production LL-37 stimulated keratinocytes. Human keratinocytes were grown to confluence and treated with 3.2 μM LL-37 or LL-37 and a 4x molar excess of GM-111101 for 6 h. Supernatants were collected and placed in a sterile 96-well plate. Production of IL-8 was determined by ELISA (R&D Systems, Minneapolis, MN) in accordance with manufacturer's instructions. Co-addition of GM-1111 significantly inhibited IL-8 release into medium. *$P<0.01$ as compared with negative control group without LL37; **$P<0.05$ as compared with positive control group without GM-111101 treatment.

drug-free emollient (control) or emollient with 1% GM-1111 either immediately (t = 0) or 12 h after the first injection (t = 12 h). Emollient application was repeated after each of the intradermal LL-37 injections. Cutaneous inflammation from intradermal LL-37 was significantly reduced by topical 1% GM-1111 (Figure 7). Whether applied at t = 0 or t = 12 h after the first LL-37 injection, topical GM-1111-containing emollient significantly reduced both erythema (t = 0, Figure 7B; t = 12 h, Figure 7C) and PMN infiltration (t = 0, Figures 7E, 7G and Figure 6C; t = 12 h, Figures 7F, 7G and Figure 6D) relative to untreated or vehicle only animals receiving the intradermal LL-37. The SAGE-containing emollient also significantly reduced the area of erythema (Figure 7H) and redness score [4.6±0.3 after LL-37 alone, 1.6±0.4 after LL-37+ SAGE (t = 0) and 1.5±0.5 after LL-

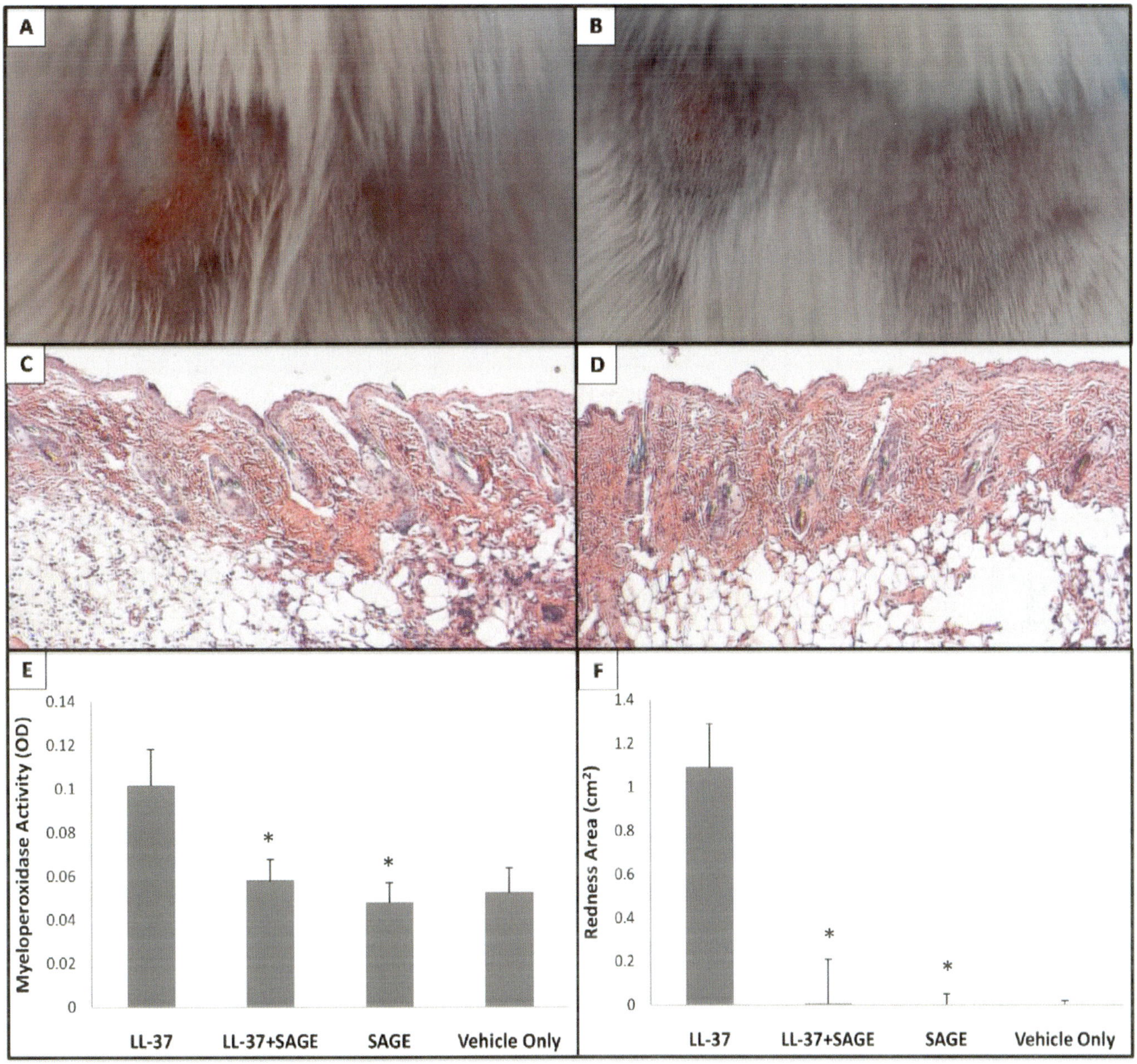

Figure 5. SAGE co-injection inhibits erythema and PMN infiltration from intradermal LL-37. Balb/c mice were shaved to expose an area of skin on the back. Twenty four hours later, mice were intradermally injected with 40 μl of vehicle (nanopure water), LL-37 (at 320 μM concentration in water), SAGE GM-1111 (1,280 μM in water), or LL-37+ GM 1111 mix (peptide +4 molar equivalents of SAGE) placed intradermally into the shaved skin using a 31-gauge needle and 0.5 ml insulin syringe. Injections were repeated every 12 h thereafter. Forty-eight hours after the initial injection (four injections in total), animals were lightly anesthetized with isoflurane, the area of injected skin was photographed, the intensity of erythema was assessed as a redness score (from 1 to 5, with 5 as the most red), and the area of erythema was measured with micrometer calipers. The injected skin was then biopsied for histopathologic staining and to assess PMN infiltration through measurement of myeloperoxidase (MPO) activity. **A**. Gross picture of LL-37 injected skin region. **B**. Co-injection model of LL-37 and SAGE GM-1111. **C**. H&E-stained cross-sectional view of a LL-37 injected skin sample. **D**. H&E-stained cross-sectional view of a LL-37 mixed with GM-1111- injected skin region. **E**. MPO activity measurement of LL-37 injection with different treatments. **F**. Area of erythema from LL-37 injection. *$P<0.05$ vs intradermal LL-37 alone; $n=6$ per group

37+ SAGE ($t=12$ h), both $P<0.05$ vs LL-37 alone], and decreased MPO activity within biopsies of injected skin (Figure 7G). Anti-inflammatory effects were not evident using 1% concentration of 53 kDa HA in the emollient in place of the GM-1111 (Figure 8). Confocal microscopy was performed on LL-37 injected mouse skin after topical treatment with emollient containing fluorescent-labeled GM-1111 (Figure 9). In the presence of irritant disruption of the stratum corneum, labeled SAGE penetrated deeply into inflamed skin. These results support our hypothesis that the SAGE GM-1111, but not HA, would be topically effective in a pharmaceutically acceptable emollient to treat the cathelicidin peptide-mediated elements of inflammation associated with rosacea.

S100 calgranulins have not been previously reported as pathobiologically important in rosacea, but their presence would not be surprising in light of the prominent PMN infiltration in this disease [1]. Immunohistochemical staining for the RAGE ligand S100A8 confirmed the presence of this mouse homologue for the

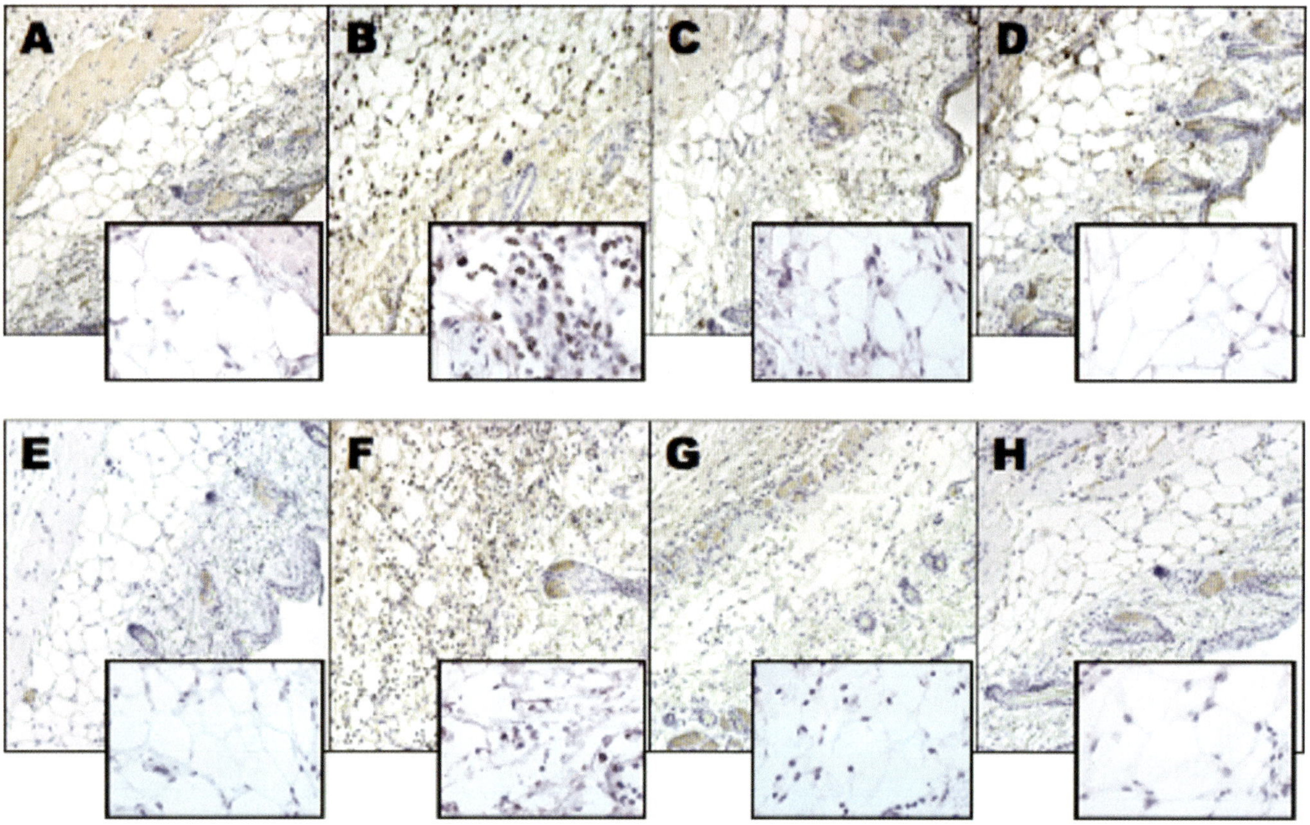

Figure 6. Topical SAGE reduces PMN infiltration and S100 calgranulin accumulation from intradermal LL-37. LL-37, PBS and LL-37 and SAGE-injected mouse skin was stained with antibody to mouse Gr-1 to examine neutrophil infiltration, and also for S100A8 calgranulin, the major RAGE-binding calgranulin present in murine PMNs [17] as described in Methods. **A.** Staining of normal control skin for the PMN antigen Gr-1. **B.** Staining of LL-37 injected skin for the PMN antigen Gr-1. **C.** Staining of skin injected with LL-37 plus GM-1111 (applied at t = 0) for the PMN antigen Gr-1. **D.** Staining of skin injected with LL-37 plus GM-1111 (applied at t = 12 h) for the PMN antigen Gr-1. **E.** Staining of normal control skin for the RAGE ligand S100A8. **F.** Staining of LL-37 injected skin for the RAGE ligand S100A8. **G.** Staining of skin injected with LL-37 plus GM-1111 (applied at t = 0) for the RAGE ligand S100A8. **H.** Staining of skin injected with LL-37 plus GM-1111 (applied at t = 12 h) for the RAGE ligand S100A8. Figures and insets are shown at 20x and 40x magnification, respectively.

human leukocyte S100 calgranulin S100A12 [17] in LL-37-injected skin (Figures 6E vs 6F). Importantly, topical GM-1111 treatment reduced S100A8 staining expression compared to LL-37 alone (Figures 6G and 6H vs 6F).

SAGEs inhibit cutaneous inflammation from croton oil

As another model, we employed croton oil, which is commonly used to study PMN-mediated skin inflammation in screening anti-inflammatory compounds for dermatologic use [18]. Croton oil contains the phorbol ester tetradecyl phorbol acetate (TPA), which activates protein kinase C in skin cells, producing abundant chemotaxins which can signal PMN influx. Cutaneous inflammation from croton oil has also recently been linked in part to recruitment of inflammatory cells by HMGB-1 released from TPA-exposed keratinocytes [19]. When painted on the ear, croton oil produces intense redness (Figure 10A bottom), accompanied by edema (Figure 10C) and intradermal increase in MPO activity (Figure 10E), indicative of PMN infiltration, compared to the control ear (Figures 10A top, B and E). Topical application of GM-1111 significantly decreased phorbol-induced ear edema (Figure 10D), MPO activity (Figure 10E), increase in erythema (Figure 10F), and increase in ear thickness (Figure 10G). This indicates that topical SAGEs may have utility in treating other dermatoses that are in part or completely mediated by PMNs.

Discussion

Herein we show that novel sulfated glycosaminoglycan ethers have broad anti-inflammatory activity. The SAGE GM-1111 avidly bound to the leukocyte adhesion molecule P-selectin, the Mac-1 integrin and the pro-inflammatory pattern recognition receptor RAGE. This SAGE also potently inhibited P-selectin, blocked catalytic activity of the cationic PMN protease HLE, and inhibited the interaction of RAGE with its disparate ligands, including the AGE product CML-BSA, the S100 calgranulin S100b and the nuclear alarmin HMGB-1. Furthermore, GM-1111 demonstrated the ability to block leukocytes from using RAGE as an alternative adhesion ligand. The activities exemplified by GM-1111 (Table 1 and Figures 2 and 3) are generally demonstrated by a wide range of SAGEs with distinct structures and distinctive structure-activity profiles [6]. In aggregate, these activities would be predicted to be broadly anti-inflammatory. We confirmed this to be the case using a recently reported model of human rosacea [3]. LL-37 avidly bound to SAGE (Figure 4A) and addition of GM-1111 to medium blocked the ability of LL-37 to induce IL-8 expression by cultured human keratinocytes (Figure 4B). Further, co-injection of GM-1111 with LL-37 inhibited development of erythema (Figures 5A vs B and F) and skin infiltration of PMNs (Figure 5C vs 5D and 5E) in response to intradermal LL-37 peptide. Topical GM-1111 was also effective at

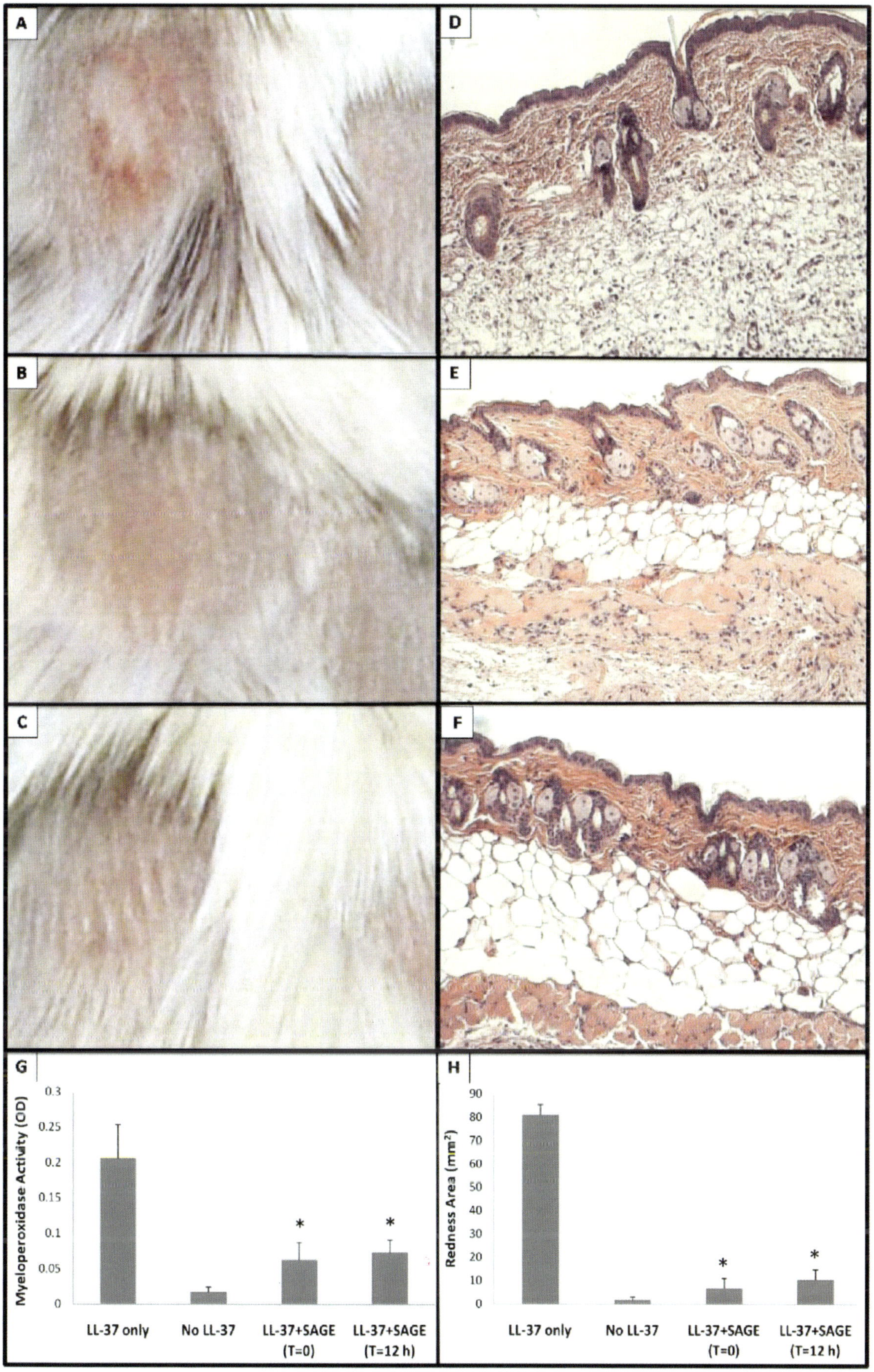
A
B
C
D
E
F
G
Myeloperoxidase Activity (OD)
0.3
0.25
0.2
0.15
0.1
0.05
0
*
*
LL-37 only
No LL-37
LL-37+SAGE (T=0)
LL-37+SAGE (T=12 h)
H
Redness Area (mm²)
90
80
70
60
50
40
30
20
10
0
*
*
LL-37 only
No LL-37
LL-37+SAGE (T=0)
LL-37+SAGE (T=12 h)

Figure 7. Topical SAGE reduces LL-37-induced inflammation. Balb/c mice were injected intradermally as described in Figure 5, and treated topically with GM-1111-1 (1% w/w) in a triglyceride-based emollient. **A–C**. Gross pictures of LL-37 injected skin region: **A**, no treatment; **B**, GM-1111 treatment immediately (t = 0) after LL-37 injection; **C**, GM-1111 treatment beginning at t = 12 h after LL-37 injection. **D**. H&E-stained cross-sectional view of a LL-37 injected skin sample. **E**. H&E-stained cross-sectional view of GM-1111 treatment at t = 0 in LL-37 injected skin region. **F**. H&E-stained cross-sectional view of GM-1111 at t = 12 h treatment in LL-37 injected skin region. **G**. MPO activity measurement of LL-37 injection with different treatments. **H**. Area of erythema from LL-37 injection. *P<0.05 vs intradermal LL-37 alone; n = 6 per group.

ameliorating LL-37 induced skin inflammation (Figure 7), and similarly reduced inflammatory edema and PMN infiltration in response to dermal application of croton oil (Figure 10). Thus, topical SAGEs are the first mechanistically based approach for treating rosacea that intersects with currently understood pathogenic mechanisms in this disease [3], and may also be therapeutic for other leukocyte mediated skin disorders.

Cathelicidin peptides are polycationic antimicrobial peptides important for innate immunity of skin and other organs [5]. In humans, the major cathelicidin peptide is LL-37, which is produced by proteolytic processing of its precursor hCAP18 (human cationic antimicrobial protein 18). In addition to being antimicrobial, antifungal and antiviral, LL-37 is chemoattractant through activation of the formyl peptide receptor-like 1 (FPRL1) receptor on leukocytes, and can induce keratinocyte IL-8 and IL-18 secretion through activation of the epidermal growth factor receptor or the p38 and ERK1/2 MAP kinase pathways, respectively [5]. Through FPRL1, LL-37 also activates endothelial cells, resulting in angiogenesis [20]. These activities account for the erythema, telangiectases and PMN infiltration of rosacea [3].

The polyanionic glycosaminoglycan heparin has been previously reported to inhibit LL-37 binding to lipopolysaccharide [21]

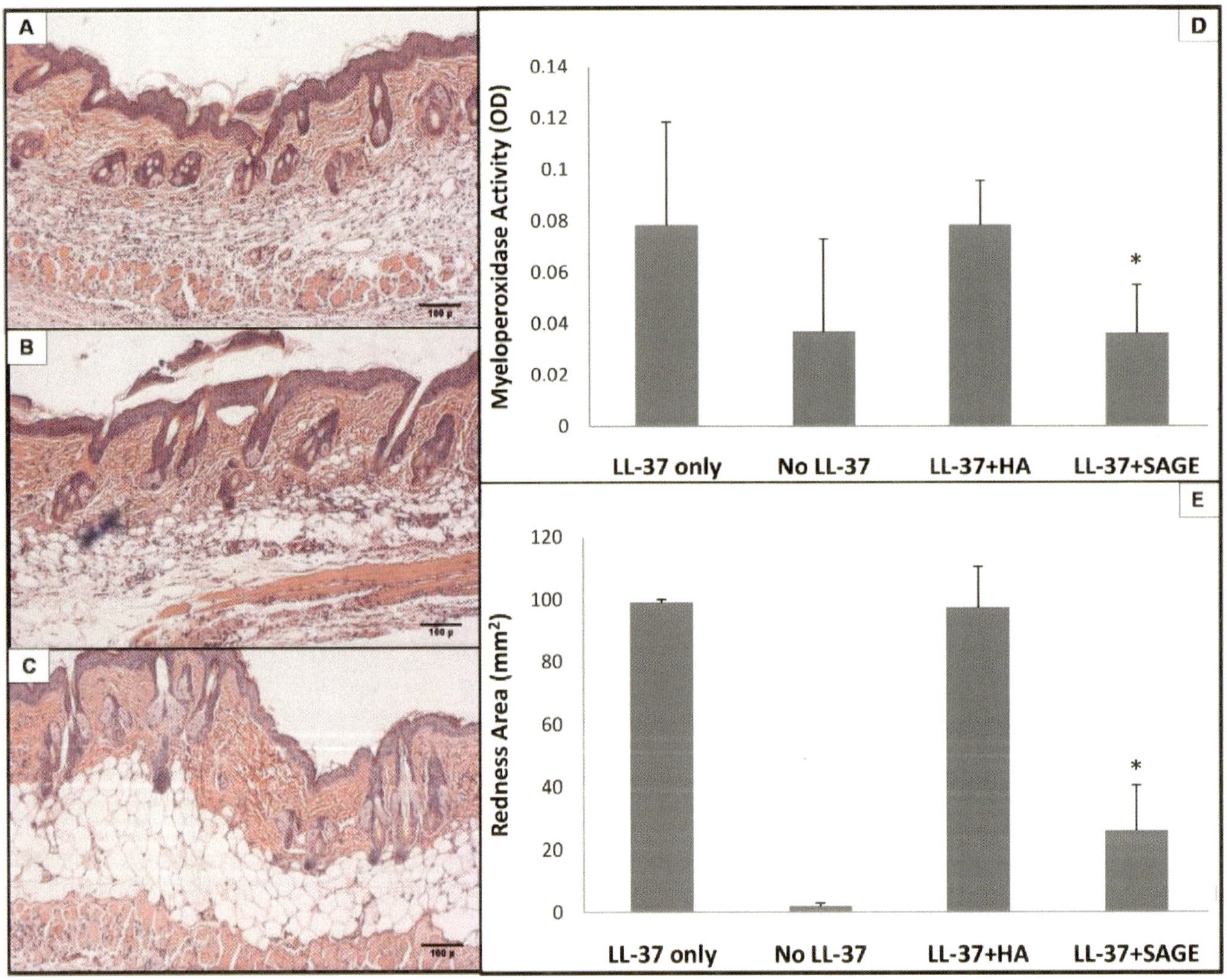

Figure 8. HA emollient does not reduce LL-37-induced inflammation. Experiments were performed as in Figure 7, but with immediate (t = 0) application of 1% w/w HA-containing emollient (53 kDa HA) or 1% w/w GM-1111 emollient. *P<0.05 vs LL-37 alone. **A**. H&E-stained cross-sectional view of LL-37 injected skin. **B**. H&E-stained section of LL-37 injected skin treated with topical HA emollient alone. **C**. H&E-stained section of LL-37 injected skin treated with topical emollient containing 1% SAGE GM-1111. **D**. MPO activity measurement of LL-37 injection with different treatments. **E**. Area of erythema from LL-37 injection. Erythema scores after LL-37 injection were: 5.1±0.1 after LL-37 alone; 4.9±0.44 after LL-37+ HA; 2.3±0.7 after LL-37+ SAGE (P<0.05 LL-37 alone vs LL-37+ SAGE). *P<0.05 vs intradermal LL-37 alone; n = 6 per group.

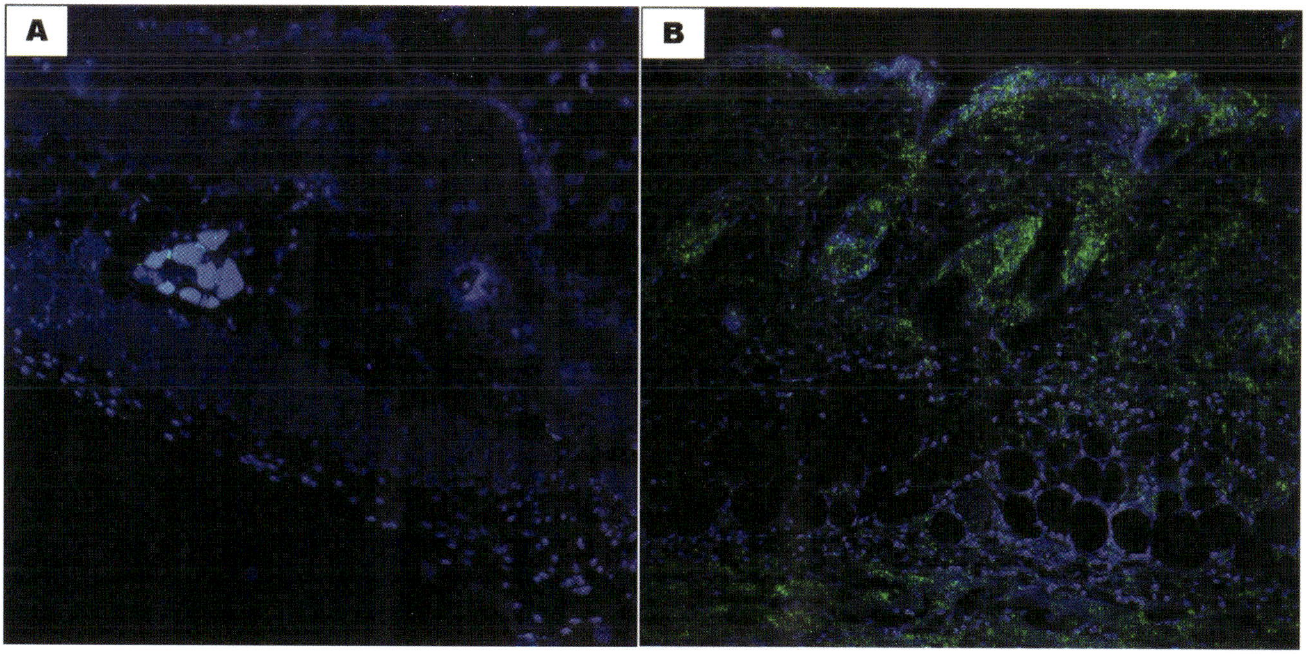

Figure 9. Topical SAGE penetrates into inflamed mouse skin. Balb/c mice were injected intradermally with LL-37 every 12 h for 48 h as in Figure 7. Control emollient [3% (w/w) methylcellulose] or emollient containing Alexa Fluor 633-labeled GM-1111 was applied topically to the injected skin after the last two LL-37 injections. Under low light conditions, skin was harvested 12 h after the last emollient application, fixed in paraformaldehyde and embedded in paraffin. Slides were deparaffinized with xylene, stained with DAPI (1:100 dilution in fluorescent mounting medium) and imaged using an FV1000 confocal microscope. The skin surface is oriented at the top of each image. **A**. Skin from controls demonstrates blue DAPI ($\lambda_{ex}=358$ nm; $\lambda_{em}=461$ nm) image but no SAGE fluorescence. **B.** Skin treated with Alexa Fluor 633-labeled GM-1111 demonstrates fluorescence ($\lambda_{ex}=633$ nm; $\lambda_{em}=647$ nm; false colored green in the image) consistent with SAGE penetration into LL-37-inflamed skin.

and thereby reduce the antibacterial effects of LL-37 [22]. Heparin also neutralizes the toxicity of other cationic peptides, including eosinophil major basic protein and eosinophil cationic protein [23,24]. This led us to hypothesize that the SAGEs could charge neutralize and reduce the biologic effects of exuberantly expressed LL-37 in humans with rosacea. The data from *in vitro* (Figure 4) and *in vivo* (Figures 5 and 7) experiments support this hypothesis. GM-1111 not only bound LL-37 (Figure 4A) and inhibited LL-37 when co-mixed with it prior to intradermal injection (Figure 5), but also when applied topically to the skin (Figure 7). Because LL-37 is also overexpressed in psoriatic skin, where it has been proposed to form complexes with human self-DNA to activate plasmacytoid dendritic cells and the processes that lead to lesions of psoriasis [5,25], GM-1111 or other SAGEs

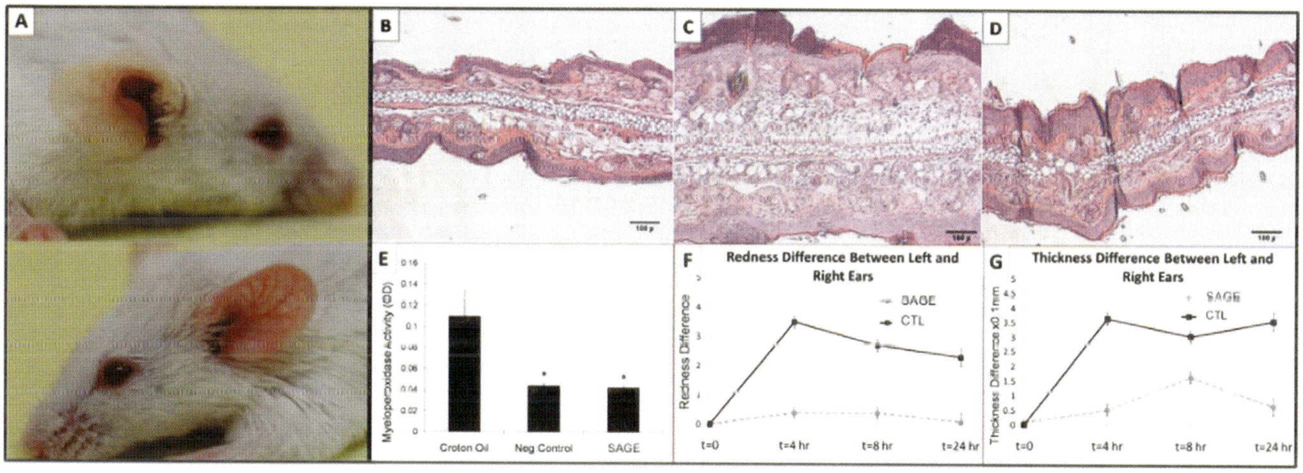

Figure 10. Topical SAGE reduces ear edema from croton oil. GM-1111 (1%) was applied topically in the croton oil model. **A**. Normal control right ear (top) and croton oil painted left ear (bottom). **B**. H&E section of control normal ear. **C**. H&E-stained cross-sectional view of a croton oil painted ear with vehicle treatment. **D**. H&E-stained cross-sectional view of croton oil painted ear with SAGE treatment. **E**. MPO activity measurement in ears. **F**. Ear thickness differences between left (croton oil) and right (normal) ears. **G**. Redness difference between right and left ears. *$P<0.05$ vs croton oil with vehicle emollient alone (negative control).

might also prove therapeutically useful in other common inflammatory skin diseases.

In addition to blocking cathelicidin peptides, SAGEs are also potent inhibitors of RAGE with at least four of its disparate ligands (Table 1 and Figure 3). The pathogenic role of RAGE in skin diseases has only recently been explored. However, RAGE is already known to be centrally important in photo-ageing [9], the S100 calgranulins S100A7 and S100A17 are highly upregulated in psoriatic skin [26], and HMGB-1 has been recently reported to mediate cutaneous inflammation from topical croton oil [19]. Our finding that S100A8, the mouse homologue for human S100A12 [17], is increased in LL-37-injected skin (Figure 6) suggests that S100 calgranulins also may have a prominent role in the cutaneous inflammation seen in patients with rosacea.

RAGE is a promiscuous pattern recognition receptor from the immunoglobulin superfamily and plays a prominent role in magnifying inflammation [27,28]. Once ligated, RAGE mediates post-receptor signaling including activation of nuclear factor-κB (NF-κB), leading to a profound inflammatory response [27,28]. Through a prominent NF-κB-responsive consensus sequence in its promoter, RAGE activation also leads to even greater RAGE expression [27,28]. Furthermore, RAGE interacts with the leukocyte Mac-1 integrin (CD11b/CD18) and p150,95 (CD11c/CD18) to facilitate leukocyte inflammatory cell recruitment [13]. Attraction of leukocytes to inflammation is additionally augmented by interaction of the RAGE ligands S100 calgranulins and HMGB-1 [13,27–29].

Structurally, RAGE is comprised of three immunoglobulin-like regions: a distal "V" type domain, followed by two "C" type domains, a short transmembrane domain and a cytoplasmic tail required for signaling [27,28]. The extracellular domain of RAGE has been used in detailed analyses of RAGE-ligand interactions [30] and the crystal structure of the receptor [31]. SAGEs likely inhibit RAGE-ligand interaction in part through interactions with the V domain, which consists of a large hydrophobic cavity rimed on its surface with basic amino acids to form a cationic center [30]. This is supported by a crystal structure for RAGE which reveals an elongated molecule with a large basic patch and a large hydrophobic patch, both highly conserved [31], which might offer attractive sites for binding of both acidic anionic and alkyl groups, respectively, of SAGEs. The dramatic differences among structurally similar SAGEs [6] and ligand specific structure-activity relationships strongly suggest that charge alone is only a small contributor to overall anti-inflammatory effects. Binding of polyanions such as SAGEs to this cationic region might be expected to not only inhibit binding of AGEs, which ligate RAGE at its V domain, but also, dependent upon the nature of substituent alkyl groups, to produce steric interference with the binding of other ligands such as S100/calgranulins and HMGB-1 which require adjacent C1 and/or C2 regions for full RAGE ligation [32].

A major issue with the use of sulfated polysaccharides such as SAGEs for topical treatment of skin diseases is their availability to the dermis. Literature on the bioavailability of sulfated polysaccharides across skin is conflicting, with some groups reporting little penetration but others suggesting transdermal absorption of heparin and unfractionated heparin as a result of their detergent properties [33–39]. In the most recently published work, fluorescent-labeled unfractionated heparin was found to adhere to keratinocytes in culture, and within 48 hours, almost half of topically applied labeled heparin was found to transcutaneously penetrate the skin of hairless rats mounted onto a Franz static diffusion cell [40]. Whereas SAGEs might permeate normal skin in humans less well than in mice, inflammation could serve to greatly increase SAGE penetration (Figure 9), as seen with other drugs used for serious skin diseases [41] and similar to the well-recognized enhancement of antibiotic penetration into cerebrospinal fluid in the presence of a disrupted blood-brain barrier in meningitis. Various techniques have been developed to enable transdermal delivery of low molecular weight (~5,000 Da) heparin, including penetration enhancers [42,43], liposomal formulation [43,44], iontophoresis [45,46] and low frequency ultrasound [45,47,48]. These strategies might also facilitate dermal penetration of similarly sized SAGEs to enable their effective topical use in skin disorders.

The chemistry and function of HA have been well explored in cutaneous biology, and bacterial and animal-derived HA continue to be an important component for the cosmetics, pharmaceutical and medical device industries. Our research suggests that simple chemical modifications of HA can generate novel anionic polysaccharides with broad anti-inflammatory activities. SAGEs have the additional advantage of being non-animal derived, thus circumventing the risks of adulteration and sourcing problems inherent in animal-derived sulfated polysaccharides [15]. Our observations suggest that SAGEs in topical application may prove to be a safe and useful treatment not only for rosacea, but also other inflammatory skin diseases.

Materials and Methods

Materials

Polyclonal goat anti-human RAGE (Cat# AF1145), recombinant HMGB-1, recombinant human P-selectin/Fc chimera, and recombinant human RAGE/Fc chimera were purchased from R&D Systems (Minneapolis, MN). Rabbit polyclonal IgG antibody to LL-37 (Cat# sc-50423) was from Santa Cruz Biotechnology (Santa Cruz, CA), and peroxidase-linked goat anti-rabbit polyclonal IgG (Cat# A0545) was from Sigma Aldrich (St. Louis, MO). Human S100b calgranulin was from Calbiochem (San Diego, CA). Alexa Fluor® 633 hydrazide was from Molecular Probes (Eugene, OR). The AGE product CML-BSA was from MBL International (Woburn, MA). Protein A, horse radish peroxidase (HRP)-conjugated rabbit polyclonal anti-goat IgG (Cat# 31402), carbonate-bicarbonate buffer and bovine serum albumin blocker (10x) were from Piercenet (Rockford, IL). Calcein AM, Dulbecco's modified Eagle's medium (DMEM), EpiLife medium, ethylenediamine tetraacetic acid (EDTA), fetal bovine serum (FBS), HEPES, non-essential amino acids, penicillin/streptomycin/L-glutamine solution, RPMI-1640 without L-glutamine, sodium bicarbonate, and tetramethyl benzidine chromogen (TMB) single solution chromogen were from Invitrogen (Carlsbad, CA). High-bind 96-well microplates were from Corning Life Sciences (Corning, NY), and heparin binding plates were from BD Biosciences (Bedford, MA). U937 monocytes and nHDF cells were purchased from American Type Culture Collection (Manassas, VA). nHEK cells were obtained from Invitrogen (Madison, WI). Antibodies for immunohistochemistry were sourced as identified in figure legends. All other chemicals not specified were from Sigma-Aldrich (St. Louis, MO). HA was obtained commercially from a recombinant *B. subtilis* expression system (Novozymes Biopolymers, Bagsvaerd, Denmark) or from streptococcal fermentation (LifeCore, Chaska, MN).

Animal Care and Use

All animal protocols were approved by the University of Utah institutional animal care and use committee (IACUC). Approved protocols include 08-06002, 08-06005 and 08-11008.

Characterization of SAGEs

A variety of SAGEs were prepared with four parameters varied: molecular weight, type of ether modification, substitution degree of ether modification, and degree of sulfation. These data are reported elsewhere [6]. Ether substitution degree (SD) of SAGE was determined by ^{1}H NMR, and for GM-1111 was estimated to be SD = 1, or ~1 alkyl group per disaccharide unit. After sulfation, GM-1111 was dissolved in water, dialyzed, and lyophilized to give a white powder shown by ^{1}H NMR to have a sulfation SD of 1.0–1.5. Fluorescent-labeled GM-1111 was synthesized by conjugation with Alexa Fluor 633 hydrazide.

Molecular weight was determined with gel permeation chromatography using a Waters 515 HPLC pump, Waters 410 differential refractometer, Waters 486 tunable absorbance detector, and Ultrahydrogel 250 or 1000 columns (7.8 mm i.d X 130 cm) (Milford, MA). Eluent was 200 mM phosphate buffer (pH 6.5): MeOH = 80:20 (v/v), and flow rate was 0.3 or 0.5 mL/min. The system was calibrated with standard HA samples from Dr. U. Wik (Pharmacia, Uppsala, Sweden). Average molecular weight of GM-1111 was ~5,000–6,000 Da.

Formulation of GM-1111 emollient

A 1% (w/w) emollient was prepared in Spectrum Transdermal Ointment (Lotioncrafters, Olga, WA), a commercially available proprietary ointment comprised of cetyl ricinoleate, carnuba wax, *D*-α-tocopheryl acetate, shea butter, caprylic triglyceride, lecithin and beeswax. GM-1111 (100 mg) was dissolved in 2.0 g of nanopure water, ointment was added to give 10.0 g, the mixture blended thoroughly and the emulsion processed through an ointment mill. Control emollient was made with 2 g water without active ingredient. Sodium hyaluronate emollient was prepared with 100 mg of 53 kDa HA (Novozymes, Bagsvaerd, Denmark) following an analogous protocol. Each formulation was stored at 4°C.

Cell culture

U937 monocytes were grown in suspension at 37°C in 5% CO_2-95% air in RPMI-1640 supplemented with 10% heat inactivated FBS, 2 mM L-glutamine, 1 mM sodium pyruvate, 0.1 mM MEM non-essential amino acids, 100 units/ml penicillin and 100 mg/ml streptomycin. nHDF cells were grown in DMEM supplemented with 10% FBS and penicillin-streptomycin. nHEK cells were grown in EpiLife medium supplemented with 0.06 mM Ca^{2+}, 1% EpiLife defined growth supplement and penicillin-streptomycin. Experiments were performed with cells from passages 1-5.

Factor XII activation assay

Five μl of pooled normal human plasma was incubated with 100 μl of GM-1111 ranging from 0.1-1000 μg/ml in 0.05M HEPES containing 0.05% TritonX-100 for 5 min at 25°C. Amidolytic activity was determined with 0.5 mM H-D-CHT-Gly-Arg-*p*NA by following the change of optical density (OD) for 30 min at 405 nm [16]. The OD obtained at 30 min was plotted against the concentrations of the activator.

Cell surface binding assays

The effect of GM-1111 on binding of U937 monocytes to P-selectin or RAGE was studied using calcein labeled cells incubated in micro plates coated with P-selectin-Fc or RAGE-Fc chimeras. These methods have been reported in detail [10].

Inhibition of human leukocyte elastase (HLE)

Inhibition of HLE by SAGEs was determined using the specific chromogenic substrate suc-Ala-Ala-Val-*p*NA, according to methods previously described [10].

Solid phase binding assays

Three types of ELISAs were performed: one to study the binding of vascular adhesion molecules and LL-37 to GM-1111, and another to study binding between RAGE and its ligands, including CML-BSA, HMGB-1 and S100b. A competitive ELISA was also performed to study the ability of GM-1111 to inhibit/compete RAGE binding to its ligands. These ELISAs have been reported in detail [10].

In vitro cytotoxicity and anticoagulant assays

nHDF cells were seeded (4,000/100 μl medium) in each well of 96-well flat-bottomed microplates, and incubated at 37°C in 5% CO_2 for 12 hours. Medium was changed with complete medium containing GM-1111 at final concentrations of 10 to 10^6 ng/ml to each well. At 48 hours, 20 μl MTS (CellTiter96® Aqueous One assay; Promega, Madison, WI) was added to each well, and cells were further incubated for 2 h. Absorbance of the samples was measured at 490 nm using a 96-well plate reader to determine cytotoxicity. Cytotoxicity was assessed similarly in nHEK cells. Automated amidolytic assays for anti-Xa and anti-IIa activity were performed by BioCascade, Arlington, WI.

Skin irritation tests in mice

SAGEs were tested *in vivo* to assess dermal irritation potential. GM-1111 was prepared at 0.1, 1 and 10 mg/ml. Formic acid (10%) and PBS were used as positive and negative control, respectively. Balb/c mice (n = 6 per group), free from skin irritation, trauma, or adverse clinical signs prior to study, were randomized and grouped for test conditions. Backs of animals were clipped free of fur. Each mouse received four parallel epidermal abrasions with a sterile needle at the bottom area of the test site, while the upper area of the test site remained intact. Under isofluroane anesthesia, two 0.5-ml samples of the test solution were applied to the entire test site under a double gauze layer to an area of skin approximately 2.5 cm^2. Patches were backed with plastic, covered with a non reactive tape and the test site wrapped with a bandage. After 24 h exposure to the agent, the bandage and soaked test gauze were removed and test sites were wiped with tap water to remove remaining test compound. At 24 and 72 h after application, test sites were examined for dermal reactions in accordance with the FHSA- recommended Draize scoring criteria [14]. Primary Irritation Index (P.I.I.) of test article was calculated following test completion. A material producing a P.I.I. score of greater than or equal to 5.00 would be considered positive and be classed as a primary irritant to skin.

Peptide synthesis

LL-37 was prepared by the core peptide facility at the University of Utah, containing the amino acid sequence: LLGDFFRKSKEKIGKEFKRIVQRIKDFLRNLVPRTES. Synthetic peptides were purified to >95% by HPCL and sequence was confirmed by mass spectrometry.

LL-37-mediated skin inflammation models

To study the effect of SAGE in rosacea, we used a previously reported disease model produced by intradermal injection of LL-37 [3]. Balb/c mice were shaved prior to study to expose skin on the back. Twenty-four hours later, 40 μl of vehicle (nanopure water), LL-37 (320 μM), SAGE (1,280 μM), or LL-37+ SAGE mix (peptide + 4x molar concentration of SAGE) was injected intradermally into the shaved skin using a 0.5 ml syringe and 31-gauge insulin needle in a manner to raise an intact dermal bleb, identifying that administration was at the lower epidermis or dermis. To standardize results, all intradermal injections were performed by a single investigator with experience performing intradermal injections on the human volar forearm with needle bevel facing upward. SAGE and LL-37 were mixed together in PBS and allowed to incubate 15 min at room temperature before injection. Injections were repeated every 12 h thereafter. Forty-eight hours after the initial injection (four injections in total), animals were anesthetized with isofluorane. Injected skin was photographed to record severity of erythema and edema. Mice were euthanized with CO_2, and injected skin was excised for hematoxylin and eosin staining and immunochemistry. From the center of excised skin, a 6 mm punch biopsy was obtained, weighed, snap frozen in liquid N_2 and stored at -80 C for measurement of tissue MPO.

To study topical SAGE in this model, mice were injected with LL-37 as described above. GM-1111 was then applied topically as a 1% concentration in 50 µl of emollient, either immediately after the first LL-37 injection or 12 h thereafter, with repeated application every 12 h after each LL-37 injection. After application, emollient was massaged into the affected area of skin with a gloved finger rubbed 32 consecutive times in a counter-clockwise direction. Control animals were treated similarly with emollient alone. To standardize treatment, all topical medication applications were performed by a single investigator after the individual performing intradermal injections had finished the injections and left the laboratory area. After four LL-37 intradermal injections, mice were photographed and biopsied as above.

Croton oil inflammation model

As another model of PMN-mediated skin inflammation, we employed croton oil [18]. Croton oil (0.8% solution in acetone) was painted (10 µl each side) on one ear of Balb/c mice, with the other ear as a control. Fifteen minutes later, GM-1111 was then dosed topically as a 1% concentration in 50 µl of emollient applied to each side of the croton-oil treated ear. After application, emollient was massaged into each side of the ear with a gloved finger rubbed 32 consecutive times in a counter-clockwise direction. Control animals were treated in a similar fashion with emollient alone. To standardize treatment, all topical medication applications were performed by a single investigator after the individual performing croton oil applications had left the laboratory area. After 4, 8 and 24 h, ear thickness was measured near the top of the ear distal to the cartilaginous ridges. Change in ear thickness from control was taken as an edema index. Following 24 h measurements, mice were euthanized with CO_2 and 6 mm ear punch biopsies taken, weighed, frozen and stored at −80°C for determination of MPO activity. A single investigator performed all measurements and biopsies in order to standardize the procedure. Remaining ears were removed, embedded and frozen for hematoxylin and eosin stains and immunohistochemistry.

MPO assay

Tissue MPO activity was measured using the method of Suzuki et al. [49] modified by Young et al. [50]. Biopsies were placed in 0.75 ml of 80 mM PBS (pH 5.4) containing 0.5% hexadecyltrimethyl-ammonium bromide (HTAB). Each sample was homogenized for 45 s at 4°C with a Tissue Tearor Homogenizer (Model 985-370; Biospec Products, Bartlesville, OK). Homogenate was transferred to a microcentrifuge tube with an additional 0.75 ml HTAB in PBS. The 1.5 ml sample was centrifuged at 12,000×*g* for 15 min at 4°C. Triplicate 30 µl samples of the resulting supernatant were added to 96-well microtiter plates. For MPO assay, 200 µl of a mixture containing 100 µl of 80 mM PBS (pH 5.4), 85 µl of 0.22 M PBS (pH 5.4), and 15 µl of 0.017% hydrogen peroxide were added to each well. To this, 20 µl of 18.4 mM tetramethylbenzidine HCl in 8% aqueous dimethylformamide (DMF) was added to start the reaction. Microtiter plates were incubated at 37°C for 3 min, and placed on ice. The reaction was stopped with the addition of 30 µl of 1.46 M sodium acetate. MPO activity was assessed at 630 nm and expressed as optical density (OD)/biopsy.

Immunohistochemistry

LL-37, PBS and LL-37 and SAGE-injected mouse skin was stained with antibody to mouse Gr-1 to examine neutrophil infiltration, and also for S100A8 calgranulin, the major RAGE-binding calgranulin present in murine PMNs [17]. Slides were deparaffinized and hydrated through Citrisolv and graded ethanol washes. Endogenous peroxidase activity was blocked with 1% H_2O_2 in PBS with 0.1% Tween-20 (PBST) for 20 min. Antigen retrieval was performed by microwaving in 1% antigen unmasking solution (Vector Laboratories) for 20 min followed by incubation at room temperature for 30 min. Immunostaining was performed using the Vectastain Elite ABC peroxidase kit (Vector Laboratories). Briefly, non-specific antibody binding was minimized by incubating sections for 90 min in diluted normal blocking serum. Sections were incubated overnight at 4°C in a humidified chamber with primary goat anti-mouse calgranulin A antibodies (Santa Cruz #sc-8113) at a 1:200 dilution and rat anti-mouse Gr-1 (R&D Systems #RB6-8C5) at a 1:500 dilution. Following overnight incubation, slides were washed in PBST for 9 min, incubated 2 h with biotinylated secondary antibody diluted to 5 µg/ml in PBST, followed by Vectastain Elite ABC Reagent (Vector) diluted in PBST for 30 min. Between incubations, sections were washed for 12 min in PBST. Immunoreactivity was detected by incubating with the DAB peroxidase substrate kit (Vector Laboratories) for 1–2 min. Sections were then washed in nanopure water and counterstained with hematoxylin before dehydration and mounting with coverslips.

Statistical Analysis

All experiments were performed in triplicate or quadruplicate for *in vitro* tests. Results are expressed as means ± standard error of the mean (SEM). Significant differences between samples were calculated by comparison of means using the Aspin−Welch test. In experiments with multiple groups or treatments, a one-way analysis of variance (ANOVA) followed by Student-Newman-Keuls *post hoc* test was used to analyze for group differences. Significance was declared at $P<0.05$.

Author Contributions

Conceived and designed the experiments: GDP NVR TPK. Performed the experiments: JZ XX NVR BA LM WJR. Analyzed the data: XX LM. Contributed reagents/materials/analysis tools: JZ XX NVR. Wrote the paper: TPK NVR GDP GK.

References

1. Powell FC (2005) Rosacea. N Engl J Med 352: 793–803.
2. Elewski BE, Draelos Z, Breno B, Jansen T, Layton A, et al. (2010) Rosacea—global diversity and optimized outcome: proposed international consensus from the Rosacea International Expert Group. J Europ Academ Dermatol Venereology doi:10.1111/j.1468-3083.2010.03751.x.
3. Yamasaki K, Di Nardo A, Bardan A, Murakami M, Ohtake T, et al. (2007) Increased serine protease activity and cathelicidin promotes skin inflammation in rosacea. Nat Med 13: 975–980.
4. Bevins CL, Liu F-T (2007) Rosacea: skin innate immunity gone awry? Nat Med 13: 904–906.

5. Kenshi Y, Gallo RL (2008) Antimicrobial peptides in human skin disease. Eur J Dermatol 18: 11–21.
6. Prestwich G, Zhang J, Kennedy TP, Rao N, Xu X (2010) Alkylated semi-synthetic glycosaminoglycosan ethers, and methods for making and using thereof. U.S. Patent 7,855,187B1.
7. Wang L, Brown JR, Varki A, Esko JD (2002) Heparin's anti-inflammatory effects require glucosamine 6-*O*-sulfation and are mediated by blockade of L- and P-selectins. J Clin Invest 110: 127–136.
8. Fryer A, Huang Y-C, Rao G, Jacoby D, Mancilla E, et al. (1997) Selective O-desulfation produces nonanticoagulant heparin that retains pharmacologic activity in the lung. J Pharmacol Exp Ther 282: 208–219.
9. Lohwasser C, Neureiter D, Weigle B, Kirchner T, Schuppan D (2006) The receptor for advanced glycation end products is highly expressed in the skin and upregulated by advanced glycation end products and tumor necrosis factor-alpha. J Invest Dermatol 126: 291–299.
10. Rao NV, Argyle B, Xu X, Reynolds PR, Walenga JM, et al. (2010) Low anticoagulant heparin targets multiple sites of inflammation, suppresses heparin-induced thrombocytopenia, and inhibits interaction of RAGE with its ligands. Am J Physiol Cell Physiol 299: C97–C110.
11. Foell D, Wittkowski H, Vogl T, Roth J (2007) S100 proteins expressed in phagocytes: a novel group of damage-associated molecular pattern molecules. J Leukoc Biol 81: 28–37.
12. Klune JR, Dhupar R, Cardinal J, Billiar TR, Tsung A (2008) HMGB1: endogenous danger signaling. Mol Med 14: 476–484.
13. Chavakis T, Bierhaus A, Al-Fakhri N, Schneider D, Witte S, et al. (2003) The pattern recognition receptor (RAGE) is a counterreceptor for leukocyte integrins: a novel pathway for inflammatory cell recruitment. J Exp Med 10: 1507–1515.
14. Bosshard E (1985) Review on skin and mucous-membrane irritations tests and their application. Food Chem Toxicol 23: 149–154.
15. Kishimoto TK, Viswanathan K, Ganguly T, Elankumaran S, Smith S, et al. (2008) Contaminated heparin associated with adverse clinical events and activation of the contact system. N Engl J Med 358: 2457–2467.
16. Silverberg M, Dunn JT, Garen L, Kaplan AP (1980) Autoactivation of human Hageman factor. Demonstration using a synthetic substrate. J Biol Chem 255: 7281–7286.
17. Fuellen G, Foell D, Nacken W, Sorg C, Kerkhoff C (2003) Absence of S100A12 in mouse: implications of RAGE-S100A12 interaction. Trends Immunol 24: 622–624.
18. Bralley EE, Greenspan P, Hargrove JL, Wicker L, Hartle DK (2008) Topical anti-inflammatory activity of *Polygonum cuspidatum* extract in the TPA model of mouse ear inflammation. J Inflammation 5: 1–7. doi:10.1186/476-9255-5-1.
19. Mittal D, Sacchaeri F, Venereau E, Pusteria T, Bianchi ME, et al. (2010) TLR4-mediated skin carcinogenesis is dependent on immune and radioresistant cells. EMBO J 29: 2242–2252.
20. Koczulla R, von Degenfeld G, Kupatt C, Krotz F, Zahler S, et al. (2003) An angiogenic role for the human peptide antibiotic LL-37/hCAP-18. J Clin Invest 111: 1665–1672.
21. Ogata M, Fletcher MF, Kloczewiak M, Loiselle PM, Zanzot EM, et al. (1997) Effect of anticoagulants on binding and neutralization of lipopolysaccharide by the peptide immunoglobulin conjugate $CAP18_{106-138}$-immunoglobuin G in whole blood. Infect Immun 65: 2160–2167.
22. Baranska-Rybak W, Sonesson A, Nowicki R, Schmidtchen A (2006) Glycosaminoglycans inhibit the antibacterial activity of LL-37 in biological fluids. J Antimicrob Chemotherapy 57: 260–265.
23. Barker RL, Gundel RH, Gleich GJ, Checkel JL, Loegering DA, et al. (1991) Acidic polyamino acids inhibit human eosinophil granule major basic protein toxicity. Evidence of a functional role for ProMBP. J Clin Invest 88: 798–805.
24. Fryer AD, Jacoby DB (1992) Function of pulmonary M_2 muscarinic receptors in antigen-challenged guinea pigs is restored by heparin and poly-L-glutamate. J Clin Invest 90: 2292–2298.
25. Nestle FO, Kaplan DH, Barker J (2009) Psoriasis. N Engl J Med 361: 496–590.
26. Wolf R, Howard OMZ, Dong H-F, Voscopoulos C, Boeshans K, et al. (2008) Chemotactic activity of S100A7 (psoriasin) is mediated by RAGE and potentiates inflammation with highly homologous but functionally distinct S100A15. J Immunol 181: 1499–1506.
27. Schmidt AM, Yan SD, Yan SF, Stern DM (2001) The multiligand receptor RAGE as a progression factor amplifying immune and inflammatory responses. J Clin Invest 108: 949–955.
28. Alexiou P, Chatzopoulou M, Pegklidou K, Demopoulos VJ (2010) RAGE: a multiland receptor unveiling novel insights in health and disease. Curr Med Chem 17: 2232–2252.
29. Orlova VV, Choi EY, Xie C, Chavakis E, Bierhaus A, et al. (2007) A novel pathway way of HMGB1-mediated inflammatory cell recruitment that requires Mac-1 integrin. EMBO J 26: 1129–1139.
30. Matsumoto S, Yoshida T, Murata H, Harada S, Fujita N, et al. (2008) Solution structure of the variable-type domain of the receptor for advanced glycation end products: new insight into AGE-RAGE interaction. Biochem 47: 12299–12311.
31. Park H, Boyington JC (2010) The 1.5 Å crystal structure of human receptor for advanced glycation endproducts (RAGE) ectodomains reveals unique features determining ligand binding. J Biol Chem doi/10/1074/jbc.M110/169276.
32. Xie J, Reverdatta S, Frolov A, Hoffmann R, Burz DS, et al. (2008) Structural basis for pattern recognition by the receptor for advanced glycation end products (RAGE). J Biol Chem 282: 27255–27269.
33. Schraven E, Trottnow D (1973) Perkutane Resorption von Heparin-^{35}S aus einer speziell zubereiteten Öl-in-Wasser-Emulsion. Arzneim-Forsch/Drug Res 23: 274–275.
34. Schaefer H, Zesch A (1976) Die Penetration von Heparin in die menschliche Haut. Pharmazie 31: 251–254.
35. Zesch A, Schaefer H (1976) Penetration, Permeation und Resorption von Heparin in-vivo-Untersuchungen an der menschlichen Haut. Arzneim-Forsch/ Drug Res 26: 1365–1368.
36. Zimmermann RE (1982) Untersuchungen zur transkutanen Heparinapplikation. Therapiewoche 32: 6157–6164.
37. Stuttgen G, Panse P, Bauer E (1990) Permeation of the human skin by heparin and mucopolysaccharide polysulfuric acid ester. Arzneim-Forsch/Drug Res 40: 484–489.
38. de Moerlosse P, Gavillet O, Salomon D, Minazio P, Reber G (1992) Heparin-related activity in peripheral venous blood after percutaneous application of various glycosaminoglycan containing creams. Blood Coag Fibrinol 3: 827–878.
39. Bonina FP, Montenegro L (1994) Vehicle effects on in vitro heparin release and skin penetration from different gels. Int J Pharm 102: 19–24.
40. Parisel C, Saffar L, Gattegno L, Andre V, Abdul-Malak N, et al. (2003) Interactions of heparin with human skin cells: Binding, location, and transdermal penetration. J Biomed Mater Res 67A: 517–523.
41. Meingassner JG, Aschauer H, Stuetz A, Biollich A (2005) Pimecrolimus permeates less than tacrolimus through normal, inflamed, or corticosteroid-pretreated skin. Exp Dermatol 14: 752–757.
42. Karande P, Jain A, Mitragotri S (2004) Discovery of transdermal penetration enhancers by high-throughput screening. Nat Biotech 22: 192–197.
43. Betz G, Nowbakht P, Imboden R Imanidis G (2001) Heparin penetration into and permeation through human skin from aqueous and liposomal fomulations in vitro. Int J Pharm 228: 147–159.
44. Song Y-K, Kim C-K (2006) Topical delivery of low-molecular-weight heparin with surface-charged flexible liposomes. Biomaterials 27: 271–280.
45. Lanke SSS, Kolli CS, Strom JG, Banga AK (2009) Enhanced transdermal delivery of low molecular weight heparin by barrier perturbation. Int J Pharm 365: 26–33.
46. Pacini S, Punzi T, Gulisano M, Cecchi F, Vannucchi S, Ruggiero M (2006) Transdermal delivery of heparin using pulsed current iontophoresis. Pharmaceutical Res 23: 114–120.
47. Mitragotri S, Kost J (2001) Transdermal delivery of heparin and low-molecular weight heparin using low-frequency ultrasound. Pharmaceutical Res 18: 1151–1156.
48. Ogura M, Paliwwal S, Mitragotri S (2008) Low-frequency sonophoresis: Current status and future prospects. Adv Drug Del Rev 60: 1218–1223.
49. Suzuki K, Ota H, Sasagawa S, Sakatani T, Fujikura T (1983) Assay method for myeloperoxidase in human polymorphonuclear leukocytes. Anal Biochem 132: 345–352.
50. Young JM, Spires DA, Bedord CJ, Wagner B, Ballaron SJ, et al. (1984) The mouse ear inflammatory response to topical arachidonic acid. J Invest Dermatol 82: 367–371.

Permissions

All chapters in this book were first published in PLOS ONE, by The Public Library of Science; hereby published with permission under the Creative Commons Attribution License or equivalent. Every chapter published in this book has been scrutinized by our experts. Their significance has been extensively debated. The topics covered herein carry significant findings which will fuel the growth of the discipline. They may even be implemented as practical applications or may be referred to as a beginning point for another development.

The contributors of this book come from diverse backgrounds, making this book a truly international effort. This book will bring forth new frontiers with its revolutionizing research information and detailed analysis of the nascent developments around the world.

We would like to thank all the contributing authors for lending their expertise to make the book truly unique. They have played a crucial role in the development of this book. Without their invaluable contributions this book wouldn't have been possible. They have made vital efforts to compile up to date information on the varied aspects of this subject to make this book a valuable addition to the collection of many professionals and students.

This book was conceptualized with the vision of imparting up-to-date information and advanced data in this field. To ensure the same, a matchless editorial board was set up. Every individual on the board went through rigorous rounds of assessment to prove their worth. After which they invested a large part of their time researching and compiling the most relevant data for our readers.

The editorial board has been involved in producing this book since its inception. They have spent rigorous hours researching and exploring the diverse topics which have resulted in the successful publishing of this book. They have passed on their knowledge of decades through this book. To expedite this challenging task, the publisher supported the team at every step. A small team of assistant editors was also appointed to further simplify the editing procedure and attain best results for the readers.

Apart from the editorial board, the designing team has also invested a significant amount of their time in understanding the subject and creating the most relevant covers. They scrutinized every image to scout for the most suitable representation of the subject and create an appropriate cover for the book.

The publishing team has been an ardent support to the editorial, designing and production team. Their endless efforts to recruit the best for this project, has resulted in the accomplishment of this book. They are a veteran in the field of academics and their pool of knowledge is as vast as their experience in printing. Their expertise and guidance has proved useful at every step. Their uncompromising quality standards have made this book an exceptional effort. Their encouragement from time to time has been an inspiration for everyone.

The publisher and the editorial board hope that this book will prove to be a valuable piece of knowledge for researchers, students, practitioners and scholars across the globe.

List of Contributors

Leslie Burdett Hart and Lori H. Schwacke
Division of Biostatistics and Epidemiology, Department of Medicine, Medical University of South Carolina, Charleston, South Carolina, United States of America
National Oceanic and Atmospheric Administration, National Ocean Service, Hollings Marine Laboratory, Charleston, South Carolina, United States of America

Suzanne M. Lane, Todd Speakman and Eric S. Zolman
National Oceanic and Atmospheric Administration, National Ocean Service, Hollings Marine Laboratory, Charleston, South Carolina, United States of America

Silin Pang, Huali Wu, Qian Wang, Minxuan Cai and Jing Shang
New Drug Screening Center, China Pharmaceutical University, Nanjing, China
State Key Laboratory of Natural Medicines, China Pharmaceutical University, Nanjing, China

Weimin Shi
Shanghai First People Hospital, Shanghai, China

Teri K. Rowles
National Oceanic and Atmospheric Administration, National Marine Fisheries Service, Office of Protected Resources, Silver Spring, Maryland, United States of America

Dave S. Rotstein
National Oceanic and Atmospheric Administration, National Marine Fisheries Service, Office of Protected Resources, Silver Spring, Maryland, United States of America
Marine Mammal Pathology Services, Olney, Maryland, United States of America

Randall S. Wells, Jason Allen and Aaron Barleycorn
Chicago Zoological Society, c/o: Mote Marine Laboratory, Sarasota, Florida, United States of America

Brian C. Balmer
Chicago Zoological Society, c/o: Mote Marine Laboratory, Sarasota, Florida, United States of America
University of North Carolina Wilmington, Department of Biology and Marine Biology, Wilmington North Carolina, United States of America

Megan Stolen
Hubbs-SeaWorld Research Institute, Melbourne Beach, Florida, United States of America

Wayne McFee
Coastal Marine Mammal Stranding Assessments Program, National Oceanic and Atmospheric Administration, National Centers for Coastal Ocean Science, Center for Coastal Environmental Health and Biomolecular Research, Charleston, South Carolina, United States of America

Tracey Goldstein
Wildlife Health Center, School of Veterinary Medicine, University of California, Davis, California, United States of America

Balvinder Rehal and April Armstrong
Department of Dermatology, University of California Davis, Davis, California, United States of America

Detlef Becker, Elise Langer, Martin Seemann, Gunda Seemann, Isabel Fell, Joachim Saloga, Stephan Grabbe and Esther von Stebut
Department of Dermatology, University Medicine, Johannes Gutenberg University, Mainz, Germany

David Wong, Bory Kea and David Fiorentino
Department of Dermatology, Stanford University School of Medicine, Stanford, California, United States of America

Rob Pesich and Patrick Brown
Department of Biochemistry, Stanford University School of Medicine, Stanford, California, United States of America

Brandon W. Higgs, Wei Zhu and Yihong Yao
MedImmune, Translational Sciences, One MedImmune Way, Gaithersburg, Maryland, United States of America

Silin Pang, Huali Wu, Qian Wang, Minxuan Cai and Jing Shang
New Drug Screening Center, China Pharmaceutical University, Nanjing, China
State Key Laboratory of Natural Medicines, China Pharmaceutical University, Nanjing, China

Weimin Shi
Shanghai First People Hospital, Shanghai, China

Brett D. Thombs
Department of Psychiatry, McGill University, Montréal, Québec, Canada
Department of Epidemiology, Biostatistics, and Occupational Health, McGill University, Montréal, Québec, Canada

Department of Medicine, McGill University, Montréal, Québec, Canada
School of Nursing, McGill University, Montréal, Québec, Canada
Lady Davis Institute for Medical Research, Jewish General Hospital, Montréal, Qu ébec, Canada
Division of Rheumatology, Jewish General Hospital, Montre´ al, Que´bec, Canada
Department of Psychiatry, Jewish General Hospital, Montréal, Québec, Canada

Lisa R. Jewett
Department of Psychiatry, McGill University, Montréal, Québec, Canada
Lady Davis Institute for Medical Research, Jewish General Hospital, Montréal, Qu ébec, Canada

Marie Hudson and Murray Baron
Department of Medicine, McGill University, Montréal, Québec, Canada
Lady Davis Institute for Medical Research, Jewish General Hospital, Montréal, Qu ébec, Canada
Division of Rheumatology, Jewish General Hospital, Montre´ al, Que´bec, Canada

Vanessa L. Malcarne
Department of Psychology, San Diego State University, San Diego, California, United States of America

Yunying Chen, Sara Lind Enoksson, Catharina Johansson, Annika Scheynius and Mikael C. I. Karlsson
Clinical Allergy Research Unit, Department of Medicine Solna, Karolinska Institutet and Karolinska University Hospital Solna, Stockholm, Sweden

Maria A. Karlssonand and Lena Lundeberg
Dermatology Unit, Department of Medicine Solna, Karolinska Institutet and Karolinska University Hospital Solna, Stockholm, Sweden

Gunnar Nilsson
Clinical Immunology and Allergy Unit, Department of Medicine Solna, Karolinska Institutet and Karolinska University Hospital Solna, Stockholm, Sweden

Takeshi Satoh, Aurelien Sarde, Celine Trouillet and Frederic Geissmann
School of Medicine, Centre for Molecular and Cellular Biology of Inflammation (CMCBI), King's College London, London, United Kingdom

Alexander Smith, Sophie Mian and Ghulam Mufti
Haematology Department, King's College London, London, United Kingdom

Hui-chun Lu and Franca Fraternali
Randall Division of Molecular Biophysics, King's College London, London, United Kingdom

Jean-Francois Emile
Hopital Ambroise-Pare, Pathology department, AP-HP, Paris, France

Jean Donadieu
Centre de Référence de l'Histiocytose, Hopital d'Enfants Armand Trousseau, Pediatric Hematology Unit, AP-HP, Paris, France

Wei He, Fei Zhu and Xinyu Zhao
Injury Control Research Center, Obesity and Body Composition Research Center, School of Public Health, Zhejiang University, Hangzhou, China

Shankuan Zhu
Injury Control Research Center, Obesity and Body Composition Research Center, School of Public Health, Zhejiang University, Hangzhou, China
Injury Research Center, Medical College of Wisconsin, Milwaukee, Wisconsin, United States of America

Xiaoguang Ma
Injury Research Center, Medical College of Wisconsin, Milwaukee, Wisconsin, United States of America
Department of Epidemiology and Biostatistics, Arnold School of Public Health, University of South Carolina, Columbia, South Carolina, United States of America

Min Zheng
Department of Dermatology, Second Affiliated Hospital, Zhejiang University, Hangzhou, China,

Zhao Chen
Division of Epidemiology and Biostatistics, Mel and Enid Zuckerman College of Public Health, University of Arizona, Tucson, Arizona, United States of America

Steven B. Heymsfield
Pennington Biomedical Research Center, Baton Rouge, Louisiana, United States of America

Suvi-Päivikki Sinikumpu, Laura Huilaja, Päivi M. Hägg, Erika Wikström and Kaisa Tasanen
Department of Dermatology, Medical Research Center, University of Oulu and Oulu University Hospital, Oulu, Finland

Markku Koiranen, Juha Auvinen and Markku Timonen
Institute of Health Sciences, Faculty of Medicine University of Oulu, Oulu, Finland

Jari Jokelainen
Institute of Health Sciences, Faculty of Medicine University of Oulu, Oulu, Finland
Unit of General Practice, Oulu University Hospital, Oulu, Finland

Yang Lili, Wei Yi, Yang Ji and Li Ming
Departments of dermatology, Zhongshan Hospital, Fudan University, Shanghai, China,

Sun Yue and Shi Weimin
Departments of dermatology, Shanghai First People's Hospital, Shanghai Jiaotong University, Shanghai, China

Knut M. Wittkowski, Jennifer Belasco, John Gray and James G. Krueger
The Rockefeller University, New York, New York, United States of America

Craig Leonardi
St. Louis University Medical School, St. Louis University, St. Louis, Missouri, United States of America

Alice Gottlieb
Tufts Medical Center, Tufts University, Boston, Massachusetts, United States of America,

Alan Menter
Baylor Institute of Research, Dermatology Research Center, Baylor University Medical Center, Baylor University, Dallas, Texas, United States of America

Gerald G. Krueger and Razieh Soltani-Arabshahi
University of Utah, Salt Lake City, Utah, United States of America

Paul W. Tebbey, Liz Horn and for the International Psoriasis Council
International Psoriasis Council, Dallas, Texas, United States of America

Malgorzata Romanowska, Louise Reilly and John Foerster
Division of Experimental Medicine, University of Dundee, Dundee, United Kingdom

Colin N. A. Palmer
Biomedical Research Institute, University of Dundee, Dundee, United Kingdom

Mattias C. U. Gustafsson
Department of Laboratory Medicine, Division of Medical Microbiology, Lund University, Lund, Sweden

Thilo Jakob and Stefan F. Martin
Allergy Research Group, Department of Dermatology, University Freiburg Medical Center, Freiburg, Germany

Eva Oswald
Allergy Research Group, Department of Dermatology, University Freiburg Medical Center, Freiburg, Germany
Molecular Dermatology, Department of Dermatology, University Freiburg Medical Center, Freiburg, Germany
Faculty of Biology, University of Freiburg, Freiburg, Germany

Alina Sesarman and Claus-Werner Franzke
Molecular Dermatology, Department of Dermatology, University Freiburg Medical Center, Freiburg, Germany

Cassian Sitaru
Molecular Dermatology, Department of Dermatology, University Freiburg Medical Center, Freiburg, Germany
BIOSS Centre for Biological Signalling Studies, Freiburg, Germany

Leena Bruckner-Tuderman
Molecular Dermatology, Department of Dermatology, University Freiburg Medical Center, Freiburg, Germany
BIOSS Centre for Biological Signalling Studies, Freiburg, Germany
Freiburg Institute for Advanced Studies, Freiburg, Germany

Ute Wölfle
Competence Centre Skintegral, Department of Dermatology, University Freiburg Medical Center, Freiburg, Germany

Joanna Ponińska and Rafał Płoski
Department of Medical Genetics, Medical University of Warsaw, Warsaw, Poland

Bolesław Samoliński, Aneta Tomaszewska, Filip Raciborski, Piotr Samel-Kowalik, Artur Walkiewicz, Agnieszka Lipiec, Barbara Piekarska, Jarosław Komorowski, Edyta Krzych-Fałta, Andrzej Namysłowski and Jacek Borowicz
Department of Prevention of Environmental Hazards and Allergology, Medical University of Warsaw, Warsaw, Poland

Sławomir Majewski
Department of Dermatology and Venereology, Medical University of Warsaw, Warsaw, Poland

Søren Meisner
Stoma Care Clinic, Bispebjerg University Hospital, Copenhagen, Denmark

Paul-Antoine Lehur
Institute of Digestive Diseases, University Hospital of Nantes, Nantes, France

Brendan Moran
Pelican Cancer Foundation, North Hampshire Hospital, Basingstoke, United Kingdom

Lina Martins
London Health Sciences Centre, London, Ontario, Canada

Gregor Borut Ernst Jemec
Department of Dermatology, Health Sciences Faculty, Roskilde Hospital, University of Copenhagen, Copenhagen, Denmark

Rebeca Manso
Pathology Department, Fundación Jiménez Díaz, Madrid, Spain

Socorro María Rodríguez-Pinilla
Pathology Department, Fundación Jiménez Díaz, Madrid, Spain
Molecular Pathology Programme, Lymphoma Group, CNIO, Madrid, Spain

Gorka Ruiz de Garibay
Molecular Pathology Programme, Lymphoma Group, CNIO, Madrid, Spain
Clinical Immunology Department, Hospital Clı´nico de San Carlos, Madrid, Spain

Maria del Mar López
Molecular Pathology Programme, Lymphoma Group, CNIO, Madrid, Spain
Biotechnology Programme, Monoclonal Antibodies Unit, CNIO, Madrid, Spain

Margarita Sánchez-Beato
Molecular Pathology Programme, Lymphoma Group, CNIO, Madrid, Spain
Oncology-Haematology Area, Instituto Investigacio´n Sanitaria, Hospital Universitario Puerta de Hierro-Majadahonda, Madrid, Spain

Miguel Ángel Piris
Molecular Pathology Programme, Lymphoma Group, CNIO, Madrid, Spain
Pathology Department, Hospital Universitario Marque´s de Valdecilla, Universidad de Cantabria, IFIMAV, Santander, Spain

Luis Lombardia
Clinical Research Programme, Molecular Diagnostics Clinical Research Unit, CNIO, Madrid, Spain

Luis Requena
Dermatology Department, Fundacio´n Jimenez Dı´az, Madrid, Spain

Lydia Sánchez
Biotechnology Programme, Immunohistochemistry Unit, CNIO, Madrid, Spain

Amy P. Abernethy
Department of Medicine, Duke University Medical Center, Durham, North Carolina, United States of America

April K. S. Salama
Department of Medicine, Duke University Medical Center, Durham, North Carolina, United States of America
Duke Cancer Institute, Duke University Medical Center, Durham, North Carolina, United States of America

Nicole de Rosa, Randall P. Scheri, Scott K. Pruitt and Douglas S. Tyler
Duke Cancer Institute, Duke University Medical Center, Durham, North Carolina, United States of America
Department of Surgery, Duke University Medical Center, Durham, North Carolina, United States of America

James E. Herndon II
Duke Cancer Institute, Duke University Medical Center, Durham, North Carolina, United States of America
Department of Biostatistics and Bioinformatics, Duke University Medical Center, Durham, North Carolina, United States of America

Jennifer Marcello
Department of Biostatistics and Bioinformatics, Duke University Medical Center, Durham, North Carolina, United States of America

Thérèse Kearns and Ross M. Andrews
Child Health Division, Menzies School of Health Research, Charles Darwin University, Darwin, Northern Territory, Australia

Bart J. Currie
Child Health Division, Menzies School of Health Research, Charles Darwin University, Darwin, Northern Territory, Australia
Preventable Chronic Conditions, Northern Territory Department of Health and Families, Darwin, Northern Territory, Australia

Danielle Clucas
Department of Paediatrics, The University of Melbourne, Melbourne, Victoria, Australia,

Christine Connors
Preventable Chronic Conditions, Northern Territory Department of Health and Families, Darwin, Northern Territory, Australia

Jonathan R. Carapetis
Telethon Institute for Child Health Research, Centre for Child Health Research, University of Western, Perth, Western Australia, Australia

Grace Joshy
National Centre for Epidemiology and Population Health, The Australian National University, Canberra, Australia

Rosemary J. Korda
National Centre for Epidemiology and Population Health, The Australian National University, Canberra, Australia
Australian Centre for Economic Research on Health, The Australian National University, Canberra, Australia

Emily Banks
National Centre for Epidemiology and Population Health, The Australian National University, Canberra, Australia
The Sax Institute, Sydney, Australia

Adrian Bauman and Tien Chey
Sydney School of Public Health, The University of Sydney, Sydney, Australia

Hidde P. Van Der Ploeg
Sydney School of Public Health, The University of Sydney, Sydney, Australia
Department of Public and Occupational Health, EMGO Institute for Health and Care Research, VU University Medical Centre, Amsterdam, the Netherlands

Idan Cohen, Keren Leibson and Sara Sivan
The Morris Kahn Laboratory of Human Genetics, National Institute for Biotechnology in the Negev, Ben Gurion University, Beer-Sheva, Israel
Department of Molecular Genetics and Virology, Ben-Gurion University, Beer-Sheva, Israel

Ohad S. Birk
The Morris Kahn Laboratory of Human Genetics, National Institute for Biotechnology in the Negev, Ben Gurion University, Beer-Sheva, Israel
Department of Molecular Genetics and Virology, Ben-Gurion University, Beer-Sheva, Israel
Genetics Institute, Soroka Medical Center, Beer-Sheva, Israel

Ran Taube
Department of Molecular Genetics and Virology, Ben-Gurion University, Beer-Sheva, Israel

Ramon Y. Birnbaum
Department of Bioengineering and Therapeutic Sciences, University of California San Francisco, San Francisco, California, United States of America
Institute for Human Genetics, University of California San Francisco, San Francisco, California, United States of America

Yasuaki Kobayashi and Masaharu Nagayama
Research Institute for Electronic Science, Hokkaido University, Sapporo, Japan
CREST, Japan Science and Technology Agency, Tokyo, Japan

Junichi Kumamoto and Mitsuhiro Denda
CREST, Japan Science and Technology Agency, Tokyo, Japan
Shiseido Research Center, Shiseido Co., Ltd., Yokohama, Japan

Yumi Sanno and Akihiko Sakai
Graduate School of Science and Technology, Kanazawa University, Kanazawa, Japan

Moe Tsutsumi and Makiko Goto
Shiseido Research Center, Shiseido Co., Ltd., Yokohama, Japan

Hiroyuki Kitahata
Department of Physics, Graduate School of Science, Chiba University, Chiba, Japan

Satoshi Nakata
Graduate School of Science, Hiroshima University, Higashi-Hiroshima, Japan

Jianxing Zhang
Center for Therapeutic Biomaterials, University of Utah, Salt Lake City, Utah, United States of America
Department of Medicinal Chemistry, University of Utah, Salt Lake City, Utah, United States of America

Index